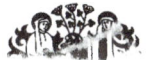

ARDS
ACUTE RESPIRATORY
DISTRESS IN ADULTS

ARDS

Acute Respiratory Distress in Adults

Edited by

Timothy W. Evans

and

Christopher Haslett

With a Foreword by Thomas L. Petty MD

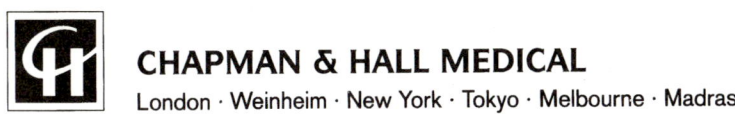

CHAPMAN & HALL MEDICAL
London · Weinheim · New York · Tokyo · Melbourne · Madras

Published by Chapman & Hall, 2–6 Boundary Row, London SE1 8HN, UK

Chapman & Hall, 2–6 Boundary Row, London Se1 8HN, UK

Chapman & Hall GmbH, Pappelallee 3, 69469 Weinheim, Germany

Chapman & Hall USA, 115 Fifth Avenue, New York NY 10003, USA

Chapman & Hall Japan, ITP-Japan, Kyowa Building, 3F, 2-2-1 Hirakawacho, Chiyoda-ku, Tokyo 102, Japan

Chapman & Hall Australia, 102 Dodds Street, South Melbourne, Victoria 3205, Australia

Chapman & Hall India, R. Seshadri, 32 Second Main Road, CIT East, Madras 600 035, India

Distributed in the USA and Canada by Singular Publishing Group Inc. 4284 41st Street, San Diego, California 92105

First edition 1996
© 1996 Chapman & Hall

Typeset in 10/12 Palatino by Photoprint, Torquay, Devon

Printed in Great Britain by Cambridge University Press, Cambridge

ISBN 0 41256910 8

A catalogue record for this book is available from the British Library

Library of Congress Catalog Card Number: 96–83464

∞ Printed on acid-free text paper, manufactured in accordance with ANSI/NISO Z39, 48–1992 (Permanence of Paper).

CONTENTS

CONTRIBUTORS

ELIZABETH L. ARONSEN MD
Special Faculty Instructor, National Jewish
    Center for Immunology and Respiratory
    Medicine,
4500 E. 9th Avenue,
Suite 600S,
Denver CO 80220,
USA

DAVID BIHARI FRCP
Staff Specialist,
Intensive Care Unit,
St George Hospital,
Gray Street,
Kogarah NSW 2217,
Australia

EDWARD J. CAMPBELL MD
Clinical Investigator, Department of Veterans
    Affairs, Salt Lake Veterans Affairs
    Medical Center, and Associate Professor of
    Medicine, Division of Respiratory, Critical
    Care, and Occupational Pulmonary
    Medicine,
University of Utah Health Sciences Center,
50 North Medical Drive,
Salt Lake City UT 84132,
USA

DAVID CICCOLELLA MD
Assistant Professor of Medicine and
    Director, Asthma Center,
Pulmonary and Critical Care Division,
Temple University School of Medicine,
3401 N. Broad Street,
Philadelphia PA 19103
USA

BRYAN CORRIN MD, FRCPath
Professor of Thoracic Pathology,
National Heart & Lung Institute,
Royal Brompton Hospital,
Sydney Street,
London SW3 6NP,
UK

NICHOLAS P. CURZEN BM, MRCP
MRC Training Fellow, and Honorary
    Registrar in ITU and Cardiology,
National Heart & Lung Institute,
Royal Brompton Hospital,
Sydney Street,
London SW3 6NP,
UK

DANIEL DE BACKER MD
Senior Fellow,
Department of Intensive Care,
Erasme University Hospital,
Route de Lennik 808,
B-1070 Brussels,
Belgium

GREGORY P. DOWNEY MD, FRCP(C)
Associate Professor of Medicine and
    Program Director,
Division of Respirology,
1 Kings College Circle,
University of Toronto,
Ontario,
Canada M5S 1A8

IAN DRANSFIELD PhD
Senior Lecturer in Medical Cell Biology,
Respiratory Medicine Unit,
Department of Medicine (RIE),
Rayne Laboratory,
University of Edinburgh Medical School,
Teviot Place,
Edinburgh EH8 9AG,
UK

TIMOTHY W. EVANS MD, FRCP, PhD
Reader in Critical Care Medicine, National
    Heart & Lung Institute, and Consultant in
    Thoracic and Intensive Care Medicine,
Royal Brompton Hospital,
Sydney Street,
London SW3 6NP,
UK

PHILLIP FACTOR DO
Assistant Professor of Medicine, University
    of Illinois at Chicago, and Associate
Director, Intensive Care Unit,
Michael Reese Hospital and Medical Center,
2929 S. Ellis Avenue,
Chicago IL 60616–3390,
USA

KONRAD J. FALKE MD
Professor of Anaesthesiology and Surgical
    Intensive Care, and Chairman,
Klinik für Anaesthesiologie und operative
    Intensivmedizin,
Virchow-Klinikum,
Humboldt Universität zu Berlin,
Augustenburger Platz 1,
D-13353 Berlin,
Germany

JACK GAULDIE PhD
Professor and Chairman, Department of
    Pathology,
McMaster University,
Health Sciences Centre, Room 2N16,
1200 Main Street West,
Hamilton,
Ontario,
Canada L8N 3Z5

HERWIG GERLACH MD
Senior Staff Anaesthesiologist and Head
    Physician,
Virchow-Klinikum,
Humboldt Universität zu Berlin,
Augustenburger Platz 1,
D-13353 Berlin,
Germany

RAVI S. GILL BM, FRCA
Senor Registrar in Anaesthetics,
Queen Alexandra Hospital,
Southwick Hill Road,
Cosham,
Portsmouth PO6 3LY,
UK

ERIC H. GLUCK MD
Associate Professor of Medicine and Chief
    of Pulmonary and Critical Care Medicine,
The Chicago Medical School,
3001 Green Bay Road,
North Chicago,
Illinois 60064,
USA

MARK J.D. GRIFFITHS BSC, MRCP
Wellcome Research Fellow,
Adult Intensive Care Unit,
Royal Brompton Hospital,
Sydney Street,
London SW3 6NP,
UK

E. ROBERT GROVER FRCA
Clinical Research Physician,
Department of Cardiovascular/Critical Care
    Medicine,
The Wellcome Foundation,
Langley Court,
South Eden Park Road,
Beckenham BR3 3BS,
UK

JOHN M.C. GUTTERIDGE PhD, DSC, FIBiol
Professor of Biochemistry
Oxygen Chemistry Laboratory,
National Heart & Lung Institute,
Royal Brompton Hospital,
Sydney Street,
London SW3 6NP,
UK

DAVID M. HANSELL MRCP, FRCR
Consultant Radiologist and Honorary Senior
  Lecturer,
Department of Radiology,
Royal Brompton Hospital,
Sydney Street,
London SW3 6NP,
UK

PATRICIA L. HASLAM PhD, MRCPath
Senior Lecturer,
Cell Biology Unit, Cardiothoracic Surgery,
National Heart & Lung Institute,
Imperial College School of Medicine,
Dovehouse Street,
London SW3 6LY,
UK

CHRISTOPHER HASLETT FRCP, FRCP (Edin)
Professor of Respiratory Medicine,
Chairman of the Department of Medicine
  (RIE) and Director of the Rayne
  Laboratories,
University of Edinburgh,
Royal Infirmary,
Lauriston Place,
Edinburgh EH3 9YW,
UK

BRIAN F. KEOGH FRCA
Consultant in Anaesthesia and Intensive
  Care,
Royal Brompton Hospital,
Sydney Street,
London SW3 6NP,
UK

STEVEN L. KUNKEL MD
Professor of Pathology,
Division of Pulmonary and Critical Care
  Medicine,
University of Michigan Medical Center,
3916 Taubman Center,
1500 E. Medical Center Drive,
Ann Arbor MI 48109–0360,
USA

DAVID G. McCORMACK MD, FRCP(C), FCCP
Associate Professor of Medicine, University
  of Western Ontario,
The Alan C. Burton Vascular Biology
  Laboratory,
Victoria Hospital,
375 South Street,
London,
Ontario
Canada N6A 4G5

PETER D. MACNAUGHTON MD, MRCP, FRCA
Consultant in Anaesthetics and Intensive
  Care,
Derriford Hospital,
Derriford Road,
Plymouth PL6 8DH,
UK

JOHN J. MARINI MD
Professor of Medicine, University of
  Minnesota, and Director of Pulmonary
  and Critical Care Medicine,
St Paul Ramsey Medical Center,
640 Jackson Street,
St Paul MN 55101–2595,
USA

MICHAEL A. MATTHAY MD
Professor of Medicine and Anesthesia, and
  Senior Member, Cardiovascular Research
  Institute,
505 Parnassus, M-917,
University of California,
San Francisco CA 94143–0130,
USA

ROBERT J. MEYER MD
Assistant Professor of Medicine, Pulmonary
    and Critical Care,
Oregon Health Sciences University,
3181 S.W. Sam Jackson Park Road, UHN-67,
Portland OR 97201–3098,
USA

ALAN H. MORRIS MD
Professor of Medicine, Adjunct Professor of
    Medical Informatics, University of Utah,
    and Director of Research,
Pulmonary Division,
LDS Hospital,
8th Avenue and C Street,
Salt Lake City UT 84143,
USA

JOHN F. MURRAY MD, FRCP
Professor of Medicine, University of
    California San Francisco, and Senior
    Member, Cardiovascular Research
    Institute,
UCSF Campus Box 0841,
University of California,
San Francisco CA 94143–0841,
USA

MOLLY L. OSBORNE MD, PhD
Associate Professor of Medicine, Pulmonary
    and Critical Care,
Department of Veterans Affairs,
Medical Center,
3710 Southwest US Veterans Hospital Road,
Portland OR 97207,
USA

CAROLINE A. OWEN MD, PhD
Research Assistant Professor of Medicine,
Division of Respiratory, Critical Care, and
    Occupational Pulmonary Medicine,
Department of Internal Medicine,
University of Utah Health Sciences Center,
50 North Medical Drive,
Salt Lake City UT 84132,
USA

DIRK PAPPERT MD
Senior Staff Anaesthesiologist and Head
    Physician,
Virchow-Klinikum,
Humboldt Universität zu Berlin,
Augustenburger Platz 1,
D-13353 Berlin,
Germany

POLLY E. PARSONS MD
Associate Professor, Pulmonary and Critical
    Care Medicine, University of Colorado
School of Medicine, and Director, MICU,
Department of Medicine, #4000,
Denver General Hospital,
777 Bannock Street,
Denver CO 80204,
USA

NIGEL A.M. PATERSON MB, FRCP(C)
Professor of Medicine, University of Western
    Ontario,
The Alan C. Burton Vascular Biology
    Laboratory,
Victoria Hospital,
375 South Street,
London,
Ontario
Canada N6A 4G5

PETER D. POTGIETER FCA (SA)
Director of ICU,
King Fahad National Guard Hospital,
PO Box 22490,
Riyadh 11426,
Kingdom of Saudi Arabia

GREGORY J. QUINLAN PhD
Research Fellow,
Oxygen Chemistry Laboratory,
National Heart & Lung Institute,
Royal Brompton Hospital,
Sydney Street,
London SW3 6NP,
UK

ROLF ROSSAINT MD
Senior Staff Anaesthesiologist and Head
Physician,
Virchow-Klinikum,
Humboldt Universität zu Berlin,
Augustenburger Platz 1,
D-13353 Berlin,
Germany

JOHN M. SHANNON PhD
Associate Professor,
National Jewish Center for Immunology and
Respiratory Medicine,
1400 Jackson Street,
Denver CO 80206,
USA

WILLIAM J. SIBBALD MD, FRCP(C)
Professor of Medicine, University of Western
Ontario, Critical Care Trauma Centre and
The Alan C. Burton Vascular Biology
Laboratory,
Victoria Hospital,
375 South Street,
London,
Ontario,
Canada N6A 4G5

KENNETH M. SIM FRCA
Consultant Anaesthetist,
Queen Victoria Hospital,
East Grinstead,
Sussex RH19 3DZ
UK

PATRICIA J. SIME MB CHB, MRCP (UK)
Parker B. Francis Pulmonary Research
Fellow,
McMaster University,
Health Sciences Centre, Room 4H21,
1200 Main Street West,
Hamilton,
Ontario,
Canada L8N 3Z5

DANIEL R. SMITH MD
Staff Pulmonologist,
East Tenessee Pulmonary Associates,
Oak Ridge,
Tennessee TN37830,
USA

S. CRAIG STOCKS PhD
Wellcome Travelling Research Fellow,
Institut für Immunbiologie,
Albert Ludwigs Universität Freiburg,
Stefan Meier Strasse 8,
D 79104 Freiburg,
Germany

ROBERT M. STRIETER MD
Associate Professor of Internal Medicine,
Division of Pulmonary and Critical Care
Medicine,
University of Michigan Medical Center,
3916 Taubman Center,
1500 E. Medical Center Drive,
Ann Arbor MI 48109–0360,
USA

JACOB I. SZNAJDER MD
Associate Professor of Medicine, University
of Illinois at Chicago, and Head, Section
of Pulmonary and Critical Care Medicine,
Michael Reese Hospital and Medical Center,
2929 S. Ellis Avenue
Chicago IL 60616–3390,
USA

GALEN B. TOEWS MD
Professor of Internal Medicine and Chief,
Division of Pulmonary and Critical Care
Medicine,
University of Michigan Medical Center,
3916 Taubman Center,
1500 E. Medical Center Drive,
Ann Arbor MI 48109–0360,
USA

JOHN S. TURNER MMed, MD (Capetown),
  FCP(SA)
Critical Care Specialist,
Harfield House,
Wilderness Road,
Claremont 7700,
South Africa

JEAN-LOUIS VINCENT MD, PhD
Clinical Director, Department of Intensive
  Care, and Professor of Intensive Care
  Medicine,
Erasme University Hospital,
Route de Lennik 808,
B-1070 Brussels,
Belgium

G. SCOTT WORTHEN MD
Associate Professor of Medicine, University
  of Colorado School of Medicine, and
  Senior Staff Physician, Department of
  Medicine,
National Jewish Center for Immunology and
  Respiratory Medicine,
1400 Jackson Street,
Denver CO 80206,
USA

FOREWORD

Great progress has been made since the first description of the acute respiratory distress syndrome by the Denver group in 1967 (*Lancet*). Although we introduced the term 'adult respiratory distress syndrome' in our second and more detailed description of the syndrome (*Chest*, 1971), this was probably a mistake for the simple reason that children also suffer the same syndrome following acute lung insults.

Today, the syndrome of acute respiratory distress in adults (ARDS) is recognized as a worldwide problem, but the prevalence of disease varies in different parts of the world. A huge amount of research has focused on the mechanisms of acute lung injury and yet the exact sequence of events and mediators in inflammatory cascade, which result in acute respiratory failure from ARDS, is not known but many possibilities exist. The definition of ARDS has been gradually modified in recent years and investigators around the world are now collaborating in order to establish more uniform concepts in identification, risk factors and mechanisms of lung injury, which someday will result in improved approaches to management. Already, at least some centers are showing improved outcomes in ARDS, achieving an approximate 60% survival rate. In the past, most large series documented only about a 40% survivability taking all causes of ARDS. This apparent progress is likely attributable to more meticulous and disciplined care than any specific pharmacologic attack on the basic mechanism resulting in ARDS. A range of pulmonary impairment from none to moderate is found in survivors, yet most can function normally on recovery.

Editors Evans and Haslett have produced a truly comprehensive review of all aspects of ARDS that promises to be informative to all students of this interesting clinical state. Hopefully, this volume will point us in the right direction for future progress. I believe that it will.

Thomas L. Petty MD
Professor of Medicine
Denver, Colorado, USA

ABBREVIATIONS

AA — arachidonic acid

A-aDO_2 — alveolar–arterial oxygen gradient

AAG — alkylacylglycerol

aFGF — acidic fibroblast growth factor

ALI — acute lung injury

APACHE — acute physiological and chronic health evaluation

ARDS — syndrome of acute respiratory distress in adults

ARF — acute respiratory failure

ATP — adenosine triphosphate

BAL — bronchoalveolar lavage

cAMP — cyclic adenosine monophosphate

CaO_2 — arterial oxygen content

CAVH — continuous arteriovenous hemofiltration

CAVH-D — CAVH with countercurrent dialysis

CcO_2 — capillary oxygen content

cDNA — complementary deoxyribonucleic acid

CEA — carcinoembryonic antigen

CFV — continuous flow ventilation

CHFV — combined high frequency ventilation

CI — cardiac index

C_L — lung compliance

CLSE — calf lung surfactant extract

cNOS — constitutive nitric oxide synthase

CO — cardiac output

CO_2 — carbon dioxide

CSF — colony stimulating factor

CT — computed tomography

C_T — total compliance

CTAP — connective tissue activating peptide

Cth — total thoracic compliance

CvO_2 — mixed venous oxygen content

Cw — chest wall compliance

DAD — diffuse alveolar damage

DG — diglyceride

DO_2 — oxygen diffusing capacity

DPPC — dipalmitoylphosphatidylcholine

DTPA — diethylenetriaminepentaacetic acid

ECCO_2R — extracorporeal carbon dioxide removal

ECGE — extracorporeal gas exchange

ECM — extracellular matrix

ECMO — extracorporeal membrane oxygenation

EC-SOD — extracellular superoxide dismutase

EDCF — endothelium derived contracting factor

EDRF — endothelium derived relaxing factor

EGF — epidermal growth factor

ENA — epithelial-neutrophil activating factor

ET — endothelin

EVLW — extravascular lung water

FE_{CO_2} — fractional expired carbon dioxide concentration

FE_{O_2} — fractional expired oxygen concentration

FGF — fibroblast growth factor

F_{IO_2}	fractional inspired oxygen concentration	iNOS	inducible nitric oxide synthase
FMLP	formyl methionyl leucine phenylalanine	$_\gamma$IP	INF-γ-inducible peptide
FRC	functional residual capacity	IPF	idiopathic pulmonary fibrosis
G-CSF	granulocyte colony stimulating factor	IRAP	interleukin-1 receptor antagonist
GM-CSF	granulocyte-macrophage colony stimulating factor	IRDS	infantile respiratory distress syndrome
GRP	gastrin releasing peptide	IRV	inverse ratio ventilation
GSH	glutathione	ITPV	intratracheal pulmonary ventilation
H & E	hematoxylin and eosin	iu	international units
Hb	hemoglobin saturation	IVGE	intravascular gas exchange
HCl	hydrochloric acid	IVOX	intravascular oxygenator, intravenacaval oxygenation
HDL	high density lipoproteins		
HETE	hydroxyeicosotetraenoic acid	KGF	keratinocyte growth factor
HFJV	high frequency jet ventilation	LAD	leukocyte adhesion deficiency
HFO	high frequency oscillation	LBP	LPS binding protein
HFPPV	high frequency positive pressure ventilation	LD	lethal dose
		LDL	low density lipoproteins
HGF/SF	hepatocyte growth factor/ scatter factor	LELF	lung epithelial lining fluid
		LFPPV-ECCO$_2$R	Low frequency, positive pressure ventilation with extracorporeal CO_2 removal
HLE	human leukocyte elastase		
Ho	null hypothesis		
H_2O_2	hydrogen peroxide		
HOCl	hypochlorous acid	LIS	lung injury score
HPV	hypoxic pulmonary vasoconstriction	LPC	lysophosphatidylcholine
		LPS	lipopolysaccharide
HR	heart rate	LT	leukotriene
HRCT	high resolution computed tomography	MAP	mean airway pressure, microtubule associated protein
ICAM	intercellular adhesion molecule		
		MCP	mononuclear chemotactic peptide
ICD	International Classification of Diseases	M-CSF	macrophage colony stimulating factor
ICU	intensive care unit		
I/E	ratio of inspiratory time to expiratory time	MEK	MAP ERK kinase
		MIP	macrophage inflammatory protein
Ig	immunoglobulin		
IGF	insulin-like growth factor	MODS	multiple organ dysfunction syndrome
IL	interleukin		
IMO	intravenous membrane oxygenator	MOF	multiple organ failure
		MRI	magnetic resonance imaging
INF	interferon		

mRNA	messenger ribonucleic acid	P_{ECO_2}	expired carbon dioxide tension
MSOF	multiple systems organ failure	PEEP	positive end expiratory pressure
LNAME	N^ω-nitro-L-arginine	PEEPi	intrinsic PEEP (end expiratory alveolar pressure)
NANC	nonadrenergic noncholinergic		
LNMMA	N^G-monomethyl-L-arginine	PET	positron emission tomography
NAP	neutrophil activating peptide	PF	platelet factor
NCA	nonspecific crossreacting antigen	PG	phosphatidylglycerine, prostaglandin
NHE	N^+H^+ exchange	PHA	phytohemagglutinin
NHLI	National Heart and Lung Institute	pHa	arterial pH
		pHi	intramucosal pH
NK	natural killer	PI	phosphatidylinositol
NNNMU	N-nitroso-N-methylurethane	PIP	peak inspiratory pressure
NO	nitric oxide	PKC	protein kinase C
NO_2	nitrogen dioxide	PLA	phospholipase A
N_2O	nitrous oxide	PLC	phospholipase C
NOS	nitric oxide synthase	PMA	phorbol myristate acetate
O_2	oxygen	PMN	polymorphonuclear neutrophil
O_2^-	superoxide anion		
OA	okadaic acid	P_{O_2}	partial pressure of oxygen
O_2ER	oxygen extraction	Ppeak	peak airway pressure
OFR	oxygen free radical	PPH	primary pulmonary hypertension
OSF	organ system failure		
PA	phosphatidic acid	PPHN	pulmonary hypertension of the newborn
Pa_{CO_2}	arterial carbon dioxide tension		
		p.p.m.	parts per million
PAF	platelet activating factor	PPV	positive predictive value
PAI	plasminogen activator inhibitor, protein accumulation index	PS	phosphatidylserine
		Pset	maximum airway pressure
		PUMP	punctuated metalloproteinase
Pa_{O_2}	arterial oxygen tension		
PAOP	pulmonary artery occlusion pressure	Pv_{O_2}	venous oxygen tension
		PVR	pulmonary vascular resistance
PAP	pulmonary artery pressure		
Paw	airway pressure	$\dot{Q}$	perfusion
PC	phosphatidylcholine	$\dot{Q}_{O_2}$	systemic oxygen delivery
PCIRV	pressure controlled inverse ratio ventilation	$\dot{Q}s/\dot{Q}t$	right to left shunt fraction
		$\dot{Q}t$	thermodilution cardiac output
PCV	pressure controlled ventilation		
PDGF	platelet derived growth factor	ROS	reactive oxygen species
		RQ	respiratory quotient
PE	phosphatidylethanolamine	Sa_{O_2}	arterial oxygen saturation

SAPS	simplified acute physiological score	TNF	tumor necrosis factor
SCR	short consensus repeat	t-PA	tissue-type plasminogen activator
SDS	sodium dodecyl sulfate	Tx	thromboxane
setPEEP	positive end expiratory pressure setting	u-PA	urokinase-type plasminogen activator
SIRS	systemic inflammatory response syndrome	$\dot{V}$	ventilation
		V_A	alveolar volume
SM	sphingomyelin	$\dot{V}_A$	alveolar ventilation
SOD	superoxide dismutase	VAP_{CO_2}	venoarterial P_{CO_2} gradient
SP	surfactant protein	VC	vital capacity
S_{VO_2}	mixed venous oxygen saturation	VCAM	vascular cell adhesion molecule
SVR	systemic vascular resistance	V_D	dead space gas volume
		V_D/V_T	physiological dead space fraction
TBAR	thiobarbituric acid reactivity	V_E	expired minute volume
TGF	transforming growth factor	VLA	very late antigen
TGI	tracheal gas insufflation	VLDL	very low density lipoproteins
TIMP	tissue inhibitor of metalloproteinases	V_{O_2}	oxygen consumption
T_I/T_T	inspiratory time fraction (duty cycle)	$\dot{V}/\dot{Q}$	ventilation-perfusion ratio
		VR	ventilatory rate
T_LCO	carbon monoxide transfer factor	V_T	tidal volume

PART ONE

INTRODUCTION AND OVERVIEW

John F. Murray

The editors of this text on the syndrome of acute respiratory distress in adults (ARDS) have insisted, quite rightly, that the first chapter should begin with some introductory comments and a definition of the subject that the rest of the book is about. The easy part of the assignment is the introduction, which will take the form of an historical overview and a brief examination and evaluation of some of the pathogenetic concepts that have evolved as medical scientists have tried to understand the origins of this fascinating but elusive disorder. Defining it, however, is not as easy as it sounds, because there is no uniformly accepted definition of the syndrome, and the various definitions that have been used by workers in the field since the term was introduced in 1971 have differed considerably. In this chapter I will discuss the reasons for this apparent impasse, and I will describe two definitions: one that I and my colleagues proposed in 1988, and another that emerged from two American–European consensus conferences in 1992. Nevertheless, as has been the fashion, I suspect that other authors will employ their own definitions or use ones that have been championed by someone else.

HISTORICAL OVERVIEW

In 1967, Ashbaugh and coworkers [1] published their now celebrated article in which they described 12 patients with striking but similar clinical, physiologic, radiographic and pathologic abnormalities that differentiated them from nearly 300 other patients who had also been treated for respiratory failure in the intensive care units of Colorado General Hospital and Denver General Hospital. All 12 patients had severe dyspnea, tachypnea, cyanosis that was refractory to oxygen administration, decreased respiratory system compliance, and diffuse alveolar infiltrations on their chest radiographs. Pathologic findings in seven patients who died included atelectasis, vascular congestion and hemorrhage, severe pulmonary edema and hyaline membranes. Four years later, Petty and Ashbaugh [2] designated this constellation of abnormalities the adult respiratory distress syndrome. There is no doubt that these two articles attracted a considerable amount of attention and that they catalyzed much of the work that soon followed. But there is also no doubt that patients with similar clinical, radiographic and pathologic features to those reported by Ashbaugh and Petty had been described before by other authors.

Not surprisingly, the original observations were made by military surgeons who cared for previously healthy soldiers who had been severely wounded in battle. Because ARDS is now an established complication of multiple traumatic injuries, especially those associated with shock, it was inevitable that the disorder would occur in sufficient numbers to be identified as an entity among the countless casualties of successive wars. (The interested

ARDS Acute Respiratory Distress in Adults. Edited by Timothy W. Evans and Christopher Haslett. Published in 1996 by Chapman & Hall, London. ISBN 0 412 56910 8

reader is referred to the review by Simeone [3] about the pulmonary complications of nonthoracic wounds, which was written during the Vietnam war when the disorder was becoming a frequent and serious problem. During the second world war, what is now called ARDS was called 'wet lung' by Burford and Burbank [4] for 'want of a better term', and further characterized by Brewer and coworkers [5] during the same conflict. It was recognized at the time that 'wet lung' was not restricted to victims of thoracic injuries, but also occurred in casualties of wounds to other parts of the body from blast injuries, abdominal trauma or fractures of long bones [3]. Even during the first world war, Pasteur [6] described 'massive collapse' of the lungs of soldiers who had sustained thoracic injuries, which when called 'pulmonary contusion' is considered today a member of the ARDS family. Moreover, pulmonary edema in victims of gunshot wounds to the head was also clearly identified and reported during the first world war [7].

There are no good data on the prevalence of 'wet lung' among the millions of casualties of the second world war, but when the disorder occurred, it was recognized as a serious problem with a high mortality rate [5], and seemed chiefly to accompany severe traumatic injuries, those likely to be associated with shock. In this regard, it is of considerable interest to read the comprehensive report by Moon [8] on the pathologic findings in persons who died with or of shock from causes other than battlefield trauma. This review of the autopsy reports of 122 patients, all personnel of the US army, who died of a variety of acute and severe medical and surgical disorders, including accidental or surgical trauma, burns, fulminating infections, anoxia, low atmospheric pressure, heat stroke, abdominal emergencies and miscellaneous conditions, reads like a catalog of today's precipitating conditions of ARDS [9]. At autopsy, a similar pattern of visceral abnormalities was found, regardless of the cause of death. It should come as no surprise that the pathologic findings in the lungs were those that characterize the syndrome, notably pulmonary hyperemia and edema, and atelectasis.

Not much was written about pulmonary edema as a complication of nonthoracic traumatic injuries during the Korean war, but during the Vietnam war the disorder became a problem of considerable magnitude. The newly introduced system of rapid evacuation by helicopter and vigorous fluid resuscitation rescued hundreds of critically wounded personnel, who undoubtedly would have died on the battlefield had they received comparable injuries in previous conflicts. In nearby hospitals these desperately ill patients often developed what became known as 'shock lung', from its obvious traumatic origins, and after one particularly long and bloody battle the condition was so prevalent that it was called 'Da-nang lung' [10]. The lesson from this brief review is not that ARDS has been known by other names for a long time, but that it can be thought of as a consequence, albeit a deleterious one, of the remarkable improvements that were made during the last few decades in the early treatment of medical and surgical catastrophes; because of these advances, many patients – who formerly would have died – live long enough to develop the delayed complications of devastating illness. It is in large part owing to these extraordinary medical accomplishments that the syndrome has become more common than it used to be, and hence it has attracted much deserved recognition. Moreover, modern techniques have allowed ARDS to be better characterized clinically, radiographically, physiologically and pathologically than it was, and this knowledge has created familiarity and acceptance; and finally, the disorder has been given a catchy name that almost everyone has heard of even though they are a little vague about it.

DEFINITION

ARDS is not the only subject that has proved difficult to define precisely. When Associate Justice Potter Stewart was unable to formulate a coherent definition of *'obscenity'* in a case heard before the United States Supreme Court in 1964, his frank declaration [11] 'but I know it when I see it' solved the problem and became the most widely quoted judicial pronouncement on the subject. This statement is apposite to ARDS. All physicians know that a patient has the disorder 'when (they) see it'; the problem lies in providing a coherent definition of what they are seeing in terms that everyone accepts.

There seems to be general agreement that ARDS is a form of acute lung injury. Most people also agree that the syndrome represents a form of injury that is particularly severe and that arises principally from involvement of the lung parenchyma (i.e. chiefly the pulmonary capillaries, overlying respiratory epithelium and neighboring structures), as opposed to disorders of the conducting airways (e.g. asthma or bronchiolitis) or large blood vessels (e.g. pulmonary embolism). Why then has ARDS been so difficult to define?

A large part of the problem lies in the fact that the syndrome occurs in multiple and extremely varied clinical settings. Moreover, in many of these in which the cause of the lung injury is known, the clinical, radiographic, physiologic and even pathologic abnormalities are similar to those that occur in settings in which the cause is unknown. Beginning with Petty and Ashbaugh [2], all causes – known and unknown – have been lumped together under the large umbrella term of ARDS. Subsequently, most definitions were operational and relied on three features of the disorder [12]: (1) **hypoxemia**, although the level of severity varied from one series to another; (2) **diffuse radiographic infiltrations**, although the type and magnitude were seldom specified; and (3) **decreased respiratory system compliance**, although this was not easily measured and required that the patient be mechanically ventilated and, for best results, either paralyzed or heavily sedated. Some investigators have attempted to exclude overhydration and cardiogenic causes of pulmonary edema by specifying that the pulmonary artery occlusion pressure must be measured and be normal, but the values that were considered 'normal' varied from 12 mmHg or less [13] to 18 mmHg or less [14]. Other definitions were even broader and included 'acute respiratory failure due to noncardiogenic pulmonary edema' [15].

ARDS nearly always begins early and progresses swiftly in patients with certain known risk factors, such as sepsis, hypotension or multiple traumatic injuries, who are often seriously ill from the underlying condition. Their chest radiographs show diffuse alveolar-type densities, which reflect the presence and extent of increased permeability pulmonary edema, and which in severe cases may be nearly confluent. Physiologic complications include hypoxemia from right to left shunting of blood, decreased pulmonary compliance and low end expiratory lung volume, all of which are related to filling of alveolar spaces with protein-rich edema fluid and to atelectasis secondary to increased surface forces. These complications are caused by injury to the respiratory epithelium, particularly type I pneumocytes, and the adjacent microvascular endothelium (Table 1.1). Hyaline membranes, intra-alveolar hemorrhage and 'congestive atelectasis' are characteristic histologic findings in the lungs of patients who die within a few days of the onset of the syndrome [17,18] (Chapter 4).

In certain types of new onset ARDS, including heroin pulmonary edema, air embolism and near drowning, if the patient survives the first day or two, the lung injury quickly resolves and recovery is usually complete [19,20]. By contrast, other patients with the acute syndrome, especially that form associated with sepsis, do not improve clinically

Table 1.1 Characteristics of parenchymal lung injury

Type	Acute	Chronic
Clinical	Identifiable risk factor(s)	Frequent complications of multiple organs
	Sudden onset	Rapid evolution
Radiographic	Alveolar infiltrations	Organizing infiltrations
Physiologic	Permeability pulmonary edema	Increased vascular resistance
	Hypoxia (right to left shunt)	Hypoxia ($\dot{V}/\dot{Q}$ mismatch, ? diffusion)
	Low lung volume (edema, atelectasis)	Low lung volume (infiltration)
	Decreased compliance (increased surface forces)	Decreased compliance (increased tissue forces)
Pathologic	Injury epithelium	Type II cell hyperplasia
	Injury endothelium	Fibroblast infiltration
	Hyaline membranes	Connective tissue deposition
	Edema/hemorrhage	Remodeling

$\dot{V}/\dot{Q}$ = ventilation–perfusion ratio.
Reproduced with permission from Murray *et al.*, An expanded definition of the adult respiratory distress syndrome, published by American Journal of Respiratory and Critical Care Medicine, 1988 [16].

even though the increased permeability pulmonary edema, the hallmark of diffuse, acute microvascular endothelial-epithelial injury, subsides [21]. Instead of healing, the damaged lung parenchyma rapidly organizes and a chronic phase evolves that is associated with ongoing respiratory failure requiring continuous mechanical ventilation, and that is frequently exacerbated by nosocomial infections, other iatrogenic complications and the syndrome known as multiple organ failure [22] (Chapter 18). Most deaths occur in this sequence [23] (Chapter 2). Prominent pathologic findings in the chronic stage are those of evolving parenchymal lung damage and include hyperplasia of the type II alveolar pneumocytes, infiltration by fibroblasts, deposition of connective tissue and remodeling of the parenchyma [24].

Another feature that is beginning to receive the attention it deserves derives from the intuitively obvious fact that there is no inherent reason why the lung damage should be of equal severity in every afflicted patient. Because the type, magnitude and duration of a given insult to the lungs undoubtedly vary in the different conditions that are known to cause or to be associated with acute parenchymal lung injury, it follows that the clinical, radiographic and physiologic consequences of such an injury vary as well. The results of at least three large prospective series of patients at risk for developing ARDS have shown that there is a continuum of response and that more patients develop 'mild to moderate' than 'severe' acute lung injury [25–27]. Where ARDS lies within this continuum is arbitrary and, as mentioned, variable according to different definitions. But there is a consensus among most authors that when the term ARDS is used, the injury should be widespread and severe.

Based on these considerations, my colleagues and I [16] proposed an expanded definition that takes into account three key features of ARDS that have already been mentioned: (1) that in many but not all patients the acute injury evolves into a chronic phase; (2) that most authorities believe the abnormalities are severe; and (3) that there are a multiplicity of causes, some known and some unknown.

ACUTE VERSUS CHRONIC

The clinical, radiographic, physiologic and pathologic abnormalities already noted and listed in Table 1.1 indicate that the syndrome may have both acute and chronic phases, an important observation that has been stressed by others [15]. The factors responsible for the transformation are unknown, but the process occurs remarkably fast, often within 3–7 days as judged by pathologic findings [18]. The change from acute to chronic has major prognostic implications because much of the mortality occurs in the latter variety [23].

SEVERITY

The expanded definition incorporates the belief that the syndrome is an especially severe form of acute lung injury, and that

Table 1.2 Components and individual values of the lung injury score

Component	Value
1. Chest roentgenogram score	
No alveolar consolidation	0
Alveolar consolidation confined to 1 quadrant	1
Alveolar consolidation confined to 2 quadrants	2
Alveolar consolidation confined to 3 quadrants	3
Alveolar consolidation in all 4 quadrants	4
2. Hypoxemia score	
Pao_2/Fio_2 – ≥ 300	0
Pao_2/Fio_2 – 225–299	1
Pao_2/Fio_2 – 175–224	2
Pao_2/Fio_2 – 100–174	3
Pao_2/Fio_2 – < 100	4
3. PEEP score (when ventilated)	
PEEP – ≤ 5 cmH$_2$0	0
PEEP – 6–8 cmH$_2$0	1
PEEP – 9–11 cmH$_2$0	2
PEEP – 12–14 cmH$_2$0	3
PEEP – ≥ 15 cmH$_2$0	4
4. Respiratory system compliance score (when available)	0
Compliance – ≥ 80 ml/cmH$_2$0	1
Compliance – 60–79 ml/cmH$_2$0	2
Compliance – 40–59 ml/cmH$_2$0	3
Compliance – 20–39 ml/cmH$_2$0	4
Compliance – ≤ 19 ml/cmH$_2$0	

The final value is obtained by dividing the aggregate sum by the number of components that were used.

	Score
No lung injury	0
Mild to moderate	0.1–2.25
Severe lung injury (ARDS)	> 2.5

Pao_2/Fio_2 = arterial oxygen tension to inspired oxygen concentration ratio; PEEP = positive end expiratory pressure.
Reproduced with permission from Murray *et al.* [16].

other milder forms also occur. To allow a quantitive distinction, we formulated a 'lung injury score' (Table 1.2) that enables an assessment of severity to be made from information that is usually readily available (or should be).

CAUSES

In 1975, I argued [28] that it was important to separate the various causes of ARDS because their specific etiologies may affect our understanding of their pathogenesis, pathophysiology and response to treatment; others, however, argued in favor of continuing the policy of lumping all causes into a single entity [29]. In our defense of the expanded definition [16], we cited two examples, one concerning early diagnosis and the other concerning treatment, to emphasize the importance of making etiologic distinctions. The causes can be separated into two broad categories (Table 1.3): in one category the lungs are injured as a **direct** consequence of the causative disease, which is usually known, and in the other category the lungs are damaged as an **indirect** byproduct of the systemic reactions, which are for the most part unknown, unleashed by a disorder that often originates in extrathoracic organs. For direct injuries, we suggested designating 'caused by' and then stating the responsible condition, and for the indirect injuries, we suggested using 'associated with' followed by the name of the underlying disorder.

The definition recommended by the 1992 American–European Consensus Conference [30] incorporates the same general principles but includes two modifications. (1) In the abbreviated term ARDS, the consensus definition proposed to substitute 'acute' for 'adult' to recognize the fact that the disorder is not limited to adults but may occur in children; however, this emphasis on acute fails to acknowledge that the syndrome often progresses into a prolonged chronic phase with important clinical implications. (2) All patients with acute lung injury and a $Pa_{O_2}/F_{IO_2} < 200$ are considered to have ARDS, with certain exclusions, regardless of the extent of their radiographic abnormalities and without making any allowance for the effect of positive end expiratory pressure on arterial P_{O_2}. Subclassification into direct and indirect pathogenetic categories, as described earlier, was also recommended [30].

PATHOGENESIS

The early designations of what is now termed ARDS incorporated the major pathologic or physiologic findings from which one was supposed to infer something about pathogenesis. During the first world war, for example, Pasteur [6] used 'massive collapse' to describe what was found at death; several years later, this terminology was changed to 'pulmonary atelectasis' to support the concept that bronchial obstruction and weakened respiratory forces were responsible. The term 'wet lung' of the second world war highlighted the presence of severe pulmonary edema and accompanying hypoxia. None of these terms,

Table 1.3 Three part definition of parenchymal lung injury

Part	Definition
1	Acute or chronic, depending on course
2	Mild to moderate or severe (ARDS) lung injury, depending on lung injury score
3	Caused by (direct): aspiration pneumonitis fat embolism drug (e.g. heroin, paraquat) ingestion toxic gas (e.g. phosgene, smoke) inhalation infectious (e.g. influenza A, *Pneumocystis carinii*) agents or associated with sepsis multiple blood transfusions acute pancreatitis disseminated intravascular coagulation

Reproduced with permission from Murray *et al.* [16].

however, shed much light on specific pathogenic mechanisms.

In part because so little was known about pathogenesis, during the Vietnam war the term 'shock lung' was used to emphasize the fact that hypotension, usually from battlefield injuries but also from other (nonmilitary) disorders as well, led to the syndrome. One of the consequences of the Vietnam medical experience was the establishment of special units for the intensive clinical investigation of shock, in which the importance of pulmonary complications of a variety of nonthoracic disorders was confirmed [31]. But as pointed out by Fishman [32], despite increased clarification by clinical observations and pathologic descriptions, the term shock lung was a 'distinctive nonentity' insofar as providing any insights into pathogenesis. Unfortunately, calling the disorder ARDS does not help much either.

It has been recognized for a long time, however, that the pulmonary complications of shock of various causes and of nonthoracic injuries may be multifactorial in origin, and that these mechanisms, singly or in concert, may produce the same pathologic abnormalities. For example, fat emboli were often present in the lungs of victims of the syndrome in the second world war, and subsequently it was speculated that microemboli of tissue products and aggregates of transfused blood might play a role. Other possible causative mechanisms were sudden compression of the lungs, various 'toxins' and high concentrations of inhaled oxygen. In the Vietnam war the routine practice of administering enormous quantities of fluid intravenously undoubtedly caused or contributed to the development of pulmonary edema in many casualties.

As described in the previous section, current descriptions of the syndrome cast an inclusive net over the many different disorders associated with a particular constellation of clinical, radiographic, physiologic and pathologic abnormalities. This emphasizes

Table 1.4 Direct causes of ARDS (with examples of each to illustrate different pathogenetic mechanisms)

Infectious agents
  Influenza pneumonia
  AIDS associated histoplasmosis
  Pneumocystis carinii pneumonia
  Falciparum malaria

Toxic chemicals
  Phosgene inhalation
  Massive aspiration of gastric juice
  Salicylate overdose
  Heroin pulmonary edema
  Near drowning

Thoracic trauma
  Lung contusion
  Blast injury (explosion, lightning)

Embolized substances
  Fat embolism
  Leukoagglutinin reaction
  Aggregated blood products
  Amniotic fluid embolism
  Air embolism

the reasoning underlying the classification proposed in the previous section that separates the syndrome into direct and indirect causes. If one accepts this breakdown, examination of a list of causes of the direct form of ARDS (Table 1.4) provides a straightforward explanation of the pathogenesis of this variety of diffuse parenchymal lung injury.

By contrast, the mechanisms that underlie the indirect variety of ARDS have defied elucidation despite a large amount of careful work that has been periodically reviewed [15,33,34]. It is clearly no longer tenable to think in terms of a 'final common pathway' of the diffuse lung injury that culminates in the syndrome [35]. The 1970s were dominated by studies of mediators such as complement fragments, platelet activating factor, prostaglandins and leukotrienes. The 1980s were the decade of the neutrophil and its products, proteolytic enzymes and reactive species of oxygen. The 1990s, at least so far, belong to the cytokines and two of the cells that release them: macrophages and endothelial cells. The cellular networking system and the humoral mediators that cause and regulate inflammation of the lung parenchyma are extraordinarily complex and there is considerable overlap and redundancy. A partial list of some of the candidate mediators that may contribute to acute parenchymal lung injury and set the process in motion is provided in Table 1.5.

Table 1.5 Inflammatory mediators that may serve as indirect causes of ARDS

Chemotactic factors
  Complement fragments
  Oxidized lipids
  Alveolar macrophage-derived
    (e.g. interleukin 8)
  Metabolites of arachidonic acid

Toxic oxygen metabolites
  Superoxide anion (O_2^-)
  Hydrogen peroxide (H_2O_2)
  Hydroxyl radical ($\cdot OH$)
  Products of lipid peroxidation
  Myeloperoxidase–halide–hydrogen peroxide
    products
    Hypohalous acid
    Halogenated amines

Inflammatory hormones
  Monokines and lymphokines (e.g. interleukins,
    tumor necrosis factor, endothelin)
  Growth factors

Proteolytic enzymes
  Leukocyte granular proteases
  Kallikrein

Vasoactive substances
  Metabolites of arachidonic acid
  Amines
  Kinins
  Platelet activating factors
  Nitric oxide

Coagulation/fibrinolysis factors

Adhesion molecules
  Integrins
  Selectins

Reproduced with permission from Flick, Pulmonary Edema and Acute Lung Injury in Textbook of Respiratory Medicine published by W.B. Saunders Company, 1994 [9].

Although none of these has been conclusively established as playing a role, the search continues because of the promise that identification of one or more key components will be therapeutically beneficial. These and other possible causes of ARDS are discussed in detail elsewhere in this book.

SUMMARY

This brief review of the evolution of knowledge about ARDS is woefully incomplete, but so is our understanding of many important aspects of the condition that, as emphasized, are likely to differ depending on the cause. We have learned a lot about the syndrome during the last 20 years but we still lack essential information that can be translated into effective prevention and control. The subsequent chapters in this book provide an essential framework of knowledge into which new concepts and data can be integrated into improved therapy.

ACKNOWLEDGEMENTS

Supported by Pulmonary Vascular SCOR Grant (HL19155) from the National Heart, Lung, and Blood Institute.

REFERENCES

1. Ashbaugh, D.G., Bigelow, D.B., Petty, T.L. and Levine, B.E. (1967) Acute respiratory distress in adults. *Lancet*, **ii**, 319–23.
2. Petty, T.L. and Ashbaugh, D.G. (1971) The adult respiratory distress syndrome: clinical features, factors influencing prognosis and principles of management. *Chest*, **60**, 233–9.
3. Simeone, F.A. (1968) Pulmonary complications of nonthoracic wounds: a historical perspective. *J. Trauma*, **8**, 625–48.
4. Burford, T.H. and Burbank, B. (1945) Traumatic wet lung; observations on certain fundamen-

tals of thoracic trauma. *J. Thorac. Cardiovasc. Surg.*, **14**, 415–24.

5. Brewer, L.A. III, Burbank, B., Samson, P.C. and Schiff, C.A. (1946) The 'wet lung' in war casualties. *Ann. Surg.*, **123**, 343–62.

6. Pasteur, W. (1914) Massive collapse of the lung. *Br. J. Surg.*, **1**, 587–601.

7. Moutier, F. (1918) Hypertension et mort par oedème pulmonaire aigu chez les blessés cranioencéphaliques. (Relation de ces faits aux recherches récentes sur les fonctions des capsules surrénales.) *Presse Méd.*, **108**, 108-126.

8. Moon, V.H. (1948) The pathology of secondary shock. *Am. J. Pathol.*, **24**, 235–73.

9. Flick, M.R. (1994) Pulmonary edema and acute lung injury, in *Textbook of Respiratory Medicine*, 2nd edn (eds J.F. Murray and J.A Nadel), W.B. Saunders, Philadelphia, p. 1742.

10. Ackroyd, F.W. (1968) Discussion, in Pulmonary Effects of Nonthoracic Trauma (eds B. Eiseman and D.G. Ashbaugh), *J. Trauma*, **8**, 676–7.

11. *Jacobellis v. Ohio*, 378 US 184, 1964, p. 197.

12. Petty, T.L. (1982) Adult respiratory distress syndrome: definition and historical perspective. *Clin. Chest Med.*, **3**, 3–7.

13. Fowler, A.A., Hamman, R.F., Good, J.T. *et al.* (1983) Adult respiratory distress syndrome: risk with common predispositions. *Ann. Intern. Med.*, **98**, 593–7.

14. Simmons, R.S., Berdine, G.G., Seidenfeld, J.J. *et al.* (1987) Fluid balance and the adult respiratory distress syndrome. *Am. Rev. Respir. Dis.*, **135**, 924–9.

15. Rinaldo, J.E. and Rogers, R.M. (1982) Adult respiratory distress syndrome: changing concepts of lung injury and repair. *N. Engl. J. Med.*, **306**, 900–9.

16. Murray, J.F., Matthay, M.A., Luce, J.M. and Flick, M.R. (1988) An expanded definition of the adult respiratory distress syndrome. *Am. Rev. Respir. Dis.*, **138**, 720–3.

17. Lamy, M., Fallat, R.J., Koeniger, E. *et al.* (1976) Pathologic features and mechanisms of hypoxemia in adult respiratory distress syndrome. *Am. Rev. Respir. Dis.*, **114**, 267–84.

18. Bachofen, M. and Weibel, E. (1977) Alterations of the gas exchange apparatus in adult respiratory insufficiency associated with septicemia. *Am. Rev. Respir. Dis.*, **116**, 589–615.

19. Clark, M.C. and Flick M.R. (1984) Permeability pulmonary edema caused by venous air embolism. *Am. Rev. Respir. Dis.*, **129**, 633–5.

20. Cohen, D.S., Matthay, M.A., Cogan, M.G. and Murray, J.F. (1992) Pulmonary edema associated with salt water near-drowning: new insights. *Am. Rev. Respir. Dis.*, **146**, 794–6.

21. Holter, J.F., Weiland, J.E., Pacht, E.R. *et al.* (1986) Protein permeability in the adult respiratory distress syndrome. Loss of size selectivity of the alveolar epithelium. *J. Clin. Invest.*, **78**, 1513–22.

22. Bone, R.C., Balk, R., Slotman, G. *et al.* (1992) Adult respiratory distress syndrome: sequence and importance of development of multiple organ failure. *Chest*, **101**, 320–6.

23. Montgomery, A.B. Stager, M.A., Carrico, C.J. and Hudson, L.D. (1985) Causes of mortality in patients with the adult respiratory distress syndrome. *Am. Rev. Respir. Dis.*, **132**, 485–9.

24. Bachofen, M. and Weibel, E.R. (1982) Structural alterations of lung parenchyma in the adult respiratory distress syndrome. *Clin. Chest Med.*, **3**, 35–56.

25. Weinberg, P.F., Matthay, M.A., Webster, R.O. *et al.* (1984) Biologically active products of complement and acute lung injury in patients with the sepsis syndrome. *Am. Rev. Respir. Dis.*, **130**, 791–6.

26. Weigelt, J.A., Norcross, J.F., Borman, K.R. and Snyder W.H. (1985) Early steroid therapy for respiratory failure. *Arch. Surg.*, **120**, 536–40.

27. Luce, J.M., Montgomery, A.B., Marks, J.D. *et al.* (1988) Ineffectiveness of high dose methylprednisolone in preventing parenchymal lung injury and improving mortality in patients with septic shock. *Am. Rev. Respir. Dis.*, **138**, 62–8.

28. Murray, T.L. (1975) The adult respiratory distress syndrome (may it rest in peace). [Editorial.] *Am. Rev. Respir. Dis.*, **111**, 716–8.

29. Petty, T.L. (1975) The adult respiratory distress syndrome. Confessions of a lumper. [Editorial.] *Am. Rev. Respir. Dis.*, **111**, 713–5.

30. Bernard, G.R. Artigas, A, Brigham, K.L. *et al.* (1994) Report of the American–European Consensus Conference on acute respiratory distress syndrome: definitions, mechanisms, relevant outcomes, and clinical trial coordination. *Am. Rev. Respir. Dis.*, **149**, 818–24.

31. Hardaway, R.M., James, P.M., Anderson, R.W. *et al.* (1967) Intensive study and treatment of shock in man. *JAMA*, **199**, 779–90.

32. Fishman, A.P. (1973) Shock lung. A distinctive nonentity. *Circulation*, **47**, 921–3.

33. Murray, J.F. (1977) Conference report: Mechanisms of acute lung injury. *Am. Rev. Respir. Dis.*, **115**, 1071–8.

34. Fein, A., Wiener-Kronish, J, Niederman, M. and Matthay, M.A. (1986) Pathophysiology of the adult respiratory distress syndrome. What have we learned from human studies? *Crit. Care Clin.*, **2**, 143–67.

35. Repine, J.E. (1992) Scientific perspectrives on adult respiratory distress syndrome. *Lancet*, **339**, 466–9.

EPIDEMIOLOGY

Molly L. Osborne and Robert J. Meyer

> Uncontrolled septicemia leads to frothy pulmonary edema that resembles serum, not the sanguineous transudative edema fluid of ... congestive heart failure.
>
> *William Osler, 1927* [1].

DEFINITION

The definition of the syndrome of acute respiratory distress in adults (ARDS) was first limited to acute lung injury, but has now been expanded to include the diffuse alveolar-capillary damage that occurs as a component of the systemic inflammatory response and multiple system organ failure. When Ashbaugh *et al.* described ARDS in 1967, they recognized that the clinical syndrome had been described almost twenty years earlier as 'congestive atelectasis' [2], but characterized ARDS more precisely as 'severe dyspnea, hypoxemia, and diffuse bilateral pulmonary infiltrates following acute lung injury in previously healthy persons' [3]. In recent years it has become clear that ARDS is really the pulmonary manifestation of systemic, multiple organ failure usually associated with sepsis and widespread, uncontrolled intravascular inflammation [4]. ARDS is usually a component of this systemic inflammatory response syndrome, which is mediated largely by widespread damage to the vascular endothelium. Importantly, patients with ARDS can progress to multiple organ dysfunction syndrome, which is defined as altered organ function in an acutely ill patient such that homeostasis cannot be maintained without intervention (Chapter 18).

The diagnostic criteria for ARDS have evolved over the last twenty-five years (Chapter 1). Initially, clinical, radiographic and physiologic signs were assessed [5]. Specifically, severe dyspnea, tachypnea, intercostal retractions and cyanosis refractory to oxygen, diffuse bilateral pulmonary infiltrates on chest radiography, reduced lung and chest wall compliance, increased alveolar to arterial oxygen tension difference, improvements in pulmonary oxygen transport with positive end expiratory pressure (PEEP), and high minute ventilation requirements were all considered to be important features of the syndrome. To help standardize grading of these defects a four component scoring system for acute lung injury was subsequently developed; that is described further by Murray (Chapter 1). To describe parenchymal lung injury more fully, its chronicity and the underlying cause (or associated condition) were added [6]. Recently, a consensus conference of North American and European investigators defined ARDS as bilateral pulmonary infiltrates and an arterial oxygen tension to inspired oxygen concentration ratio ($Pa_{O_2}/F_{I_{O_2}}$) < 200 in the absence of left heart failure and/or interstitial lung disease [7].

Thus, although no universally accepted definition exists, most authorities agree that ARDS is the pulmonary manifestation of the

ARDS Acute Respiratory Distress in Adults. Edited by Timothy W. Evans and Christopher Haslett. Published in 1996 by Chapman & Hall, London. ISBN 0 412 56910 8

systemic inflammatory response syndrome, which may then lead to multiple organ failure. Consensus criteria that define acute lung injury have been identified, and are similar to clinical definitions [8] in that a predisposing condition, gas exchange abnormalities, abnormal chest radiograph and level of pulmonary artery occlusion pressure are considered important.

INCIDENCE

The incidence of ARDS worldwide is currently estimated at about 5–7 per 100 000 individuals, much lower than initially reported. Twenty years ago the National Heart and Lung Institute's (NHLI) task force on respiratory diseases estimated that about 75 cases of ARDS per 100 000 individuals occurred in the USA per year [9]. However, more recent figures from the USA, England and the Canary Islands suggest a tenfold lower incidence, from 5.3 to 7.1 in the USA [10], 4.5 in England [11] and 1.5–3.5 in the Canary Islands [12], although an incidence of 88.6 cases per 100 000 individuals has been reported in Germany [13].

Estimates of incidence must be interpreted carefully, particularly as no universally accepted definition of ARDS exists. In a recent study employing the current code from the International Classification of Diseases (ICD), ICD-9, in a computer search strategy corroborated by chart review, the search greatly overestimated the incidence of ARDS. The positive predictive value (PPV) was only 20% [14]. This overestimation was minimized in a more sophisticated search strategy which utilized additional ICD-9 codes as exclusion criteria, e.g. congestive heart failure, connective tissue diseases, HIV related diseases, and primary or metastatic pulmonary malignancies (PPV = 66%). The methods used to determine incidence must therefore be examined for each study in order to determine how representative the data are. Firm data were lacking twenty years ago when figures for the incidence of ARDS were first published. The NHLI task force then stated that 'valid statistical data to document the magnitude of the health problem due to respiratory distress syndrome are virtually unobtainable' [9]. By contrast, the recent figures cited above from Spain, England and the USA were obtained from three prospective studies of several hundred ARDS patients meeting the (then) current diagnostic criteria for acute lung injury [10,12,15,], and a single large retrospective study [11]. However, even some of these studies may have had methodologic flaws. For example, the study from the Canary Islands excluded from the definition of ARDS patients under 15 years of age (the numerator of the incidence rate), yet did not exclude such individuals from the population estimate (the denominator of the incidence rate). Since the mean age of the population of the Canary Islands was reported to be 30.2 years, the incidence rate of ARDS in the population over 15 years is certainly higher, and is probably higher in the population as a whole. Interestingly, the recent data demonstrating a high incidence of ARDS in Germany also came from a prospective study of a large population (3.44 million), but the definition of acute respiratory failure as intubation and mechanical ventilation for more than 24 hours in patients over 14 years of age may also have been inadequate [13]. This broad definition almost certainly included patients with respiratory failure from causes other than ARDS, thereby overestimating the incidence.

The overall number of patients at risk who subsequently develop ARDS is not known. However, one study reported the incidence of ARDS associated with eight conditions thought to predispose to respiratory failure, and demonstrated a wide variation in incidence rates (Table 2.1) [15]. This variation may reflect the spectrum of intravascular inflammation and subsequent breakdown of alveolar capillary integrity. For example, cardiopulmonary bypass, burn and fracture may have a limited effect on activation of

Table 2.1 Incidence by predisposed group

Risks for predisposition	No. of patients at risk	No. of patients with the syndrome	Incidence rate (per 100)
Cardiopulmonary bypass	237	4	1.7
Burns	87	2	2.3
Bacteremia	239	9	3.8
Hypertransfusion	197	9	4.6
Fracture	38	2	5.3
Pneumonia in intensive care	84	10	11.9
Disseminated intravascular coagulation	9	2	22.2
Pulmonary aspiration	45	16	35.6

Source: Fowler *et al.* [15].

intravascular inflammatory mediators, in contrast to pneumonia, aspiration and disseminated intravascular coagulation.

DEMOGRAPHICS

The demographics of patients with ARDS suggest that an acute inciting event triggers lung injury rather than exacerbations of chronic, underlying diseases. The time course for the development of lung injury after the onset of a predisposing clinical disorder is rapid, usually less than 24 hours [16]. According to a noninterventional multicenter registry of patients with ARDS, the average patient is relatively young (49 ± 2 years old), male (3:2 males to females), white (3:1 whites to blacks) and a nonsmoker (2:1 nonsmokers to smokers) [17]. Similar demographic data have been obtained from other studies [18,19]. The demographics of health care utilization demonstrate that patients with ARDS not only require high intensity acute care, but also long term hospitalization. In general, the mean length of stay in an intensive care unit is 12 days, and the mean length of hospitalization one month [19]. Survivors require longer hospital care than nonsurvivors. The data from the noninterventional multicenter registry demonstrated that, after the third day, survivors with ARDS had higher mean arterial blood pressure and arterial pH than nonsurvivors, despite the more frequent use

of vasopressors in the nonsurvivors [17]. The average time to hospital discharge in survivors is 47 days, and the average time to death in nonsurvivors 16 days [15,17]. Several important demographic variables have not been tabulated for patients with ARDS, including occupation, socioeconomic status, nutritional status, alcohol consumption, previous health care utilization, medication use, body mass, functional status, fitness and education. No data have been published on the periodicity of hospitalizations for ARDS.

PREDISPOSING FACTORS

Most research suggests that the major risk factors associated with the development of ARDS are (in order of decreasing frequency) sepsis (40–60%), trauma (20–35%), nosocomial and gastric aspiration pneumonia (10–20%), massive transfusion (9%) and pancreatitis (7%). The percentages in parentheses show the variation from study to study (Figure 2.1) [15,17,20,21]. A significant difference in incidence was found between patients with one as opposed to several risk factors (5.8 versus 24.6 per 100 patients) [15].

Sepsis is of particular concern as the most common predisposing factor for ARDS. Although bacteremia alone carries a relatively low risk of causing progressive lung injury (5–20%), when a systemic response or organ failure ensues 25–40% of patients develop

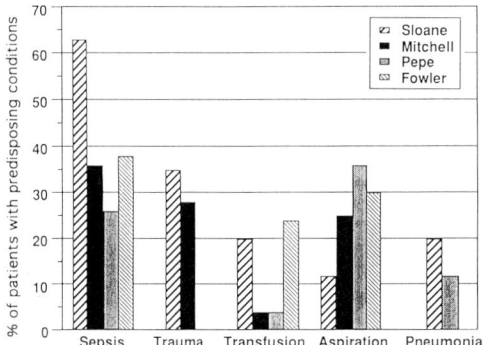

Figure 2.1 Summary of the results of four studies that investigated the relative frequency of predisposing factors in the occurrence of ARDS. The factors illustrated, most especially sepsis, are clearly important disposing conditions in the development of ARDS across these studies, despite differences in definitions of the predisposing factors and the settings between the studies.

ARDS [22]. In Gram-negative sepsis this is probably due to the ability of endotoxin to stimulate the inflammatory cascade at both cellular and subcellular levels.

PREDICTORS OF ARDS

A great deal of research has focused on identifying early predictors of acute lung injury in at risk patients, yet no such factors have been identified and validated. These would be invaluable in the early identification of patients, as well as for epidemiological research aimed at developing therapeutic strategies.

Historically, research focused on many indicators of acute systemic inflammation, including the complement system, activation of the coagulation and the fibrinolytic system, the kinin–kallikrein system and endothelial cell activation [23]. Ultimately, levels of many of these mediators of inflammation lacked the sensitivity and specificity necessary to predict the development of ARDS. Thus, complement activation alone is insufficient to produce acute lung injury, and the terminal complement complex sC5b–9 does not discriminate between patients at risk for and patients with

ARDS [24,25]. Also, levels of von Willebrand factor antigen, produced in vascular endothelial cells and released during endothelial cell injury, do not predict the development of ARDS [26].

Many other inflammatory mediators are currently under investigation. Tumor necrosis factor (TNF)α, a cytokine produced by stimulated monocytes and macrophages, may play a role in multiple disease processes including sepsis and acute lung injury. The intravascular administration of TNFα reproduces the physiologic manifestations of shock seen with the infusion of endotoxin [27]. However, several studies have been unable to associate levels of TNFα in serum or bronchoalveolar lavage (BAL) fluid with the onset of ARDS [28,29]. The authors speculated that the inconsistencies in the TNFα measurements they observed, using five different methods, might account for inconsistencies in the published literature regarding the relationship between TNFα and disease processes [29].

Desmosine, a protein crosslink between elastin chains in the lung, is released from elastin by the action of elastase from activated neutrophils. When elastin breakdown occurs in the circulation, it can pass directly out of the system in urine and an elevated urinary desmosine excretion has been shown to identify patients with ARDS with a high degree of sensitivity and specificity [30].

A recent study investigated whether or not a variety of antioxidants, measured sequentially in serum, could predict the development of ARDS at the time an initial diagnosis of sepsis was made, 6–24 hours before the development of clinical acute lung injury [31]. Specifically, increases in both manganese superoxide dismutase and catalase activity appeared to predict the development of ARDS in septic patients.

Finally, a recent study reported finding elevated levels of interleukin 8 (IL-8), a neutrophil chemotactic factor, in BAL fluid from six of seven patients who subsequently developed ARDS, compared with measurements from a similar at risk group ($P = 0.0006$) [32]. One caution in interpreting these data is that one individual from the ARDS group had a BAL IL-8 level in excess of 50-fold above the other patients in this group, substantially skewing the mean of the reported data. However, median levels were still different, and further studies of IL-8 as a marker for the development of ARDS appear to be warranted.

Nevertheless, no marker has been demonstrated to have sufficient sensitivity and specificity to predict reliably the development of ARDS in an at risk population.

NATURAL HISTORY

Despite advances in knowledge and the intensive care of patients with ARDS, the fatality rate in patients with ARDS remains in the order of 50–70% [33–35]. However, several recent studies, including a careful longitudinal study, suggest that the fatality rate is decreasing, although it varies from study to study, again reflecting different study populations and disease definitions. Thus, when fatality rates were examined at a single institution using the same criteria for ARDS over a 10 year period between 1983 and 1992, overall mortality decreased significantly from 53.7% to 39.5% (Table 2.2) [20]. Correcting for confounding variables, such as age, gender, risk group, injury severity score (in trauma patients) and enrollment in experimental protocols, did not eliminate the observed decline. Similarly, a multicenter registry recently reported a decline in overall case fatality rate, yet the lower rate of 54% was still relatively high [36]. Finally, a fall in mortality from 89% 10 years ago to 55% has been demonstrated in patients with severe lung injury (as defined by the extracorporeal membrane oxygenation (ECMO) trial in the 1970s) [37]. No obvious differences in etiology, acute physiological and chronic health evaluation (APACHE) II score, organ system failure or the incidence of sepsis were found between survivors and nonsurvivors.

PREDICTORS OF MORTALITY

In general, predictors of mortality reflect patients' clinical characteristics, the severity of lung injury and the development of acute multiorgan system failure.

Clinical characteristics, such as age, clearly have an impact on mortality in ARDS [17,36], in that a study has shown patients from 16 to 49 years of age to have a death rate of 37%, patients 50–59 years of age a rate of 62%, and patients over 60 years of age a mortality rate of 75% [17]. The presence of an underlying chronic disease such as hematological malignancy or cirrhosis in patients who develop ARDS leads to a mortality in excess of 90% [38]. By contrast, data from the multicenter ARDS registry suggest there is no significant difference in mortality in surgical versus nonsurgical patients, smoking versus nonsmoking patients, or all cancer versus versus noncancer patients [17].

The nature of predisposing conditions leading to ARDS also impacts on mortality [17]. As previously stated, sepsis is the most common clinical disorder in which ARDS develops and predicts a poor outcome. Between 20

Table 2.2 Fatality rates by year and risk group

	1983	1984	1985	1986	1987	1988	1989	1990	1991	1992
Total *n*	67	98	87	71	69	90	73	109	87	76
All risks	53.7	67.4	69.0	56.3	62.3	58.9	56.2	47.7	48.3	39.5
Sepsis	71.4	66.7	76.9	66.7	63.6	65.7	68.2	56.8	59.4	30.0
Trauma	42.9	55.0	71.4	48.0	48.0	31.8	50.0	31.0	25.0	43.7

and 40% of patients with the sepsis syndrome subsequently develop ARDS [39], and 70–90% of these, particularly those with Gram-negative sepsis, will die [40,41]. Mortality in patients with sepsis from either a pulmonary or a nonpulmonary source is higher (72%) than in patients with aspiration (52%) or primary pneumonia alone (48%) [42]. There are also predictors of low mortality, for example, a 10% mortality in patients who develop ARDS as a result of the fat embolism syndrome [43].

Severity of ARDS is a reliable indicator of mortality, in that patients with the best static lung compliance and the most substantial and prompt improvement in arterial oxygenation at the initiation of ventilatory support are most likely to recover [5] (Chapter 15). However, more recent indicators of parenchymal lung injury, such as the acute lung injury score, have not predicted outcome accurately [44]. These two observations might be reconciled if severity of ARDS is reflected best by physiological response to treatment, rather than the extent of acute inflammation.

The development of acute multiorgan system failure is associated with increased mortality in patients with ARDS and in patients with septic shock. The nonpulmonary organ dysfunction present at the time of intensive care unit (ICU) admission but before the development of acute lung injury seems to have a positive predictive value for mortality [42]. In that study, logistic regression analysis identified three variables that had an excellent combined power for predicting mortality:

1. systemic hypotension (< 100 mmHg systolic pressure at the time of ICU admission);
2. chronic liver disease;
3. nonpulmonary organ system dysfunction developing between hospital admission and admission to the ICU (odds ratio 9.5).

In the patients who developed nonpulmonary organ system dysfunction between hospital and ICU admission, mortality was 88%, but it was only 49% in those patients in which nonpulmonary organ system dysfunction was absent. Importantly, an intact epithelial barrier function seems to be critical for the resolution of alveolar edema in ARDS [44,45] (Chapter 20).

Indices that have not reliably predicted outcome in ARDS include lung injury score on day 1, measured levels of mediators of acute inflammation (e.g. leukotriene B_4, leukotriene D_4, neuropeptides, TNFα, IL-6, IL-8), and markers of endothelial activation and injury (vWF-antigen, E-selectin) [28,44]. Nevertheless, inflammatory mediators and markers of endothelial cell activation and injury continue to be of great interest to researchers in the context of mortality. Thus, high levels of a neutrophil chemotaxin, neutrophil activating peptide 1/IL-8, are correlated with a high mortality in patients with ARDS [46], and plasma P-selectin levels, markers of endothelial activation, may be greater in ARDS patients who do not survive [47]. Such findings need confirmation before they can become clinically useful.

DIRECT CAUSES OF MORTALITY

Direct causes of mortality from ARDS have not changed since the early 1980s [18]. An analysis from Seattle in 1980 demonstrated that the case fatality rate of ARDS was high (68%) and the cause of death most often the sepsis syndrome/multiple organ dysfunction (34%) rather than respiratory failure (16%) [37]. Ten years later the overall case fatality rate at the same hospital was lower at 51%, yet the causes of death remained unchanged (Table 2.3). Uncorrectable respiratory failure was the cause of death in only a minority of patients. The authors concluded that sepsis syndrome with multiple organ failure continues to be the major cause of death in patients with ARDS despite advances in antibacterial therapy [18].

Table 2.3 Direct cause of death in patients with ARDS

Cause	*Steinberg* et al. *[18]*		*Montgomery* et al. *[36]*	
	Number	*%*	*Number*	*%*
Sepsis	25	46	11	34
Respiratory	8	15	5	16
Heart	4	7	6	19
Central nervous system	10	19	7	22
Liver	4	7	0	–
Gastrointestinal	2	4	0	–
Other	1	2	3	9
Total	54	100	32	100

LONG TERM SEQUELAE

Significant respiratory impairment, although infrequent, has been well described in patients who recover from ARDS, and correlates with severity of lung injury [48] (Chapter 15). Physiological markers of severity such as low total thoracic compliance, elevated initial mean pulmonary artery pressure, duration of $F_{IO_2} > 0.6$, and maximal level of positive end expiratory pressure have been shown to correlate with abnormal pulmonary function test results performed more than one year after the onset of ARDS [49]. In particular, support with $F_{IO_2} > 0.6$ for more than 24 hours appeared to be a sensitive and specific predictor of an abnormally reduced diffusion capacity for carbon monoxide when assessed one year following ARDS. At this time, about 48% of patients had mild respiratory impairment according to pulmonary function testing, 15% had moderate and 4% severe impairment (Figure 2.2) [50].

Prolonged positive pressure ventilation, high F_{IO_2}, increased age, positive smoking history and the severity of hypoxemia during ARDS were shown to correlate strongly with pulmonary impairment after recovery [51]. Although open lung biopsies taken from patients with more unfavorable physiologic measures (poor compliance and poor blood gas response to PEEP) have the greatest cellular and fibrotic changes when assessed during acute ARDS [5], follow up data have revealed no correlation between severity graded by open lung biopsy and lung function carried out one year later [50,52].

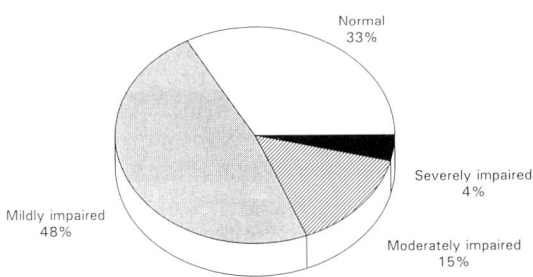

Figure 2.2 Degree of pulmonary limitation at 1 year following the occurrence of ARDS. Of the 27 patients studied, 81% had no or mild impairment as measured by standard pulmonary function testing, with the clear minority having severe impairment. (Reproduced with permission from Ghio *et al.*) [50].

EFFECTS OF TREATMENT ON OUTCOME

ARDS is a product of modern medicine in that successful medical interventions in sepsis, multiple trauma, gastric aspiration and inhalational injuries may cause some patients to survive only to develop acute lung injury. ARDS represents an unduly severe pulmonary inflammatory response that causes damage to the vascular endothelial-epithelial

Table 2.4 Non-pharmacologic strategies in the management of ARDS

Strategy	Status	References
Preventive PEEP	No role in preventing ARDS	53
Inverse ratio ventilation	Improves mechanics/oxygenation in subsets of patients; no clear survival benefit	54
Extracorporeal oxygenation	No clear data to support its use in the management of ARDS	55
Extracorporeal CO_2 removal	No demonstrable survival advantage	56
High frequency ventilation	May be useful in defined subsets of patients; no proven survival advantage	57, 58

Table 2.5 Pharmacologic agents in the treatment/prevention of ARDS

Strategy	Statuis	References
Corticosteroids	No role in early disease, ? in late	59, 60, 61
Exogenous surfactant	Possible role; no proven survival benefit	62, 63, 64, 65
Nitric oxide	Improves $\dot{V}/\dot{Q}$ match; no proven survival benefit	66
Ketoconazole	Possibly as a preventative; needs confirmation	67, 68
Monoclonal antibodies	Possible role in specific subsets; no proven overall benefit	69, 70
Non-steroidals	Mixed results; no proven survival benefit	71
Prostaglandin E1	Improved hemodynamics but no survival benefit	72, 73

barrier, and in advanced cases leads to fibrosis. Although many treatment strategies have evolved, there is little proof that intervention beyond careful routine intensive care has a significant impact on outcome. Most clinicians and researchers strongly believe that to reduce mortality and morbidity early treatment must be instituted. The treatment strategies under active investigation, both pharmacologic and nonpharmacologic, are summarized in Tables 2.4 and 2.5 [53–58].

Because adequate outcome data are lacking, physicians must provide intensive care for most patients with ARDS, even though such efforts will ultimately fail in the majority. Predictions of outcome based on the currently available severity of illness scoring systems are not useful in this regard because individual patients with similar scores will have a wide range of outcomes depending on the underlying diagnosis. So, while such scoring systems are useful for population based

prediction models, they do not predict outcomes in individual patients. Therefore, the development of good outcomes data in respiratory distress syndrome is of paramount importance (Chapter 22). Because the numbers of patients with ARDS are small, such outcomes data would best be acquired via the analysis of large regional, national or international registries. Such registries allow for the linkage of epidemiologic databases, for enumeration of treatment outcomes and determination of cost effectiveness [17]. Reliable outcomes data in patients with ARDS would allow for better discrimination between patients in whom intensive treatment has a reasonable chance of benefit and those in whom such care would likely be futile, e.g. less than 1% chance of survival [74]. With the burgeoning costs of medical care, such data could be instrumental in increasing the cost effectiveness of the medical care of patients with ARDS.

SUMMARY

ARDS remains a devastating disease, with an unacceptably high mortality rate. Although the incidence of ARDS does not appear to be as high as once thought (about 5–7 per 100 000 individuals), it still represents a significant clinical problem [10–12]. The development of clear epidemiological measures of disease occurrence, clinical predictors and preventive strategies has been hampered in the past by the lack of agreement on a suitable definition for the syndrome, but this appears to have been resolved [7]. Despite many promising trials, there is no definitive therapy for ARDS, although the general improvement in intensive care, particularly a strict protocol for ventilatory management, appears to have had some impact on survival [56]. Mortality rates are apparently declining but are quite high overall at 50–70% [33–35]. Promising therapies and modes of ventilation continue to be investigated, and it is certain that ARDS will continue to be a subject of intensive laboratory and clinical research.

REFERENCES

1. Osler, W. (1927) *The Principles and Practice of Medicine*, 10th edn, Appleton, New York.
2. Jenkins, M.T., Jones, R.F., Wilson, B. *et al.* (1950) Congestive atelectasis – a complication of intravenous fluids. *Ann. Surg.*, **132**, 327–47.
3. Ashbaugh, D.G., Bigelow, D.B., Petty, T.L. and Levine, B.E. (1967) Acute respiratory distress in adults. *Lancet*, **ii**, 319–23.
4. Bone, R.C. (1991) Multiple system organ failure and the sepsis syndrome. *Hosp. Pract.*, **Nov. 15**, 101–26.
5. Petty, T.L. and Newman, J.H. (1978) Adult respiratory distress syndrome. *West. J. Med.*, **128**, 399–407.
6. Murray, J.F., Matthay, M.A., Luce, J.M. *et al.* (1988) An expanded definition of the adult respiratory distress syndrome. *Am. Rev. Respir. Dis.*, **138**, 720–3.
7. Bernard, G.R., Artigas, A. and Brigham, K.L. *et al.* (1994) The American–European consensus conference on ARDS. Definitions, mechanisms, relevant outcomes, and clinical trials coordination. *Am. J. Respir. Crit. Care Med.*, **149**, 818–24.
8. Carmichael, L.C., Dorinsky, P.M., Bernard, G.R. *et al.* (1993) Survey of diagnosis and therapy of adult respiratory distress syndrome. *Am. Rev. Respir. Dis.*, **147**, A347.
9. Ashbaugh, D.G., Chairman, National Heart and Lung Institute's Task Force (1972) *Respiratory Diseases: Task Force Report on problems, Research Approaches, Needs*, DHEW publication NIH # 74–432, US Government Printing Office, Washington, pp. 167–80.
10. Thomsen, G.E., Morris, A.H., Canino, D. *et al.* (1993) Incidence of the adult respiratory distress syndrome in Utah. *Am. Rev. Respir. Dis.*, **147**, A347.
11. Webster, N.R., Cohen, A.T. and Nunn, J.F. (1988) Adult respiratory distress syndrome – how many cases in the UK? *Anaesthesia*, **43**, 923–6.
12. Villar, J. and Slutsky, A.S. (1989) The incidence of the adult respiratory distress syndrome. *Am. Rev. Respir. Dis.*, **140**, 814–6.
13. Lewandowski, K., Meta, J., Preiss, H. *et al.* (1993) Incidence, severity and mortality of acute respiratory failure in Berlin/Germany: a prospective multicenter trial in 72 intensive care units. *Am. Rev. Respir. Dis.*, **147**, A349.
14. Earle, L.A., Grimm, A.M., Hopkins L.E. *et al.* (1993) Identifying patients with adult respiratory distress syndrome by utilizing a search strategy employing ICD-9 codes. *Am. Rev. Respir. Dis.*, **147**, A348.
15. Fowler, A.A., Hamman, R.F., Good, J.T., *et al.* (1983) Adult respiratory distress syndrome: risk with common predispositions. *Ann. Intern. Med.*, **98**, 593–7.
16. Weinberg, P.F., Matthay, M.A., Webster, R.O. *et al.* (1984) Biologically active products of complement and acute lung injury in patients with sepsis syndrome. *Am. Rev. Respir. Dis.*, **130**, 176–6.
17. Sloane, P.J., Gee, J.H., Gottlieb, J.E. *et al.* (1992) A multicenter registry of patients with acute respiratory distress syndrome. *Am. Rev. Respir. Dis.*, **146**, 419–26.
18. Steinberg, K.P., McHugh, L.G. and Hudson, L.D. (1993) Causes of mortality in patients with the adult respiratory distress syndrome (ARDS): an update. *Am. Rev. Respir. Dis.*, **147**, A347.
19. Humphrey, H., Hall, J., Sznajder, I. *et al.* (1990) Improved survival in ARDS patients associated with a reduction in pulmonary capillary wedge pressure. *Chest*, **97**, 1176–80.

20. Mitchell, D.R., Milberg, J.A., Steinberg, K.P. *et al.* (1993) Trends in adult respiratory distress syndrome (ARDS) fatality rates from 1983–1992. *Am. Rev. Respir. Dis.*, **147**, A348.

21. Pepe, P.E., Potkin, R.T., Reus, D.H. *et al.* (1982) Clinical predictors of the adult respiratory distress syndrome. *Am. J. Surg.*, **144**, 124–30.

22. Niederman, M.S. and Fein, A.M. (1990) Sepsis syndrome, the adult respiratory distress syndrome, and nosocomial pneumonia. *Clin. Chest Med.*, **11**, 633–56.

23. Bengtsson A. (1993) Cascade system activation in shock. *Acta Anaesthesiol. Scand.*, **37**, (Suppl. 98): 7–10.

24. Webster, R.O., Larsen, G.L., Mitchell, B.C. *et al.* (1982) Absence of inflammatory lung injury in rabbits challenged intravascularly with complement-derived chemotactic factors. *Am. Rev. Respir. Dis.*, **125**, 335–40.

25. Parsons, P.E. and Giclas, P.C. (1990) The terminal complement complex (sC5b–9) is not specifically associated with the development of the ARDS. *Am. Rev. Respir. Dis.*, **141**, 98–103.

26. Moss, M., Ackerson, L., Gillespie, M.K. *et al.* (1993) Von Willebrand factor antigen levels do not predict the development of the adult respiratory distress syndrome. *Am. Rev. Respir. Dis.*, **147**, A345.

27. Tracey, K.J., Butler, B., Lowery, S.F. *et al.* (1986) Shock and tissue injury induced by human recombinant cachectin. *Science*, **234**, 470–4.

28. Hyers, T.M., Tricomi, S.M., Dettenmeier, P.A. *et al.* (1991) Tumor necrosis factor levels in serum and bronchoalveolar lavage fluid of patients with the adult respiratory distress syndrome. *Am. Rev. Respir. Dis.*, **144**, 268–71.

29. Parsons, P.E., Moore, F.A., Moore, E.E. *et al.* (1992) Studies on the role of tumor necrosis factor in adult respiratory distress syndrome. *Am. Rev. Respir. Dis.*, **146**, 694–700.

30. Tenholder, M.F., Rajagopal, K.R., Phillips, Y.Y. *et al.* (1991) Urinary desmosine excretion as a marker of lung injury in the adult respiratory distress syndrome. *Chest*, **100**, 1385–90.

31. Leff, J.A., Parsons, P.E., Day, C.E. *et al.* (1993) Serum antioxidants as predictors of adult respiratory distress syndrome in patients with sepsis. *Lancet*, **341**, 777–80.

32. Donnelly, S.C., Strieter, R.M., Kunkel, S.L. *et al.* (1993) Interleukin-8 and development of adult respiratory distress syndrome in at-risk patient groups. *Lancet*, **341**, 643–7.

33. St John, R.C. and Dorinsky, P.M. (1993) Immunologic therapy for ARDS, septic shock, and multiple-organ failure. *Chest*, **103**, 932–43.

34. Cunningham, A.J. (1991) Acute respiratory distress syndrome – two decades later. *Yale J. Biol. Med.*, **64**, 387–402.

35. Brannen, A.L., Godfrey, L.J. and Goetter, W.E. (1989) Prediction of outcome from critical illness: a comparison of clinical judgment with a prediction rule. *Arch. Intern. Med.*, **149**, 1083–6.

36. Montgomery, A.B., Stager, M.A., Carrico, C.J. *et al.* (1985) Causes of mortality in patients with the adult respiratory distress syndrome. *Am. Rev. Respir. Dis.*, **132**, 485–9.

37. Suchyta, M.R., Clemmer, T.P., Orme, J.F.Jr *et al.* (1991) Increased survival of ARDS patients with severe hypoxemia (ECMO criteria). *Chest*, **99**, 951–5.

38. Osborne, M.L. (1992) Physician decisions regarding life support in the intensive care unit. *Chest*, **101**, 217–24.

39. Wiener-Kronish, J.P., Gropper, M.A. and Matthay, M.A. (1990) The adult respiratory distress syndrome: definition and prognosis, pathogenesis and treatment. *Br. J. Anaesth.*, **65**, 107–29.

40. Seidenfeld, J.J., Pohl, D.F., Bell, R.C. *et al.* (1986) Incidence, site, and outcome of infections in patients with the adult respiratory distress syndrome. *Am. Rev. Respir. Dis.*, **134**, 12–16.

41. Kaplan, R.L., Sahn, S.A. and Petty, T.L. (1979) Incidence and outcome of the respiratory distress syndrome in gram-negative sepsis. *Arch. Intern. Med.*, **139**, 867–9.

42. Matthay, M.A., Szaflarski, N., Modin, G. *et al.* (1993) Prospective study of 123 patients with acute lung injury: predictors of mortality. *Am. Rev. Respir. Dis.*, **147**, A348.

43. Schonfeld, S.A., Ploysongsang, Y., Di Lisio, R. *et al.* (1983) Fat embolism prophylaxis with corticosteroids. *Ann. Intern. Med.*, **99**, 438–43.

44. Matthay, M.A. (1994) Function of the alveolar epithelial barrier under pathologic conditions. *Chest*, **105** (suppl.), 67S-74S.

45. Matthay, M.A. and Wiener-Kronish, J.P. (1990) Intact epithelial barrier function is critical for the resolution of alveolar edema in humans. *Am. Rev. Respir. Dis.*, **142**, 1250–7.

46. Miller, E.J., Cohen, A.B., Nagao S. *et al.* (1992) Elevated levels of NAP-1 interleukin-8 are present in the airspaces of patients with the adult respiratory distress syndrome and are associated with increased mortality. *Am. Rev. Respir. Dis.*, **146**, 427–32.

47. Ishizaka, A., Sakamaki, F., Handa, M. *et al.* (1993) Significance of the soluble form of P-selectin in the plasma of patients with acute lung injury. *Am. Rev. Respir. Dis.,* **147**, A345.

48. Ashbaugh, D.G., Petty, T.L., Bigelow, D.B. *et al.* (1969) Continuous positive-pressure breathing (CPPB) in adult respiratory distress syndrome. *J. Thorac. Cardiovasc. Surg.,* **57**, 31–41.

49. Elliott, C.G., Rasmusson, B.Y., Crapo, R.O. *et al.* (1987) Prediction of pulmonary function abnormalities after adult respiratory distress syndrome (ARDS). *Am. Rev. Respir. Dis.,* **135**, 634–8.

50. Ghio, A.J., Elliot, C.G., Crapo, R.O. *et al.* (1989) Impairment after adult respiratory distress syndrome. *Am. Rev. Respir. Dis.,* **139**, 1158–62.

51. Suchyta, M.R., Jensen, R.L., Elliott, C.G. *et al.* (1993) Respiratory impairment after ARDS. *Am. Rev. Respir. Dis.,* **147**, A348.

52. Suchyta, M.R., Elliott, C.G., Colby, T. *et al.* (1991) Open lung biopsy does not correlate with pulmonary function after the adult respiratory distress syndrome. *Chest,* **99**, 1232–7.

53. Pepe, P.E., Hudson, L.D., Carrico, C.J. (1984) Early application of positive end-expiratory pressure to patients at risk for the adult respiratory distress syndrome. *N. Engl. J. Med.,* **311**, 281–6.

54. Tharrat, R.S., Allen, R.P. and Albertson, T.E. (1988) Pressure controlled inverse ratio ventilation in severe adult respiratory distress syndrome. *Chest,* **94**, 755–62.

55. Zopol, W.M., Snider, M.T., Hill, J.D. *et al.* (1979) Extracorporeal membrane oxygenation in severe acute respiratory failure. *JAMA,* **242**, 2193–6.

56. Morris, A.H., Clemmer, T.P., Orme, J.F.Jr *et al.* (1989) Clinical trial of extracorporeal CO_2 removal. *Chest,* **96** (suppl. 2), 138S (abstract).

57. Carlon, C.G., Howland, W.S., Ray, C. *et al.* (1983) High-frequency jet ventilation: a prospective randomized evaluation. *Chest,* **84**, 551–9.

58. MacIntyre, N.R., Follet, J.V., Dietz, J.L. *et al.* (1986) Jet ventilation at 100 breaths per minute in adult respiratory failure. *Am. Rev. Respir. Dis.,* **134**, 897–901.

59. Bernard, G.R., Luce, J.M., Sprung, C.L. *et al.* (1987) High-dose corticosteroids in patients with the adult respiratory distress syndrome. *N. Engl. J. Med.,* **317**, 1565–70.

60. Bone, R.C., Fisher, C.J., Clemmer, T.P. *et al.* (1987) A controlled clinical trial of high-dose methyl-prednisolone in the treatment of severe sepsis and septic shock. *N. Engl. J. Med.,* **317**, 653.

61. Chinn, A., Meduri, G.U., Leeper, K. *et al.* (1993) High dose corticosteroids (HDC) for rescue treatment of fibroproliferation in late ARDS. *Am. Rev. Respir. Dis.,* **147**, A349.

62. Jobe, A. and Ikegami, M. (1987) Surfactant for the treatment of respiratory distress syndrome. *Am. Rev. Respir. Dis.,* **136**, 1256–75.

63. Lewis, J.F. and Jobe, A.H. (1993) Surfactant and the adult respiratory distress syndrome. *Am. Rev. Respir. Dis.,* **147**, 218–33.

64. Weg, J., Reines, H., Balk, R. *et al.* (1991) Safety and efficacy of an aerosolized surfactant (Exosurf) in human sepsis induced ARDS. *Chest,* **100**, 137S.

65. Wiedemann, H., Baughman, R., deBoisblanc, B. *et al.* (1992) A multi-centered trial in human sepsis induced ARDS of an aerosolized synthetic surfactant (Exosurf). *Am. Rev. Respir. Dis.,* **145**, A184 (abstract).

66. Rossaint, R., Falke, K.J., Lopez, F. *et al.* (1993) Inhaled nitric oxide for the adult respiratory distress syndrome. *N. Engl. J. Med.,* **328**, 399–405.

67. Yu, M. and Tomasa, G. (1993) A double-blind, prospective, randomized trial of ketoconazole, a thromboxane synthetase inhibitor, in the prophylaxis of adult respiratory distress syndrome. *Crit. Care Med.,* **21**, 1635–42.

68. Slotman, G.J., Burchard, K.W., D'Arezzo, A. *et al.* (1984) Ketoconazole prevents acute respiratory failure in critically ill surgical patients. *J. Trauma,* **28**, 648–54.

69. Warren, H.S., Danner, R.L. and Munford, R.S. (1992) Anti-endotoxin monoclonal antibodies. *N. Engl. J. Med.,* **326**, 1153–7.

70. Parrillo, J.E. (1993) Pathogenetic mechanisms of septic shock. *N. Engl. J. Med.,* **328**, 1471–7.

71. Goldstein, G. and Luce, J. (1990) Pharmacologic treatment of the adult respiratory distress syndrome. *Clin. Chest Med.,* **11**, 773–87.

72. Shoemaker, W.C. and Appel, P.L. (1986) Effects of prostaglandin E1 in adult respiratory distress syndrome. *Surgery,* **99**, 275–83.

73. Bone, R.C., Slotman, G., Maunder, R. *et al.* (1989) Randomized double-blind, multicenter study of prostaglandin E1 in patients with adult respiratory distress syndrome. *Chest,* **96**, 114–9.

74. Schneiderman L.J., Jecker N.S. and Jonsen A.R. (1990) Medical futility: its meaning and ethical implications. *Ann. Intern. Med.,* **112**, 949–54.

Nicholas P. Curzen, Christopher Haslett and Timothy W. Evans

Lung injury can result from a wide range of acute or chronic pulmonary and extrapulmonary pathologies (Figure 3.1). Acute lung injury in adults can produce a spectrum of clinical presentation, at the extreme end of which is the syndrome of acute respiratory distress (ARDS). Since its original description as a disease entity [1], ARDS has been the subject of intensive research, but the limitations of this abbreviation in describing such a diverse clinical condition and group of patients have become increasingly apparent. As the epidemiology, aetiology, natural history and pathology of acute lung injury have been researched, it has become harder to define what condition is defined by the term 'ARDS' [2,3]. It has also become apparent that studies utilizing strict clinical definitions of the condition exclude subgroups of patients. Thus, it has been estimated that only 5% of patients with a risk factor for ARDS develop the full syndrome [4]. In particular, enhancing our understanding of the condition, the development of effective therapeutic interventions, and if possible preventing its occurrence will depend on the acquisition of information about those patients who initially have a milder form of acute lung injury which progresses to 'full blown' ARDS. In many patients who develop ARDS, particularly those whose predisposing factor was distant to the lung, such as sepsis, severe burns or pancreatitis, clinically overt lung disease may not become apparent for several hours or days. Whilst subclinical lung damage can occur earlier, this 'latent period' may provide special opportunities for defining very early disease mechanisms, which may provide better predictive indices of those patients at very high risk of developing full blown ARDS and help identify key processes that could be targeted therapeutically with the aim of attenuating or even aborting the lung injury process. Again, however, there is the problem of defining the risk period, particularly as some patients may already have a degree of subclinical ARDS (Figure 3.2). There is also the problem of timing events in the risk period and comparing studies where patients with widely varying predisposing conditions may be identified at different times, and often late in the risk period. Whilst it is clear that systemic, and possibly pulmonary, inflammatory events are occurring and progressing rapidly in the risk period, there have been few detailed studies of the very early risk period in patients with well defined risk factors. However, one such series of studies has shown clear evidence that patients with altered pulmonary levels of interleukin 8 (IL-8) [5] and blood levels of soluble L-selectin [6] and neutrophil elastase [7] within 90 minutes of multiple trauma, pancreatitis or perforated viscus represent a very high risk group for ARDS. These observations suggest that neutrophil chemotaxis, endothelial inter-

ARDS Acute Respiratory Distress in Adults. Edited by Timothy W. Evans and Christopher Haslett. Published in 1996 by Chapman & Hall, London. ISBN 0 412 56910 8

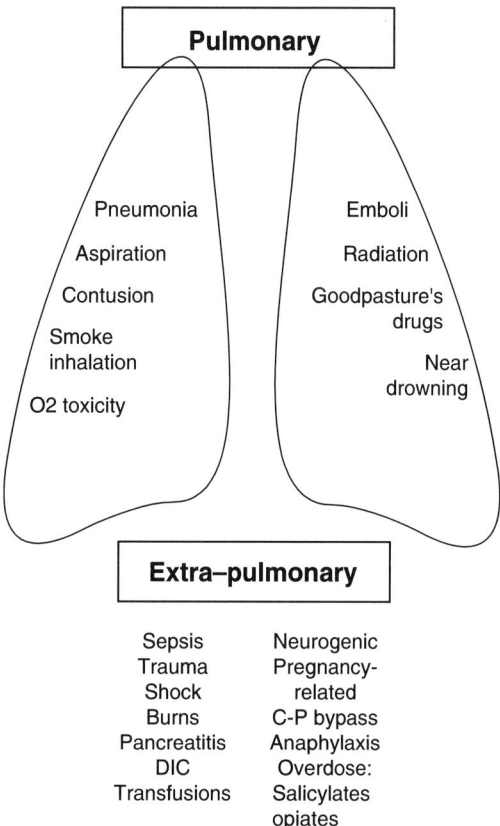

Pulmonary

Pneumonia
Aspiration
Contusion
Smoke inhalation
O2 toxicity

Emboli
Radiation
Goodpasture's drugs
Near drowning

Extra–pulmonary

Sepsis	Neurogenic
Trauma	Pregnancy-
Shock	related
Burns	C-P bypass
Pancreatitis	Anaphylaxis
DIC	Overdose:
Transfusions	Salicylates
	opiates

Figure 3.1 Pulmonary and extrapulmonary conditions associated with acute lung injury. DIC = disseminated intravascular coagulopathy; C-P = Cardiopulmonary.

action and enzyme secretion very early in the risk period may represent some of the earliest events in a process which results in clinically overt ARDS 24–48 hours later.

Lung injury is common: 35% of patients with sepsis have mild to moderate lung injury, and 25% severe lung injury or fully developed ARDS [8], with a mortality in the latter group of between 50 and 75%. Lung injury is rarely an isolated process, so much so that ARDS is now considered to be only the pulmonary component of a multisystem vascular disorder [9,10] in which there is dysfunction not only of gas exchange but also of peripheral oxygen delivery and uptake,

which can lead to multiple organ failure (MOF) [11]. Thus, respiratory failure may be the cause of death in as few as 16% of patients [12], most of the remainder being attributable to MOF. It seems therefore that ARDS represents only the extreme manifestation of a spectrum of lung injury (Figure 3.3). Secondly, it is increasingly apparent that lung injury represents only the pulmonary manifestation of a wide ranging systemic vascular insult producing several, overlapping, recognizable clinical syndromes (Figure 3.4).

DIVERSITY OF ACUTE LUNG INJURY

PATHOGENESIS

The fact that in many cases of ARDS the lung appeared to become a major target for secondary injury after initial distant insults, such as pancreatitis, led to the early concept that lung injury may be the result of 'humoral factors' generated by these distant events. It is now commonly believed that important inflammatory mediators create an acute inflammatory response in the microvessels of the lung (and other organs) and that locally released inflammatory cell products damage the endothelial cells and epithelial cells of the alveolar-capillary in membrane. This results in ultrastructural changes within the cells leading to increased permeability [13] (Chapters 15 and 20), and the release of a wide range of vasoactive agents, including nitric oxide (NO) (Chapter 30), eicosanoids and endothelins, which modulate vascular tone at a local level [14]. Activation of platelets [15] and the complement [16] and coagulation [17,18] cascades leads to the formation of microthrombi [19]. The overall result is a loss of structural and functional vascular integrity.

Thus inflammatory injury to the lung microvessels is a central early pathogenetic event. There is much evidence that neutrophils are specifically implicated in the pathogenesis of most cases of ARDS. Histological

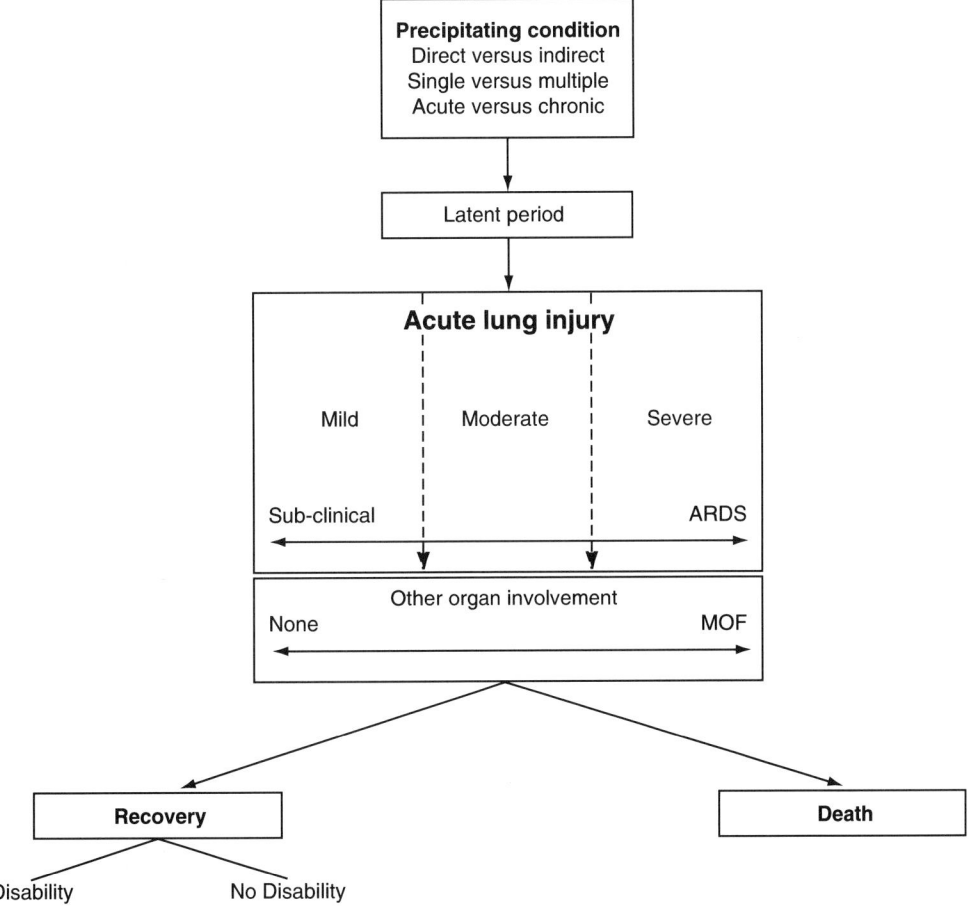

Figure 3.2 Spectrum of disease. Acute lung injury occurs following a diverse range of insults. It produces a range of clinical manifestations from mild to severe, and is often associated with systemic vascular dysfunction resulting in failure of other organs. The outcome is also necessarily variable. MOF = multiple organ failure.

specimens in early ARDS reveal an intense inflammatory infiltrate [20] (Chapter 4) that is predominantly neutrophilic in nature. Analysis of bronchoalveolar lavage (BAL) fluid from ARDS patients shows an increase in neutrophils [21] as well as their secretory products, such as elastase [22] and collagenase [23], and positive correlations between neutrophil count in BAL fluid and the progression and/or severity of ARDS have been observed [24,25]. However, ARDS can occur in neutropenic patients [26]. It is possible that the lung tissues of such patients contain sufficient neutrophils to initiate the pathological process. Given the redundancy of the inflammatory response, however, it is perhaps more likely that other cells, particularly monocytes, which possess much of the histotoxic potential of the neutrophil, take the lead role. Nevertheless, here, as in other chapters, neutrophils are exemplified as the archetypal acute inflammatory cell, although all the processes discussed are also applicable to monocytes.

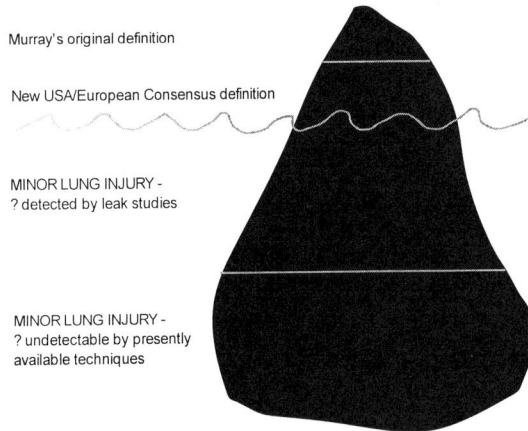

Figure 3.3 Iceberg of acute lung injury. It has become clear that clinically obvious cases of acute lung injury are only the tip of a larger group with vascular inflammatory injury.

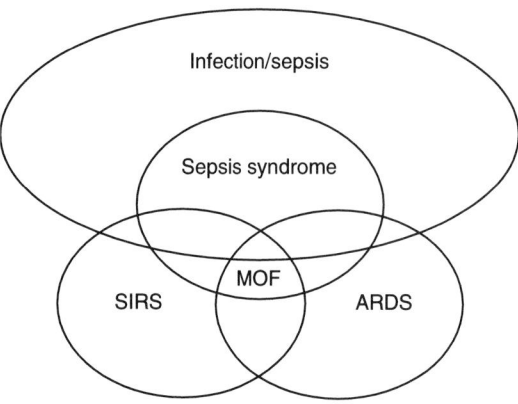

Figure 3.4 Clinical syndromes associated with lung injury. MOF = multiple organ failure; SIRS- = systemic inflammatory response syndrome.

Even in the healthy state there is a special relationship between neutrophils and pulmonary microvessels, and this may have some relevance to the pathogenesis of acute lung injury. A subpopulation of neutrophils – the 'marginated pool' – is always temporarily sequestered in lung capillaries. These cells, which are released into the circulation by exercise or adrenaline, may account for up to 50% of neutrophils in the vascular compartment. The pulmonary marginated neutrophil pool is likely to derive from a special rheological relationship between neutrophils and pulmonary capillaries. The mean diameter of the lung capillary is 5.5 μm whereas that of the neutrophils is 7.5 μm; thus most neutrophils are required to squeeze through lung capillaries with an ease proportional to their size and deformability.

Therefore systematically generated inflammatory mediators are likely to act first upon this resident pool before recruitment of circulatory neutrophils occurs. Experiments *in vitro* have clearly demonstrated that neutrophil mediated cell injury or extracellular matrix degradation can only occur where the neutrophil is closely applied to its 'target' surface (Figure 3.5). This creates a restrictive environment which would tend to greatly increase the local concentration of injurious neutrophil release products while at the same time excluding their antagonists (particularly large molecular size antiproteinases). Such a restricted microenvironment would also maximize the opportunity for very reactive agents, such as some oxidants (Chapter 11), to injure endothelial cells, and cell contact would also bring neutrophil surface-fixed proteinases (Chapter 10) directly to bear on the endothelial cell surface.

In the pulmonary capillary this interaction is likely to be promoted by at least two mechanisms: an increased adhesive interaction between neutrophils and endothelial cells (Chapter 9) and a reduction in neutrophil deformability (Chapter 8). It is of great interest that a number of important cytokines and chemokines not only upregulate neutrophils and endothelial adhesion molecules but also profoundly reduce neutrophil deformability. Many inflammatory mediators have the capacity to act upon the neutrophil–microvascular interaction and by the time lung inflammation is established all the inflam-

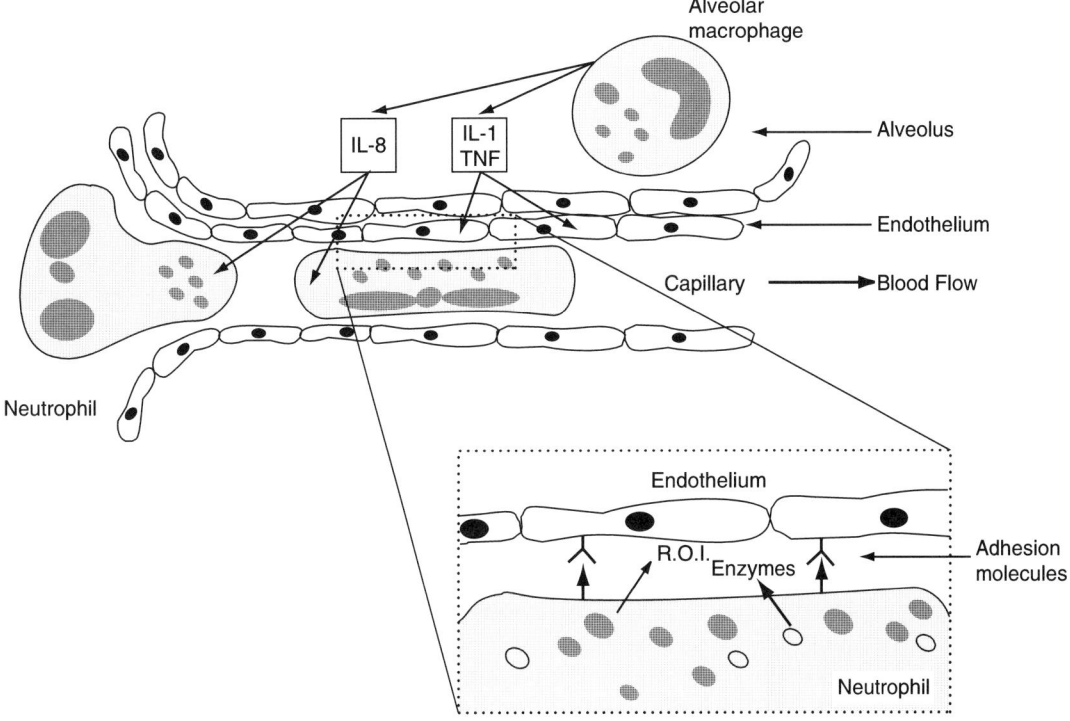

Figure 3.5 (a) Neutrophil interaction with pulmonary capillaries. (b) Expanded diagram of adhesive microenvironment (R.O.I. = reactive oxygen intermediates).

matory cascades depicted in Figure 3.5 are likely to be operational and to exert amplifications effects. However, there is now ample evidence for the central importance of cytokines and chemokines (Chapter 7) and at the initiation of the lung process which ultimately progresses to ARDS, IL-8 may be of particular significance [5].

Insults to the epithelial side of the alveolar–capillary barrier cause damage to the type I, and to a lesser extent II pneumocytes, followed by hypertrophy of surviving type II cells as well as a remarkably early and rapid proliferation of fibroblasts in the interstitial tissue [26,27]. In some cases, quantification of the surfactant pool following lung injury is technically difficult and has yielded inconsistent results [28–30]. However, changes in the surfactant composition of BAL samples

appear to be sensitive markers of early acute lung injury [31,32], almost certainly reflect altered metabolic activity in type II cells.

Positive correlations between the neutrophil count in BAL fluid and the progression and/or the severity of illness have been identified [24,25]. Thus, of 50 patients with a range of severity of respiratory failure or risk factors for ARDS, 13 met the full diagnostic criteria for the syndrome at first assessment. Nine of the remainder went on to develop ARDS and 28 did not. In all cases, plasma neutrophil elastase complex correlated with worsening arterial hypoxia and the protein content of BAL fluid. The BAL fluid itself contained elastase complex, the level of which correlated with the neutrophil count and protein content. Patients at risk of, or with, ARDS therefore have a spectrum of respiratory failure to which intravascular and intra-alveolar neutrophil elastase release and capillary permeability are related. This suggests that the clinical state currently recognized as ARDS is not a distinct pathophysiological entity. Thus, a partial understanding of the underlying inflammatory process activated following pulmonary insults does not assist in predicting the clinical manifestation resulting from different types of insult: single versus multiple; local versus systemic; acute or chronic; direct or indirect.

PATHOPHYSIOLOGY

These processes result in endothelial and epithelial damage associated with characteristic pathophysiological sequelae of impaired gas exchange, ventilation ($\dot{V}$) and perfusion ($\dot{Q}$) mismatch, the intra-alveolar leakage of protein-rich fluid, reduced pulmonary compliance, and pulmonary hypertension [33]. Clinically, the picture varies from mild respiratory impairment to overwhelming alveolar edema. While this sequence of disease progression has been confirmed in postmortem studies of patients dying with ARDS [34,35], little information is available about those with acute lung injury who survive. Attempts have therefore been made to achieve an objective clinical assessment of the degree of lung injury, using noninvasive techniques to assess the integrity of the alveolar-capillary membrane. Radiolabeling of red blood cells and transferrin has allowed a distinction to be made between patients with ARDS and those with pulmonary edema secondary to cardiac or renal failure (Chapter 15) [36]. This technique represents a qualitative measure of the permeability of the endothelium to protein, but has provided inconsistent results when quantitation assessments have been made. Furthermore, such a protein accumulation index (PAI) does not predict which patients will develop ARDS from those who will not in an adult population [37]. There is, however, some correlation between the severity of respiratory failure and PAI when other factors were taken into account, indicating a spectrum of injury severity in the patient population.

Clinical hemodynamic studies have emphasized the universal finding of elevated pulmonary vascular resistance (PVR) in patient groups with respiratory failure [38]. However, in full blown ARDS, pulmonary hypertension can contribute to pulmonary edema formation [10], and impaired right ventricular performance [39] has been associated with increased mortality [40]. The changes in PVR in acute lung injury are the result of several factors, both physical (thromboemboli, positive end expiratory pressure ventilation, edema fluid) and functional (elevated vascular tone) (Chapter 17) [41,42]. One of the most important components in the alteration of vascular tone is the disruption of physiological hypoxic pulmonary vasoconstriction (HPV) [43]. This response normally results in the diversion of blood away from hypoxic alveoli with the result that $\dot{V}/\dot{Q}$ mismatch is prevented. The mechanism by which it occurs has not yet been fully elucidated, but since HPV persists in both isolated animal lungs [44,45] and following pulmonary transplant [46] it is thought to be mediated via intrinsic mechanism(s). Most evidence suggests that it is endothelium dependent, although cultured pulmonary artery smooth muscle cells can exhibit an independent contractile response to hypoxia [47]. Thus, HPV represents a beneficial homeostatic control mechanism that is disrupted in acute lung injury [48], which is highly significant in determining oxygenation because the alveolar edema and atelectasis that occur induce large increases in physiological dead space. Indeed, patients with ARDS investigated using the multiple inert gas technique display a degree of intrapulmonary shunting that would explain the observed alveolar–arterial P_{O_2} gradient, regardless of any reduction in lung diffusing capacity [49].

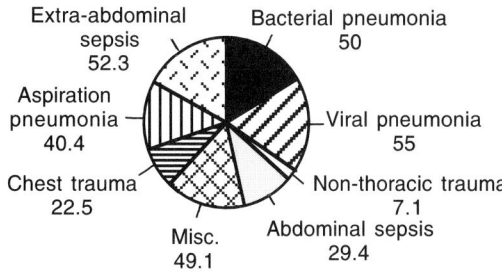

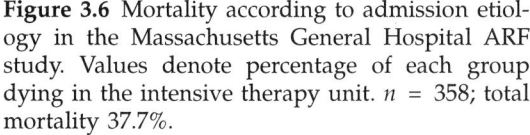

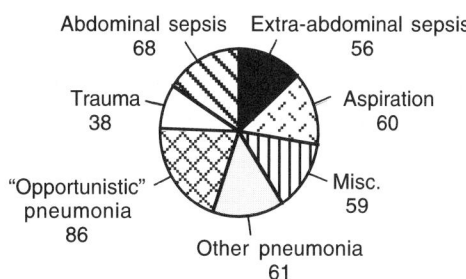

Figure 3.6 Mortality according to admission etiology in the Massachusetts General Hospital ARF study. Values denote percentage of each group dying in the intensive therapy unit. *n* = 358; total mortality 37.7%.

Figure 3.7 Mortality according to admission etiology in the European Collaborative ARDS Study. Values denote percentage mortality in each group. *n* = 583; overall mortality 59%.

CLINICAL EPIDEMIOLOGICAL CORRELATES BETWEEN INSULT AND OUTCOME

There is evidence that the major determinants of survival in patients with ARDS are the associated clinical condition and risk factors, as well as coexisting organ failure [10,50]. It is also clear [51–53] that survival is age dependent. Further analysis of the association between initiating condition and subsequent clinical course and prognosis promises to have considerable value in future preventative and management strategies. Several large studies have initiated this difficult process. Thus, 491 patients admitted to the respiratory and surgical intensive care units of a large general hospital in the United States were classified according to chest radiographic appearance, ventilatory mode and requirement and state of oxygenation (in relation to the inspired oxygen) [54]. Categories of acute respiratory failure (ARF) were defined as: at risk; mild; moderate; severe. The overall mortality was 38.8% in the 358 patients classified as having some degree of ARF at entry. Mortality was dependent on the condition considered to have precipitated the respiratory failure, ranging from 55% for viral pneumonia to 9.1% for nonthoracic trauma (Figure 3.6). In 133 patients who were not hypoxemic at the time of admission to the

intensive care unit and whose radiographic abnormalities were mild, the mortality was 6% in those who did not develop ARF, 24.3% in those who moved into the 'mild' ARF group, and 46.3% and 91.7% respectively in those who went on to the 'moderate' or 'severe' ARF categories. Again there was considerable variation in mortality according to the admission diagnosis, for example 2.6% in those with nonthoracic trauma and 42.9% in those with extra-abdominal sepsis.

In the European Collaborative Study [55] 583 patients were included on the basis of a set of strict diagnostic criteria for severe hypoxic respiratory failure. Overall, sepsis was the most common precipitating condition. The overall mortality was 59% in this study, but it again suggested that mortality varies according to the initiating pathology. Thus, those with 'opportunistic' pneumonias had a mortality of 86%, compared with 38% for trauma victims (Figure 3.7).

Outcome in acute lung injury therefore depends in part on the underlying primary pathology and precipitating event. However, other evidence has demonstrated that the presence and number of complications that develop during the course of the illness also have a major influence. Not surprisingly, the absence of complications, such as shock, pulmonary infection and acute renal failure, in the European study was associated with a lower mortality, which has important implications when acute lung injury is regarded as a clinical spectrum. The early identification of those at high risk of either the most severe forms of acute lung injury or other organ system failure, and an aggressive approach to the manipulation of their disease, using both standard supportive care and also newer therapies directed at the underlying pathological process at a cellular and molecular level (Chapter 30), may be possible in the future.

CURRENT DEFINITION

There are now several ways to approach the diagnosis of ARDS. Traditionally, there has been a requirement for bilateral diffuse pulmonary infiltrates on chest radiography; arterial hypoxemia and a high gradient between this value and the level of inspired oxygen; the exclusion of 'cardiogenic' pulmonary edema by a normal pulmonary artery occlusion pressure (PAOP); and a reduction in pulmonary compliance. The problems associated with making these measurements are numerous, as they are subject to considerable subjective interpretation. In addition, some criteria are necessarily rather arbitrary, such as the degree of change of the arterial/alveolar gradient required, or the definition of a normal PAOP [56,57]. As a result of these difficulties, an attempt to modify the definition of ARDS has been made [58]. Probably most important of all, a scoring system was introduced that allows for the inclusion of patients with a range of lung injury from mild to severe (Table 1.2). The scoring system has several advantages. Firstly, it provides a tool by which the degree of injury can be assessed and reviewed, which is valuable for the study of the individual patient and for the study of different patient populations. Secondly, it minimizes the need for 'cut off' values for inclusion parameters such as the degree of hypoxemia. Thirdly, it removes PAOP as part of the score because this, although frequently

useful as adjunctive information in the clinical setting, is an unreliable guide to the origin of interstitial pulmonary fluid. Fourthly, as part of the definition there is a requirement to classify the stage which the condition has reached temporally. Finally, there is an attempt to summarize the disorders that are causing or contributing to the lung injury.

The problems surrounding the definition and classification of acute lung injury and ARDS have been recently reviewed by the American–European Consensus Conference on ARDS [59]. The conclusions of most relevance were as follows.

1. ARDS should be the abbreviation for the 'acute' respiratory distress syndrome because the condition can be identified in children.
2. The term 'acute lung injury' refers to the spectrum of presentation, and ARDS describes those patients at the most severe end of this spectrum. The arbitrary nature of 'cut off' values for the definition of ARDS was recognized.
3. The clinical condition should be classified by the description of the precipitating cause.

CONCLUSION

ARDS is not a distinct entity. It is rather the most extreme clinical manifestation of the pathophysiological response to acute lung injury. Furthermore, acute lung injury is now regarded as only one manifestation of a diverse multisystem vascular injury that also has a spectrum of clinical presentation and outcome (Figure 3.2). The importance of this concept is that it encourages the early identification of patients with mild acute lung injury and their aggressive treatment to prevent progression to ARDS and its various complications: a progression that we know from epidemiological studies is associated with worsening prognosis. As well as seeking to treat the patient with established ARDS in a more effective manner (armed with the knowledge that the majority of survivors have little loss of long term pulmonary function [55,60]), we are now faced with the task of manipulating the underlying pathological process causing the pulmonary and systemic vascular damage and dysfunction.

ACKNOWLEDGEMENTS

N.P.C. is an MRC Training Fellow.

REFERENCES

1. Ashbaugh, D.G., Bigelow, D.B., Petty, T.L. and Levine, B.E. (1967) Acute respiratory distress syndrome in adults. *Lancet*, **ii**, 319–23.
2. Beale, R., Grover, E.R., Smithies, M. and Bihari, D. (1993) Acute respiratory distress syndrome ('ARDS'): no more than a severe acute lung injury? *B.M.J.*, **307**, 1335–9.
3. Oh, T.E. (1992) Defining adult respiratory distress syndrome. *Br. J. Hosp. Med.*, **47**, 350–3.
4. Baumann, W.R., Jung, R.C., Koss, M. *et al.* (1986) Incidence and mortality of adult respiratory distress syndrome: a prospective analysis from a large metropolitan hospital. *Crit. Care Med.*, **14**, 1–4.
5. Donnelly, S.C., Streiter, R.M., Kunkel, S.L. *et al.* (1993) Interleukin-8 and development of adult respiratory distress syndrome in at-risk patient groups. *Lancet* **341**, 643–7.
6. Donnelly, S.C., Haslett, C., Dransfiled, I. *et al.* (1994) Role of selectins in development of adult respiratory distress syndrome. *Lancet* 92:**344**, 215–9.
7. Donnelly, S.C., MacGregor, I. Zamani, A. *et al.* (1995) Plasma elastase levels and the development of adult respiratory distress syndrome (ARDS). *Am. J. Resp. Crit. Care Med.* **155**, 1428–33.
8. Weinberg, P.F., Matthay, M.A. and Webster, R.O. (1984) Biologically active products of complement and acute lung injury in patients with the sepsis syndrome. *Am. Rev. Respir. Dis.*, **130**, 791–6.
9. Mizer, L., Weisbrode, S. and Dorinsky, P.M. (1989) Neutrophil accumulation and structural changes in non-pulmonary organs following phorbol myristate acetate-induced acute lung injury. *Am. Rev. Respir. Dis.*, **139**, 1017–26.
10. Bone, R.C., Balk, R. and Slotman, G. (1992) Adult respiratory distress syndrome and importance of multiple organ failure. *Chest*, **101**, 320–6.
11. Griffiths, M.J.D. and Evans, T.W. (1994) Adult respiratory distress syndrome, in *Respiratory Medicine*, 2nd edn (eds R.A.L. Brewis, G.J. Gibson and D.M. Geddes), Baillière Tindall, London, pp. 605–29.
12. Montgomery, A.B., Stager, M.A., Carrico, C.J. and Hudson, L.D. (1985) Causes of mortality in patients with the adult respiratory distress syndrome. *Am. Rev. Respir. Dis.*, **132**, 485–9.
13. Phillips, P. and Tsan, M-F. (1992) Cytoarchitectural aspects of endothelial barrier function in response to oxidants and inflammatory mediators, in *Lung Vascular Injury* (eds A. Johnson and T.J. Ferro), Marcel Dekker, New York.
14. Curzen, N.P., Griffiths, M.J.D. and Evans, T.W. (1994) The role of the endothelium in modulating the vascular response to sepsis. *Clin. Sci.*, **86**, 359–74.
15. Heffner, J.E., Sahn, S.A. and Repine, J.E. (1987) The role of platelets in the adult respiratory distress syndrome. Culprits or bystanders? *Am. Rev. Respir. Dis.*, **135**, 482–92.
16. Till, G.O., Johnston, J.K., Kunkel, R. and Ward, P.A. (1982) Intravascular activation of complement and acute lung injury. Dependency on neutrophils and toxic oxygen metabolites. *J. Clin. Invest.*, **69**, 1126–35.
17. Hellgren, M., Edberg, N. and Eklund, J. (1984) Blood coagulation and fibrinolytic factors and their inhibitors in critically ill patients. *Intensive Care Med.*, **10**, 23–8.
18. Bone, R.C., Francis, P.B. and Pierce, A.K. (1976) Intravascular coagulations associated with adult respiratory distress syndrome. *Am. J. Med.*, **61**, 585–9.
19. Tomashefski, J.F. Jr, Davies, P., Boggis, L. *et al.* (1983) The pulmonary vascular lesions of the adult respiratory distress syndrome. *Am. J. Pathol.*, **112**, 112–16.
20. Tate, R.M. and Repine, J.E. (1983) Neutrophils and the adult respiratory distress syndrome. *Am. Rev. Respir. Dis.* **128**, 552–9.
21. Lee, C.T., Fein, A., Lippman, M. *et al.* (1981) Elastolytic activity in pulmonary lavage fluid from patients with adult respiratory distress syndrome. *N. Engl. J. Med.*, **304**, 192–6.
22. Christner, P., Fein, A., Golberg, S. *et al.* (1985) Collagenase in the lower respiratory tract of patients with adult respiratory distress syndrome. *Am. Rev. Respir. Dis.*, **131**, 690–5.
23. Braude, S., Apperley, J., Krauz, T. and Gold-

man, J.M. (1985) Adult respiratory distress syndrome after allogeneic bone marrow transplantation, evidence for a neutrophil-independent mechanism. *Lancet*, **i**, 1239–42.

24. Rocker, G.M., Wiseman, M.S., Dearson, D. and Shale, D.J. (1989) Diagnostic criteria for the adult and natural history respiratory distress syndrome: time for reappraisal. *Lancet*, **i**, 120–3.

25. Sinclair, D.G., Broude, S., Haslam, P.L. *et al.* (1994) Pulmonary endothelial permeability in patients with severe lung injury: clinical correlates. *Chest*, **106**, 535–9.

26. Reide, U.N., Joachim, H., Hassenstein, S. *et al.* (1978) The pulmonary blood barrier of human shock lungs (a clinical, ultrastructural and morphometric study). *Pathol. Res. Pract.*, **162**, 41–72.

27. Hill, J.D., Ratcliff, J.L., Parrott, J.C.W. *et al.* (1976) Pulmonary pathology in acute respiratory insufficiency: lung biopsy as a diagnostic tool. *J. Thorac. Cardiovasc. Surg.*, **71**, 64–9.

28. Holm, B., Notter, R., Siegle, J. and Matalon, S. (1985) Pulmonary physiological and surfactant changes during injury and recovery from hypoxia. *J. Appl. Physiol.*, **59**, 1402–9.

29. Young, S.L., Crapo, J.P., Kremers, S.L. and Brumley, G.W. (1982) Pulmonary surfactant lipid production in oxygen-exposed rat lungs. *Lab. Invest.*, **46**, 570–6.

30. Gross, N. (1991) Altered surfactant subtypes in an experimental form of radiation pneumonitis. *Am. J. Physiol.*, **260**, L302–10.

31. Gregory, T., Longmore, W., Moxley, M. *et al.* (1991) Surfactant chemical composition and biophysical activity in acute respiratory distress syndrome. *J. Clin. Invest.*, **88**, 1976–81.

32. Haslam, P.H., Hughes, D.A., McNaughton, P.D. *et al.* (1994) Surfactant replacement therapy in patients with late stage adult respiratory distress syndrome. *Lancet*, **343**, 1009–11.

33. Zapol, W.M. and Snider, M.T. (1977) Pulmonary hypertension in severe acute respiratory failure. *N. Engl. J. Med.*, **296**, 476–480.

34. Murray, J.F. (1977) Conference report. Mechanisms of acute respiratory failure. *Am. Rev. Respir. Dis.*, **115**, 1071–8.

35. Snow, R.L., Davies, P., Pontoppidan, H. *et al.* (1982) Pulmonary vascular remodelling in adult respiratory distress syndrome. *Am. Rev. Respir. Dis.*, **126**, 887–92.

36. Rocker, G.M., Morgan, A.G., Pearson, D. *et al.* (1987) Pulmonary vascular permeability to transferrin in the pulmonary oedema of renal failure. *Thorax*, **42**, 620–3.

37. Hunter, D.N., Morgan, C.J. and Evans, T.W. The use of radionuclide techniques in the asessment of alveolar – capillary membrane permeability on the intensive care unit. *Intensive Care Med.*, **16**, 363–71.

38. Zapol, W.M., Snider, M.T., Rie, M.A. *et al.* (1985) Pulmonary circulation during adult respiratory distress syndrome, in *Acute Respiratory Failure* (eds W.M. Zapol and K.J. Falke), Marcel Dekker, New York, 24, pp. 241–73.

39. Sibbald, W.J. and Driedger, A.A. (1983) Right ventricular function in disease states: pathophysiological considerations. *Crit. Care Med.*, **11**, 339–45.

40. Bernard, G.R., Rinaldo, J., Harris, T. *et al.* (1985) Early predictors of ARDS reversal in patients with established ARDS. *Am. Rev. Respir. Dis.*, **131**, 143.

41. Leeman, M. (1991) The pulmonary circulation in acute lung injury: a review of some recent advances. *Intensive Care Med.*, **17**, 254–60.

42. Fox, G.A. and McCormack, D.G. (1992) A new look at the pulmonary circulation in acute lung injury. *Thorax*, **47**, 743–7.

43. Curzen, N.P., Griffiths, M.J.D. and Evans, T.W. (1995) Pulmonary vascular control mechanisms in acute lung injury, in *Clinical Pulmonary Hypertension* (ed. A.H. Morice), Portland Press, London, pp. 171–202.

44. Hauge, A. (1968) Role of histamine in hypoxic pulmonary hypertension in the rat. I. Blockade or potentiation of endogenous amine, kinins and ATP. *Circ. Res.*, **22**, 371–83.

45. Hauge, A. and Melmon, K.L. (1968) Role of histamine in hypoxic pulmonary hypertension in the rat. II. Depletion of histamine, serotonin, and catecholamines. *Circ. Res.* **22**, 385–92.

46. Robin, E.D., Theodore, J., Burke, C.M. *et al.* (1987) Hypoxic pulmonary vasoconstriction persists in the human transplanted lung. *Clin. Sci.*, **72**, 283–7.

47. Murray, T.R., Chen, L., Marshall, B.E. and Macarak E.J. (1990) Hypoxic contraction of cultured pulmonary vascular smooth muscle cells. *Am. J. Respir. Cell Mol. Biol.*, **3**, 457–65.

48. Weir, E.K., Milczoch, J., Reeves, J.T. and Grover, R.F. Endotoxin and prevention of hypoxic pulmonary vasoconstriction. *J. Lab. Clin. Med.*, **68**, 975–83.

49. Dantzker, D.R., Brook, C.J., Dehart, P. *et al.* (1979) Ventilation – perfusion distributions in

the adult respiratory distress syndrome. *Am. Rev. Respir. Dis.*, **120**, 1039–52.

50. Fowler, A.A., Hamman, R.F., Zerbe, G.O. *et al.* (1985) Adult respiratory distress syndrome: prognosis after onset. *Am. Rev. Respir. Dis.*, **132**, 472–8.

51. Sloane, P.J., Gee, M.H., Gottleib, J.E. *et al.* (1992) A multicentre registry of patients with acute respiratory distress syndrome. *Am. Rev. Respir. Dis.*, **146**, 419–26.

52. Pepe, P.E., Potkin, R.T., Holtman Reus, D. *et al.* (1982) Clinical predictors of the adult respiratory distress syndrome. *Am. J. Surg.*, **144**, 124–30.

53. Mancebo, J. and Artigas A. (1987) A clinical study of the adult respiratory distress syndrome. *Crit. Care Med.*, **15**, 243–6.

54. Frikker, M.J., Lynch, K., Pontoppidan, H. *et al.* (1992) The adult respiratory distress syndrome: aetiology, progression and survival, in *Adult Respiratory Distress Syndrome* (eds A. Artigas, F. Lemaire, P.M. Suter and W.M. Zapol), Churchill Livingstone, Edinburgh, Chapter 1.

55. Artigas, A., Carlet, J., Chastang, C. *et al.* (1992) Adult respiratory distress syndrome: clinical presentation, prognostic factors and outcome, in *Adult Respiratory Distress Syndrome* (eds A.Artigas, F. Lemaire, P.M. Suter and W.M. Zapol), Churchill Livingstone, Edinburgh, Chapter 47.

56. Simmons, R.S., Berdine, G.G., Seidenfeld, J.J. *et al.* (1987) Fluid balance and the adult respiratory distress syndrome. *Am. Rev. Respir. Dis.*, **135**, 924–9.

57. Fowler, A.A., Hamman, R.F., Good, J.T. *et al.* (1983) Adult respiratory distress syndrome: risk with common predispositions. *Ann. Intern. Med.*, **98**, 593–7.

58. Murray, V.F., Matthay, M.A., Luce, J.M. *et al.* (1988) Pulmonary perspectives: an expanded definition of the adult respiratory distress syndrome. *Am. Rev. Respir. Dis.* **138**, 720–3.

59. Bernard, G.R., Artigas, A., Brigham, K.L. *et al.* (1994) Report of the American – European Consensus conference on ARDS: definitions, mechanisms, relevant outcomes and clinical trial coordination. *Intensive Care Med.*, **20**, 225–32.

60. Alberts, W.M., Priest, G.R. and Moser, K.M. (1983) The outlook for survivors of ARDS. *Chest*, **84**, 272–4.

DIFFUSE ALVEOLAR DAMAGE 4

Bryan Corrin

At the time that the Denver team of Ashbaugh, Petty and colleagues were crystallizing their ideas on what they first referred to as acute respiratory distress in adults (ARDS) [1], and later termed the adult respiratory distress syndrome [2–4], Liebow was describing the pathology of the condition. The name that Liebow coined for the nonspecific changes of acute alveolar injury was diffuse alveolar damage (DAD) [5–6], a term that will be adhered to in this chapter. Previously, pathologists such as Moon had described similar changes in the lungs of patients dying of shock [7].

CAUSES

Liebow's concept of DAD corresponds to the Denver workers' ideas on ARDS, namely that quite different insults to the lung result in a common pattern of injury. Some injurious agents reach the lungs directly via the airways, e.g. oxygen in high concentrations, gases such as phosgene and metallic fumes such as those of mercury and cadmium. Other agents noxious to the lungs reach their target organ via the bloodstream, having been injected or ingested: paraquat and cytotoxic chemotherapeutic agents are examples of these. Other agents responsible for DAD penetrate the chest wall to damage the lungs, e.g. ionizing radiation. More complex mechanisms, which are dealt with later, underlie the DAD of shock. Often in clinical practice, damaged lungs that require rest have to be forcibly ventilated and subjected to injurious concentrations of oxygen, to the patient's ultimate detriment.

PATHOLOGY

The gross appearance of the lungs in DAD has been well summarized in the term congestive atelectasis. At autopsy the lungs are heavy, dark and airless (Figure 4.1). The appearances resemble those encountered in the infantile respiratory distress syndrome (IRDS). This pathological similarity underlies the clinical and radiological similarities of IRDS and ARDS that led the Denver workers to adopt the latter term.

Microscopically the term congestive atelectasis is equally applicable, the alveoli being collapsed and their capillaries engorged (Figure 4.2). Generally, the blood within the distended capillaries is unremarkable, but occasionally changes in the platelets and leukocytes are evident (see below).

Although congestive atelectasis is the classic pathology of DAD/ARDS, other changes are sometimes encountered. One of these is that the lungs are not collapsed but filled with hemorrhagic edema fluid [7,9–11], giving rise to such simple terms as wet lung, or, because this change was commonly encountered shortly after one of the battles of the Vietnam war, Da-Nang lung.

The similarity between IRDS and ARDS

ARDS Acute Respiratory Distress in Adults. Edited by Timothy W. Evans and Christopher Haslett. Published in 1996 by Chapman & Hall, London. ISBN 0 412 56910 8

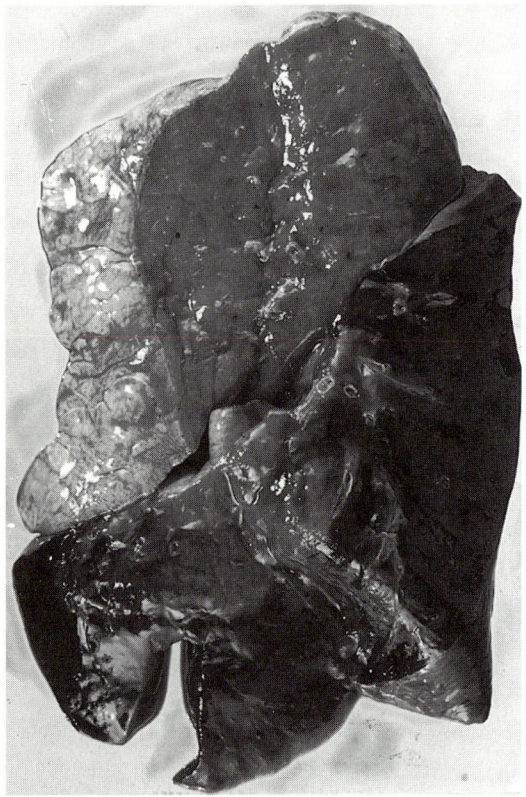

Figure 4.1 Congestive atelectasis in a 15 year old boy who died of septic shock due to peritonitis. The lower lobe is dark and airless due to congestion and collapse.

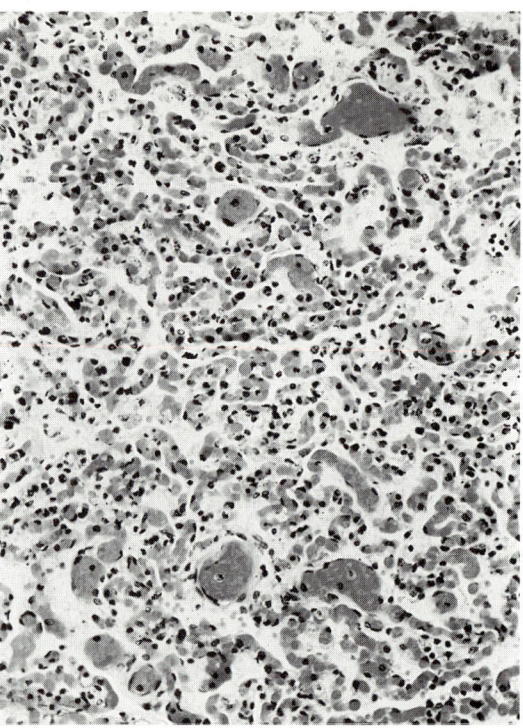

Figure 4.2 Microscopy of the lung shown in Figure 4.1. The capillaries are engorged and the alveoli collapsed. H & E ×190. (Reproduced with permission from Corrin [8]).

extends to what is now recognized to be an advanced rather than an initial feature, namely the formation of hyaline membranes (Figures 4.3 and 4.4). Hyaline membranes are the histological hallmark of DAD and whenever they are encountered it may be assumed that the alveolar epithelium has undergone necrosis. When it is recalled that it is the tight junctions between alveolar epithelial cells that keep the normal alveolus dry [14,15], it is evident that segmental epithelial loss will lead to escape of interstitial fluid into the air space, displacing and denaturing the surface active layer and so leading to collapse [16].

The pathology of 'shock lung' requires special consideration. The term shock is here used collectively for the state of circulatory collapse that complicates severe trauma, hemorrhage, sepsis or conditions such as acute pancreatitis and aortic dissection. The consequences of shock in organs such as the lungs are remarkably uniform, despite its varied causes.

The pathology of shock lung stems from events in the microvasculature of the lung. Although often showing nothing other than engorgement, it is sometimes evident that the alveolar capillaries contain increased numbers of platelets or neutrophil leukocytes.

At times it is noticeable that in patients dying of shock the alveolar capillaries are silted up with numerous platelets, occasionally interspersed with strands of fibrin or globular hyaline microthrombi [17] (Figure

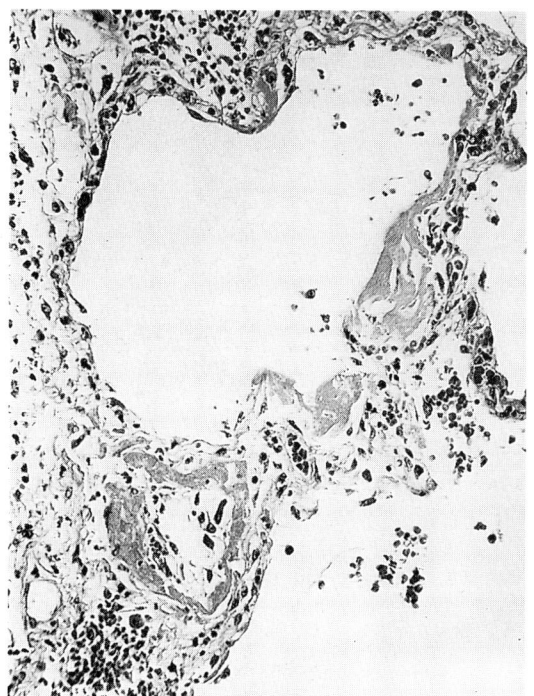

Figure 4.3 Hyaline membranes line the alveolar walls in a case of suicidal paraquat poisoning. Material kindly supplied by Dr D. Melcher. H & E ×190. (Reproduced with permission from Corrin and Vijeyaratnam [12]; published by S. Karger AG, Basel.)

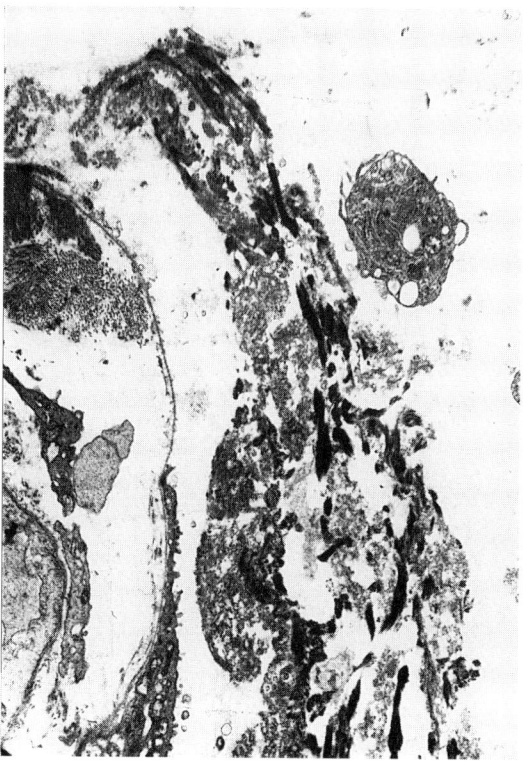

Figure 4.4 Diffuse alveolar damage with the alveolar wall (left) partially denuded of its epithelium. Closely applied to the otherwise base basement membrane is a mixture of a fibrin and cell debris which is seen at the light microscopic level as a hyaline membrane. Electron micrograph, ×5300, provided by Miss A. Dewar. (Reproduced with permission from Addis [13].)

4.5). These are the changes of disseminated intravascular coagulation and are found throughout the vascular system [18]. Megakaryocytes, normally found in small numbers within pulmonary capillaries [19–24], are often increased in shock [8,25] and other conditions associated with disseminated intravascular coagulation [26]. This indicates their premature release from the bone marrow and entrapment in the alveolar capillaries. That this should be augmented in consumptive coagulopathy is easily understood. Platelet fragmentation with release of biogenic agents such as histamine and 5-hydroxytryptamine may well contribute to the increased capillary permeability seen in shock [27–29].

It is likely that changes in the leukocytes, notably the neutrophils, are of greater importance than platelet entrapment. In septic shock particularly, but also in other forms of shock, increased numbers of neutrophils are sometimes found in the pulmonary capillaries (Figure 4.6), while electron microscopy has demonstrated their fragmentation within the alveolar capillary lumen (Figure 4.7) [30–33]. Initially, emphasis was placed on the subsequent release of lysosomal enzymes as being important in the generation of lung injury, but while the importance of this cannot be gainsaid it is doubtful whether it is significant early on. Before the neutrophils

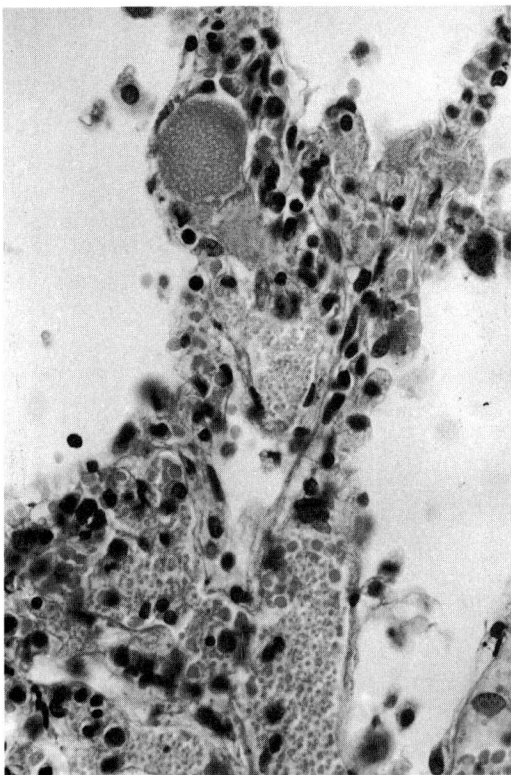

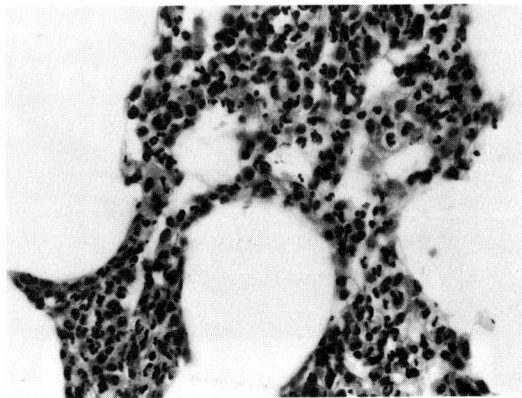

Figure 4.6 Hemorrhagic shock. The alveolar capillaries show gross sequestration of neutrophil polymorphonuclear leukocytes. H & E ×400.

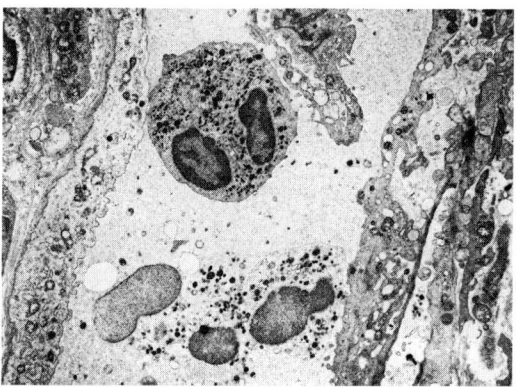

Figure 4.5 In a fatal case of septic shock the alveolar capillaries show platelet aggregation and a globular hyaline microthrombus (top). H & E ×560. (Reproduced with permission from Corrin [8].)

Figure 4.7 Adult respiratory distress syndrome. Neutrophil polymorphonuclear leukocytes sequestrated in the alveolar capillaries show disruption with release of their granules. Electron micrograph ×3500, (by courtesy of Miss A. Dewar.)

actually disintegrate it is likely that they are activated to secrete the agents that are so effective in antibacterial defense, namely reactive oxygen species [34]. Release of these in amounts greater than can be inactivated by protective enzymes such as superoxide dismutase is known to damage host cells as well as invading organisms. Excessive oxygen radical production results in oxidation of lipids and protein sulfhydryl groups and DNA damage [35]. In shock, blood leukocytes are activated throughout the circulation, adhere to each other and arrive in the lungs as microemboli, staying to release their products in this, the first capillary bed many of them encounter in the activated state. Although shock is a multisystem disorder, the lungs are

by far the most common organs to show changes at autopsy [36–38]. Such neutrophil activation is probably mediated by the complement cascade mechanism involving either the classic or alternative pathway and release of chemotactic factors such as C5a [39–40], although this is not universally accepted [41]. Other possible mediators contributing to neutrophil activation include granulocyte macrophage colony stimulating factor, tumor necrosis factor α, lipopolysaccharide, interleukin 8 and intercellular adhesion molecule 1 [42–45].

Although platelet and neutrophil accumulation in the lung is impressive when encountered, these features are often not obvious in shock although the lungs are clearly damaged: the changes then apparent are merely those of congestion and collapse, the latter attributable to surfactant deficiency caused both by exudates inactivating preformed surfactant and type II cell damage compromising its replacement. Whilst these changes are difficult to explain in isolation, platelet and neutrophil activation is widespread in shock and as the pulmonary capillary bed is the first downstream of the systemic veins, lung injury is perhaps easier to understand. An appreciation that products of both activated and disintegrating platelets and neutrophils circulate within the blood helps in understanding the multisystem endothelial damage that is found in shock, whilst the position of the lungs in the circulation is probably responsible for the fact that they are the organs which most commonly show pathological changes in patients dying of shock [36–38].

Whereas changes in the formed elements of the blood are only occasionally evident in the alveolar capillaries, an almost universal finding in shock lung is capillary congestion. Only recently has a plausible explanation for this evolved. A factor that causes vascular dilatation has recently been detected as coming from the vascular endothelium and acting on the medial muscle coat of the vessel. At first termed endothelium derived relaxing factor, this factor is now known to be nitric oxide, a remarkably simple chemical that has long been recognized to be poisonous [46]. Fortunately, its half life in the vessel wall is very short, timed in seconds rather than minutes. The enzyme responsible for its production (from L-arginine), nitric acid synthase, is found in endothelium and can be induced in the vascular medial smooth muscle. Both the constitutive and inducible forms of the enzyme are activated by bacterial lipopolysaccharide [47,48] and it therefore seems likely that in septic shock bacterial products act directly on the vessel wall, resulting in the production of excess amounts of nitric oxide. Even momentarily increased levels of nitric oxide might be expected to cause arterial dilatation and hence capillary congestion. Important as neutrophil activation undoubtedly is in acute lung injury, it would appear that in septic shock circulating bacterial products such as lipopolysaccharide cause vascular dilatation and possibly increased permeability by direct action on the blood vessels [47,48].

REPAIR OF DAMAGED LUNGS

A basic process of repair that is common to alveolar injury, irrespective of its etiology, begins within a few days. The stem cell concerned in epithelial regeneration is the type II pneumocyte [49–52]. These cells first proliferate and then differentiate into type I pneumo-

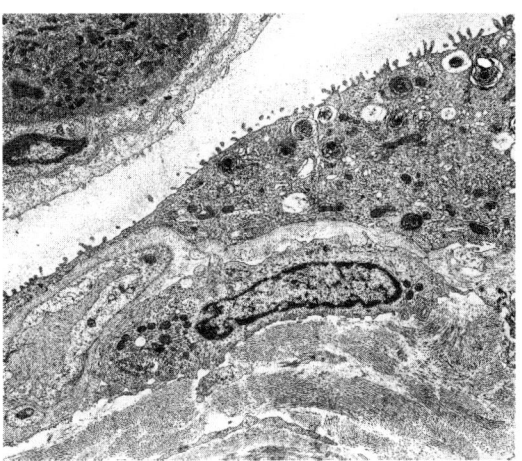

Figure 4.8 An alveolar epithelial cell having the squamous form of a type I cell but the microvilli and lamellar bodies of a type II cell. Such intermediate cells are indicative of epithelial regeneration. Electron micrograph ×5700, (by courtesy of Miss A. Dewar.)

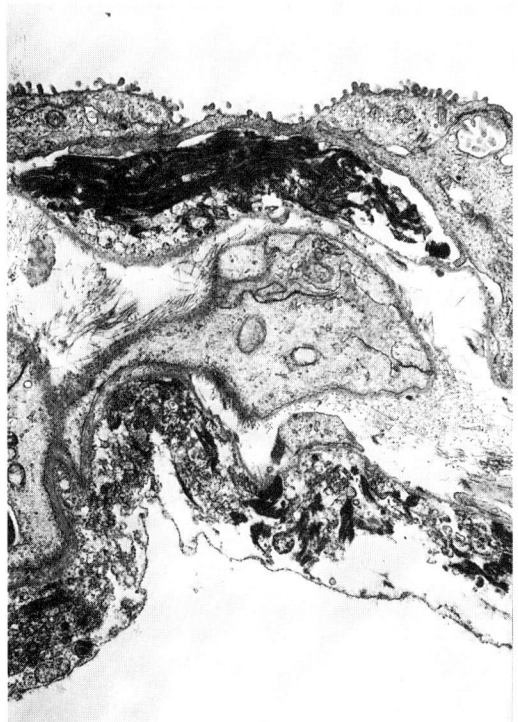

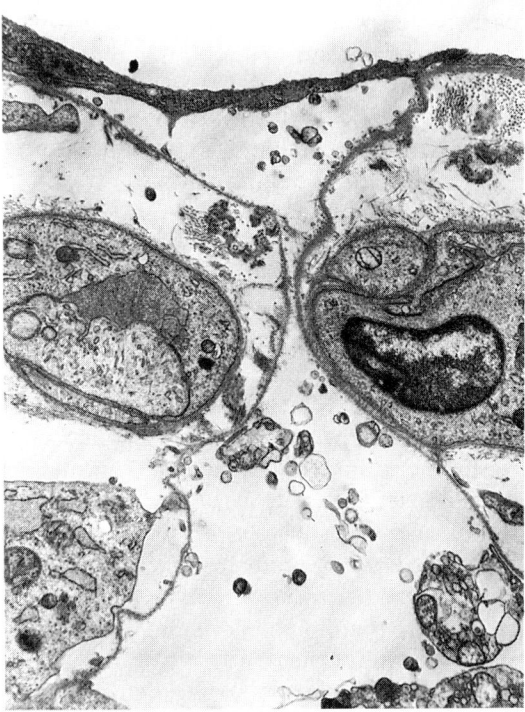

Figure 4.9 Diffuse alveolar damage: repair stage. At the top a hyaline membrane is being incorporated into the alveolar wall by regenerating alveolar epithelial cells. Electron micrograph ×6000 (by courtesy of Miss A. Dewar.)

Figure 4.10 Diffuse alveolar damage: repair stage. Regenerating epithelial cells bridge the mouth of a collapsed alveolus, permanently sealing off this former air space. Electron micrograph ×7000. (Reproduced with permission from Addis [13].)

cytes, thereby re-epithelializing the denuded basement membranes. The type II pneumocytes appear as a row of cuboidal cells lining the alveoli, or plump pleomorphic spindle cells with prominent nucleoli may be seen, representing cell forms intermediate between types II and I pneumocytes (Figure 4.8). Sometimes there is squamous metaplasia instead of orderly differentiation into type I pneumocytes.

In contrast to the type I epithelial cells, which have no regenerative powers and are replaced by differentiation of proliferating type II cells, endothelial cells are replaced by lateral spread of their own kind. An effete endothelial cell is first undermined by its healthy neighbours and is only cast off when

these have completely covered the basement membrane [53]. Therefore, although segments of bare basement membrane have been described on the vascular side of the air–blood barrier [54], they are not seen to the same extent as on the epithelial side. Nevertheless, thrombosis superimposed on such endothelial damage is described [54] and subsequent organization of such thrombi is probably responsible for the extensive vascular remodeling that has been described in the reparative phase of DAD. This consists of fibrocellular intimal thickening that narrows the lumen of small vessels throughout the lung and can be visualized as decreased background filling on *postmortem* arteriograms [55].

Interstitial connective tissue cells also take part in the proliferative process. Fibroblasts proliferate, leading to the deposition of collagen and the development of interstitial fibrosis [56,57]. An increase in lung collagen can be detected in patients with ARDS surviving longer than 14 days and this progressively increases with the duration of the disease [58]. Sometimes this leads to clinically debilitating fibrotic lung disease in survivors.

Interactions between fibroblasts and the alveolar epithelium through gaps in the basement membrane have been described, suggesting that the regenerating epithelial cells play a role in the underlying process of fibrosis [59–62]. Indeed, fibrogenic cytokines such as tumor necrosis factor α can be detected in the regenerating alveolar epithelium and are probably secreted into the subjacent connective tissue to promote interstitial fibrosis [44].

Fibroblasts also migrate into alveolar exudates through defects in the epithelial basement membrane and form collagen within the air spaces [57,63]. As epithelial cells grow over the newly formed connective tissue, a new basement membrane is laid down, thereby incorporating the alveolar collagen into the interstitium [57]. Hyaline membranes may also be incorporated into the alveolar walls in a similar way (Figure 4.9) [64].

Another way in which repair may result in permanent shrinkage of the lung is one in which regenerating epithelial cells bridge the mouths of collapsed alveoli (Figure 4.10) so that these air spaces can never re-expand, a process termed atelectatic induration [65,66].

These processes can be well established in as short a time as two weeks, by which time the lung is contracted and firm and has a fine sponge-like pattern on its cut surface representing microcystic change and irregular scarring. With small air cysts alternating with solid areas of fibrosis and foci of squamous metaplasia there is a resemblance to the bronchopulmonary dysplasia seen in the late stages of IRDS [67,68]. The changes are similar to the end stage of any fibrotic process but are reached remarkably quickly.

REFERENCES

1. Ashbaugh, D.G., Bigelow, D.B., Petty, T.L. and Levine, B.E. (1967) Acute respiratory distress in adults. *Lancet*, **ii**, 319–23.
2. Ashbaugh, D.G., Petty, T.L., Bigelow, D.B. and Harris, T.M. (1969) Continuous positive-pressure breathing (CPPB) in adult respiratory distress syndrome. *J. Thorac. Cardiovasc. Surg.*, **57**, 31–41.
3. Petty, T.L. and Ashbaugh, D.G. (1971) The adult respiratory distress syndrome. Clinical features, factors influencing prognosis and principles of management. *Chest*, **60**, 233–9.
4. Petty, T.L. (1975) The adult respiratory distress syndrome – confessions of a 'lumper'. *Am. Rev. Respir. Dis.*, **111**, 713–5.
5. Liebow, A.A. (1967) New concepts and entities in pulmonary disease, in International Academy of Pathology monograph No.8, *The Lung*, Williams & Wilkins, Baltimore, pp. 332–65.
6. Katzenstein, A.A., Bloor, C.M. and Liebow, A.A. (1976) Diffuse alveolar damage – the role of oxygen, shock and related factors. *Am. J. Pathol.*, **85**, 210–22.
7. Moon, V.H. (1948) The pathology of secondary shock. *Am. J. Pathol.*, **24**, 235–73.
8. Corrin, B. (1980) Lung pathology in septic shock. *J. Clin. Pathol.*, **33**, 891–4.
9. Martin, A.M., Soloway, H.B. and Simmons, R.L. (1968) Pathologic anatomy of the lungs following shock and trauma. *J. Trauma*, **8**, 687–99.
10. Bredenburg, C.E., James, P.M., Collins, *et al.* (1969) Respiratory failure in shock. *Ann. Surg.*, **169**, 392–403.
11. Nash, G., Foley, F.D. and Langlinais, P.C. (1975) Pulmonary interstitial edema and hyaline membranes in adult burn patients. *Hum. Pathol.*, **5**, 149–60.
12. Corrin, B. and Vijeyaratnam, G.S. (1975) Experimental models of interstitial pneumonia: paraquat, iprindole. *Prog. Respir. Res.*, **8**, 107–20.
13. Addis, B.J. (1990) Diffuse alveolar damage, in *The Lungs* (ed. B. Corrin), Churchill Livingstone, Edinburgh, pp. 55–68.
14. Schneeberger-Keeley, E.E. and Karnovsky, M.J.

(1968) The ultrastructural basis of alveolar-capillary membrane permeability to peroxidase used as a tracer. *J. Cell Biol.*, **37**, 781–93.

15. Schneeberger, E.E. and Karnovsky, M.J. (1971) The influence of intravascular fluid volume on the permeability of newborn and adult mouse lungs to ultrastructural protein tracers. *J. Cell Biol.* **49**, 319–34.

16. Petty, T.L., Reiss, O.K., Paul, G.N. *et al.* (1977) Characteristics of pulmonary surfactant in adult respiratory distress syndrome associated with trauma and shock. *Am. Rev. Respir. Dis.*, **15**, 531–6.

17. Bleyl, U. and Rossner, J.A. (1976) Globular hyaline microthrombi – their nature and morphogenesis. *Virchows Arch. [A]*, **370**, 113–28.

18. Bone, R.C., Francis, P.B. and Pierce, A.K. (1976) Intravascular coagulation associated with the adult respiratory distress syndrome. *Am. J. Med.*, **61**, 585–9.

19. Brill, R. and Halpern, M.M. (1948) The frequency of megakaryocytes in autopsy sections. *Blood*, **3**, 286–91.

20. Tinggaard Pedersen, N. (1974) The pulmonary vessels as a filter for circulating megakaryocytes in rats. *Scand. J. Haematol.*, **13**, 225–31.

21. Tinggaard Pedersen, N. (1978) Occurrence of megakaryocytes in various vessels, and their retention in the pulmonary capillaries of man. *Scand. J. Haematol.*, **21**, 379–5.

22. Trowbridge, E.A., Martin, J.F. and Slater, D.N. (1982) Evidence for a theory of physical fragmentation of megakaryocytes, implying that all platelets are produced in the pulmonary circulation. *Thromb. Res.*, **28**, 461–75.

23. Slater, D.N., Trowbridge, E.A. and Martin J.F. (1983) The megakaryocyte in thrombocytopenia: a microscopic study which supports the theory that platelets are produced in the lungs. *Thromb. Res.*, **31**, 163–76.

24. Sharma, G.K. and Talbot, I.C. (1986) Pulmonary megakaryocytes: 'missing link' between cardiovascular and respiratory disease? *J. Clin. Pathol.*, **39**, 969–76.

25. Crow, J. (1982) Pulmonary haematoxyphil bodies. *J. Clin. Pathol.*, **35**, 690–1.

26. Soares, F.A. (1992) Increased numbers of pulmonary megakaryocytes in patients with arterial pulmonary tumour embolism and with lung metastases seen at necropsy. *J. Clin. Pathol.*, **45**, 140–2.

27. Hardaway, R.M. (1973) Disseminated intravascular coagulation as possible cause of acute respiratory failure. *Surg. Gynecol. Obstet.*, **137**, 1–5.

28. Haynes, J.B., Hyers, T.M., Giclas, P.C. *et al.* (1980) Elevated fibrin(ogen) degradation products in adult respiratory distress syndrome. *Am. Rev. Respir. Dis.*, **122**, 841–7.

29. Sankey, E.A., Crow, J., Mallett, S.V. *et al.*, (1993) Pulmonary platelet aggregates – possible cause of sudden peroperative death in adults undergoing liver transplantation. *J. Clin. Pathol.*, **46**, 222–7.

30. Blaisdell, F.W., Lim, R.C. and Stallone, R.J. (1970) The mechanism of pulmonary damage following traumatic shock. *Surg. Gynecol. Obstet.*, **130**, 15–22.

31. Clowes, G.H.A. (1974) Pulmonary abnormalities in sepsis. *Surg. Clin. North Am.*, **54**, 993–1013.

32. Connell, R.S., Swank, R.L. and Webb M.C. (1975) The development of pulmonary ultrastructural lesions during haemorrhagic shock. *J. Trauma.* **15**, 116–29.

33. Sandritter, W., Mittesmayer, C., Riede, U.N. *et al.* (1978) Shock lung syndrome. *Ann. Thorac. Surg.* **162**, 7–23.

34. Williams, J.H., Patel, S.K., Hatakeyama, D. *et al.* (1993) Activated pulmonary vascular neutrophils as early mediators of endotoxin-induced lung inflammation. *Am. J. Respir. Cell Molec. Biol.*, **8**, 134–44.

35. Rinaldo, J.E. and Rogers, R.M. (1982) Adult respiratory distress syndrome: changing concepts of lung injury and repair. *N. Engl. J. Med.*, **306**, 900–9.

36. McGovern, V.J. (1971) Shock. *Pathol. Annu.*, **6**, 279–98.

37. McGovern, V.J. (1972) The pathophysiology of gram-negative septicaemia. *Pathology*, **4**, 265–71.

38. McGovern, V.J. (1980) Hypovolaemic shock with particular reference to the myocardial and pulmonary lesions. *Pathology*, **12**, 63–72.

39. Craddock, P.R., Hammerschmidt, D.E., White, J.G. *et al.* (1977) Complement (C5a)-induced granulocyte aggregation *in vitro*: a possible mechanism of complement-mediated leukostasis and leukopenia. *J. Clin. Invest.*, **60**, 260–4.

40. Tate, R.M. and Repine, J.E. (1983) Neutrophils and the adult respiratory distress syndrome. *Am. Rev. Respir. Dis.*, **128**, 552–9.

41. Cardozo, C., Edelman, J., Jagirdar, J. and

Lesser, M. (1991) Lipopolysaccharide-induced pulmonary vascular sequestration of polymorphonuclear leukocytes is complement independent. *Am. Rev. Respir. Dis.*, **144**, 173–8.

42. Stephens, K.E., Ishizaka, A., Larrick, J.W. and Raffin, T.A. (1988) Tumor necrosis factor causes increased pulmonary permeability and edema. *Am. Rev. Respir. Dis.*, **137**, 1364–70.

43. Johnson, J., Brigham, K.L., Jesmok, G. and Meyrick, B. (1991) Morphologic changes in lungs of anesthetized sheep following intravenous infusion of recombinant tumor necrosis factor-alpha. *Am. Rev. Respir. Dis.*, **144**, 179–86.

44. Nash, J.R.G., Mclaughlin, P.J., Hoyle, C. and Roberts D. (1991) Immunolocalization of tumour necrosis factor-alpha in lung tissue from patients dying with adult respiratory distress syndrome. *Histopathology*, **19**, 395–402.

45. Wegner, C.D., Wolyniec, W.W., Laplante, A.M. *et al.* (1992) Intercellular adhesion molecule-1 contributes to pulmonary oxygen toxicity in mice – role of leukocytes revised. *Lung*, **170**, 267–79.

46. Moncada, S., Palmer, R.M.J. and Higgs, E.A. (1991) Nitric oxide: physiology, pathophysiology and pharmacology. *Pharmacol. Rev.*, **43**, 109–42.

47. Fleming, I., Gray, G.A., Schott, C. and Stoclet, J. (1991) Inducible but not constitutive production of nitric oxide by vascular smooth muscle cells. *Eur. J. Pharmacol.*, **200**, 375–6.

48. Lui, S.F., Adcock, I.M., Old, R.W. *et al.* (1993) Lipopolysaccharide treatment in vivo induces widespread tissue expression of inducible nitric oxide synthase mRNA. *Biochem. Biophys. Res. Commun.*, **196**, 1208–13.

49. Evans, M.J., Cabral, L.J., Stephens, R.J. and Freeman, G. (1973) Renewal of alveolar epithelium in the rat following exposure to NO_2. *Am. J. Pathol.*, **70**, 175–98.

50. Evan, M.J., Cabral, L.J., Stephens, R.J. and Freeman, G. (1975) Transformation of alveolar type 2 cells to type 1 cells following exposure to NO_2. *Exp. Mol. Pathol.*, **22**, 142–50.

51. Adamson, I.Y.R. and Bowden, D.H. (1974) The type 2 cells as progenitor of alveolar epithelial regeneration. *Lab. Invest.*, **30**, 25–42.

52. Adamson, I.Y.R. and Bowden, D.H. (1975) Derivation of type 1 epithelium from type 2 cells in the developing rat lung. *Lab. Invest.*, **32**, 736–45.

53. Reidy, M.A. and Schwartz, S.M. (1981) Endothelial regeneration. III. Time course of intimal changes after small defined injury to rat aortic endothelium. *Lab. Invest.*, **44**, 301.

54. Kapanci, Y., Weibel, E.R., Kaplan, H.P. and Robinson, F.R. (1969) Pathogenesis and reversibility of the pulmonary lesions of oxygen toxicity in monkeys. II Ultrastructural and morphometric studies. *Lab. Invest.*, **20**, 101–18.

55. Tomashefski, J.F., Davies, P. Boggis, C. *et al.* The pulmonary vascular lesions of the adult respiratory distress syndrome. *Am. J. Pathol.*, **112**, 112–6.

56. Bachofen, M. and Weibel, E.R. (1974) Basic pattern of tissue repair in human lungs following unspecific injury. *Chest*, **65** (suppl.), 14s–19s.

57. Fukuda, Y., Ishizaki, M., Masud, Y. *et al.* (1987) The role of intraalveolar fibrosis in the process of pulmonary structural remodeling in patients with diffuse alveolar damage. *Am. J. Pathol.*, **126**, 171–82.

58. Zapol, W.M., Trelstad, R.L., Coffey, J.W. *et al.* (1979) Pulmonary fibrosis in severe acute respiratory failure. *Am. Rev. Respir. Dis.*, **119**, 547–54.

59. Brody, A.R. and Craighead, J.E. (1976) Interstitial associations of cells lining air spaces in human pulmonary fibrosis. *Virchows Arch. [A]*, **372**, 39–49.

60. Brody, A.R., Soler, P. Basset, F. *et al.* (1981) Epithelial–mesenchymal associations of cells in human pulmonary fibrosis and in BHT-oxygen-induced fibrosis in mice. *Exp. Lung Res.*, **2**, 207–20.

61. Adamson, I.Y.R., Young, L. and Bowden, D.H. (1988) Relationship of alveolar epithelial injury and repair to the induction of pulmonary fibrosis. *Am. J. Pathol.*, **130**, 377–83.

62. Adamson, I.Y.R., Hedgecock, C. and Bowden, D.H. (1990) Epithelial cell–fibroblast interactions in lung injury and repair. *Am. J. Pathol.*, **137**, 385–92.

63. Fukuda, Y., Ferrans, V.J., Schoenberger, C.I. *et al.* (1985) Patterns of pulmonary structural remodeling after experimental paraquat toxicity. *Am. J. Pathol.*, **452**, 452–75.

64. Katzenstein, A.A. (1985) Pathogenesis of 'fibrosis' in interstitial pneumonia: an electron microscopic study. *Hum. Pathol.*, **16**, 1015–24.

65. Burkhardt, A. (1986) Pathogenesis of pulmonary fibrosis. *Hum. Pathol.*, **17**, 971–3.

66. Burkhardt, A. (1989) Alveolitis and collapse in the pathogenesis of pulmonary fibrosis. *Am. Rev. Respir. Dis.*, **140**, 513–24.

67. Churg, A., Golden, J., Fligiel, S. and Hogg, J.C. (1983) Bronchopulmonary dysplasia in the adult. *Am. Rev. Respir. Dis.*, **127**, 117–20.

68. Wohl, M.E.B. (1990) Bronchopulmonary dysplasia in adulthood. *N. Engl. J. Med.*, **323**, 1834–6.

PART TWO

BASIC MECHANISMS

Christopher Haslett

PARADOXES: DETRIMENTAL AND BENEFICIAL EFFECTS OF INFLAMMATION, ITS CAPACITY FOR PROGRESSION AND RESOLUTION

It is now accepted that the inflammatory process plays an important role in the pathogenesis of a wide variety of inflammatory diseases that comprise a heavy burden of morbidity and untimely deaths in the developed world. In the lung these include chronic bronchitis and emphysema, asthma, interstitial lung diseases and syndromes of acute respiratory distress in adults (ARDS) and neonates. Most of these diseases are characterized by the persistent accumulation of inflammatory cells which is associated with chronic lung injury and fibrosis. As discussed in Chapter 13, there appears to be a close link between the intensity of inflammation and acute lung injury in ARDS but there is also a rapid and sometimes massive fibrotic reaction (p.216).

Nevertheless, it is also clear that inflammatory responses in the lung do not always progress relentlessly down the pathway to lung destruction and fibrosis. ARDS provides some remarkable clinical examples of the capacity of the lung (under poorly understood circumstances) to recover from massive inflammatory lung injury (Chapter 12) and perhaps even from some forms of lung scarring (Chapter 13). Despite what we know of the complex pathology of established ARDS (Chapter 4), there are several reports demonstrating that of those patients who survive ARDS there is a significant subgroup who appear to make a full functional recovery (Chapter 15). This is a testament to the potential for resolution of inflammation and for the lung to repair and to reconstitute injured tissue, at least to a significant degree. In the author's experience there is the remarkable example of a 20 year old woman who developed ARDS, required several days mechanical ventilation, suffered major complications including repeated pneumothoraces, Gram-negative septicemia, Gram-negative bacterial pneumonia and massive blood loss due to stress peptic ulceration. Nevertheless, she was successfully weaned from the ventilator and improved very slowly over 3 months. Less than 2 years later she had made a full recovery and is now a successful club middle-distance runner, training with Olympic athletes!

Perhaps if we can understand how inflammation normally resolves and injured lungs become repaired, a better understanding of the circumstances whereby resolution and repair fail and progressive lung disease develops may be gained. Moreover, it may ultimately become possible to manipulate biological pathways in the lung in order to favor those promoting resolution rather than persistence of lung inflammation. It will be

ARDS Acute Respiratory Distress in Adults. Edited by Timothy W. Evans and Christopher Haslett. Published in 1996 by Chapman & Hall, London. ISBN 0 412 56910 8

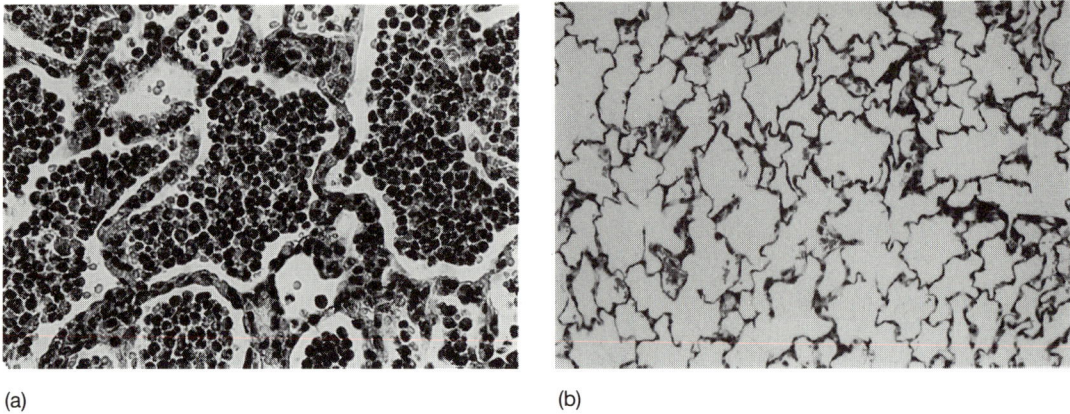

(a)   (b)

Figure 5.1 (a) Histological section of experimental streptococcal pneumonia at 48 hours after the onset of disease (× c.400). There are large numbers of extravasated neutrophils and monocytes in the alveolar spaces. (b) By 5 days the inflammatory response has completely resolved.

difficult in ARDS itself to dissect out the mechanisms of inflammatory resolution, but there is a simpler and equally dramatic example of the potential for resolution of acute pulmonary inflammation. In the preantibiotic era, the massive pulmonary inflammatory response to streptococcal invasion of the lung (which resulted in the pathological features of lobar pneumonia) probably saved the lives of more than 80% of affected individuals [1]. Yet, remarkably in this 'beneficial' inflammatory response, more than 95% of those who survived displayed resolution of the lung inflammation with no evidence of lung destruction or scarring [2]. Contemporary studies of experimental streptococcal pneumonia (Figure 5.1) confirm this historical perspective and clearly demonstrate complete resolution of lung inflammation despite the massive accumulation of neutrophils and inflammatory macrophages. These examples serve as a stimulus for the following discussion of possible mechanisms involved in the resolution of inflammation.

In his treatise on acute inflammation [3]. Hurley considered that the acute inflammatory response might terminate through the development of chronic inflammation, sup-

puration and scarring, or by resolution. It is reasonable to suppose that all the alternatives to resolution are nonideal and could contribute to disease processes, particularly in the lung whose function depends on the integrity of delicate gas exchanging membranes. However, until very recently little research effort has been directed at the cellular and molecular mechanisms underlying the normal resolution of inflammation. The remainder of this chapter therefore considers some of the processes that are likely to occur in the resolution of inflammation, and speculates how a better understanding of these mechanisms will help elucidate the pathogenesis of inflammatory disease and suggest novel anti-inflammatory therapy.

In order for tissues to return to normal during the resolution of inflammation, all of the processes occurring during its evolution must be reversed. Thus, in the simplest model of a self-limited inflammatory response, such as might occur in response to the instillation of bacteria into the alveolar airspace, these must include removal of the inciting stimulus and dissipation of the mediators so generated; cessation of granulocyte emigration from blood vessels; restoration of normal microvascular permeability; limitation of granulocyte secretion of potentially histotoxic and proinflammatory agents; cessation of the emigration of monocytes from blood vessels and their maturation into inflammatory macrophages; and, finally, removal of extravasated fluid, proteins, bacterial and cellular debris, granulocytes and macrophages. Experiments *in vitro* suggest that neutrophils and monocytes can emigrate between endothelial and epithelial cell monolayers without necessarily causing injury to these 'barrier cells'. However, it is also clear that even at sites of 'beneficial' inflammation, such as streptococcal pneumonia, there may be quite extensive endothelial and epithelial injury and even areas of complete destruction and denudation of these layers [4], but the capacity of streptococcal pneumonia to resolve implies that this injury must not be sufficient in degree or extent to inhibit the mechanisms responsible for repair. Therefore, during the resolution of inflammation there must also exist very effective mechanisms for repair of damage and reconstitution of resident tissue cells (Chapters 12 and 13). With the completion of resolution and repair events, the stage should then be set for full recovery of normal tissue architecture and function.

Each of these events will be considered, but factors relevant to the behavior of neutrophil granulocytes in the resolution of inflammation will receive most attention. The neutrophil is the archetypal acute inflammatory cell. It is essential for host defense but it is also implicated in the pathogenesis of a wide range of inflammatory diseases [5] and there is a large body of evidence implicating its direct involvement in the pathogenesis of ARDS [6]. It is usually the first cell to arrive at the scene of tissue perturbation and a number of key inflammatory events, including monocyte emigration [7] and the generation of inflammatory edema [8], appear to depend upon the initial accumulation of neutrophils. They contain a variety of agents with the capacity not only to injure tissues [9], but also to cleave matrix

proteins into chemotactic fragments with the potential to amplify inflammation by attracting more cells. They have recently been shown to contain a granule component CAP37 [10] which is a specific monocyte chemotaxin. Termination of granulocyte emigration from blood vessels and their subsequent clearance from inflamed sites are obvious prerequisites for inflammation to resolve and are important events to consider in the control of inflammatory tissue injury generally [11]. Moreover, gaining further knowledge of the mechanisms controlling the cessation of the emigration of these cells and their disposal may suggest new therapeutic opportunities for manipulating inflammation and promoting mechanisms which favor resolution rather than the persistence of inflammation.

MEDIATOR DISSIPATION

During the resolution of inflammation the powerful mediators initiating the response must somehow be removed, inactivated or otherwise rendered impotent. This aspect of mediator biology has received much less attention than mechanisms involved in their initial generation, and it is likely that different mechanisms may be utilized for different mediators. For example, thromboxane $(Tx)A_2$ and endothelial derived relaxing factor (nitric oxide, NO) are labile factors which are spontaneously unstable (Chapter 30). Platelet activating factor (PAF) and complement C5a are inhibited *in vitro* by an inactivating enzyme [12], and some chemotactic cytokines such as interleukin (IL)-8 are thought to become inactivated by binding to cells [13]. Reduction of mediator efficacy might occur by local reduction of their concentration diluted by inflammatory edema. Mediator efficacy may also be reduced by attenuation of target cell responsiveness, for example in the downregulation of receptors which occurs during desensitization of neutrophils to high concentrations of a variety of inflammatory mediators [15]. It is also likely *in situ* that locally generated factors may exert opposing influences, for example neutrophil immobilizing factor would tend to counteract the effects of chemotactic peptides. In cytokine biology much attention has been paid to agents that initiate or amplify inflammation, but, by analogy with the proteins involved in the blood coagulation cascade, the whole system must be kept under close control by very effective inhibitors and other negative influences. Some such agents have been discovered, e.g. the IL-1 receptor antagonist, yet the inhibitory 'partners' of the most newly described cytokines and chemotactic peptides have yet to be described. The final requirement for the success of most of the above mechanisms is that the production of mediators at the site must cease.

It is therefore likely that control of a single, complex function such as neutrophil chemotaxis in response to a chemotactic peptide, e.g. C5a or IL-8, is influenced at a number of points and by a number of factors including the concentration of mediators; the concentration of their inhibitors or inactivators; possible desensitizing mechanisms, and the effects of other locally generated agents with negative influences on chemotaxis. The redundancy of the inflammatory response *in vivo* must also be taken into consideration. Not only may single mediators exert multiple effects under different circumstances, but important events may be provoked by agents from different mediator families. For example C5a, leukotriene (LT) B_4 IL-8, epithelial-neutrophil activating factor (ENA)-78, and probably many more factors, are likely to exert neutrophil chemotactic effects *in vivo*. In order to gain a dynamic perspective of the resolution of inflammation it will therefore be necessary to consider how a variety of important mediators may act in concert at the inflamed site, and seek to appreciate the integrated impact of negative and positive stimuli on dynamic events *in situ*. Thus, the overall propensity for inflammation to persist would be expected to cease when the balance

of mediator effects tips towards the inhibitory rather than the stimulatory, presumably as a result of the combination of at least some of the possible mechanisms considered above.

CESSATION OF GRANULOCYTE AND MONOCYTE EMIGRATION

Until quite recently it was considered that the differential rate of emigration of granulocytes and monocytes at the inflamed site was due mainly to a slower responsiveness of monocytes to 'common' chemotactic factors such as C5a. However, in the light of new discoveries in chemokine and adhesive molecule biology it is reasonable to suggest that the emigration through microvascular endothelium of specific leukocytes in different pathological circumstances is likely to be caused by the combined effects of the local release of cell specific chemokines **and** the utilization of different components of the adhesive molecule repertoire that control inflammatory cell endothelial cell adhesion. For example, IL-8 is a specific neutrophil chemotaxin, and transcapillary neutrophil migration is likely to be mediated by the adhesive interaction between the leukocyte integrins on the neutrophil surface with adhesive molecules such as intercellular adhesion molecule (ICAM)-1 on the endothelial surface; whereas, specific chemotactic peptides such as monocyte chemotactic peptide (MCP)-1 and the use of an alternative adhesive molecule interaction between such as very late antigen (VLA)$_4$ on the monocyte surface and vascular cell adhesion molecule (VCAM)-1 on the endothelium may be utilized to achieve specific monocyte emigration. Since VCAM-1 tends to be expressed later than E-selectin by stimulated endothelial cells, sequential emigration of leukocytes may also be influenced by the time course of endothelial adhesion molecule expression.

The factors controlling cessation of inflammatory cell emigration remain obscure. Evolution and resolution of inflammation are dynamic processes, and simple histological techniques may inadequately represent these events. Because poorly understood factors such as cell removal rates may also exert major influences on the number of cells observed in 'static' histological sections, the study of neutrophil emigration kinetics requires the careful monitoring of labeled populations of cells. When intravenous pulses of radiolabeled neutrophils were used to define the emigration profiles of neutrophils from blood into acutely inflamed skin [15], joints [16] or lung [17] (Figure 5.2), it was found that neutrophil influx ceased remarkably early. By contrast, a greatly prolonged influx occurred in an inflammatory model which progressed to chronic tissue injury and scarring [18]. Indeed, in experimental strepto-coccal pneumonia, where the histological appearance at 48 hours would suggest massive and continued neutrophil influx (Figure 5.1), we were able to show that neutrophil migra-tion to the site had ceased at least 24 hours previously (Figure 5.2). Cessation of granulo-cyte emigration occurring so soon in the evolu-tion of acute inflammation may therefore represent one of the earliest resolution events, and a number of the following hypothetical mechanisms could be responsible.

1. Locally generated chemotactic factor inhibitors could inactivate neutrophil chemotactic factors.
2. 'Deactivation' or desensitization of neutro-phils to high concentrations of inflamma-tory mediators may lead to extravasated neutrophils becoming unresponsive to fur-ther chemotactic factor stimulation [19]
3. A negative feedback loop might operate whereby neutrophils which have already accumulated exert an influence that pre-vents more neutrophils entering from the bloodstream.
4. Cessation of neutrophil emigration may simply occur as a result of dissipation or removal of chemotactic factors from the inflamed site.

5. The layers of endothelial and epithelial cells, which normally permit neutrophils to emigrate during the initiation of inflam-mation [20,21], could alter to form a 'bar-rier' to further neutrophil emigration.

Which of these hypothetical events are important *in vivo* is by no means clear. In a skin model of inflammation it appeared that a desensitization mechanism [15] was operat-ing and in some forms of human disease involving persistent inflammation there have been suggestions that chemotactic factor inhibitory agents may be defective. However, in experimental arthritis there was no evi-dence for a desensitization mechanism nor for a chemotactic factor inhibitory mechanism [16]. Cessation of neutrophil emigration into the joint coincided with loss of chemoattract-ants from the joint space. Loss of chemo-attractants was not dependent upon cellular accumulation at the site, an observation pro-viding evidence against a simple negative feedback mechanism [16]. Although the mechanism responsible for the loss of chemo-taxin was not identified, these observations suggest that the local generation and removal of chemoattractants are likely to be centrally important in the persistence and cessation of neutrophil emigration.

Neutrophil surface adhesive molecules are upregulated very rapidly upon neutrophil exposure to chemotaxins such as C5a and IL-8. It is now thought that L-selectin on the surface of the neutrophil is important in the initial interaction with endothelial cells under the conditions of shear stress which exists *in vivo*, whereas the leukocyte integrins, e.g. CD11b/CD18 (Mac-1), are particularly important in the second phase of 'tight' adhe-sion necessary for capillary transmigration. (Chapter 9). Neutrophil adhesion molecules must then uncouple to permit the next stage of migration to proceed. Molecular mechan-isms controlling the 'turnon' and 'turnoff' signals of the integrins and other surface mol-

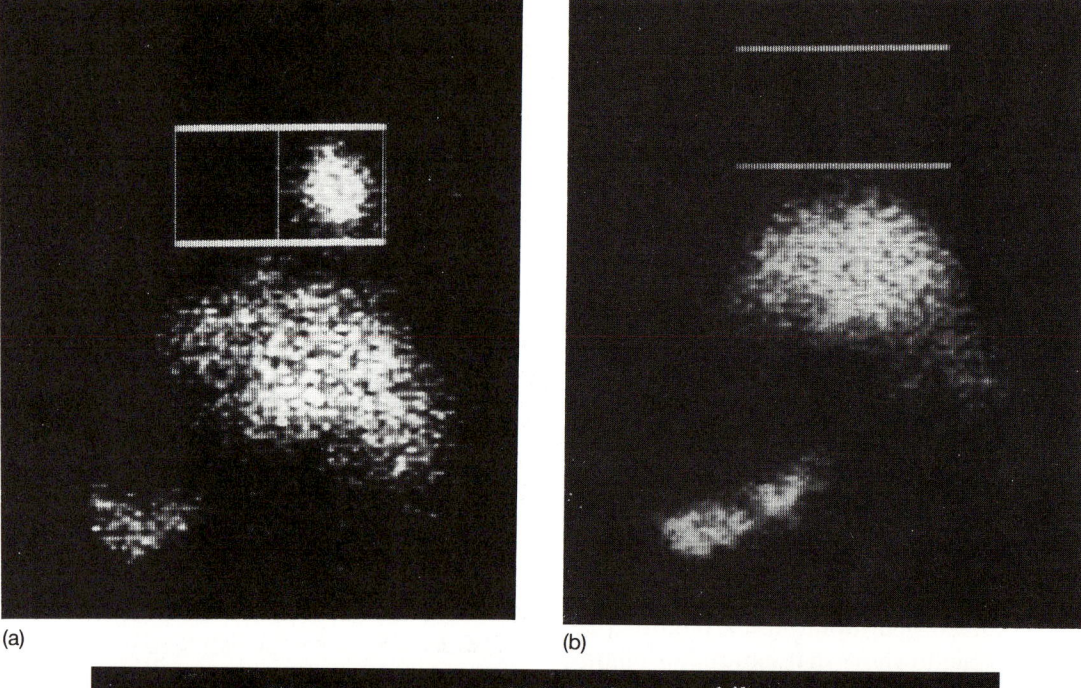

(a)　　　　　　　　　　　　　　　　　　　　(b)

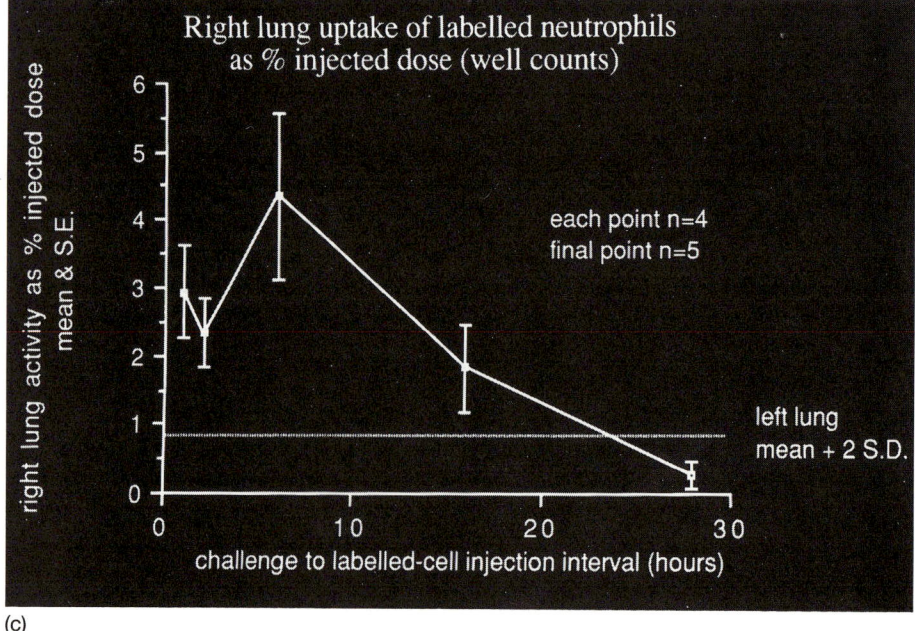

(c)

Figure 5.2 (a) External 24 hour γ-camera scintigram of a rabbit which had received intravenous ^{111}In-labeled neutrophils 6 hours after the bronschoscopic introduction of streptococcal pneumonia into the right upper lobe. There is a major emigration of labeled cells to the lung. (b) In contrast, the 24 hour scintigram of a rabbit which had received IV ^{111}In-labeled neutrophils 24 hours after streptococcal pneumonia instillation shows that neutrophil emigration to the lung has ceased. (c) Quantification of ^{111}In-labeled neutrophils scans in groups of rabbits at various times after induction of streptococcal pneumonia showing that neutrophil emigration reaches baseline within 28 hours of the initiation of pneumonia.

ecules are now the subject of detailed scrutiny [22]. The endothelium also plays an active role in these events. Neutrophil adhesion modules interact with counter receptors on the endothelium, e.g. E-selectin, ICAM-1, ICAM-2 and P-selectin [23]. It appears that endothelial P-selectin and E-selectin are involved in the initial neutrophil adhesion (P-selectin and E-selectin), whereas the link between ICAM-1 on the endothelium and Mac-1 (CD11b/CD18) integrin on the neutrophil surface is likely to be important in the second stage of adhesion and transmigration [24]. Endothelial adhesive molecules are markedly upregulated by factors such as IL-1 and tumor necrosis factor (TNF), which are generated by local cells, particularly macrophages, during the initiation of inflammation [25]. There has been no detailed *in vivo* research on changes of adhesion molecule expression during the termination of neutrophil emigration, but in experimental arthritis it is clear that the inflamed site will permit a further wave of neutrophil emigration in response to a second inflammatory stimulus [16]. Therefore any 'barriers' to cell adhesion or transmigration existing at the time of cessation of neutrophil emigration must be readily reversible, presumably by the further action of newly generated inflammatory cytokines which induce renewed expression/ activation of endothelial surface adhesive molecules together with parallel effects on neutrophil locomotion and the expression/ activation of neutrophil surface adhesive molecules. The detailed identification of mechanisms controlling the local generation and dissipation of agents which promote chemotaxis and upregulation and activation of adhesive molecules is therefore essential for understanding of the processes of termination or persistence of neutrophil emigration at inflamed sites.

Little is known about the control of monocyte emigration *in situ*, although similar principles would be applicable to the identification of mechanisms involved in the cessation of their emigration.

RESTORATION OF NORMAL MICROVASCULAR PERMEABILITY

In some experimental models lung inflammation may be generated without detectable leak of plasma proteins from the microvessels, and from classical ultrastructural studies neutrophil migration to inflamed sites is not necessarily associated with overt endothelial or epithelial injury [20,21]. Nevertheless, in 'real' acute inflammation, such as experimental pneumococcal pneumonia [4], there is clear morphological evidence of endothelial injury ranging from cytoplasmic vasculation to areas of complete denudation and fluid leakage into alveolar spaces. However, the sheets of endothelial and epithelial cells must retain their capacity for complete repair as the pneumonia resolves. Since many inflammatory diseases, such as ARDS, are characterized by severe and persistent endothelial and epithelial injury and there is evidence of at least a degree of inevitable endothelial and epithelial injury in examples of 'beneficial inflammation', this may represent a pivotal point at which the loss of the normal controls of tissue injury and repair might represent a major mechanism in the development of inflammatory disease (Chapter 13). Although the underlying processes are poorly understood, repair is likely to occur by a combination of local cell proliferation to bridge gaps and the recovery of some cells from sublethal injury. Little is known of how endothelial cells recover from sublethal injury, but epithelial cells [26] (Chapter 12) *in vitro* appear to be able to recover from hydrogen peroxide induced injury by a mechanism which requires new protein synthesis. Such cytoprotective mechanisms have received little study. Similarly, it is known that endothelial monolayers, deliberately 'wounded' *in vitro*, have a remarkable capacity to reform, yet little is known of the underlying mechanisms [27].

CONTROL OF INFLAMMATORY CELL SECRETION

Rigid control, and ultimately cessation, of neutrophil secretion of granule enzymes is likely to be important in the limitation of inflammatory tissue injury and the resolution of inflammation. Although there has been much recent study of the initiation and upregulation of phagocyte secretion *in vitro* [28], comparatively little research has been directed at downregulation mechanisms or of how these processes are controlled *in vivo*. Phagocyte secretion *in situ* is likely to be modulated by the balance between stimulatory and inhibitory mediators. The simplest mechanism for termination of secretion, that is the cell exhausting its secretory potential, is unlikely because cells removed from inflamed sites retain significant residual capacity for further secretion upon stimulation *ex vivo* [29]. Other factors that may contribute to downregulation or termination of secretion are the exhaustion of internal energy supplies, receptor downregulation, dissipation of stimuli and, finally, death or removal of the cell itself.

In a short lived, terminally differentiated cell like the neutrophil granulocyte, which normally has a blood half life of about six hours, the ultimate demise of the cell could itself represent an important mechanism in the irreversible downregulation of its secretory function. We have recently discovered that aging neutrophils die in a constitutive, predictable fashion by apoptosis, or programmed cell death (see below). During apoptosis the neutrophil retains its granule enzyme and membrane function, including the ability to exclude vital dyes, but loses the ability to secrete granule contents in response to external stimulation with inflammatory mediators [30]. The apoptotic neutrophil undergoes surface changes by which it becomes recognized as 'senescent self' by inflammatory macrophages which phagocytose the intact senescent cell. Apoptosis therefore provides a mechanism which renders the neutrophil inert and functionally isolated from inflammatory mediators in its microenvironment, thus greatly limiting the destructive potential of the effete neutrophil before it is removed by local phagocytes.

CLEARANCE PHASE OF INFLAMMATION

Once extravasated inflammatory cells have completed their defensive tasks for the host, and inciting agents, such as bacteria, have been removed, the site must then be cleared of fluid, proteins, antibodies and debris. Finally, the key cellular players of inflammation – granulocytes and inflammatory macrophages – must be removed before the tissues can return to normality.

Clearance of fluid, proteins and debris

Most fluid is probably removed via the lymphatic vessels, although reconstitution of normal hemodynamics may contribute by restoring the balance of hydrostatic and osmotic forces in favor of net fluid absorption at the venous end of the capillary. Proteolytic enzymes in plasma exudate and inflammatory cell secretions are likely to break down any fibrin clot at the inflamed site and products of this digestion are likely to be drained by the lymphatics, which become widely distended as the removal of fluid and proteins increases.

The macrophage may also play a role in this phase. It can remove fluids (which might contain a variety of proteins) by pinocytosis. In activated inflammatory macrophages, pinocytosis can occur at a rate such that 25% of the cell surface is reused each minute [31]! Inflammatory macrophages also display greatly increased phagocytic potential. They can recognize opsonized and nonopsonized particles and express cell surface receptors for a wide variety of altered and damaged cells and proteins. The critical role of macrophages in the clearance phase of inflammation was first recognized by Metchnikoff more than a century ago, and we are now just beginning to elucidate the molecular mechanisms of some of his seminal light microscopical observations.

Clearance of extravasated granulocytes

Although we have been aware for some time of the histotoxic potential of a wide variety of neutrophil contents, the fate of this cell *in situ* had not been formally studied until recently. There is no evidence that extravasated neutrophils return to the bloodstream or that lymphatic drainage provides an important disposal route, and it is generally agreed that the bulk of neutrophils meet their fate at the inflamed site. It was widely assumed that the majority of neutrophils inevitably disintegrate at the inflamed site before their fragments are removed by local macrophages [3]. However, if this was the rule, healthy tissues would inevitably be exposed to large quantities of potentially damaging neutrophil contents. Although a number of pathological descriptions have favored neutrophil necrosis as a major mechanism operating in inflammation, many of these examples have derived from histological observations of diseased tissues rather than from examples of 'beneficial', self-limited inflammation. Furthermore, there has been evidence for over a century of an alternative fate for extravasated neutrophils, again based on the classical observations of Elias Metchnikoff [32]. He was the first to catalog the cellular events of the evolution and resolution of acute inflammation in vital preparations. Rather than neutrophil necrosis as the major mechanism, he described an alternative process whereby intact, senescent neutrophils were removed by local macrophages. Over the ensuing decades there have been a number of sporadic reports in both health and disease of macrophage phagocyto-

sis of neutrophils, and of particular relevance to the resolution of inflammation is the clinical phenomenon of 'Reiter's cells' – neutrophil-containing macrophages which have been described in cytology of synovial fluid from the inflamed joints of patients with Reiter's disease and other forms of acute arthritis [33,34]. In experimental peritonitis, where it is possible to sample the inflammatory exudate with ease, it appears that macrophage ingestion of apparently intact neutrophils is the dominant mode of neutrophil removal from the inflamed site [35]. The mechanisms underlying these *in vivo* observations have only recently been addressed *in vitro*. It was found that human neutrophils harvested from peripheral blood and 'aged' overnight were recognized and ingested by inflammatory macrophages (but not by monocytes), whereas freshly isolated neutrophils were not ingested [36]. This suggested that, during aging, a time related process must have been associated with changes in the neutrophil surface, leading to its recognition as 'senescent self'. The development of improved methods for harvesting and culturing human neutrophils with minimal activation and avoiding cell losses from aggregation and clumping allowed us to study in detail the changes occurring in cultured neutrophils. It was discovered that aging granulocytes constitutively undergo apoptosis or programmed cell death and that this process is responsible for the recognition of intact senescent neutrophils by macrophages [37].

This is an appropriate point at which to consider what is known of the processes of apoptosis and necrosis in other cellular systems, and the possible relevance of these alternative neutrophil fates for our understanding of the control of inflammation.

Necrosis versus apoptosis

From the work of Wyllie and his colleagues it is now recognized that the death of nucleated cells can be classified into at least two distinct types: necrosis or accidental death, and apoptosis (programmed cell death) [38,39].

Necrosis can be observed where tissues are exposed to gross insults such as high concentrations of toxins or hypoxia. It is characterized by rapid loss of membrane function and abnormal permeability of the cell membrane, which can be measured by the failure to exclude vital dyes such as trypan blue. There is early disruption of organelles, including liposomal disintegration and irreversible damage to mitrochondria. The stimuli inducing necrosis often affect large numbers of contiguous cells and the widespread release of liposomal contents may obviously be associated with local tissue injury and the initiation or amplification of a local inflammatory response. By contrast, apoptosis occurs in situations where death is predictable, or indeed physiological, such as the removal of unwanted cells during embryological remodeling, and a number of other situations in which cell turnover is physiologically rapid, e.g. crypt cells in the gut epithelium. Recognizing the widespread importance of this process in tissue kinetics, Wyllie and his colleagues coined the term 'apoptosis' – 'the falling off, as of leaves from a tree' in ancient Greek. This had an appealing analogy with autumn: a carefully programmed and regulated event in which the loss of individual leaves from a tree occurs in a random fashion but where the overall process is not detrimental to the host.

In the wide variety of physiological and pathophysiological situations where apoptosis is now well described, the process occurs with remarkably reproducible structural changes, implying a common underlying series of cellular and molecular mechanisms [39]. During apoptosis, cells shrink and there are major changes in the cell surface, which becomes featureless, with the loss of microvillae and with the development of deep invaginations in the surface. How-

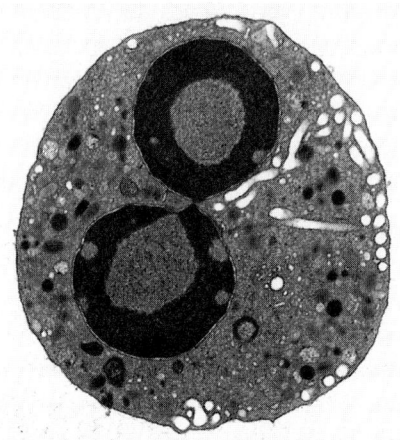

Figure 5.3 Electron micrograph (× c. 11 000) of an apoptotic human neutrophil showing the characteristic chromatin aggregation, prominent nucleolus and dilated cytoplasmic vacuoles. Note that the cell membrane is intact and the granule structure appears normal. (Micrograph taken by Jan Henson.).

ever, the membrane remains intact and organelles such as mitochondria and lysosomes remain intact until very late in the process. The endoplasmic reticulum appears to undergo characteristic, marked dilatation, which on light microscopy may give the appearance of vacuoles in the cytoplasm. The ultrastructural changes in the nucleus are most characteristic, with condensation of chromatin into dense crescent-shaped aggregates and prominence of the nuceolus (Figure 5.3). Apoptotic cells are rapidly ingested by phagocytes *in vivo*, such that in tissue sections of the remodeling embryo apoptotic cells are usually seen contained within other cells. Usually macrophages are responsible for their ingestion, but other 'semiprofessional' phagocytes, e.g. epithelia and fibroblast-like cells, can also participate, particularly in embryological remodeling. The remarkable efficiency of apoptotic cell clearance, together with the fact that it occurs randomly within cell populations renders this mode of cell death much less conspicuous than necrosis in histological sections. In embryological remodeling whole sections. In embryological remodeling whole tracts of tissue can be removed by this process over a few hours without causing local tissue injury or inciting an inflammatory response.

A key feature of apoptosis is internucleosomal cleavage of chromatin in a pattern indicative of endogenous endonuclease activation [40]. This creates low molecular sized fragments of chromatin, which are integers of the 180 base pairs of DNA associated with a nucleosome. When DNA extracted from apoptotic cells is subjected to agarose gel electrophoresis this results in a characteristic 'ladder' pattern of DNA fragments. Over the past decade a number of laboratories have been pursuing the endonuclease(s) responsible for this particular feature of apoptosis. Final characterization has remained elusive, and, while a number of candidates have been suggested [41], there is as yet no agreement on the molecular nature of the endonuclease concerned.

APOPTOSIS IN AGEING GRANULOCYTES LEADS TO THEIR PHAGOCYTOSIS BY MACROPHAGES

Neutrophils harvested from blood or from acutely inflamed human joints remain intact and continue to exclude trypan blue for up to 24 hours 'aging' in culture [37]. With time in culture there is a progressive increase in the proportion of cells exhibiting the light microscopical features of apoptosis, confirmed by electron microscopy and by the chromatin cleavage ladder pattern indicative of endogenous endonuclease activation [37]. These changes occur in parallel with an increase in the proportion of human monocyte derived macrophages ingesting cultured neutrophils in a phagocytic assay [37]. Apoptotic neutrophils are not indestructible. Beyond 24 hours in culture there is a progressive increase in the percentage of cells that fail to exclude trypan blue and spontaneous release of gran-

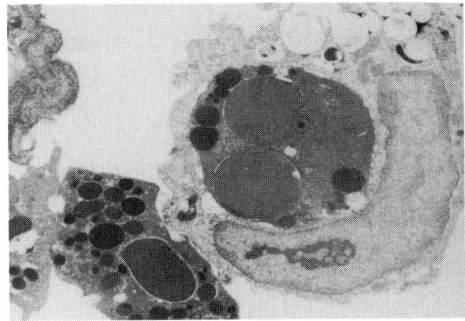

Figure 5.4 Electron micrograph of resolving experimental streptococcal pneumonia showing a macrophage which contains an apoptotic neutrophil (×9000).

ule enzymes occurs. However, when neutrophils are cultured beyond 24 hours in the presence of macrophages, the removal of apoptotic cells is so effective that no trypan blue-positive cells are seen and there is no release of granule enzyme markers into the surrounding medium [42].

The speed with which monocyte derived macrophages recognize, ingest and destroy apoptotic neutrophils *in vitro* is quite remarkable. Individual macrophages can ingest several neutrophils, which then undergo extremely rapid degradation. This may represent part of the explanation as to why the dynamic contribution of this process to cell and tissue kinetics has not been fully appreciated until recently. However, there are now several examples demonstrating clear histological evidence of a role for apoptosis in the *in vivo* removal of granulocytes in acute inflammation. These include acute arthritides [37], neonatal acute lung injury [43] and experimental pneumococcal pneumonia during its resolution phase (Figure 5.4).

Given the proinflammatory potential of neutrophils and their contents, there are now several lines of *in vitro* experimental evidence to support the hypothesis that apoptosis provides a neutrophil clearance mechanism which would limit tissue injury and tend to promote resolution rather than persistence of inflammation.

1. During the process of neutrophil apoptosis there is marked loss of a number of neutrophil functions; including chemotaxis, superoxide production and secretion of granule enzymes upon deliberate external neutrophil stimulation [30]. These data suggest that apoptosis may lead to a 'shutting off' of neutrophil functions, resulting in it becoming functionally isolated from external stimuli that would otherwise trigger responses which could damage tissue. This mechanism could be important if fully mature phagocytes are not immediately available in the vicinity of the neutrophil undergoing apoptosis.

2. Neutrophils undergoing apoptosis are very rapidly taken up by macrophages, and during phagocytosis they appear to retain their enzyme contents and are ingested while still intact, thus preventing the leakage of granule enzymes that would occur should the cell disintegrate before or during uptake by macrophages. This is emphasized by a simple model *in vitro* in which macrophages and neutrophils are cocultured. If macrophage uptake of apoptotic neutrophils is blocked (with colchicine for example) [42], rather than being ingested the apoptotic cells then disintegrate and release toxic contents such as myeloperoxidase and elastase before their cellular fragments are taken up by macrophages.

3. The usual response of macrophages to the phagocytosis of particles *in vitro* is to release proinflammatory mediators such as thromboxane, enzymes and proinflammatory cytokines. However, it has been found that even maximal uptake of apoptotic neutrophils fails to stimulate the release of proinflammatory mediators [44]. This was not simply the result of a toxic or inhibitory effect of the apoptotic neutrophil on the macrophage, because phagocytes which had ingested apoptotic cells were able to generate maximum release of potential mediators when subsequently stimulated by opsonized zymozan. Moreover, when apoptotic neutrophils were deliberately opsonized before ingestion, macrophages **did** respond by the release of thromboxane [44]. Furthermore, when granulocytes are cultured beyond apoptosis to a point when they fail to exclude trypan blue, their ingestion by macrophages induces the release of proinflammatory mediators. Thus, recognition of the senescent granulocyte in the apoptotic morphology rather than the necrotic morphology determines the lack of macrophage proinflammatory response, and this lack of macrophage response is not a function of the apoptotic particle itself, but is determined by the mechanism through which the apoptotic cell is normally ingested. These observations provided considerable impetus for research into the molecular mechanisms by which macrophages recognize and ingest apoptotic cells.

MECHANISMS WHEREBY MACROPHAGES RECOGNIZE APOPTOTIC NEUTROPHILS

Early work by Duval and colleagues [45], using various sugars to inhibit the interactions between macrophages, suggested that phagocytes possess a lectin mechanism capable of recognizing sugar residues on the apoptotic thymocyte surface exposed by loss of sialic acid. This mechanism does not appear to be involved in the macrophage recognition of apoptotic granulocytes, but these findings stimulated our early work demonstrating that recognition of apoptotic neutrophils occurred by a 'charge sensitive' mechanism, inhibitable by cationic molecules such as amino sugars and amino acids and directly influenced by minor changes of pH, in a fashion suggesting involvement of negatively charged residues on the apoptotic neutrophil surface [46]. As well as drawing attention to other recognition systems inhibited by amino sugars (which ultimately turned out to be of relevance to macrophage/apoptotic cell recognition), these data implied that low pH and the presence of cationic molecules might be expected to inhibit the clearance of apoptotic cells at inflamed sites. This was of particular interest because a number of neutrophil derived products, including elastase and myeloperoxidase, are known to be highly cationic and have been detected in significant amounts in inflamed tissues. Furthermore, in situations where inflammation is chronic or where there is abscess formation, interstitial pH may be very low.

The amino sugar inhibition pattern suggested two new lines of inquiry, which led to the definition of macrophage cell surface molecules involved in the clearance of apoptotic neutrophils. Firstly, since amino sugars are known to inhibit the functions of certain members of the integrin family, a detailed series of investigations was performed using a range of monoclonal antibodies directed against candidate integrins in the β_2 and β_3 family, leading to the implication of macrophage surface $\alpha v \beta_3$ in the recognition of apoptotic neutrophils and also apoptotic lymphocytes [47]. Secondly, this amino sugar inhibition pattern was previously described in platelet – platelet interactions occurring via thrombospondin and thrombospondin receptors on their surfaces. This led to work that now implicates CD36 on the macrophage surface [48], and it is thought that thrombospondin itself may serve as an intracellular bridging molecule between the macrophage and the apoptotic cell surface.

Recent studies in a murine system, directed at the putative ionic sites on the apoptotic cell surface that might be involved in macrophage recognition, have suggested that (as yet uncharacterized) receptors on macrophages can recognize exposed phosphatidyl serine residues on the surface of apoptotic cells [49]. These normally reside on the inner leaflet of the membrane lipid bilayer, but during apoptosis it is hypothesized that there is 'flipping' of this layer in a fashion which may be analogous to that occurring during the sickling of erythrocytes. It appears that the main difference between these two recognition systems relates to the utilization of alternative recognition mechanisms by different subpopulations of macrophages [50]. The *in vivo* significance of these observations is as yet uncertain.

CLEARANCE OF APOPTOTIC GRANULOCYTES BY CELLS OTHER THAN MACROPHAGES

It is recognized histologically in embryonic remodeling and in thymus involution that, while apoptotic cells are usually taken up by local macrophages, they may also be seen within epithelial or fibroblast-like cells. We therefore compared the ability of monolayers of fibroblasts, endothelial and epithelial cells from a variety of sources to recognize apoptotic neutrophils *in vitro*. In these experiments only the fibroblast appeared to recognize and ingest apoptotic neutrophils [51]. The fibroblast has long been recognized as a 'semiprofessional' phagocyte capable of ingesting latex beads, dye particles and mast cell granules. The significance of fibroblast phagocytosis of senescent neutrophils is uncertain, but the fibroblast appears to employ recognition mechanisms differing from the macrophage, in that they appear to utilize a sugar – lectin recognition mechanism in addition to the integrin mechanism described in the macrophage–neutrophil system [51]. More recently, Savill *et al.* have shown that renal mesangial cells, fibroblast-like cells that are also recognized as 'semiprofessional' phagocytes, also have the capacity to take up large numbers of apoptotic neutrophils [52].

The significance of these observations is uncertain. It is possible that uptake of apoptotic neutrophils by resident cells, including fibroblasts, serves as a clearance mechanism before extravasated monocytes have fully matured into inflammatory macrophages capable of recognizing and ingesting apoptotic cells. Alternatively, it may serve as a 'back up' mechanism should the macrophage disposal mechanism be overwhelmed by waves of neutrophil apoptosis. However, since the fibroblast is responsible for scar tissue matrix protein secretion it is possible that this possible clearance route is an 'undesirable' alternative, particularly if the uptake of apoptotic neutrophils should cause fibroblast replication and secretion of collagen.

More recently, there have been suggestions of an even wider and central role for apoptosis in the repair and remodeling of tissues. In resolution of experimental nephritis it has been shown [53] that the clearance of excessive numbers of mesangial cells by apoptosis is a central process in glomerular remodeling. Similarly, fibroblast apoptosis has been proposed as a key mechanism in the remodeling of pulmonary scar tissue and granulation tissue which may occur in late ARDS [54].

REGULATION OF GRANULOCYTE APOPTOSIS BY EXTERNAL MEDIATORS

Recent histological observations of resolving pulmonary inflammation have suggested that extravasated neutrophils undergo apoptosis at a slower rate than neutrophils derived from peripheral blood. In experimental pneumonia at 48 hours (Figure 5.1) large numbers of neutrophils without any significant evidence of apoptosis were seen. The use of radiolabeled pulses of neutrophils delivered intravenously during the evolution of this model suggested that neutrophil emigration from the blood to the inflamed lung had largely ceased by 16 hours (Figure 5.2). This implied that the bulk of neutrophils observed at 48 hours had been present for at least 24 hours, yet the half life of neutrophils in blood is 4–5 hours. These observations suggested that factors present at the inflamed site might have inhibited the constitutive rate of neutrophil apoptosis. We have now shown that

the rate of neutrophil apoptosis *in vitro* is inhibited by a variety of inflammatory mediators [55] including endotoxic lipopolysaccharide, C5a and granulocyte-macrophage colony stimulating factor (GM-CSF) (which is particularly potent at inhibiting the rate of neutrophil apoptosis). If, as seems likely, apoptosis, by leading to macrophage removal of unwanted cells, controls the tissue longevity of neutrophils, these might represent important mechanisms controlling the 'tissue load' of inflammatory cells *in situ*.

Intracellular mechanisms governing apoptosis are as yet poorly understood. However, there are indications that internal controls in granulocytes may differ from those in lymphoid cells. In thymocytes, elevation of intracellular calcium $[Ca^{2+}]_i$ concentration by calcium ionophores induces apoptosis, and apoptosis induced by other stimuli, such as glucocorticoids, is associated with rises in $[Ca^{2+}]_i$ [56]. However, in neutrophils spontaneously undergoing apoptosis there were no such rises in $[Ca^{2+}]_i$, and agents increasing $[Ca^{2+}]_i$ caused dramatic slowing of neutrophil apoptosis without inducing necrosis [57]. Furthermore, treatment of aging neutrophils with chelating agents, which bind intracellular calcium, is associated with an increase in the rate of neutrophil apoptosis [57]. Rises in intracellular calcium are known to occur when neutrophils are primed or activated *in vitro* and this is likely to represent at least part of the mechanism underlying the retardation of neutrophil apoptosis observed after external stimulation with inflammatory mediators. Furthermore, when neutrophils are aged in the presence of inhibitors of protein synthesis, e.g. cycloheximide, there is an acceleration of the constitutive rate of apoptosis. This is in marked contrast to corticosteroid induced thymocyte apoptosis which is inhibited by cycloheximide. These observations suggest the existence of a protein synthesis dependent, apoptosis inhibitory factor in neutrophils. It is hypothesized that external inflammatory mediators inhibit the rate of neutrophil apoptosis by causing a rise in intracellular calcium which subsequently acts on downstream processes including mRNA and protein synthesis of this putative inhibitory factor(s).

It is now clear that apoptosis in a variety of cell types can be influenced by proto-oncogene expression. The best worked out system is bcl-2 [58], the expression of which is associated with inhibition of apoptosis in a variety of cell types, but its significance in the neutrophil is uncertain. C-myc expression in fibroblasts and lymphoid cells appears to induce apoptosis [59], and more recently p53 and Rb-1 have also been implicated. It remains to be established whether the products of these genes are relevant for the control of inflammatory cell apoptosis, and it is presently unclear how the genetic controls are linked with second messenger controls and the final effector events including endonuclease activation, downregulation of cell function and cell surface changes responsible for phagocyte recognition.

A ROLE FOR GRANULOCYTE APOPTOSIS IN THE CONTROL OF INFLAMMATION?

Granulocyte apoptosis could play at least two important roles in the control of inflammation. By controlling the functional longevity and tissue removal of unwanted granulocytes and providing a pivotal point at which inflammatory cytokines and growth factors exert their controls on inflammatory cell longevity, it is likely that (together with neutrophil influx) neutrophil apoptosis and clearance are important determinants of the overall tissue load of inflammatory cells (Figure 5.5). Secondly, it is reasonable to suggest that the fate of neutrophils, whether by apoptosis or by necrosis, is an important factor in the control of inflammation. Inflammatory disease is now thought to result from a quan-

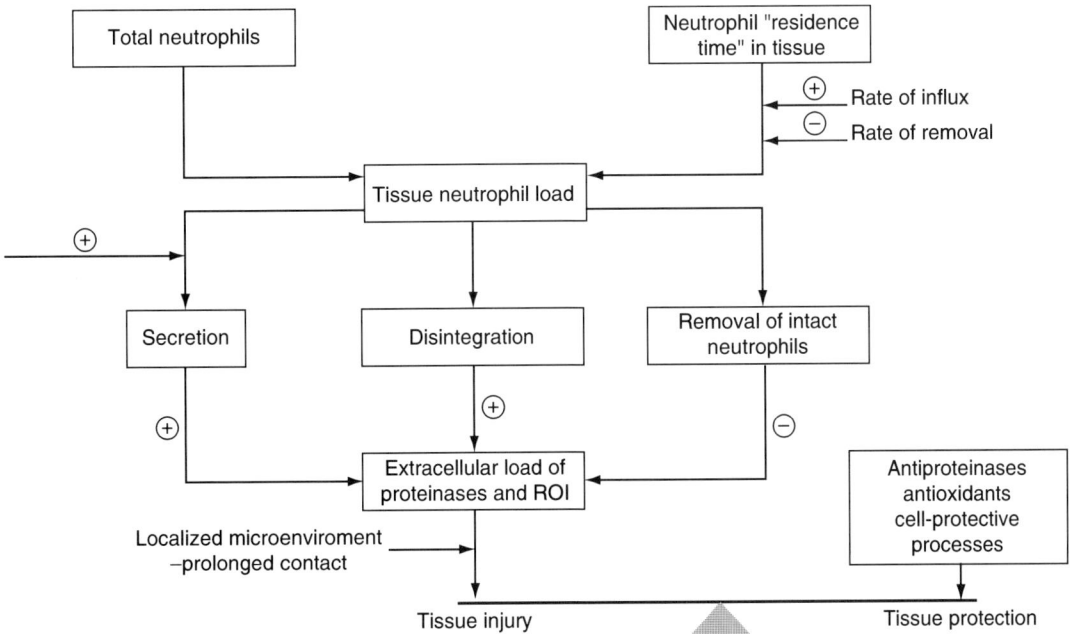

Figure 5.5 The 'balance' between the capacity of inflammatory cells to injure tissues and tissue defense mechanisms, including pivotal points at which factors involved in the emigration and clearance of granulocytes may impinge on the equation. ROI = reactive oxygen intermediate.

tative imbalance between potentially damaging inflammatory influences and their tissue protective mechanisms, as exemplified by the proteinase/antiproteinase theory of emphysema. Whether neutrophils meet their fate by a mechanism that involves removal of the whole cell or via a mechanism that results in disintegration and disgorgement of their potentially histotoxic and proinflammatory contents is likely to impinge on such an equation. Detailed consideration has been given to the observations that apoptosis may serve to keep potentially injurious granular contents within the cell membrane while at the same time the cell becomes unable to respond by degranulation in response to external stimuli. Moreover, the intact cell is removed by a novel phagocytic recognition mechanism which determines that macrophages fail to release proinflammatory mediators during macrophage recognition and phagocytosis. This is not to suggest that apoptosis is the only mechanism for removal of neutrophils at an inflamed site. While, in all the spontaneously resolving examples of inflammation we have examined in humans and in experimental models, the removal of whole granulocytes by apoptosis appears to be a major mechanism, examples of neutrophil necrosis are also seen, particularly in some inflammatory diseases, such as systemic vasculitis, where light microscopical features of neutrophils necrosis and disintegration have been described in tissues close to inflamed vessels, and called 'leukocytoclastic vasculitis'. It is possible therefore that the **balance** between the degree of neutrophil apoptosis and the degree of neutrophil necrosis at an inflamed site may represent a pivotal point in the control of tissue injury and in the propensity of an inflamed site to resolve or to progress.

Therefore, with knowledge presently available, it seems reasonable to suggest that granulocyte necrosis at inflamed sites can be regarded as a deleterious and undesirable mode of clearance, which, by contrast with apoptosis, is likely to favor persistence of inflammatory tissue injury rather than resolution of inflammation.

FATE OF MACROPHAGES

Although monocytes appear to undergo apoptosis spontaneously *in vitro* [60], as they mature into macrophages they have a very low constitutive rate of apoptosis [61], but can be induced to undergo apoptosis with a number of toxic stimuli (G.J. Bellingan *et al.*, unpublished data) including cycloheximide (although higher concentrations of cycloheximide are required to induce macrophage apoptosis compared with those that promote neutrophil apoptosis). Furthermore, during the resolution of experimental streptococcal pneumonia, while there is clear evidence of neutrophil apoptosis and ingestion by macrophages, there is no histological clue as to the fate of inflammatory macrophages during the resolution phase *in situ* (C. Haslett, unpublished observations). These observations suggest that macrophages might leave the inflamed tissue and meet their fate at a distal site. We have recently carried out studies of the fate of inflammatory macrophages during the resolution of experimental murine peritonitis and have found that inflammatory macrophages have a short tissue resistance time, compared with resident macrophages, and that they exit the inflamed peritoneum to be cleared in the draining lymph nodes [62]. Whether their final demise involves apoptosis and clearance by specialized local phagocytes is as yet uncertain.

RESOLUTION MECHANISMS AND THE CONTROL OF INFLAMMATION

On preliminary evidence a speculative scheme can be proposed whereby a stereotyped sequence of inflammatory events results in the resolution of inflammation. Injury to endothelial and epithelial cell 'barriers' is minimized, but is associated with leak of fluid and protein; reconstitution of normal microvascular permeability occurs by the reforming of cell junctions and the regeneration of cell sheets; neutrophil influx ceases early in the evolution of acute inflammation and relates to cessation of local chemoattractant generation and dissipation; monocytes mature into inflammatory macrophages to remove proteins and other debris; neutrophil secretion is restricted and the aged cell undergoes apoptosis, which controls neutrophil longevity and determines the macrophage removal of the intact senescent cell without stimulating macrophage release of proinflammatory mediators; excess tissue macrophages are removed by unknown processes.

There are several steps in the above scheme which could go awry and lead to circumstances favoring the development of persistent inflammation. For example, if the macrophage fails to develop the appropriate receptors for removing apoptotic cells, neutrophils would eventually become necrotic and disgorge their damaging contents, or alternatively they may be taken up by local fibroblasts, possibly with a profibrotic response. Once a chronic inflammatory state begins to develop there is evidence that local pH falls. This would tend to inhibit macrophage recognition of apoptotic neutrophils, as would the continued accumulation of inflammatory cell cationic products, such as elastase, etc., which would contribute to the inhibition of macrophage clearance of apoptotic neutrophils.

Hurley [3] recognized that there were several mechanisms other than resolution whereby acute inflammation could terminate. These included chronic inflammation, scarring and abscess formation. By comparison with resolution, all of these termination events must clearly be regarded as detrimental to organ function. As we begin to learn more about the mechanisms involved in the resolution of inflammation, it may be possible to 'divert' inflammatory processes towards resolution rather than one of the other less desirable pathways. More specifically, with increasing knowledge of apoptosis and its internal mechanisms it may be possible to use this 'controlled' process of cell suicide or programmed cell death to remove specific inflammatory cells by the mechanisms 'which nature intended' at particular pathogenetic stages when they are critical to the disease process.

ACKNOWLEDGEMENTS

This work was supported by the Medical Research Council of Great Britain in the form of a Programme Grant and a number of preceding project grants and Fellowships. Further support was obtained from the National Asthma Campaign and the British Lung Foundation.

Thanks are due to close colleagues who participated in the work and who were a constant source of stimulation. These include John Savill in particular, Moira Whyte, Laura Meagher and Ian Dransfield.

REFERENCES

1. Heffron, R. (1939) Pneumonia: with special reference to pneumococcus lobar pneumonia. xv 1086p Commonwealth Fund NY.
2. Robertson, O.H. and Uhley, C.G. (1938) Changes occurring in the macrophage system of the lungs in pneumococcus lobar pneumonia. *J. Clin. Invest.*, **15**, 115–30.
3. Hurley, J.V. (1983) Termination of acute inflammation. 1. Resolution, in *Acute Inflammation*, 2nd edn, Churchill Livingstone, London, pp. 109–17.
4. Larsen, G.L., McCarthy, K., Webster, R.O. *et al.* (1980) A differential effect of C5a and C5a des arg in the induction of pulmonary inflammation. *Am. J. Pathol.*, **100**, 179–92.
5. Weiss, S.J. (1989) Tissue destruction by neutrophils. *N. Engl. J. Med.*, **320**, 365–76.
6. Donnelly, S.C. and Haslett C. (1992) Cellular mechanisms of acute lung injury: implications for future treatment in the adult respiratory distress syndrome. *Thorax*, **47**, 260–3.
7. Doherty, D.E., Downey, G.P., Worthen, G.S. *et al.* (1988) Monocyte retention and migration in pulmonary inflammation. *Lab. Invest.*, **59**, 200–13.

8. Wedmore, C.V. and Williams, T.J. (1981) Control of vascular permeability by polymorphonuclear leukocytes in inflammation. *Nature*, **289**, 646–50.

9. McColl, S.R. and Showall, H.J. (1994) Neutrophil-derived inflammatory mediators, in *Immunopharmacology of Neutrophils* (ed. P.G. Helliwell and T.J. Williams), Academic Press, London, pp. 95–105.

10. Spitznagel, J.K. (1990) Antibiotic proteins of neutrophils. *J. Clin. Invest.*, **86**, 1851–4.

11. Haslett, C. (1992) Resolution of acute inflammation and the role of apoptosis in the tissue fate of granulocytes. *Clin. Sci.*, **83**, 639–48.

12. Berenberg, J.L. and Ward, P.A. (1973) Chemotactic factor of inactivator in normal human serum. *J. Clin. Invest.*, **52**, 1200–7.

13. Kunkel, S.L., Standiford, T., Kasaahara, K. and Strieter, R.M. (1991) Interleukin-8: the major neutrophil chemotactic factor in the lung. *Exp. Lung Res.*, **17**, 17–23.

14. Henson, P.M., Schwartzmann, N.A. and Zanolari, B. (1981) Intracellular control of human neutrophil secretion. II. Stimulus specificity of desensitisation induced by six different soluble and particulate stimuli. *J. Immunol.*, **127**, 754–9.

15. Colditz, I.G. and Movat, H.Z. (1984) Desensitisation of acute inflammatory lesions to chemotaxins and endotoxin. *J. Immunol.*, **133**, 2163–8.

16. Haslett, C., Jose, P.J., Giclas, P.C. *et al.* (1989) Cessation of neutrophil influx in C5a-induced acute experimental arthritis is associated with loss of chemoattractant activity from joint spaces. *J. Immunol.*, **142**, 3510–17.

17. Clark, R.J., Jones, H.A., Rhodes, C.G. and Haslett, C. (1989) Non-invasive assessment in self-limited pulmonary inflammation by external scintigraphy of [111]indium-labelled neutrophil influx and by measurement of the local metabolic response with positron emission tomography. *Am. Rev. Respir. Dis.*, **139**, A58.

18. Haslett, C., Shen, A.S., Feldsien, D.C. *et al.* (1989) [111]Indium-labelled neutrophil flux into the lungs of bleomycin-treated rabbits assessed non-invasively by external scintigraphy. *Am. Rev. Respir. Dis.*, **140**, 756–63.

19. Ward, P.A. and Becker, E.L. (1967) The deactivation of rabbit neutrophils by chemotactic factor and the nature of the activatable esterase. *J. Exp. Med.*, **127**, 693–709.

20. Hurley, J.V. (1963) An electron microscopic study of leukocyte emigration and vascular permeability in rat skin. *Aust. J. Exp. Biol. Med. Sci.*, **41**, 171–9.

21. Milks, L. and Cramer, E. (1984) Transepithelial electrical resistance studies during *in vitro* neutrophil migration. *Fed. Proc.*, **43**, 477.

22. Springer, T.A. (1990) Adhesion receptors of the immune system. *Nature*, **346**, 425–34.

23. Hynes, R.O. (1992) Integrins: versatility, modulation and signalling in cell adhesion. *Cell*, **69**, 11.

24. Lawrence, M.B. and Springer, T.A. (1991) Leukocytes roll on a selectin at physiologic flow rates: distinction form and prerequisite for adhesion through integrins. *Cell*, **65**, 859–73.

25. Pober, J.S. and Cotran, R.S. (1990) Cytokines and endothelial cell biology. *Physiol. Rev.*, **70**, 427–51.

26. Parsons, P.E., Sugahara, K., Cott, G.R. *et al.* (1987) The effect of neutrophil migration and prolonged neutrophil contact on epithelial permeability. *Am. J. Pathol.*, **129**, 302–12.

27. Haudenschild, C.L. and Schwartz, S.M. (1979) Endothelial regeneration. II. Restitution of endothelial continuity. *Lab. Invest.*, **41**, 407–18.

28. Henson, P.M., Henson, J.E., Fittschen, C., *et al.* (1988) Phagocytic cells: degranulation and secretion, in Gallin J.I. ed. *Inflammation, Basic Principles and Clinical Correlates* (ed. J.I. Gallin), Raven Press, New York, pp. 363–90.

29. Zimmerli, W., Seligmann, B. and Gallin, J.I. (1986) Exudation primes human and guinea pig neutrophils for subsequent responsiveness to the chemotactic peptide *N*-formyl methionyl leucyl phenylamine and increases complement C3bi receptor expression. *J. Clin. Invest.*, **77**, 925–33.

30. Whyte, M.K.B., Meagher, L.C., MacDermott, J. and Haslett, C. (1993) Down-regulation of neutrophil function by apoptosis: a mechanism for functional isolation of neutrophils from inflammatory mediator stimulation. *J. Immunol.*, **150**, 5123–34.

31. Steinmann, R.M., Brodie, S.E. and Cohn, Z.A. (1976) Membrane flow during pinocytosis – a sterological analysis. *J. Cell. Biol.*, **68**, 665–87.

32. Metchnikoff, E. (1968) *Lectures on the Comparative Pathology of Inflammation*, lecture VII, delivered at the Pasteur Institute in 1891 (translated by F.A. Starling and E.H. Starling), Dover, New York.

33. Pekin, T., Malinin, T.I. and Zwaifler, R. (1967) Unusual synovial fluid findings in Reiter's syndrome. *Ann. Intern. Med.*, **66**, 677–84.

34. Spriggs, R.S., Boddington, M.M. and Mowat, A.G. (1978) Joint fluid cytology in Reiter's syndrome. *Ann. Rheum. Dis.*, **37**, 557–60.

35. Chapes, S.K. and Haskill, S. (1983) Evidence for granulocyte-mediated macrophage activation after *C. parvum* immunization. *Cell. Immunol.*, **75**, 367–77.

36. Newman, S.L., Henson, J.E. and Henson, P.M. (1982) Phagocytosis of senescent neutrophils by human monocyte-derived macrophages and rabbit inflammatory macrophages. *J. Exp. Med.*, **156**, 430–42.

37. Savill, J.S., Wyllie, A.H., Henson, J.E. *et al.* (1989) Macrophage phagocytosis of aging neutrophils in inflammation – programmed cell death leads to its recognition by macrophages. *J. Clin. Invest.*, **83**, 865–75.

38. Kerr, J.F.R., Wyllie, A.H. and Currie, A.R. (1972) Apoptosis: a basic biological phenomenon with wide-ranging implications in tissue kinetics. *Br. J. Cancer*, **26**, 239–57.

39. Wyllie, A.H., Kerr, J.F.R. and Currie, A.R. (1980) Cell death: the significance of apoptosis. *Int. Rev. Cytol.*, **68**, 251.

40. Wyllie, A.H. (1981) Glucocorticoid-induced thymocyte apoptosis is associated with endogenous endonuclease activation. *Nature*, **284**, 555–8.

41. Pietsch, M.C., Polzar, B., Stephan, H. *et al.* (1993) Characterization of the endogenous deoxyribonuclease involved in nuclear DNA degradation during apoptosis (programmed cell death). *EMBO J.* **12**, 371–7.

42. Kar, S., Ren, Y. Savill, J.S. and Haslett, C. (1995) Inhibition of macrophage phagocytosis *in vitro* of aged neutrophils increases release of neutrophil contents. *Clin. Sci.*, **85**, 27p.

43. Grigg, J.M., Savill, J.S., Sarraf, C., Haslett, C. and Silverman, M. (1991) Neutrophil apoptosis and clearance from neonatal linings. *Lancet*, **338**, 720–722.

44. Meagher, L.C., Savill, J.S., Baker, A. *et al.* (1992) Phagocytosis of apoptotic neutrophils does not induce macrophage release of thromboxane B_2. *J. Leukoc. Biol.*, **52**, 269–73.

45. Duvall, E., Wyllie, A.H. and Morris, R.G. (1985) Macrophage recognition of cells undergoing programmed cell death. *Immunology*, **56**, 351–8.

46. Savill, J.S., Henson, P.M. and Haslett, C. (1989) Phagocytosis of aged human neutrophils by macrophages is mediated by a novel 'charge sensitive' recognition mechanism. *J. Clin. Invest.*, **84**, 1518–27.

47. Savill, J.S., Dransfield, I., Hogg, N. and Haslett, C. (1990) Macrophage recognition of 'senescent self'. The vitronectin receptor mediates phagocytosis of cells undergoing apoptosis. *Nature*, **342**, 170–3.

48. Savill, J.S., Hogg, N. and Haslett, C. (1992) Thrombospondin co-operates with CD36 and the vitronectin receptor macrophage in recognition of aged neutrophils. *J. Clin. Invest.*, **90**, 1513–29.

49. Fadok, V.A., Voelker, D.R., Campbell, P.A. *et al.* (1992) Exposure of phosphatidylserine on the surface of apoptotic lymphocytes triggers specific recognition and removal by macrophages. *J. Immunol.*, **148**, 2207–16.

50. Fadok, V., Savill, J.S., Haslett, C. *et al.* (1992) Different populations of macrophages use either the vitronectin receptor or the phosphatidylserine receptor to recognize and remove apoptotic cells. *J. Immunol.*, **149**, 4029–35.

51. Hall, S.E., Savill, J.S., Henson, P.M. and Haslett, C. (1994) Apoptotic neutrophils are phagocytosed by fibroblasts with participation of the fibroblast vitronectin receptor and involvement of a mannose/fucose-specific lectin. *J. Immunol.*, **153**, 3218–27.

52. Savill, J.S., Smith, J., Sarraf, C. *et al.* (1992) Glomerular mesangial cells and inflammatory macrophages ingest neutrophils undergoing apoptosis. *Kidney Int.*, **42**, 924–36.

53. Baker, A.J., Mooney, A., Hughes, J. *et al.* (1994) Mesangial cell apoptosis: the major mechanism for resolution of glomerular hypercellularity in experimental mesangial proliferative nephritis. *J. Clin. Invest.*, **94**, 2105–16.

54. Polunovsky, V.A., Chen, B., Henke, C. *et al.* (1993) Role of mesenchymal cell death in lung remodelling after injury. *J. Clin. Invest.*, **92**, 388–97.

55. Lee, A., Whyte, MBK and Haslett, C. (1993) Prolonged *in vitro* lifespan and functional longevity of neutrophils induced by inflammatory mediators acting through inhibition of apoptosis. *J. Leukoc. Biol.*, **54**, 283–8.

56. McConkey, D.J., Nicotera, P., Hartzell, P. *et al.* (1989) Glucocorticoids activate a suicide process in thymocytes through an elevation of cytosolic Ca^{2+} concentration. *Arch. Biochem. Biophys.*, **269**, 365–70.

57. Whyte, MKB, Meagher, L.C., Hardwick, S.J.

et al. (1993) Transient elevations of cytosolic free calcium retard subsequent apoptosis in neutrophils *in vitro. J. Clin. Invest.,* **92**, 446–55.

58. Vaux, D.L., Cory, S. and Adams, J.M. (1992) Bcl-2 gene promotes haemopoietic cell survival and cooperates with c-myc to immortalise pre-B cells. *Nature,* **335**, 440–442.

59. Evan, G.I., Wyllie, A.H., Gilbert, G.S. *et al.* (1992) Induction of apoptosis in fibroblasts by c-myc protein. *Cell,* **69**, 119–28.

60. Mangan, D.F. and Wahl, S.M. (1991) Differential regulation of human monocytes in pro-grammed cell death (apoptosis) by chemotactic factors and pro-inflammatory cytokines. *J. Immunol.,* **147**, 3408–12.

61. Bellingan, G.J., Dransfield, I. and Haslett, C. (1994) Characterization of apoptosis in the human macrophage. *Clin. Sci.,* **86**, 2p.

62. Bellingan, G.J., Caldwell, H., Howie, S.E.M *et al.* (1995) *In vivo* fate of the inflammatory macrophage during the resolution of inflammation: inflammatory macrophages do not die locally but emigrate to the draining lymph nodes. (submitted).

Polly E. Parsons

Although it cannot yet be either prevented or cured, our understanding of the pathogenesis of the syndrome of acute respiratory distress in adults (ARDS) has increased dramatically in the last 25 years. Initially the syndrome was thought to involve only the lungs and be the result of a single process, the activation of the complement cascade. Even though subsequent investigations have now shown that the injury is neither limited to the lungs nor is the pathogenesis simple, it is important to review the early studies which focused on complement activation because they both implicated the neutrophil in the development of lung injury and led to the investigations of the role of endotoxin, which remain a cornerstone for investigations today.

COMPLEMENT HYPOTHESIS

The hypothesis that complement mediated neutrophil activation caused acute lung injury arose from early observations in patients undergoing hemodialysis. In 1968 Kaplow and Goffinet demonstrated that patients developed significant neutropenia during the initiation of hemodialysis [1]. It was subsequently noted that the patients also had transient pulmonary dysfunction and that neutrophils were sequestered within the lung at the time that the peripheral neutropenia occurred [2,3]. Further studies found

that the cellophane membrane of the dialysis machine activated the complement cascade and that activated complement components were responsible for the hemodialysis associated neutropenia [4]. The link between the activation of complement and lung injury was further supported by a series of animal studies. In a sheep model the infusion of activated complement fragments resulted in pulmonary hypertension, hypoxia, increased lung lymph flow and increased lymph protein concentration [2]; and in rats the intravascular activation of complement resulted in a neutrophil dependent model of lung injury [5]. In rabbits the infusion of C5a, the complement component that was found to induce neutrophil aggregation *in vitro* [4], caused neutrophil aggregation within the pulmonary microvasculature [6]. Significantly, however, other studies in rabbits clearly showed that neutrophil aggregation alone was not associated with an increase in lung vascular permeability [7]. This occurred only if the activation of complement was accompanied by a second severe insult such as hypoxia [7].

There are multiple mechanisms by which complement activation could contribute to acute lung injury. A complete review of the complement cascade is beyond the scope of this chapter but the elements which are most likely to prove important in acute lung injury

ARDS Acute Respiratory Distress in Adults. Edited by Timothy W. Evans and Christopher Haslett. Published in 1996 by Chapman & Hall, London. ISBN 0 412 56910 8

will be briefly reviewed. Activation of both the classical and alternative pathways results in the cleavage of C3. C3a acts as an anaphylatoxin, stimulating the release of histamine and the contraction of smooth muscle [8]. Histamine release could increase vascular permeability and both histamine release and smooth muscle contraction could alter pulmonary blood flow to either amplify or modulate injury. C3b amplifies complement activation by binding to C3 convertase enzymes generating C5 convertase, which then cleaves C5 [9]. C3b and C3bi are both recognized by the receptor CR1, which is present on the surface of many cell types, including neutrophils and monocytes, and may modulate complement activation and cell injury by increasing the cleavage of C3b [10]. iC3b is also recognized by the receptor CD11b/CD18. The cleavage of C5 produces C5a, which effects several neutrophil functions including chemotaxis, adherence and the release of toxic mediators, such as oxidants, proteases and arachidonate metabolites [11]. C5a may also promote the conversion of xanthine dehydrogenase to xanthine oxidase, further enhancing oxidant mediated injury [11]. This could be particularly important as a major source for xanthine dehydrogenase is the endothelium. Within the lung C5a also stimulates the generation of arachidonate metabolism [11]. C5b binds through a series of sequential steps to C6, C7, C8 and C9 to form the terminal component of complement, C5b–9 or the membrane attack complex. This complex increases the permeability of cell membranes by creating pores and *in vitro* has also been found to stimulate the release of oxidants from neutrophils and monocytes [12].

The potential importance of complement components in the development of acute lung injury has been demonstrated in a series of animal studies. Mice that are specifically deficient in C5 develop attenuated lung injury in response to pneumococcal sepsis, burns and hyperoxia when compared with controls [13–15], although they have an enhanced response to intratracheal pseudomonas bacteria [16]. Furthermore, when antibodies to C5a were administered to baboons with severe *Escherichia coli* sepsis, C5a levels were decreased [17], pulmonary dysfunction was abrogated and survival improved [17,18]. Similarly, in a rodent model of acute lung injury induced by the concomitant infusion of *E. coli* and platelet activating factor (PAF), pretreatment with recombinant soluble C receptor 1, which affects complement activation by regulating C3 and C5 convertase, significantly decreased lung permeability. In this model the deposition of both C3 and C5b–9 on pulmonary vascular endothelium was decreased but neutrophil accumulation within the lung was not affected [19].

In the light of animal studies showing that complement activation could cause neutrophil dependent lung injury it seemed likely that a similar process could be responsible for the development of ARDS. Initial studies using bioassays to detect circulating complement activity and levels in patients at risk of, and with, ARDS suggested a strong correlation between complement and severe lung injury [20,21]. However, subsequent studies in which complement activation was quantitated using immunoassays failed to show a cause and effect relationship, as activated fragments of complement were detectable in both critically ill patients at risk of ARDS, but who did not develop the syndrome as well as those with established lung injury [22–24]. As with the animal studies, these clinical investigations indicated that complement activation alone did not cause acute lung injury and cast doubt on whether there was any relationship between the two. Nevertheless, Langlois and Gawryl reported recently that in septic patients circulating levels of the terminal component of complement (Soluble C5b–9, sC5b–9) predicted the development of ARDS [25]. In a later study that measured multiple components of complement including sC5b–9 in multiple groups of patients, of sC5b–9 lev-

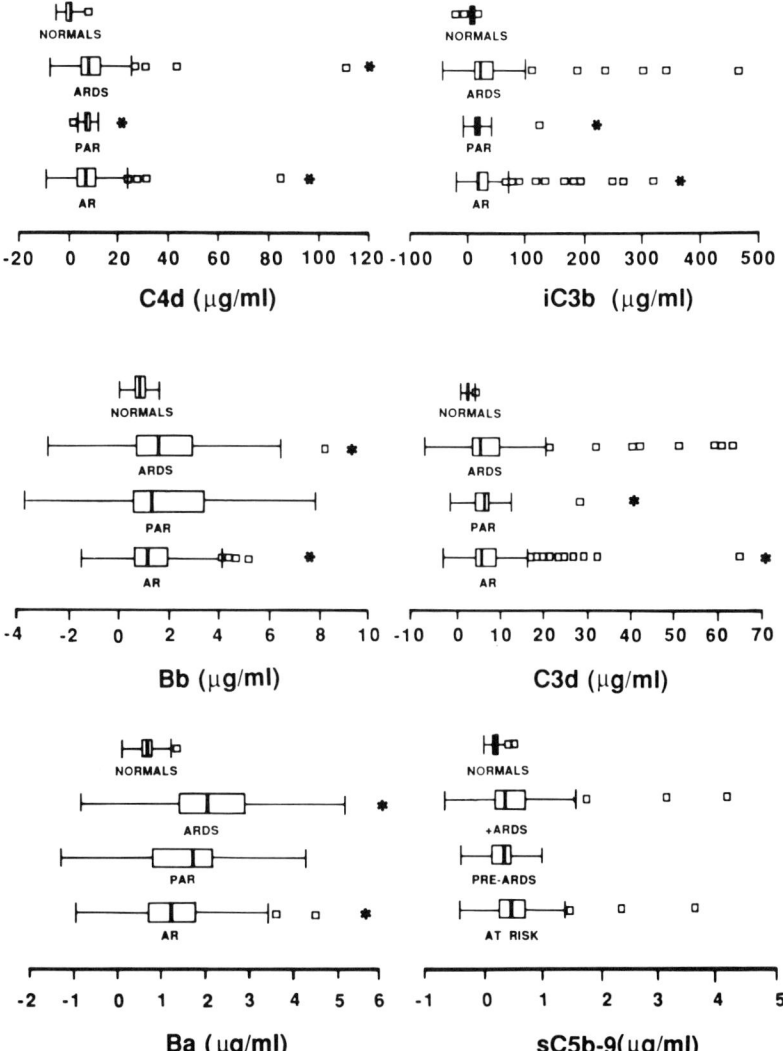

Figure 6.1 Complement fragment measurements in three groups of patients (ARDS; PAR, samples drawn from patients at risk for ARDS prior to the development of the syndrome; AR, samples drawn from patients at risk who never developed ARDS). * = $P < 0.05$ compared with normals. sC5b-9 levels are not significantly different from normals. (Reproduced with permission from Parsons and Giclas [26].)

els did not differentiate patients at risk from patients with ARDS and were not necessarily adequate markers for complement activation (Figure 6.1). However, 100% of patients with ARDS and 99% of those at risk had some evidence for complement activation (Table 6.1), indicating that complement was ubiquitously activated in critically ill patients [26].

ENDOTOXIN

The role of endotoxin in the pathogenesis of ARDS has been investigated since 1974, when the infusion of pseudomonas into sheep was first shown to produce increased pulmonary vascular permeability [27], a finding reproduced by an infusion of *E. coli* endotoxin in

Table 6.1 The complement cascade is activated in patients at risk for ARDS as well as patients with ARDS

	(+) Complement activation	(–) Complement activation
At risk ($n = 75$)	74	1
ARDS ($n = 23$)	23	0

sheep [28]. These observations suggested that endotoxin rather than, or perhaps in addition to, complement activation was the critical mediator in the development of acute lung injury.

Endotoxin refers to the lipopolysaccharide (LPS) component of the cell walls of Gram-negative bacteria and is comprised of three major components: an oligosaccharide chain referred to as the O antigen, which is species specific; a core polysaccharide; and the lipid A region which both anchors the complex to the cell and accounts for the majority of the biological activity. In contrast to the species specificity of the O antigen, the core–lipid A complex is virtually identical antigenically for all Gram-negative bacteria.

Endotoxin is associated with numerous direct and indirect effects that could potentially initiate and propagate both lung and systemic injuries. This chapter will focus on the effects of LPS which eventually lead to the accumulation of neutrophils within the alveolar space. This process includes the recruitment and retention of neutrophils within the lung, the migration of neutrophils through the vascular endothelium and the alveolar epithelium and the release of toxic mediators. Many of these processes will be elaborated upon in other chapters but since LPS may initiate the inflammatory cascade that results in lung injury they will be introduced here.

LPS AND NEUTROPHILS

The neutrophil has been implicated in the development of ARDS in humans since initial histopathological studies demonstrated sig-

nificant neutrophil accumulation within the lungs of both patients at risk of, and with, the established syndrome [29,30] (Chapter 4). Additional supporting evidence for the importance of the neutrophil has accumulated over time in both animal models and humans. Animal models of acute lung injury, including complement activation as described above, and phorbol myristate acetate [31], endotoxin [32,33] tumor necrosis factor (TNF) [34,35] or interleukin (IL)-1 [36,37] infusion, have been shown to be neutrophil dependent (Chapter 8). Bronchoalveolar lavage (BAL) fluid from patients with ARDS is characterized by the presence of large numbers of neutrophils [38], and radiolabeled autologous neutrophils intravenously infused into patients with ARDS accumulate in the lung [39]. Neutrophil influx into the lungs is associated with alterations in pulmonary gas exchange and capillary permeability [40]. In the light of these data the discussion of the role of endotoxin in acute lung injury will concentrate on a neutrophil dependent mechanism, although there may be other pathways via which acute lung injury occurs. For example, a small number of patients with profound neutropenia and sepsis have developed ARDS [41]. Although these cases do not exclude a pathogenic role for neutrophils in the majority of patients, they do suggest that there may be more than one way to produce acute lung injury.

Within the systemic circulation the major effects of endotoxin include complement activation and the priming and stimulation of both neutrophils and monocytes. Endotoxin itself activates both the classical and alternate pathways of complement [42] but this requires larger quantities of endotoxin than are thought to be available during the pathogenesis of an acute inflammatory response, such as may occur in ARDS [43]. The priming of neutrophils, which requires only nanogram concentrations of endotoxin, is a potentially important phenomenon in ARDS. Following exposure to a priming stimulus, which does not itself cause neutrophil activation, neutrophil responsiveness can be significantly enhanced (Chapter 8). Priming agents include endotoxin as well as TNF, interleukins, colony stimulating factors and PAF. These mediators prime for numerous neutrophil responses, including stimulated superoxide production, secretion and adherence. After priming, the neutrophils respond to any secondary stimulus in a similar fashion. The most commonly considered secondary stimuli are formyl methionyl leucine phenylalanine (FMLP) and complement fragments. The mechanism by which priming occurs remains obscure.

However, in the absence of plasma or serum the concentration of LPS which stimulates neutrophils [44] is orders of magnitude greater than has been measured in patients at risk of [45,46] or with ARDS [24]. The mechanism for the enhancement of the LPS effect by serum or plasma is not completely understood but is due at least in part to the acute phase protein LPS binding protein (LBP) [47,48]. LBP has been shown to enhance several LPS stimulated responses, including TNF release from macrophages [47], the upregulation of adherence glycoprotein CD18 on neutrophils [49] and neutrophil adherence [44]. Recently, the glycerophospatidylinositol-linked glycoprotein, CD14, was identified as a receptor for the LPS–LBP complexes [50]. CD14 is present on the surface of monocytes [50], neutrophils [51] and macrophages [52]. Endotoxin itself, as well as FMLP, can stimulate an increase in the expression of both CD14 and CD11b/CD18 on neutrophil surfaces [53]. CD14 also exists as a soluble form, sCD14, which is involved in endothelial and epithelial interactions with LPS by a mechanism which is still being determined [54].

Evidence from both whole animal and isolated, perfused lung studies indicates that neutrophil priming may be an important mechanism in the development of acute lung injury. In rabbits the infusion of either low dose endotoxin or FMLP produced no lung injury, while the concomitant infusion of the two produced a significant rise in permeability suggesting a synergistic mechanism [55]. When neutrophils were preincubated with endotoxin in plasma prior to the infusion into rabbits, neutrophil sequestration within the lung was enhanced, indicating that endotoxin exerted a primary effect on the neutrophil [56]. These results have been confirmed in an isolated perfused lung model [57].

The role of endotoxin induced neutrophil priming has been more difficult to evaluate in patients at risk for and with ARDS. Endotoxin is present in the blood in patients at risk for ARDS [45,46] and appears to be associated with the development of the syndrome, as shown in Figure 6.2 [47]. Whether or not circulating neutrophils from at risk patients and patients with established ARDS are activ-

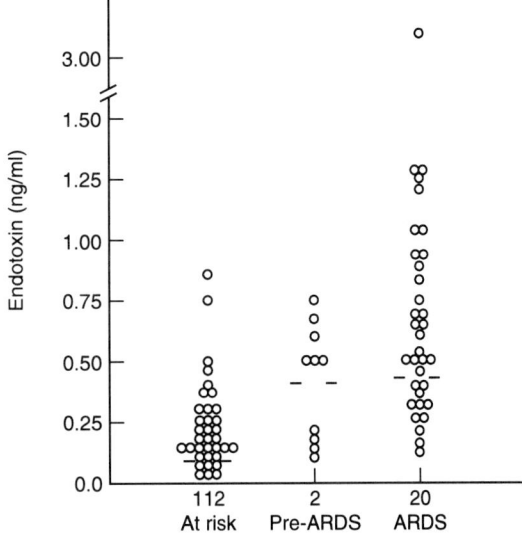

Figure 6.2 Endotoxin levels in three groups of patients: ARDS, pre-ARDS (samples obtained from patients at risk for ARDS prior to the development of the syndrome) and at risk (samples drawn from patients at risk who never developed the syndrome). Numbers displayed on the horizontal axis represent samples in which there was no detectable endotoxin. Endotoxin levels were significantly greater in both the ARDS and pre-ARDS group compared with the at risk group. (Reproduced with permission from Parsons *et al.* [24].)

ated remains an area of controversy. For example, in one study of neutrophils isolated from patients, chemotaxis, chemiluminescence and superoxide release were increased in neutrophils from ARDS patients compared with neutrophils from normal subjects, while adherence was decreased [58]; whereas in another oxidant production was increased but chemotaxis was decreased [59]. Numerous factors, including timing and site of sample collection, disease state definitions and variations in assay methodology, may in part explain the apparent discordance in the literature. In our own investigations we have found that circulating neutrophils from patients at risk for or with ARDS do not produce superoxide at baseline and are not primed for stimulated superoxide release [60]. We hypothesize that those neutrophils which have been primed or activated have been removed from the circulation, perhaps selectively retained within the lung, and not readily available for study.

During the development of acute lung injury neutrophils are recruited to and retained within the lung. This process is probably the result of a combination of the ability of the cell to deform and the adherence of neutrophils to capillary endothelium. As discussed in Chapter 8, the average diameter of a normal neutrophil is approximately 8 μm [61], while the diameter of the pulmonary capillary through which the neutrophil has to pass to transit the lung is 5.5–6 μm [62]. The importance of this size differential is further amplified by the relatively low perfusion pressure of the pulmonary capillary bed [63], such that even under baseline conditions the neutrophil has to deform to pass through the lung. LPS in the presence of serum induces actin assembly in neutrophils, increases cell stiffness and increases neutrophil retention within capillary-sized pore filters [64]. When the cells are treated with cytochalasin B, which prevents the assembly of actin, the changes in cell stiffness are also prevented, indicating that the two phenomena are clearly

related. LPS stimulates adherence by upregulating adhesion glycoproteins, such as CD11/18, on the neutrophil [47,65], as well as glycoproteins such as E-selectin on the endothelium [66].

To dissect out the relative contributions of the alterations in neutrophil morphology and adherence in neutrophil retention, Worthen and colleagues have performed a series of experiments blocking the two components. They have found that blocking CD14, a receptor on the cell surface for the binding of LPS, prevents LPS induced actin assembly, alterations in cell stiffness [64], adherence to endothelial cells [44] and retention within filters [64], whereas blocking CD18 with the monoclonal antibody 60.3 has no effect on neutrophil retention within filters even though it interferes with neutrophil adherence to surfaces [52]. These data suggest that LPS induced modulation of neutrophil deformability could be critical early in the process of neutrophil sequestration within the lung. Additional evidence to support this premise is provided by the observation that LPS stimulated alterations in neutrophil deformability [64] and adherence to endothelial cells [67] occur within minutes, whereas LPS stimulated upregulation of E-selectin occurs over 4–6 hours [66]. Thus, the effects of LPS on the endothelial cell may be more important in the prolongation of neutrophil retention within the lung rather than in the initiation of retention.

In addition to priming neutrophils and directly altering neutrophil morphology and function, LPS also stimulates neutrophils to release toxic mediators, including oxygen radicals, proteases, PAF and eicosanoids, all of which may contribute to lung injury. Oxygen radicals (Chapter 11) can directly injure the lung by inducing DNA strand breaks, lipid peroxidation and increasing the susceptibility of proteins to damage by proteases [68,69]. Oxidants can further propagate lung injury by inactivating antiproteases such as α_1-antitrypsin, stimulating the generation of thromboxane and leukotriene metabolites, and reacting with nitric oxide (NO) to form peroxynitrate [69,70]. The role of LPS in oxidant mediated injury is confounded by the ability of LPS to increase the production of antioxidants. Rats that are pretreated with endotoxin are protected from hyperoxic induced lung injury [71] and both direct and indirect evidence suggest that the protection is conferred at least in part by the increased production of antioxidants [72–74].

In patients with ARDS, oxidant–antioxidant balance is disturbed. As described above, circulating neutrophils from patients release increased quantities of oxygen metabolites. In addition, patients with ARDS have increased levels of xanthine oxidase [75], lipid peroxidation products [76] and inactivated antiproteases [69] in their blood, increased levels of inactivated antiproteases in their BAL fluid [77,78] and increased concentrations of hydrogen peroxide in their exhaled breath [79,80]. By contrast, they also have increased circulating levels of catalase [81], manganese superoxide dismutase [82] and ceruloplasmin [83] and decreased levels of glutathione [84] and vitamin E [85].

Proteases (Chapter 10) can also cause direct lung injury by damaging the constituents of the basement membrane [86] and endothelial cells [87]. The lung is rich in antiproteases, which theoretically could protect against protease mediated damage, but neutrophil dependent, protease mediated injury occurs despite the presence of antiproteases [87,88]. At least two mechanisms contribute to this apparent dichotomy. *In vitro*, neutrophils can produce focal proteolysis by excluding antiproteases from the pericellular area [88] and neutrophil elastase can decrease the functional activity of α_1-antitrypsin by binding and cleaving it. Both of these effects could occur in patients with ARDS. Neutrophil elastase levels are increased in the BAL fluid of patients [89,90] and α_1-antitrypsin activity is decreased both by oxidation and by neutrophil elastase interaction [91].

LPS also stimulates the release of both PAF and eicosanoids from neutrophils as well as other cells. PAF has numerous actions which could contribute to lung injury, including the stimulation of platelet aggregation, priming and activating neutrophils, induction of pulmonary vasoconstriction and, possibly, direct injury to endothelial cells [92]. Following the infusion of endotoxin in animals, PAF levels are increased [92] and the administration of PAF inhibitors decreases endotoxin induced alterations in pulmonary hemodynamics and permeability [92,93] in some animal models. Similarly, eicosanoids could contribute to lung injury by a number of mechanisms, including the alteration of the hypoxic vasoconstriction response (prostaglandin (PG)I_2), recruitment of neutrophils to the lung (leukotriene (LT)B_4 and thromboxane (Tx)A_2), and platelet aggregation (TxA_2). In animal models, endotoxin stimulates the release of eicosanoids [94], although studies using selective inhibitors have not always confirmed a direct relationship between eicosanoid production and lung injury [95].

There is some evidence that eicosanoids and PAF are present in patients with ARDS. LTD_4 [94,96], LTC_4 [94], are present in BAL from ARDS patients and persistent increases in urinary LTE_4 levels in ARDS patients are associated with persistent abnormalities in gas exchange and compliance [97]. PAF was found by a single group of investigators in BAL of patients with ARDS [98]. The lavage studies, although apparently convincing, are confounded by variable rates of eicosanoid clearance and metabolism.

Circulating levels of thromboxane and 6-keto prostaglandin $F_{1\alpha}$ are increased in some patients both at risk for and with ARDS [99] and neutrophil leukotriene production was found to be decreased in a single study of patients who had sustained major trauma [100]. Measurements of circulating PAF are technically difficult. In a single study using indirect measurements, PAF appeared to be increased in patients with ARDS [101], although those findings remain to be confirmed.

LPS AND MONOCYTES

Whether monocytes are important in the development of lung injury in humans is not known. Although they are usually considered to be immunomodulatory, monocytes actually share many characteristics of neutrophils in their responsivity to LPS and could, potentially contribute to injury. Like neutrophils, monocytes can be primed for oxidant production by LPS as well as other mediators [102]. Also, LPS stimulates actin assembly in monocytes, decreases cell deformability [52], increases adherence [103], and increases monocyte retention within the lung [104]. In contrast to neutrophils, however, monocyte retention is dependent on CD18 [104]. Further investigation of the potential roles of monocytes in inflammatory processes may provide clues to the development of acute lung injury in those models that appear to be neutrophil independent, such as patients with profound neutropenia and ARDS.

LPS AND THE ENDOTHELIUM

In addition to upregulating adherence glycoproteins, LPS has other effects on the endothelium that could also contribute to lung injury. In high concentrations, LPS can directly injure endothelial cells by an oxidant dependent mechanism [105]. Interactions between LPS and endothelial cells can also potentiate lung injury. LPS stimulates the release of IL-8 and other chemokines from endothelial cells [52,54,106.]. As will be described more extensively in other chapters, IL-8 is both a chemotactic and activating factor for neutrophils [107] (Chapter 7). It is produced by many cell types other than endothelial cells, including monocytes and macrophages, and it is found in large quantities within the lung. The relative contribution of these other cell types to the total produc-

tion of IL-8 is probably much greater than the contribution of the endothelial cell, but local production of IL-8 by endothelial cells could contribute to the regulation of lung injury as IL-8 may inhibit the adhesion of neutrophils to activated endothelium [106]. LPS also stimulates endothelial cells to release eicosanoids, which could further contribute to lung damage by mechanisms discussed above.

LPS IN THE ALVEOLAR SPACE

The intra-alveolar effects of LPS may contribute significantly to acute lung injury. In animal models, air space [108] as well as the intravascular administration of LPS induces neutrophil accumulation within the lung. A likely target for both modes of injury is the alveolar macrophage. It is easy to understand how the intra-alveolar administration of LPS can directly affect macrophages. As described for neutrophils and monocytes, LPS can prime alveolar macrophages for the production of toxic metabolites [52], which could serve to propagate injury. LPS also directly stimulates macrophages to release other mediators, including colony stimulating factors, PAF and TNF. Each of these can propagate injury by numerous actions, including the priming of neutrophils. The effects of TNF will be elaborated on in subsequent chapters (Chapters 7, 8) but it is important to recognize that it can stimulate macrophages to release IL-8, IL-1, prostaglandin E_2 [42] and NO [52], all of which could contribute to lung injury. Concomitantly, however, LPS also stimulates macrophages to release interferons, which may ameliorate the acute inflammatory response [52]. The intravascular administration of LPS can also cause macrophage activation [109,110], although it is not clear that the LPS itself reaches the alveolar space. In that situation it is likely that the effect of LPS is actually secondary and the result of mediators released following LPS stimulation of cells, including neutrophils, monocytes and endothelium, which extrude into the alveolus.

ENDOTOXIN TOLERANCE

The effects of LPS described above virtually all lead to the development and propagation of injury but LPS can also induce tolerance. Tolerance in this context is used to describe the situation that occurs when exposure to a sublethal dose of LPS is associated with a relative hyporesponsiveness to subsequent exposure. Two forms or phases of tolerance to endotoxin have been described. The first occurs over weeks, is associated with antibody production, and confers protection against specific O antigens [111–113]. The phase of endotoxin tolerance that is perhaps more relevant to the development of acute lung injury occurs within hours of the administration of a sublethal dose of endotoxin and is characterized by hyporesponsiveness to any subsequent exposure [111,114]. In animal models and *in vitro*, the initial response to the sublethal dose of endotoxin includes an increase in both TNF and IL-1 levels and cross-tolerance has been demonstrated for endotoxin and these two cytokines [114–117]. The hyporesponsiveness to subsequent LPS is characterized by decreased production of TNF, IL-1 and IL-6 by alveolar macrophages [113,114]. The exact mechanism by which tolerance is conferred is not known and data to support multiple mechanisms, including post-transcriptional [111,114] and post-translational [118] defects as well as a reduction in GTPase activity [119], exist.

The extent to which endotoxin tolerance could modulate the development of acute lung injury in humans is difficult to assess, but at least four studies suggest that the phenomenon may occur in humans. Isolated peripheral blood monocytes from patients with either sepsis syndrome or noninfectious shock have varying cytokine production. Thus, LPS stimulated monocytes from septic patients release less IL-1α, IL-1β, IL-6 and TNF, a finding more pronounced in patients with Gram-negative rather than Gram-positive infections. In patients with noninfectious shock only IL-1α is decreased [120]. Isolated monocytes from two children with *Haemophilus influenzae* meningitis displayed diminished LPS stimulated IL-1 release [114,121]. Alveolar macrophages isolated from patients with sepsis have been shown to have decreased TNF production in response to LPS [122] and CD14 expression is decreased on circulating monocytes from patients with sepsis [123]. McCall and colleagues [114] have recently shown that neutrophils from septic patients demonstrate apparent tolerance to endotoxin. They found that circulating neutrophils from patients with the sepsis syndrome did not increase the production of IL-1β mRNA in response to LPS, although the response to *Staphylococcus aureus* was normal. This hyporesponsiveness occurred in neutrophils from patients with Gram-positive and fungal infections as well as Gram-negative infections. Interestingly, the CD14 expression on the neutrophils was normal.

SOURCES OF ENDOTOXIN

Endotoxin therefore has the potential to serve in a pivotal role in the development of acute lung injury. The source of such endotoxin may be Gram-negative sepsis, one of the major risk factors for the development of ARDS. Even though circulating endotoxin is not demonstrable in all patients with ARDS, it is reasonable to assume that it could be present at least transiently in small amounts. Other categories of patients who develop ARDS present a dilemma. Clearly, there are those without Gram-negative infections who have measurable circulating endotoxin [24]. Such patients have provoked investigation of hypotheses such as bacterial translocation to account for the presence of endotoxin in the circulation in the absence of identifiable infection. The translocation theory suggests that bacteria from the gastrointestinal tract migrate through the mucosa to gain access to either the lymphatic system or the blood-stream. This phenomenon has been demonstrated in numerous animal models with insults, including burns, shock, following chemotherapy, and abdominal infection [124–127], and can apparently be amplified by factors including parenteral nutrition, immunosuppression, and starvation [124,128]. These models mimic the clinical characteristics of many patients at risk of ARDS, but demonstrating that bacterial trans-location occurs in humans has proved difficult. In patients who have sustained severe burns, intestinal permeability is increased and correlates with septic complications [129], and there are studies that suggest the preservation of the integrity of the gastrointestinal mucosa results in fewer infectious complications in trauma [124]. Multiple studies have been performed to determine whether alterations in gastrointestinal bacterial flora decrease the incidence of nosocomial infection, but with conflicting results. In particular, none would be able to distinguish between a decrease in infectious complications due to decreased bacterial translocation, or decreased aspiration of bacteria. To try to isolate the contribution of bacterial translocation to the development of multiple organ failure a study was performed in patients who had sustained major trauma. Catheters were inserted into the portal veins of 20 patients identified as being at high risk of developing ARDS and who required emergency laparotomy after trauma [130]. Serial blood samples were obtained, starting at the time of catheter placement, and analyzed for endotoxin. At no point was endotoxin detected in either portal or systemic blood, although six of the patients ultimately developed multiple organ failure. In another study intestinal permeability was measured in patients following trauma and found to be increased [131]. Serial endotoxin measurements in the same patients were negative both during and after the time the permeability measurements were performed. Further studies are needed to better characterize the source of endotoxin in patients with ARDS.

SUMMARY

The pathogenesis of ARDS remains complex. Since it was described originally, we have made tremendous advances, not only in our understanding of the pathogenesis of inflammation but in our appreciation that there is probably a spectrum of clinical disease that affects not only the lung but virtually every other organ. What remains poorly understood is how the inflammatory process is different in those patients with (for example) severe sepsis who develop ARDS, compared with those with apparently equally severe sepsis who are spared. This may in part be because all the possible mediators and cellular interactions that are involved in inflammation have not yet been investigated and the complexity of the process is confounded by factors such as tolerance. In this chapter, this complexity has been exemplified by endotoxin. It is likely that endotoxin is involved in the development of acute lung injury, as it can not only stimulate inflammatory cells to release mediators that both cause and propagate injury but also stimulates the retention of inflammatory cells within the lung, and may also cause injury directly. However, as described, there are both animal models of acute lung injury which do not involve LPS and there are patients with ARDS without either measurable endotoxin or an obvious source of endotoxin. The role of complement activation in ARDS is similarly complex. Although complement activation alone does not itself cause lung injury, as it is ubiquitous in critically ill patients, it would be a mistake to dismiss its potential to be involved.

REFERENCES

1. Kaplow, L. and Goffinet, J. (1968) Profound neutropenia during the early phase of dialysis. *JAMA*, **203**, 1135–7.
2. Craddock, P.R., Fehr, J., Brigham, K. *et al.* (1977) Complement and leukocyte-mediated pulmonary dysfunction in hemodialysis. *N. Engl. J. Med.*, **296**, 769–74.
3. Craddock, P.R., Fehr, J., Dalmasso, A. *et al.* (1977) Hemodialysis leukopenia: pulmonary vascular leukostasis resulting from complement activation by dialyzer cellophane membrane. *J. Clin. Invest.*, **59**, 879–88.
4. Craddock, P.R., Hammerschmidt, D.E., White, J.G. *et al.* (1977) Complement (C5a)-induced granulocyte aggregation in-vitro: a possible mechanism of complement-mediated leukostasis and leukopenia. *J. Clin. Invest.*, **60**, 260–4.
5. Till, G.O. Johnson, K.J. and Kunkel, R. (1982) Intravascular activation of complement and acute lung injury: dependency on neutrophils and toxic oxygen metabolites. *J. Clin. Invest.*, **69**, 1126–35.
6. Henson, P.M., Larsen, G.L., Webster, R.O. *et al.* (1982) Pulmonary microvascular alterations and injury induced by complement fragments: synergistic effect of complement activation, neutrophil sequestration and prostaglandins. *Ann. N. Y. Acad. Sci.*, **348**, 287–300.
7. Webster, R.O., Larsen, G.L., Mitchell, B.C. *et al.* (1982) Absence of inflammatory lung injury in rabbits challenged intravascularly with complement-derived chemotactic factors. *Am. Rev. Respir. Dis.*, **125**, 335–409.
8. Hugli, T. (1986) Biochemistry and biology of anaphylotoxins. *Complement*, **3**, 111–27.
9. Abbas, A., Lichtman, A. and Pober, J.S. (1991) The complement system, in *Cellular and Molecular Immunology* (ed. A.K. Abbas), W.B. Saunders, Philadelphia, pp. 259–82.
10. Perlmutter, D., Strunk, R. and Colten, H. (1992) Complement, in *The Lung: Scientific Foundations* (eds R. Crystal and J.B. West), Raven Press, New York, pp. 511–22.
11. Warren, J., Johnson, K. and Ward, P. (1992) Immunoglobulin- and complement-mediated immune injury, in *Lung Injury* (eds R. Crystal and J.B. West), Raven Press, New York, pp. 179–86.
12. Muller-Eberhard, H. (1984) The membrane attack complex. Springer Seminars. *Immunopathology*, **7**, 93–118.
13. Hosea, S., Brown, E., Hammer, C. and Frank, M. (1980) Role of complement activation in a model of adult respiratory distress syndrome. *J. Clin. Invest.*, **66**, 375–82.
14. Gelfand, J., Donelan, M., Hawiger, A. and Burke, J. (1982) Alternative complement pathway activation increases mortality in a model of burn injury in mice. *J. Clin. Invest.*, **70**, 1170–6.
15. Parrish, D., Mitchell, B., Henson, P.M. and Larsen, G. (1984) Pulmonary response of fifth component of complement-sufficient and deficient mice to hyperoxia. *J. Clin. Invest.*, **74**, 956–65.
16. Larsen, G., Mitchell, B., Harper, T. and Henson, P.M. (1982) The pulmonary response of C5 sufficient and deficient mice to *Pseudomonas aeruginosa*. *Am. Rev. Respir. Dis.*, **126**, 306–11.
17. Hagen, D.H., Stevens, J.H., Satoh, P.S. *et al.* (1989) Complement levels in septic primates treated with anti-C5a antibodies. *J. Surg. Res.*, **46**, 195–9.
18. Stevens, J., O'Hanley, P.T., Shapiro, J., *et al.* (1986) Effects of anti-C5a antibodies of the adult respiratory distress syndrome in septic primates. *J. Clin. Invest.*, **77**, 1812–6.
19. Rabinovic, R., Yeh, C., Hillegass, L. *et al.* (1992) Role of complement in endotoxin/platelet activity factor-induced lung injury. *J. Immunol.*, **149**, 1744–50.
20. Jacob, H., Craddock, P.R., Hammerschmidt, D. and Moldow, C. (1980) Complement-induced granulocyte aggregation – an unsuspected mechanism of disease. *N. Engl. J. Med.*, **362**, 789–94.
21. Hammerschmidt, D., Weaver, L., Hudson, L. *et al.* (1980) Association of complement activation and elevated plasma C5a with adult respiratory distress syndrome: pathophysiological relevance and possible prognostic value. *Lancet*, **i**, 947–9.
22. Duchteau, J., Haas, M., Schreyen, H. *et al.* (1984) Complement activation in patients at risk of developing the adult respiratory distress syndrome. *Am. Rev. Respir. Dis.* **130**, 1058–64.
23. Weinberg, P.F., Matthay, M.A., Webster, R.O. *et al.* (1984) Biologically active products of complement and acute lung injury in patients

with the sepsis syndrome. *Am. Rev. Respir. Dis.*, **130**, 791–6.

24. Parsons, P.E., Worthen, G., Moore, E. *et al.* (1989) The association of circulating endotoxin with the development of the adult respiratory distress syndrome. *Am. Rev. Respir. Dis.*, **140**, 294–301.

25. Langlois, P.F., and Gawryl, M.S. (1988) Accentuated formation of the terminal C5b-9 complement complex in patient plasma precedes development of the adult respiratory distress syndrome. *Am. Rev. Respir. Dis.*, **138**, 368–75.

26. Parsons, P.E., and Giclas, P.C. (1990) The terminal complement complex (sC5b-9) is not specifically associated with the development of the adult respiratory distress syndrome. *Am. Rev. Respir. Dis.*, **141**, 98–103.

27. Brigham, K., Woolverton, W., Glake, L. *et al.* (1974) Increased sheep lung vascular permeability caused by pseudomonas bacteremia. *J. Clin. Invest.*, **54**, 792–804.

28. Brigham, K., Bowers, R. and Haynes, J. (1979) Increased sheep lung vascular permeability caused by *E. coli* endotoxin. *Circulation*, **45**, 292–7.

29. Bachofen, M. and Weibel, E. (1982) Structural alterations of lung parenchyma in the adult respiratory distress syndrome. *Clin. Chest Med.*, **3**, 35–42.

30. Bachofen, M. and Weibel, E. (1977) Alterations of the gas exchange apparatus in adult respiratory insufficiency associated with septicemia. *Am. Rev. Respir. Dis.*, **116**, 589–96.

31. Shasby, D., Vanbenthuysen, K., Tate, R. *et al.* (1982) Granulocytes mediate acute edematous lung injury in rabbits and isolated rat lungs perfused with phorbol myristate acetate: role of oxygen radicals. *Am. Rev. Respir. Dis.*, **125**, 443–7.

32. Brigham, K. and Meyrick, B. (1986) State of the art: endotoxin and lung injury. *Am. Rev. Respir. Dis.*, **133**, 913–27.

33. Heflin, A. and Brigham, K. (1981) Prevention by granulocyte depletion of increased vascular permeability of sheep lung following endotoxemia. *J. Clin. Invest.*, **68**, 1253–60.

34. Beutler, B. and Cerami, A. (1986) Cachectin and tumor necrosis factor as two sides of the same biologic coin. *Nature*, **320**, 584–8.

35. Johnson, J., Brigham, K., Jesmok, G. and Meyrick, B. (1991) Morphologic changes in lungs of anesthetized sheep following infusion of recombinant tumor necrosis factor alpha. *Am. Rev. Respir. Dis.*, **144**, 179–86.

36. Dinarello, C. (1991) Interleukin-1 and interleukin-1 antagonist. *Blood*, **77**, 1627–31.

37. Fisher, E., Marano, M., Barber, A. *et al.* (1991) A comparison between the effects of interleukin-1-alpha administration and sublethal endotoxemia in primates. *Am. J. Physiol.*, **26**, R442–52.

38. Parsons, P.E., Fowler, A.A., Hyers, T. and Henson, P.M. (1985) Chemotactic activity in bronchoalveolar lavage fluid from patients with adult respiratory distress syndrome. *Am. Rev. Respir. Dis.*, **132**, 490–3.

39. Warshawski, F., Sibbald, W., Driedger, A. and Cheung, H. (1986) Abnormal neutrophil – pulmonary interaction in the adult respiratory distress syndrome: qualitative and quantitative assessment of pulmonary–neutrophil kinetics in humans with *in vivo* indium-111 neutrophil scintigraphy. *Am. Rev. Respir. Dis.*, **133**, 792–804.

40. Weiland, J., Davis, W., Holter, J. *et al.* (1986) Lung neutrophils in the adult respiratory distress syndrome. *Am. Rev. Respir. Dis.*, **137**, 218–25.

41. Ogribene, F., Martin, S., Parker, M. *et al.* (1986) ARDS in patients with severe neutropenia. *N. Engl. J. Med.*, **315**, 547–51.

42. Morrison, D. and Ryan, J. (1987) Endotoxin and disease mechanisms. *Annu. Rev. Med.*, **38**, 417–32.

43. Morrison, D. and Ulevitch, R. (1978) The effects of bacterial endotoxin on host mediation systems. *Am. Rev. Respir. Dis.*, **93**, 527–617.

44. Worthen, G., Avdi, N., Vukajlovich, S. and Tobias, P. (1993) Neutrophil adherence induced by lipopolysaccharide. *J. Clin. Invest.*, **90**, 2526–35.

45. Brandtzaeg, P., Kierulf, P., Gaustad, P. *et al.* (1989) Plasma endotoxin as a predictor of multiple organ failure and death in meningococcal disease. *J. Infect. Dis.*, **159**, 195–204.

46. Donner, R.L., Elin, R.J., Hossein, S.M. *et al.* (1991) Endotoxin in human septic shock. *Chest*, **99**, 169–75.

47. Tobias, P., Soldau, K. and Ulevitch, R. (1986) Isolation of a lipopolysaccharide-binding acute phase reactant from rabbit serum. *J. Exp. Med.*, **164**, 777–93.

48. Schumann, R., Leony, S., Flaggs, G. *et al.* (1990) Structure and function of lipopolysac-

charide binding protein. *Science*, **249**, 1429–31.

49. Wright, S., Ramos, R., Hermanowski-Vasatka, A. *et al.* (1991) Activation of the adhesive capacity of CR3 on neutrophils by endotoxin: dependence on lipopolysaccharide-binding protein and CD14. *J. Exp. Med.*, **173**, 1281–6.

50. Wright, S.D., Ramos, R.A., Tobias, P.S. *et al.* (1990) CD14 a receptor for complexes of lipopolysaccharide (LPS) and LBP-binding protein. *Science*, **249**, 1431–3.

51. Ulevitch, R. (1993) Recognition of bacterial endotoxins by receptor-dependant mechanisms. *Adv. Immunol.*, **53**, 267–89.

52. Henson, P.M., Doherty, D.E., Riches, D.W.H. *et al.* (1994) LPS and cytokines, in *Endotoxin and the Lung* (ed. K.L. Brigham), Marcel Dekker, New York, pp. 267–304.

53. Weingarten, R., Sklar, L., Mathison, J. *et al.* (1993) Interaction of lipopolysaccharide with neutrophils in blood via CD14. *J. Leukoc. Biol.*, **53**, 518–24.

54. Pujin, J., Schurer-Maly, C., Leturcq, D. *et al.* (1993) Lipopolysaccharide activation of human endothelial and epithelial cells is mediated by lipopolysaccharide-binding protein and soluble CD14. *Proc. Natl Acad. Sci. USA*, **90**, 2744–8.

55. Worthen, G., Hasslet, C., Rees, A. *et al.* (1987) Neutrophil-mediated pulmonary vascular injury. Synergistic effect of trace amounts of lipopolysaccharide and neutrophil stimuli on vascular permeability and neutrophil sequestration within the lung. *Am. Rev. Respir. Dis.*, **136**, 19–28.

56. Hasslet, C., Worthen, G., Giclas, P. *et al.* (1987) The pulmonary vascular sequestration of neutrophils in endotoxemia is initiated by an effect of endotoxin on the neutrophil in the rabbits. *Am. Rev. Respir. Dis.*, **136**, 9–18.

57. Anderson, B., Poggetti, R., Shanley, P. *et al.* (1991) Primed neutrophils injure rat lung through a platelet-activating factor-dependent mechanism. *J. Surg. Res.*, **50**, 510–4.

58. Zimmerman, G., Renzetti, A. and Hill, H. (1983) Functional and metabolic activity of granulocytes from patients with ARDS. *Am. Rev. Respir. Dis.*, **127**, 290–300.

59. Fowler, A.A., Fisher, B., Center, R. and Carchman, R. (1983) Development of ARDS, progressive alteration of neutrophil chemotactic and secretory processes. *Am. J. Pathol.*, **116**, 427–35.

60. Parsons, P.E., Worthen, G.S., Moore, F.A. *et al.* (1990) Activity levels of circulating neutrophils in acute lung injury. *Am. Rev. Respir. Dis.*, A359.

61. Schmid-Shonbein, G., Shih, Y. and Chien, S. (1985) Morphometry of human leukocytes. *Blood*, **56**, 866–71.

62. Guntheroth, W., Lachter, D. and Kawaburi, I. (1982) Pulmonary microcirculation: tubules rather than sheet and post. *J. Appl. Physiol.*, **53**, 510–5.

63. Parsons, P.E., Worthen, G. and Henson, P.M. (1991) Injury from inflammatory cells, in *The Lung: Scientific Foundations* (eds. R. Crystal and J.B. West), Raven Press, New York, pp. 1981–92.

64. Erzurum, S., Downey, G., Schwab, B. *et al.* (1992) Cell mechanics of neutrophils: induction of stiffness and actin by lipopolysaccharide. *J. Immunol.*, **149**, 154–62.

65. Tonnesen, M.G., Anderson, D.C., Springer, T.A. *et al.* (1989) Adherence of neutrophils to cultured human microvascular endothelial cells. Stimulation by chemotactic peptides and lipid mediators and dependence upon the Mac-1, LFA-1, p150, 95 glycoprotein family. *J. Clin. Invest.*, **83**, 637–46.

66. Bevilacqua, M. and Nelson, R. (1993) Selectins. *Clin. Invest.*, **91**, 379–87.

67. Hoover, R., Briggs, R. and Karnovsky, M. (1978) The adhesive interaction between polymorphonuclear leukocytes and endothelial cells *in-vitro*. *Cell*, **14**, 427–30.

68. Davies, K. and Goldberg, A. (1987) Proteins damaged by oxygen radicals are rapidly degraded in extracts of red blood cells. *J. Biol. Chem.*, **262**, 8227–34.

69. Repine, J.E. and Parsons, P.E. (1994) Oxidant-antioxidant balance in endotoxin induced oxidative injury and tolerance to oxidative injury, in *Endotoxin and the Lung*, (ed. K.L. Brigham), Marcel Dekker, New York, pp. 207–28.

70. Beckman, J. and Crow, J. (1993) Pathogenic implications of nitric oxide, superoxide and peri-oxynitrate formation. *Biochem. Soc. Trans.*, **21**, 330–4.

71. Frank, L., Yam, J., Roberts, R. (1978) The role of endotoxin in protection of adult rats from oxygen-induced lung injury. *J. Clin. Invest.*, **61**, 269–75.

72. Clerch, L. and Massaro, D. (1993) Tolerance of

rats to hyperoxia: lung antioxidant enzyme gene expression. *J. Clin. Invest.*, **91**, 499–508.

73. Frank, L., Summerville, J. and Massaro, D. (1980) Protection from oxygen toxicity with endotoxin: role of the endogenous antioxidant enzymes of the lung. *J. Clin. Invest.*, **65**, 1104–10.

74. Frank, L. (1982) Protection from pulmonary oxygen toxicity by pre exposure of rats to hypoxia: role of the lung anti-oxidant system. *J. Appl. Physiol.*, **53**, 475–82.

75. Grum, C., Ragsdale, R., Ketai, L. and Simon, R. (1987) Plasma xanthine oxidase activity in patients with ARDS. *J. Crit. Care*, **2**, 22–6.

76. Deby, C. (1989) Differences in tocopherol – lipid ratios in ARDS and non-ARDS patients. *Intensive Care Med.*, **15**, 877–93.

77. Lee, C., Fein, A., Lippman, M. *et al.* (1981) Elastolytic activity in pulmonary lavage fluid from patients with adult respiratory distress syndrome. *N. Engl. J. Med.*, **304**, 192–6.

78. Cochrane, C., Spragg, R., Revak, S. *et al.* (1983) The presence of neutrophil elastase and evidence of oxidation activity in bronchoalveolar lavage fluid of patients with adult respiratory distress syndrome. *Am. Rev. Respir. Dis.* **127**, 25–7.

79. Baldwin, S., Simon, R., Grum, C. *et al.* (1986) Oxidant activity in expired breath of patients with adult respiratory distress syndrome. *Lancet*, **i**, 11–4.

80. Sznajder, J., Fraiman, A., Hall, J. *et al.* (1989) Increased hydrogen peroxide in the expired breath of patients with acute hypoxemic respiratory failure. *Chest*, **96**, 606–12.

81. Leff, J., Parsons, P., Day, C.E. *et al.* (1992) Increased hydrogen peroxide scavenging and catalase activity in serum from septic patients who subsequently develop ARDS. *Am. Rev. Respir. Dis.*, **146**, 985–9.

82. Leff, J., Parsons, P., Day, C. *et al.* (1993) Serum antioxidants as predictors of adult respiratory distress syndrome. *Lancet*, **341**, 777–80.

83. Krsek-Staples, J., Kew, R. Webster, R. (1992) Ceruloplasmin and transferrin levels are altered in serum and bronchoalveolar lavage fluid of patients with adult respiratory distress syndrome. *Am. Rev. Respir. Dis.*, **145**, 1009–15.

84. Bernard, G. (1991) *N*-acetylcysteine in experimental and clinical acute lung injury. *Am. J. Med.*, **91**, 54S–59S.

85. Richard, C., Lemonnier, F., Thibault, M. and Auzepy, P. (1990) Vitamin E deficiency and lipoperoxidation during adult respiratory distress syndrome. *Crit. Care Med.*, **18**, 4–9.

86. Janoff, A. and Zelig, J. (1968) Vascular injury and lysis of basement membrane in-vitro by neutral proteases of human leukocytes. *Science*, **161**, 702–6.

87. Smedley, L., Tonneson, M.G., Sandhaus, R. *et al.* (1986) Neutrophil-mediated injury to endothelial cells: enhancement by LPS and the essential role of neutrophil elastase. *J. Clin. Invest.*, **17**, 1233–43.

88. Campbell, E. and Campbell, M. (1988) Pericellular proteolysis by substrate opsonization. *J. Cell Biol.*, **106**, 667–76.

89. Wewers, M.D., Herzyk, D.J. and Gadek, J.E. (1988) Alveolar fluid neutrophil elastase activity in the adult respiratory distress syndrome is complexed to alpha-2 macroglobulin. *J. Clin. Invest.*, **82**, 1260–7.

90. McGuire, W., Spragg, R., Cohen, A. and Cochrane, C. (1982) Studies on the pathogenesis of the adult respiratory distress syndrome. *J. Clin. Invest.*, **69**, 543–53.

91. Cochrane, C., Spragg, R. and Revak, S. (1983) Pathogenesis of the adult respiratory distress syndrome. Evidence of oxidant activity in bronchoalveolar lavage fluid. *J. Clin. Invest.*, **71**, 754–61.

92. Chang, S.W., Fedderson, C.O., Henson, P.M. and Voelkel, N.F. (1987) Platelet activating factor mediates hemodynamic changes and lung injury in endotoxin-treated rats. *J. Clin. Invest.*, **79**, 1498–1509.

93. Christmar, B.W., Lefferts, P.L., Blair, I.A. and Snapper, J.R. (1990) Effect of platelet-activating factor receptor antagonism on endotoxin-induced lung dysfunction in awake sheep. *Am. Rev. Respir. Dis.*, **142**, 1272–8.

94. Stephenson, A.H., Lonigro, A.J., Hyers, T.M. *et al.* (1988) Increased concentrations of leukotrienes in bronchoalveolar lavage fluid of patients with ARDS or at risk for ARDS. *Am. Rev. Respir. Dis.*, **138**, 714–9.

95. Chang, S.W., Westcott, J.Y., Pickett, W.C. *et al.* (1989) Endotoxin-induced lung injury in rats: role of eicosinoids. *J. Appl. Physiol.*, **66**, 2407–18.

96. Matthay, M.A., Eschenbacher, W.L. and Goetzl, E.J. (1984) Elevated concentrations of leukotriene D_4 in pulmonary edema fluid of patients with the adult respiratory distress syndrome. *J. Clin. Immunol.*, **4**, 479–83.

97. Bernard, G.R., Korley, V., Chee, P. *et al.* (1991) Persistent generation of peptide leukotrienes in patients with adult respiratory distress syndrome. *Clin. Exp. Pharm. Physiol.*, **19**, 509–15.

98. Matasumoto, K., Taki, F. Kondoh, Y. *et al.* (1992) Platelet activating factor in broncho-alveolar lavage of patients with the adult respiratory distress syndrome. *Clin. Exp. Pharm. Physiol.*, **19**, 509–15.

99. Deby-Dupontp, G., Braun, M., Lamy, M. *et al.* (1987) Thromboxane and prostacyclin release in adult respiratory distress syndrome. *Intensive Care Med.*, **13**, 167–74.

100. Schonfeld, W., Knoller, J., Joka, T. *et al.* (1992) Leukotriene generation in patients with multiple injuries. *J. Trauma*, **33**, 799–806.

101. Fink, A., Gera, D., Zung, A. *et al.* (1990) Adult respiratory distress syndrome: role of leukotriene C_4 and platelet activating factors. *Crit. Care Med.*, **18**, 905–10.

102. Pabst, M., Hedegaard, H. and Johnston, R. (1982) Cultured human monocytes require exposure to bacterial products to maintain an optimal oxygen radical response. *J. Immunol.*, **128**, 123–8.

103. Doherty, D., Zagarella, L., Henson, P.M. and Worthen, G. (1989) Lipopolysaccharide stimulates monocyte adherence by effects on both the monocyte and the endothelial cell. *J. Immunol.*, **143**, 3673–9.

104. Doherty, D. and Worthen, G. (1991) Lipopolysaccharide-induced monocyte lung retention adhesion complex and cell stiffness. *Am. Rev. Respir. Dis.*, **143**, A583.

105. Brigham, K., Meyrick, B., Berry, L. *et al.* (1979) Antioxidants protect cultured bovine lung endothelial cells from injury by endotoxin. *Circ. Res.*, **45**, 291–7.

106. Gimbrone, M., Obin, M., Brock, A. *et al.* (1989) Endothelial interleukin-8: a novel inhibitor of leukocyte-endothelial interactions. *Science*, **246**, 1601–3.

107. Kuntel, S., Standiford, T., Kasahara, K. and Strieter, R. (1991) Interleukin-8 (IL-8): the major neutrophil chemotactic factor in the lung. *Exp. Lung Res.*, **17**, 17–23.

108. Rinaldo, J., Moore, S., Lee, R. and Dauber, J. (1987) Shifts in subfraction of alveolar macrophages *in vivo* during endotoxin-induced alveolitis. *J. Leukoc. Biol.*, **42**, 230–8.

109. Chang, J. and Lesser, M. (1984) Quantitation of leukocytes in bronchoalveolar lavage samples from rats after intravascular injection of endotoxin. *Am. Rev. Respir. Dis.*, **129**, 72–5.

110. Cardozo, C., Edelman, J. Jagirdar, J. and Lesser, M. (1991) Lipopolysaccharide-induced pulmonary vascular sequestration of polymorphonuclear leukocytes is complement independent. *Am. Rev. Respir. Dis.*, **144**, 173–8.

111. Mathison, J., Virca, G., Wolfson, E. *et al.* (1990) Adaptation to bacterial lipopolysaccharide controls lipopolysaccharide-induced tumor necrosis factor production in rabbit macrophages. *J. Clin. Invest.*, **85**, 1108–18.

112. Greisman, S., Hornick, R., Carozza, F. and Woodward, T. (1964) Endotoxin tolerance. *J. Clin. Invest.*, **43**, 986–99.

113. Mathison, J., Walfson, E. and Ulevitch, R. (1988) Participation of tumor necrosis factor in the mediation of gram negative bacterial lipopolysaccharide-induced injury in rabbits. *J. Clin. Invest.*, **81**, 1925–37.

114. McCall, C., Grosso-Wilmouth, L., LaRue, K. *et al.* (1993) Tolerance to endotoxin-induced expression of the interleukin-I beta gene in blood neutrophils of humans with the sepsis syndrome. *J. Clin. Invest.*, **91**, 853–61.

115. Sanchez-Cantu, L., Rode, H. and Christou, N. (1989) Endotoxin tolerance is associated with reduced secretion of tumor necrosis factor. *Arch. Surg.*, **124**, 1432–5.

116. Alexander, H., Sheppard, B., Jensen, J. *et al.* (1991) Treatment with recombinant human tumor necrosis factor-alpha protects rats against the lethality, hypotension, and hypothermia of gram negative sepsis. *J. Clin. Invest.*, **88**, 34–9.

117. Neta, R., Oppenheim, J., Schreiber, R. *et al.* (1991) Role of cytokines (interleukin 1, tumor necrosis factor, and transforming growth factor B) in natural and lipopolysaccharide-enhanced radioresistance. *J. Exp. Med.*, **173**, 1177–82.

118. Zuckerman, S., Evans, G., Snyder, Y. and Roeder, W. (1989) Endotoxin–macrophage interaction: post transnational regulation of tumor necrosis factor expression. *J. Immunol.*, **143**, 1223–7.

119. Coffee, L., Halushka, P., Ashton, S., *et al.* (1992) Endotoxin tolerance is associated with altered GTP-binding protein function. *J. Appl. Physiol.*, **73**, 1008–13.

120. Munoz, C., Carlet, J., Fitting, C. *et al.* (1991) Dysregulation of *in vitro* cytokine production

by monocytes in sepsis. *J. Clin. Invest.*, **88**, 1747–54.

121. Heliminen, M. and Vesikari, T. (1990) Inter-leukin-1 production in bacterial meningitis. *J. Infect. Dis.*, **22**, 105–8.

122. Simpson, S., Modi, H., Balk, R. *et al.* (1991) Reduced alveolar macrophage production of tumor necrosis factor during sepsis in mice and men. *Crit. Care Med.*, **19**, 1060–6.

123. Kim, J., Balk, R., Bone, R. and Casey, L. (1992) Down-regulation of human monocyte expression of CD14 in septic patients and by lipo-polysaccharide (LPS). *Am. Rev. Respir. Dis.*, **145**, A314.

124. Moore, F., Moore, E., Jones, T. *et al.* (1989) Ten versus TPN following major abdominal trauma-reduced septic mortality. *J. Trauma*, **29**, 916–23.

125. Wells, C., Rutstein, O., Pruett, T. *et al.* (1986) Intestinal bacteria translocates into experi-mental intra-abdominal abscesses. *Arch. Surg.*, **121**, 102–7.

126. Baker, J., Deitch, E., Berg, R. *et al.* (1988) Hemorrhagic shock induces bacterial trans-location from the gut. *J. Trauma*, **28**, 896–906.

127. Deitch, E., Winterton, J. and Berg, R. (1987) The gut as a portal of entry for bacteremia. *Ann. Surg.*, **205**, 681–92.

128. Alverdy, J., Aoys, E. and Moss, G. (1988) Total parental nutrition promotes bacterial trans-location from the gut. *Surgery*, **104**, 185–90.

129. Ziegler, T., Smith, R., O'Dwyer, S. *et al.* (1988) Increased intestinal permeability associated with infection in burn patients. *Arch. Surg.*, **123**, 1313–9.

130. Moore, F., Moore, E., Poggetti, R. *et al.* (1991) Gut bacterial translocation via the portal vein: a clinical perspective with major torso trauma. *J. Trauma*, **31**, 629–38.

131. Roumen, R., Hendriks, T., Wevers, R. and Goris, J. (1993) Intestinal permeability after severe trauma and hemorrhagic shock is increased without relation to septic complica-tions. *Arch. Surg.*, **128**, 453–7.

CYTOKINES AND LUNG INJURY

7

Daniel R. Smith, Robert M. Strieter and Steven L. Kunkel

Pulmonary inflammation represents a consequence of local tissue responses to a variety of direct or indirect stimuli. Many clinical entities, including trauma, infection, ischemia-reperfusion injury, as well as the syndrome of acute respiratory distress in adults (ARDS), are characterized by varying degrees of pulmonary insult and the resulting impairment of normal gas exchange. These inflammatory responses involve coordinated interactions between immune and non-immune cells and are specifically initiated, maintained and finally resolved. A variety of mediators are involved in the coordination of these activities and include lipids, such as prostaglandins; a group of small peptides, including bradykinin; and numerous polypeptides, of which a group has been classified as cytokines.

Cytokines represent a diverse category of soluble, hormone-like, polypeptides produced by immune and nonimmune cells. These proteins mediate immunologic and physiologic activities, including growth and differentiation, cytolysis, chemotaxis and a number of other immune cell interactions and activities through receptor–ligand interactions on specific cell population targets. Cytokines display concentration dependent effects, being expressed in low concentrations during normal homeostasis, with modest increases exerting local effects, and still greater elevations resulting in systemic effects. Autocrine, paracrine and endocrine effects may result from cytokine release. The area of cytokine biology is rapidly expanding, and currently over 25 specific cytokines have been isolated and characterized. Individual subpopulations of immune cells possess different capacities to elaborate and secrete specific cytokines in response to particular stimuli. Nonimmune cells, including endothelial cells, fibroblasts and epithelial cells, also demonstrate particular responses to specific signals resulting in the production of other cytokines. Furthermore, cell populations vary in their expression of receptors for individual cytokines, and, as a result, differ in their capacity to respond to specific cytokine signals.

Investigations into the interactions between various cell populations have lead to the concept of cytokine networking. Simply stated, one population of cells may respond directly to a specific stimulus by the elaboration of a specific cytokine to exert specific effects upon another population of cells. The targets may respond by producing cytokines, which may serve as feedback signals to the primary cell, or alternatively, initiate a cascade of events by affecting yet another array of target cells. Still other inflammatory effector cells, such as monocytes and polymorphonuclear neutrophils (PMN)s, may be recruited locally in

ARDS Acute Respiratory Distress in Adults. Edited by Timothy W. Evans and Christopher Haslett. Published in 1996 by Chapman & Hall, London. ISBN 0 412 56910 8

response to specific cytokine chemotactic signals. As many of the complexities of the inflammatory cytokine cascade have been elucidated, an increasing amount of evidence now suggests that nonimmune cells play crucial roles in the generation, maintenance and resolution of both local and systemic inflammatory responses.

The lungs represent a unique interface between the body and the environment, presenting an alveolar surface area of 75 square meters and only a minimal barrier of 4–8 μm between the alveolar space and the extensive microvasculature. While this configuration is ideal for gas exchange, it also increases vulnerability to noxious stimuli and pathogens. Consequently the pulmonary tissue must possess the capacity to generate brisk inflammatory responses to both inhaled and hematogenous challenges, in order to provide prompt clearance of the offending agent and avoid compromise of essential gas exchange function. This acute inflammatory response typically results in local increases in vascular permeability and a predominantly neutrophilic influx. Once successful containment of the noxious agent has occurred, inflammation should then resolve, with normal repair, tissue remodeling and return to homeostasis. However, because of the great capacity to initiate potent inflammatory responses, the lung may also be predisposed to tissue injury by excessive local reactions generated by both local or distant precipitants. In conditions such as ARDS, the overexuberant tissue inflammation may result in severe irreversible lung injury mediated primarily by elicited and activated PMNs. Other disease states, such as the granulomatous disease, sarcoidosis, can lead to the establishment of active chronic inflammation and destructive fibrosis mediated by the maintenance of other proinflammatory signals. In this chapter we examine the potential cytokine networks between immune and nonimmune cells that mediate pulmonary inflammation.

SPECIFIC CYTOKINES THAT MODULATE PULMONARY INFLAMMATION

Cytokines represent a diverse group of biologically active polypeptides that, in addition to many other activities, are instrumental in the evolution of an acute inflammatory response. In order to illustrate potentially important cytokine networks operative in pulmonary inflammation that mediate neutrophil recruitment, our discussion is focused on the early response cytokines interleukin (IL)-1 and tumor necrosis factor (TNF), the recently characterized interleukin-1 receptor antagonist (IRAP), the potent neutrophil activating/chemotactic factor, IL-8, and the mononuclear chemotactic factor, MCP-1.

TNF AND IL-1

Although biochemically unrelated, TNF and IL-1 demonstrate similar pleiotropic and overlapping effects on a variety of cellular functions [1–6]. They are primarily produced by mononuclear phagocytes and, because of their role in generating further inflammatory responses, have been termed 'early response mediators'. In modest concentrations at sites of local inflammation they are essential, and serve to regulate cellular function closely and dictate the events leading to initiation, maintenance and repair of tissue injury in the cascade of cytokine activity following the initial response. In marked contrast to the specific, controlled effects of local production of TNF and IL-1, the exaggerated systemic release of these cytokines can result in a syndrome of multiorgan injury with increased host morbidity and mortality. Thus, TNF and IL-1 have a broad spectrum of biologic activity that can influence the outcome of an inflammatory response on both the local and the systemic level. Numerous studies have noted a significant correlation between serum TNF and IL-1 levels and both the severity of ARDS and the mortality due to multiorgan failure [7–11]. Interestingly, inhibition of endogenously produced TNF during bacteria induced septic shock significantly attenuates the pathogenesis of multiorgan injury and related mortality [10,12]. Our laboratory has examined the endogenous expression and regulation of TNF from a murine model of endotoxemia and demonstrated that TNF is rapidly produced after a lethal dose (LD_{100}) infusion of endotoxin [13]. TNF levels peak within 1 hour, then rapidly decline to nearly undetectable levels by 8 hours. This observation has been substantiated by similar findings seen in a study of human volunteer subjects injected with low doses of endotoxin [14]. Thus, the early response cytokines exhibit striking dose dependent behavior; while the normal strictly regulated production is essential in initiating appropriate responses, it is also clear that overexpression of TNF and IL-1, such as in septic shock, may trigger a cascade of events ultimately leading to the accumulation of pulmonary neutrophils and acute lung injury.

IL-1 RECEPTOR ANTAGONIST

Recent studies of a naturally occurring IL-1 inhibitor have led to the isolation, purification, cloning and expression of an IL-1 receptor antagonist (IRAP) [15–20]. IRAP is a 22 kDa polypeptide that shares approximately 40% homology with IL1β and has been shown to be produced by peripheral blood monocytes or monocytic tumor cell lines in response to either endotoxin or adherent immunoglobulin (Ig)G [15,16,18]. IRAP appears to inhibit IL-1 activity at the level of competitive occupation of the IL-1 receptor without evidence for agonist activity [15,16,18]. *In vitro*, IRAP has been shown to inhibit IL-1 induced neutrophil adhesion to endothelial cells [15,16,18]. *In vivo*, IRAP has been shown to be a potent inhibitor of *Escherichia coli* mediated septic shock and lung injury [21]. Significantly, IRAP has been demonstrated to attenuate the neutrophilic alveolitis associated with the intratracheal administration of endotoxin or IL-1 [22].

Table 7.1 Cytokines with naturally occurring inhibitors

Cytokine	Specific inhibitor
IL-1 α,β	IRAP
TNF	Soluble TNF receptor
IFN-γ	Soluble IFN receptor
IL-4	Soluble IL-4 receptor

Interestingly, there is evidence suggesting that bronchogenic carcinomas may exploit these anti-inflammatory properties and elaborate IRAP as a means of impairing host immune responses [23]. These findings suggest that IRAP has an important immunomodulating influence on IL-1 dependent inflammation, representing a possible mediator of normal homeostasis, and perhaps also impacting on the pathogenesis of acute lung injury. Further investigations are under way to determine the role of IRAP in specific disease states. As illustrated in Table 7.1, a number of other naturally occurring cytokine inhibitors have been identified and may also be of equal importance in modulating the biology of inflammation.

IL-8 AND OTHER C-X-C CHEMOKINES

The primary feature of both TNF and IL-1 dependent acute inflammation in the lung is the sequestration of neutrophils and subsequent neutrophil dependent lung injury. Although TNF and IL-1 were initially reported to be chemotactic for neutrophils [24], more recent studies have definitively demonstrated that neither IL-1 nor TNF have direct chemotactic activity *in vitro* for neutrophils [25]. These findings suggest that cytokine networks are operative *in vivo*, which are dependent upon the initial expression of early response cytokines (TNF and IL-1), followed by the generation of more specific distal mediators which directly influence neutrophil activity. The isolation, purification, cloning and expression of IL-8 has led to a more comprehensive understanding of the mechan-

Table 7.2 C-X-C chemokines

IL-8
ENA-78
NAP-2
GRO-α,β,γ
PF-4
γIP-10
CTAP-III
MIP-2

isms of neutrophil chemotaxis. IL-8 belongs to a unique supergene family that includes a number of peptide homologs that have in common four conserved cysteine residues in an identical location, with the first pair of cysteines separated by one amino acid [26,27]. These have been termed the C-X-C chemokine supergene family and, in general, demonstrate significant neutrophil chemotactic activity (Table 7.2). Specific members include: neutrophil activating peptide (NAP)-2, which is formed by proteolytic processing from platelet basic protein or connective tissue activating peptide (CTAP)-III released from platelet α granules [26–28], GROα, which was originally described as a mitogen for human melanoma cells [29], and epithelial-neutrophil activating factor (ENA)-78, recently isolated from a pulmonary epithelial cell [28]. Other members of this family also include platelet factor (PF)-4 and interferon (INF)-γ inducible peptide (γIP)-10 [26,27].

IL-8, an 8.0 kDa polypeptide, is initially synthesized as a 99 amino acid precursor with a characteristic leader sequence of 22 amino acids that subsequently undergoes proteolytic N-terminal cleavage to either 77, 72 or 69 amino acid forms with identical biological activity [26,27]. In addition to being a potent chemoattractant and activating cytokine for neutrophils [26,27], it has a tenfold to 100-fold increase in potency as a lymphocyte chemotaxin [26,27]. Furthermore, IL-8 has recently been characterized as a potent stimulus for endothelial cell chemotaxis and angiogenesis [30]. IL-8 maintains its biological activity in the presence of significant changes in pH and,

in contrast to other known chemotactic factors, resists mild proteolytic degradation [26,27]. This stability suggests that the production of IL-8 at *in vivo* sites of acute inflammation may result in prolonged biological activity for the recruitment of neutrophils. IL-8, like other known neutrophil chemotactic factors, can activate neutrophils via a GTP binding protein. This process appears to be both Ca^{2+} and protein kinase C dependent [26,27].

While original investigations isolated IL-8 from peripheral blood monocytes [27,31], subsequent studies have identified the expression of this cytokine from a variety of other cellular sources. Importantly, many of these cells are analogous to the major cellular constituents of the alveolar-capillary wall, including endothelial cells [32], fibroblasts [33,34], epithelial cells [35], alveolar macrophages [36] and neutrophils [37,38]. IL-8 production by these cells is stimulus-specific. Endothelial cells, alveolar macrophages and neutrophils produce IL-8 in response to endotoxin, TNF or IL-1, whereas pulmonary fibroblasts and epithelial cells synthesize this cytokine only in response to the host derived stimuli TNF or IL-1. These findings demonstrate that nonimmune cells of the lung actually participate as effector cells in the production of a potent neutrophil activating/chemotactic factor.

MCP-1 AND OTHER C-C CHEMOKINES

Several studies have demonstrated the production of a monocyte specific cytokine by a variety of nonimmune cells, including fibroblasts [39], smooth muscle cell [40] and endothelial cells [39]. This monocyte chemotactic/activating peptide (MCP-1) has been recently purified, isolated, cloned and expressed in recombinant form [25,41]. MCP-1 belongs to a supergene family of polypeptides with structural similarities to IL-8. While both MCP-1 and IL-8 possess four cysteine residues and disulfide bridges essential for

Table 7.3 C-C chemokines

MCP-1,2,3
MIP-1α,β
RANTES
LD78/pAT464
ACT-2/pAT744
TCA-3

biological activity, the initial cysteine residues of MCP-1 and related members are, in contrast, not separated by an amino acid, leading to the designation as the C-C family [26]. MCP-1 is a 15 kDa polypeptide derived from a 99 amino acid precursor with characteristic leader sequence of 23 amino acids, with the mature form representing 76 amino acids [26,42]. Additional C-C family polypeptides (Table 7.3) include: macrophage inflammatory protein (MIP)-1 [43]; LD78/pAT464 [44], ACT-2/pAT744 [45], RANTES [46], TCA-3 [47]. The overall amino acid sequence homology between IL-8 and MCP-1 is approximately 21% [26,42]. Interestingly, MCP-1 also possesses 68% homology at the nucleotide sequence with the murine cell cycle competence gene (JE; [42]). In contrast to the C-X-C family, this group of cytokines demonstrates monocyte activating and chemotactic properties. Experimental studies have demonstrated that purified MCP-1 can induce cytostatic activity for a number of human tumor cell lines [48]. Furthermore, MCP-1 treated monocytes can generate superoxide anion and release of lysosomal enzyme in the presence of cytochalasin B [26].

The regulation of MCP-1 production differs from that of IL-8 in specific cell populations. A major difference exists between MCP-1 and IL-8 in the disparate gene expression of these cytokines by monocytes and alveolar macrophages [47]. Both alveolar macrophages and monocytes express IL-8 when stimulated with either lipopolysaccharide (LPS), TNF or IL-1, but appear not to produce MCP-1 in response to these stimuli [47]. Furthermore, it appears that monocytes, unlike alveolar macrophages,

may produce MCP-1 protein when exposed specifically to phytohemagglutinin in the presence of serum. Endothelial cells demonstrate the capacity to elaborate MCP-1 in response to either LPS, TNF or IL-1. In contrast, pulmonary fibroblasts and epithelial cells are somewhat more stimulus specific, and only respond with MCP-1 production to TNF or IL-1, but not to LPS. Although stimulated mononuclear phagocytes rarely produce MCP-1, macrophages do synthesize a variety of other potent monocyte chemotactic factors.

ACUTE PULMONARY INFLAMMATION

The common histopathologic feature of acute inflammation and injury in the lung is the presence of intrapulmonary neutrophils. During the initiation phase of acute inflammation the movement of neutrophils from the pulmonary vascular compartment to interstitium and alveolar space is an early event in the propagation of further lung inflammation. Inflammatory stimuli from either side of the alveolar-capillary membrane may result in pulmonary microvascular alterations which lead to local increases in neutrophil adhesion (Chapter 9). These adhered neutrophils, under the influence of chemoattractants, then undergo directed migration along chemotactic gradients to the inflamed area. During recruitment these neutrophils (Chapter 11), also become activated, releasing various proteases (Chapter 10) and reactive oxygen metabolites which result in acute lung injury. As the acute inflammatory process changes from the initiation to maintenance and resolution stages, the cellular composition of the inflammatory lesions changes to a predominately mononuclear cell population. Thus, the inflammatory leukocyte elicitation is dynamic, with specific chemoattractants expressed at specific temporal windows of the inflammatory response. In bacterial infection and other clinical conditions, the recruitment of inflammatory leukocytes is mediated by a number of biologically active agents, including IL-8.

Cytokine networks between immune and nonimmune cells of the alveolar-capillary membrane are necessary for cellular communication during inflammation. The subsequent events of these interactions are crucial to initiating and propagating the inflammatory response which leads to pulmonary injury. Both TNF and IL-1 are early response cytokines that are necessary not only for the initiation of acute inflammation, but are also required for persistence of the inflammatory response, leading to chronic inflammation. The exact degree that either TNF or IL-1 participates in a pulmonary immune reaction is unclear. Investigations have identified that two novel chemotactic/activating cytokines, IL-8 and MCP-1, are dependent upon the stimulation by either TNF or IL-1. The participation of either of these chemotactic/activating cytokines in the inflammatory response may be critical for the orchestration of the directed migration of inflammatory leukocytes into the lung. Upon arrival to the lung these activated leukocytes induce pulmonary injury through the release of reactive oxygen metabolites and proteolytic enzymes. Current investigation to delineate their role *in vivo* for mediating specific pulmonary diseases is ongoing.

As mentioned above, an intense inflammatory cell influx ensues during the pathogenesis of an acute pulmonary inflammation. The cellular constituents of this lesion are in dynamic evolution. This suggests that definitive signals are generated in order to recruit specific populations of immune and nonimmune cells. Several investigations have shown that IL-8 is chemotactic for either neutrophils or lymphocytes, although the concentration required for maximal neutrophil migration *in vitro* is tenfold to 100-fold greater than optimal lymphocyte elicitation [49]. Maximal *in vitro* IL-8 induced chemotactic activity for neutrophils occurs between 1 and 100 ng/ml, with a plateau in neutrophil

migration beyond 100 ng/ml. These concentrations are compatible with the quantitative levels of IL-8 produced by mononuclear phagocytes, endothelial cells, fibroblasts and epithelial cells in response to either LPS, TNF or IL-1. Thus the capacity of IL-8 to selectively elicit neutrophils during an acute inflammatory event is related to the magnitude of IL-8 expression in response to physiologic concentrations of primary response cytokines, TNF or IL-1. This selectivity for neutrophil elicitation based on the concentration effect of IL-8 is of great significance because these cells are the usual dominant leukocyte recruited to an acute inflammatory lesion. By contrast, with sequential progression to chronic inflammation, the change in absolute level of IL-8 may then favor the elicitation of predominantly lymphocytes. Although neutrophils are the principal cells in mediating host defense, they are also often involved in the immunopathology associated with various pulmonary disorders. For example, late phase asthma, asbestosis, idiopathic pulmonary fibrosis and ARDS are pulmonary diseases that commonly demonstrate a significant neutrophil component to their histopathology.

The migration of neutrophils from the pulmonary microvascular compartment into the pulmonary interstitium and alveolar space represents an important immunopathologic event because this process is also accompanied by neutrophil activation. The earliest phases of acute inflammation are associated with enhanced local vasodilatation, vascular permeability and alterations of adhesion molecule expression by endothelial cells (Chapter 9). Neutrophil migration then ensues in a multi-stage process: they must first adhere to local endothelial cells, then diapedese extravascularly along established chemotactic gradients. Although the elicitation and activation of neutrophils into the lung is a common scenario found in the initiation and maintenance phases of a variety of pulmonary diseases, the precise mechanism(s) responsible for these events remain to be determined.

Normal differential cell count from broncho-alveolar lavage for individuals without underlying pulmonary pathology is less than 1% neutrophils [50]. The alveolitis of idiopathic pulmonary fibrosis (IPF), a chronic disease limited to the lungs, demonstrates a histopathology of striking neutrophil recruitment into the pulmonary interstitium and alveolar space. The composition of cells recovered by bronchoalveolar lavage from these patients often yields 40% or more neutrophils, however the relative proportions of other inflammatory cells found in the lungs, including B lymphocytes, T lymphocytes and alveolar macrophages remain normal [51–53] (Chapter 16). This suggests that specific chemotactic factor(s) with defined specificity for neutrophils are potentially responsible for lung parenchymal cell injury. This pronounced cellular injury may lead to disorganized repair and end stage fibrosis. The alveolar macrophage has been extensively studied and incriminated as one of the primary cellular sources of the factor(s) mediating the neutrophil influx. The identification of these inflammatory mediator(s) and their production by the other cellular constituents of the alveolar-capillary membrane remains to be elucidated. IPF and asbestosis are pulmonary disorders that share many salient features, including their underlying pulmonary pathophysiology, clinical symptoms and chest roentgenograms abnormalities [53,54]. In both disease states, alveolar macrophages have been shown to elaborate a potent neutrophil chemotactic factor. This discovery is of particular importance because both pulmonary disorders are typically characterized by a predominant neutrophil alveolitis [51–53,55]. These findings suggest that a common mechanism may be responsible for the recruitment and activation of neutrophils in these two disparate clinical entities.

ARDS is also a specific pulmonary disorder that may reflect an ongoing systemic process [56]. The underlying pathophysiology of ARDS is systemic inflammation related to sepsis, shock, trauma and a host of other inciting causes [57–60]. Prominent features of these entities are characterized by the involvement of both cellular and humoral mediators of acute inflammation at the microvascular level [61]. Diffuse alveolar-capillary membrane damage results from this microvascular injury and propagates increased vascular permeability and extravascular fluid accumulation, and ultimately augmented neutrophil intravascular aggregation and transendothelial emigration. Although we have continued to gain insight into the pathogenesis of this disease process, the mechanism(s) of neutrophil recruitment and activation in ARDS remains enigmatic. The potential role of complement activation in the pathogenesis or modulation of ARDS continues to be controversial. Several studies have demonstrated that the chemotactic/activation factor(s) active in ARDS are neither C5a, C5a des arg, a split product of C3, a fragment of fibrinogen, nor a product of fibronectin. Neutralizing antibodies to these particular proteins do not significantly alter the chemotactic activity found in the bronchoalveolar lavage fluid of patients with ARDS [62]. In addition to the role of neutrophil elicitation, neutrophil activation has been demonstrated to be of significant importance in ARDS. The resulting release of reactive oxygen metabolites and proteolytic enzymes affects the integrity of surrounding cells and leads to marked impairment of pulmonary function. Abnormalities of pulmonary gas exchange in ARDS correlate with the levels of neutrophil elastase isolated from lavage fluid from patients with this disorder [63]. IPF, asbestosis and ARDS demonstrate similarity in their cellular constituents obtained from bronchoalveolar lavage. These abnormalities reflect changes from the normal predominantly alveolar macrophage population to a relative or absolute increase in neutrophils. The association of elevated numbers of neutrophils and these specific pulmonary disorders suggests that a common potent neutrophil chemotactic/activating factor(s) may be responsible.

Our laboratory has examined mechanisms of neutrophil recruitment into the lung by assessing IL-8 production by the major cellular components of the alveolar-capillary membrane. The alveolar-capillary membrane has traditionally been viewed only as a structure for gas exchange, but an understanding of a more complex role has emerged with evolutions in molecular biological techniques and investigations of individual cell components. The alveolar-capillary membrane is now viewed as a dynamic assembly of immune and nonimmune cells that, through cytokine networking, can generate significant quantities of IL-8. Importantly, the expression of IL-8 by the major cellular constituents of the alveolar-capillary membrane is stimulus specific. Mononuclear phagocytes and endothelial cells produce IL-8 in response to either LPS, TNF or IL-1, but not to IL-6. By contrast, pulmonary fibroblasts and epithelial cells express IL-8 only in response to specific host derived signals, such as TNF or IL-1. These findings are significant because cells once thought of as 'targets' to TNF and IL-1 can actively participate as effector cells in the production of a potent neutrophil chemoattractant. Additionally, the scenario for the recruitment of neutrophils to the lung may be directly attributed to IL-8 production by the cells of the alveolar-capillary membrane. Thus, during either local (pneumonia) or systemic inflammation, such as ARDS/multiorgan failure, IL-8 and other C-X-C chemokines may be present and display prominent activity (Figure 7.1). In both Gram-negative pneumonia and sepsis, the release of lipopolysaccharide stimulates alveolar or interstitial macrophages to not only produce IL-8, but also to secrete both TNF and IL-1. The newly elaborated TNF and IL-1 can then act in either an autocrine or paracrine fashion to stimulate contiguous cells, both immune and nonimmune, to express additional IL-8.

This amplification of a chemotactic signal results in brisk recruitment of neutrophils to the pulmonary interstitium or alveolar space. Once elicited to this anatomical position, neutrophil activation prompts the release of reactive oxygen metabolites and proteolytic enzymes, culminating in local pulmonary parenchymal injury. Clinical studies examining elevations in pulmonary IL-8 levels and the development and mortality in ARDS have conflicted, although most suggest a strong correlation [64,65]. Of particular interest is the recent finding that early increases in bronchoalveolar lavage fluid IL-8 content of patients at risk correlate with the subsequent development of ARDS and, importantly, also demonstrate alveolar macrophages as important sources of IL-8 prior to neutrophil influx [66]. Recent investigations have also shown that hyperoxia can lead to an induction of IL-8 gene expression with a fourfold increase in IL-8 production by mononuclear cells, as compared with normoxic conditions [67]. Of additional clinical significance, endotoxin was found to potentiate further this hyperoxic response. These findings suggest that, under conditions simulating Gram-negative bacteria induced lung injury, the addition of an oxidant stress, such as routinely administered supplemental oxygen, may have a potentiating influence on the production of potent neutrophil chemotactic cytokines such as IL-8 and result in further lung injury.

CHRONIC PULMONARY INFLAMMATION

As outlined above, the interactions between cellular and humoral mediators that result in leukocyte elicitation and activation in the lung are complex. The accumulation of lymphocytes and monocytes/macrophages, with the concomitant decline in neutrophil recruitment, characterizes the changing composition of immune cell populations recruited during the evolution of the inflammatory process. It is increasingly evident that mediation of inflammatory cell migration into the lung is

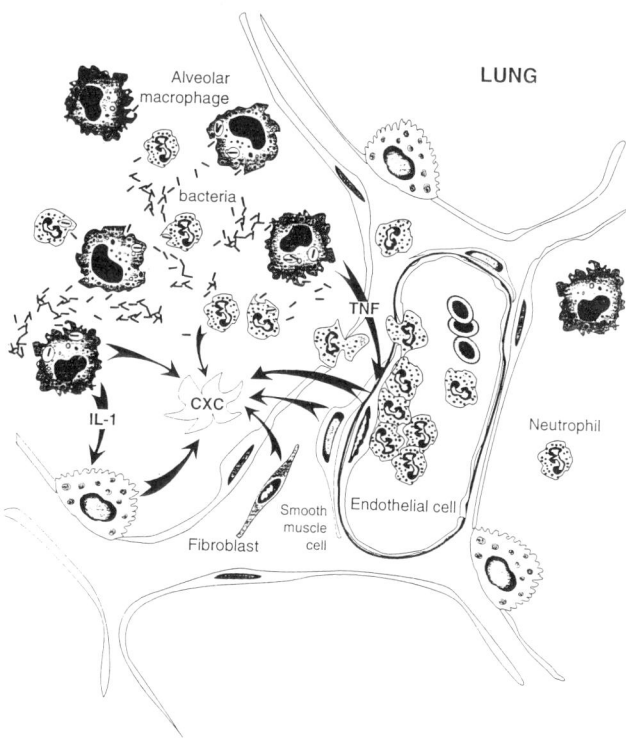

Figure 7.1 Chemokine generation via cytokine networks operative in the acute inflammation of bacterial pneumonia.

not restricted to novel neutrophil chemotactic factors, and that specific monocyte recruitment is also directed by chemoattractant proteins [41,42]. Accordingly, during evolution from acute to chronic inflammation, the elicitation of monocytes to the lung by a monocyte chemoattractant(s) may be independent from cellular sources of alveolar macrophages. The MCP-1 induced migration of monocytes into the pulmonary interstitium and alveolar space is dependent upon nonimmune pulmonary cells stimulated by host derived inflammatory cytokines, such as TNF or IL-1. These findings are relevant to *in vivo* cytokine networking leading to MCP-1 production. In the context of pulmonary inflammation, the activated alveolar or interstitial macrophage can release both TNF and IL-1, either of which can result in the production of

MCP-1. These two cytokines act specifically in a paracrine manner to stimulate pulmonary epithelial cells, fibroblasts and endothelial cells to produce MCP-1. The induction of a specific monocyte chemotactic and activating factor by pulmonary nonimmune cells may be paramount in the elicitation and maintenance phase of chronic inflammation.

SUMMARY

Cytokine networks between immune and nonimmune cells of the alveolar-capillary membrane are necessary for cellular communication during pulmonary inflammation. The subsequent events of these cellular/humoral interactions are pivotal to the initiation and propagation of the inflammatory response leading to pulmonary injury. Both

TNF and IL-1 are early response cytokines that are essential for both the initiation of acute inflammation, and the persistence of the inflammatory response culminating in chronic inflammation. The degree to which either TNF or IL-1 participates in a pulmonary immune reaction is unclear. An important aspect of acute lung injury is not only that it may be driven by local alterations in TNF or IL-1, but also that excessive systemic pro-inflammatory cytokine release may indirectly initiate pulmonary inflammation. The investigations that have identified two novel chemotactic/activating cytokines are exciting, showing that IL-8 and MCP-1 are dependent upon the stimulation by either TNF or IL-1. The participation of either of these chemotactic/activating cytokines in the inflammatory response appears to be critical for the orchestration of the directed migration of inflammatory leukocytes into the lung. After arrival in the lung, these activated leukocytes can respond to noxious stimuli or induce pulmonary injury through the release of reactive oxygen metabolites and proteolytic enzymes. Current investigations are designed to delineate their role *in vivo* for mediating specific pulmonary diseases.

ACKNOWLEDGEMENTS

We convey our special appreciation to Robin Kunkel for her excellent artwork for Figure 7.1.

This research was supported in part by National Institutes of Health grants 1P50HL46487, HL02401, HL31693, HL 50057 and DK38149.

Dr Strieter is an RJR Nabisco Research Scholar.

REFERENCES

1. Larrick, J.W. and Kunkel, S.L. (1988) The role of tumor necrosis factor and interleukin-1 in the immunoinflammatory response. *Pharmocology Research*, **5**, 129–39.
2. Kunkel, S.L., Remick, D.G., Strieter, R.M. and Larrick, J.W. (1989) Mechanisms that regulate the production and effects of tumor necrosis factor α. *Critical Reviews of Immunology*, **9**, 93–117.
3. Le, J. and Vilcek, J. (1987) TNF and IL-1: cytokines with multiple overlapping biological activities. *Laboratory Investigation*, **56**, 234–82.
4. Sherry, B. and Cerami, A. (1988) Cachectin/tumor necrosis factor exerts endocrine, paracrine, and autocrine control of the inflammatory responses. *Journal of Cell Biology*, **107**, 1269–77.
5. Dinarello, C.A. (1989) Interleukin-1 and its biologically related cytokines. *Advances in Immunology*, **44**, 153–205.
6. Cerami, A. (1992) Inflammatory cytokines. *Clinical Immunology and Immunopathology*, **62**, S3–10.
7. Shalaby, M.R., Halgunset, J., Haugen, O.A. *et al.* (1991) Cytokine-associated tissue injury and lethality in mice: a comparative study. *Clinical Immunology and Immunopathology*, **61**, 69–82.
8. Girardin, E., Grau, G.E., Dayer, J.M. *et al.* (1988) Tumor necrosis factor and interleukin-1 in the serum of children with severe infectious purpura. *New England Journal of Medicine*, **319**, 397–400.
9. Marks, J.D., Marks, C.B., Luce, J.M. *et al.* (1990) Plasma tumor necrosis in patients with septic shock: mortality rate, incidence of adult respiratory distress syndrome. *American Review of Respiratory Disease*, **141**, 94–7.
10. Tracey, K.J., Fong, Y., Hesse, D.G. *et al.* (1987) Anti-cachectin/TNF monoclonal antibodies prevent septic shock during lethal bacteremia. *Nature*, **330**, 662–4.
11. Waage, A., Halstensen, A. and Espevik, T. (1987) Association between tumor necrosis factor in serum and fatal outcome in patients with menigococcal disease. *Lancet*, **ii**, 355–7.
12. Hinshaw, L.B., Tekamp-Olson, P., Chang, A.C.K. *et al.* (1990) Survival of primates in LD$_{100}$ septic shock following therapy with antibody to tumor necrosis factor (TNF-alpha). *Circulatory Shock*, **30**, 279–92.
13. Remick, D.G., Strieter, R.M., Lynch, J.P. III *et al.* (1989) *In vivo* dynamics of murine tumor necrosis factor-α gene expression: kinetics of dexamethasone-induced suppression. *Laboratory Investigation*, **60**, 766–71.
14. Michie, H.R., Mangue, K.R., Spriggs, D.R. *et al.* (1988) Detection of circulating tumor necrosis

factor after endotoxin administration. *New England Journal of Medicine*, **318**, 1481–4.

15. Carter, D.B., Deibel, M.R., Dunn, C.J. *et al.* (1990) Purification, cloning, expression, and biological characterization of an interleukin-1 receptor anatagonist protein. *Nature*, **334**, 633–8.

16. Dinarello, C.A. (1991) Interleukin-1 and interleukin-1 antagonism. *Blood*, **77**, 1627–52.

17. Eisenberg, S.P., Evans, R.J., Arend, W.P. *et al.* (1990) Primary structure and functional expression from complementary DNA of a human interleukin-1 receptor antagonist. *Nature*, **343**, 343–6.

18. Arend, W.P. (1991) Interleukin-1 receptor antagonist – a new member of the interleukin-1 family. *Journal of Clinical Investigation*, **88**, 1445–1.

19. Hannum, C.H., Wilcox, C.J., Arend, W.P. *et al.* (1990) Interleukin-1 receptor antagonist activity of a human interleukin-1 inhibitor. *Nature*, **343**, 336–40.

20. Mazzei, G.J., Seckinger, P.L., Dayer, J.M. and Shaw, A.R. (1990) Purification and characterization of a 26-kDa competitive inhibitor of interleukin-1. *European Journal of Immunology*, **20**, 683–9.

21. Ohlsson, K., Bjork, P., Bergenfeldt, M. *et al.* (1990) IL-1ra reduces mortality from endotoxin shock. *Nature*, **348**, 550–2.

22. Ulich, T.R., Yin, S., Guo, K. *et al.* (1991) The intratracheal administration of endotoxin and cytokines: III. The interleukin-1 (IL-1) receptor antagonist inhibits endotoxin- and IL-1-induced acute inflammation. *American Journal of Pathology*, **138**, 521–4.

23. Smith, D.R., Kunkel, S.L., Standiford, T.J. *et al.* (1993) The production of interleukin-1 receptor anatagonist protein by human bronchogenic carcinoma. *American Journal of Pathology*, **14S**, 794–803.

24. Sauder, D.N., Mounessa, N.L., Katy, S.I. *et al.* (1984) Chemotactic cytokines: the role of leukocyte pyrogen and epidermal cell thymocyte-activating factor in neutrophil chemotaxis. *Journal of Immunology*, **132**, 828–37.

25. Yoshimura, T., Matsushima, K., Oppenheim, J.J. and Leonard, E.J. (1987) Neutrophil chemotactic factor produced by LPS-stimulated human blood mononuclear leukocytes: partial characterization and separation from interleukin-1. *Journal of Immunology*, **139**, 788–94.

26. Matsushima, K. and Oppenheim, J.J. (1989) Interleukin-8 and MCAF: novel inflammatory cytokines inducible by IL-1 and TNF. *Cytokine*, **1**, 2–13.

27. Baggiolini, M., Walz, A. and Kunkel, S.L. (1989) Neutrophil-activating peptide-1/interleukin-8, a novel cytokine that activates neutrophils. *Journal of Clinical Investigation*, **84**, 1045–9.

28. Walz, A., Burgener, R., Car, B. *et al.* (1991) Structure and neutrophil-activating properties of a novel inflammatory peptide (ENA-78) with homology to interleukin-8. *Journal of Experimental Medicine*, **174**, 1355–62.

29. Richmond, A.E., Balentien, E., Thomas, H.G. *et al.* (1988) Molecular characterization and chromosomal mapping of melanoma growth stimulatory activity, a growth factor structurally related to beta-thromboglobulin. *EMBO Journal*, **7**, 2025–30.

30. Koch, A.E., Polverini, P.J., Kunkel, S.L. *et al.* (1992) Interleukin-8 as a macrophage-derived mediator of angiogenesis. *Science*, **258**, 1798–801.

31. Matsushima, K., Morishita, K., Yoshimura, T. *et al.* (1988) Molecular cloning of a human monocyte-derived neutrophil chemotactic factor (MDNCF) and the induction of MDCNF mRNA by interleukin-1 and tumor necrosis factor. *Journal of Experimental Medicine*, **167**, 1883–93.

32. Strieter, R.M., Kunkel, S.L., Showell, H.J. *et al.* (1989) Endothelial cell gene expression of a neutrophil chemotactic factor by TNF-alpha, LPS, and IL-1-beta. *Science*, **243**, 1467–9.

33. Strieter, R.M., Phan, S.H., Showell, H.J. *et al.* (1989) Monokine-induced neutrophil chemotactic factor gene expression in human fibroblasts. *Journal of Biological Chemistry*, **264**, 10621–6.

34. Rolfe, M.W., Kunkel, S.L., Standiford, T.J. *et al.* (1991) Pulmonary fibroblast expression of interleukin-8: a model for alveolar macrophage-derived cytokine networking. *American Journal of Respiratory Cell and Molecular Biology*, **5**, 493–501.

35. Standiford, T.J., Kunkel, S.L., Basha, M.A. *et al.* (1990) Interleukin-8 gene expression by a pulmonary epithelial cell line: a model for cytokine networks in the lung. *Journal of Clinical Investigation*, **86**, 1945–53.

36. Strieter, R.M., Chensue, S.W., Basha, M.A. *et al.* (1990) Human alveolar macrophage gene expression of interleukin-8 by tumor necrosis factor-α, lipopolysaccharide, and interleukin-

1β. *American Journal of Respiratory Cell and Molecular Biology*, **2**, 321–6.

37. Strieter, R.M., Kashahara, K., Allen, R. *et al.* (1990) Human neutrophils exhibit disparate chemotactic factor gene expression. *Biochemical and Biophysical Research Communications*, **173**, 725–30.

38. Strieter, R.M., Kasahara, K., Allen, R.M. *et al.* (1992) Cytokine-induced neutrophil-derived interleukin-8. *American Journal of Pathology*, **141**, 397–407.

39. Strieter, R.M., Wiggins, R., Phan, S.H. *et al.* (1989) Monocyte chemotactic protein gene expression by cytokine-treated human fibroblasts and endothelial cells. *Biochemical and Biophysical Research Communications*, **162**, 694–700.

40. Valente, A.J., Graves, D.T., Vialle-Valentin, C.E. *et al.* (1988) Purification of a monocyte chemotactic factor secreted by nonhuman primate vascular cells in culture. *Biochemistry*, **27**, 4162–8.

41. Furuntani, Y., Normura, H., Notake, M. *et al.* (1989) Cloning and sequencing of the cDNA for human monocyte chemotactic and activating factor (MCAF). *Biochemical and Biophysical Research Communications*, **159**, 249–55.

42. Yoshimura, T., Yuhki, N., Moore, S. *et al.* (1989) Human monocyte chemoattractant protein-1 (MCP-1) full-length cDNA cloning, expression in mitogen-stimulated blood mononuclear leukocytes and sequence similarity to mouse competence gene JE. *FEBS Letters*, **244**, 487–93.

43. Wolpe, S.D., Davatelis, G., Sherry, B. *et al.* (1988) Macrophages secrete a novel heparin-binding protein with inflammatory and neutrophil chemokinetic properties. *Journal of Experimental Medicine*, **167**, 570–81.

44. Obaru, K., Fukuda, M., Maeda, S. and Shimada, K. (1986) A cDNA clone used to study mRNA inducible in tonsilar lymphocytes by tumor promoter. *Journal of Biochemistry (Tokyo)*, **99**, 885–94.

45. Zipfel, P.F., Balke, J., Irving, S.G. *et al.* (1989) Mitogenic activation of human T cells induces two closely related genes which share structural similarities with a new family of secreted factors. *Journal of Immunology*, **142**, 1582–90.

46. Schall, T.J., Jongstra, J., Dyer, B.J. *et al.* (1988) A human T cell-specific molecule is a member of a new gene family. *Journal of Immunology*, **141**, 1018–25.

47. Burd, P.R., Freeman, G.J., Wilson, S.D. *et al.* (1987) Cloning and characterization of a novel T cell activation gene. *Journal of Immunology*, **139**, 3126–31.

48. Matsushima, K., Larsen, C.G., DuBois, G.C. and Oppenheim, J.J. (1989) Purification and characterization of a novel monocyte chemotactic and activating factor produced by a human myelomonocytic cell line. *Journal of Experimental Medicine*, **169**, 1485–90.

49. Larsen, C.G. Anderson, A.O., Appella, E. *et al.* (1989) Neutrophil activating protein (NAP-1) is also chemotactic for T lymphocytes. *Science*, **243**, 1164–7.

50. The BAL Cooperative Group Steering Committee (1990) Bronchoalveolar lavage constituents in healthy individuals, idiopathic pulmonary fibrosis, and selected comparison groups. *American Review of Respiratory Disease*, **141**, S175–8.

51. The BAL Cooperative Group Steering Committee (1990) Bronchoalveolar lavage constituents in healthy individuals, idiopathic pulmonary fibrosis, and selected comparison groups. *American Review of Respiratory Disease*, **141**, S188–92.

52. Hunninghake, G.W., Gadek, J.E., Lawley, T.J. and Crystal, R.G. (1981) Mechanisms of neutrophil accumulation in the lungs of patients with idiopathic pulmonary fibrosis. *Journal of Clinical Investigation*, **68**, 259–8.

53. Hunninghake, G.W., Kawanami, O., Ferrans, V.J. *et al.* (1981) Characterization of the inflammatory and immune effector cells in the lung parenchyma of patients with interstitial lung disease. *American Review of Respiratory Disease*, **123**, 407–21.

54. Rebuck, A.S. and Braudi, A.C. (1983) Bronchoalveolar lavage in asbestosis. *Archives in Internal Medicine*, **143**, 956–64.

55. Hayes, A.A., Rose, A.H., Musk, A.W. and Robinson B.W. (1988). Neutrophil chemotactic factor release and neutrophil alveolitis in asbestos-exposed individuals. *Chest*, **94**, 521–5.

56. McGuire, W.W., Spregg, R.G., Cohen, A.B. and Cochran, C.G. (1982) Studies on the pathogenesis of the adult respiratory distress syndrome. *Journal of Clinical Investigations*, **69**, 543–53.

57. Fowler, A.A., Hamman, R.F., Good, J.T. *et al.* (1983) Adult respiratory distress syndrome: risk with common predispositions. *Annals of Internal Medicine*, **98**, 593–7.

58. Bell, R.C., Coalson, J.J., Smith, J.D. and Johan-

son, W.G. (1983) Multiple organ failure and infection in adult respiratory distress syndrome. *Annals of Internal Medicine*, **99**, 293–8.

59. Montgomery, A.B., Stager, M.A., Carrico, C.J. and Hudson, L.D. (1985) Causes of mortality in patients with the adult respiratory distress syndrome. *American Review of Respiratory Disease*, **132**, 485–9.

60. McManus, L.M. and Deavers, S.I. (1989) Platlet activating factor in pulmonary pathobiology. *Clinics in Chest Medicine*, **10**, 107–77.

61. Cybulsky, M.I., Chan, M.K.W. and Movar, H.Z. (1988) Acute inflammation and microthrombosis induced by endotoxin, interleukin-1, and tumor necrosis factor alpha. *Laboratory Investigation*, **58**, 365–78.

62. Parsons, P.E., Fowler, A.A., Hyers, T.M. and Henson, P.M. (1985) Chemotactic activity in bronchoalveolar lavage fluid from patients with adult respiratory distress syndrome. *American Review of Respiratory Disease*, **132**, 490–508.

63. Idell, S., Kucich, U., Fein, A. *et al.* (1985) Neutrophil elastase-releasing factors in the bronchoalveolar lavage fluid from patients with adult respiratory distress syndrome. *American Review of Respiratory Disease*, **132**, 1098–109.

64. Jorens, P.G., VanDame, J., DeBecker, W. *et al.* (1992) Interleukin-8 in the bronchoalveolar lavage fluid from patients with the adult respiratory distress syndrome (ARDS) and patients at risk for ARDS. *Cytokine*, **4**, 592–7.

65. Miller, E.J., Cohen, A.B., Nago, S. *et al.* (1992) Elevated levels of NAP-1/interleukin-8 are present in the airspaces of patients with the adult respiratory distress syndrome and are associated with increased mortality. *American Review of Respiratory Disease*, **146**, 427–32.

66. Donnelly, S.C., Strieter, R.M., Kunkel, S.L. *et al.* (1993) Interleukin-8 and development of adult respiratory distress syndrome in at-risk patient groups. *Lancet*, **341**, 643–7.

67. Metinko, A.P., Kunkel, S.L., Standiford, T.J. and Strieter, R.M. (1992) Anoxia–hyperoxia induces monocyte derived interleukin-8. *Journal of Clinical Investigation*, **90**, 791–8.

MECHANISMS OF NEUTROPHIL MEDIATED INJURY

8

G. Scott Worthen and Gregory P. Downey

The morphologic appearance of the lung in the syndrome of acute respiratory distress in adults (ARDS), in which extensive neutrophil accumulation is seen in all compartments (Chapter 4), defines this syndrome as reflecting an overwhelming inflammatory process. In the context of apparent injury to epithelial and endothelial surfaces, a model for the pathogenesis of ARDS suggests that injury by inflammatory cells plays a central role (Chapter 5).

In order for neutrophils to induce lung injury, they must be retained within the lung, migrate into the parenchyma and release injurious products. Under normal circumstances, inflammatory cells leave the bone marrow and enter the circulation in a relatively quiescent state in which they can pass though the microvasculature of the lung and other organs many times without any significant effect on those vessels or the underlying tissue. We suggest that a sequence of structural and biochemical events in the neutrophil accompanies the induction of an inflammatory response in the lung. A considerable body of work suggests that the interaction between neutrophil and lung vasculature differs from that in other organs, that migration of cells into parenchyma is associated with major structural rearrangements, and that priming of the neutrophil for enhanced secretory functions may be related to activation via recently elucidated signaling pathways in the neutrophil previously ascribed only to growth factor regulated events.

REGULATION OF NEUTROPHIL RETENTION IN THE LUNG (Figure 8.1)

Normal unstimulated neutrophils entering the lung microvascular bed from the marginating pool are retained almost exclusively within the capillaries [1]. The cells sequestered in this fashion do not pass slowly through the capillary but rather are retained at discrete sites within the lung vasculature [2], suggesting that there may be preferred sites within the lung for leukocyte sequestration. Even neutrophils which eventually transit the lung capillary may remain stationary for short periods of time ranging from seconds to as much as a few minutes. The distribution of transit times for these normal neutrophils can be affected in a number of ways by both the hemodynamics of the lung circulation [2], where increases in pulmonary artery pressure or local flow rates diminish the transit, or by exposure to chemoattractants [3], which dramatically shifts the mean transit time towards higher values. However, even after stimulation, the site (capillary) and mode (stuttering or hopping) of transit remain similar, although the magnitude of the effects is much greater in stimulated cells.

ARDS Acute Respiratory Distress in Adults. Edited by Timothy W. Evans and Christopher Haslett. Published in 1996 by Chapman & Hall, London. ISBN 0 412 56910 8

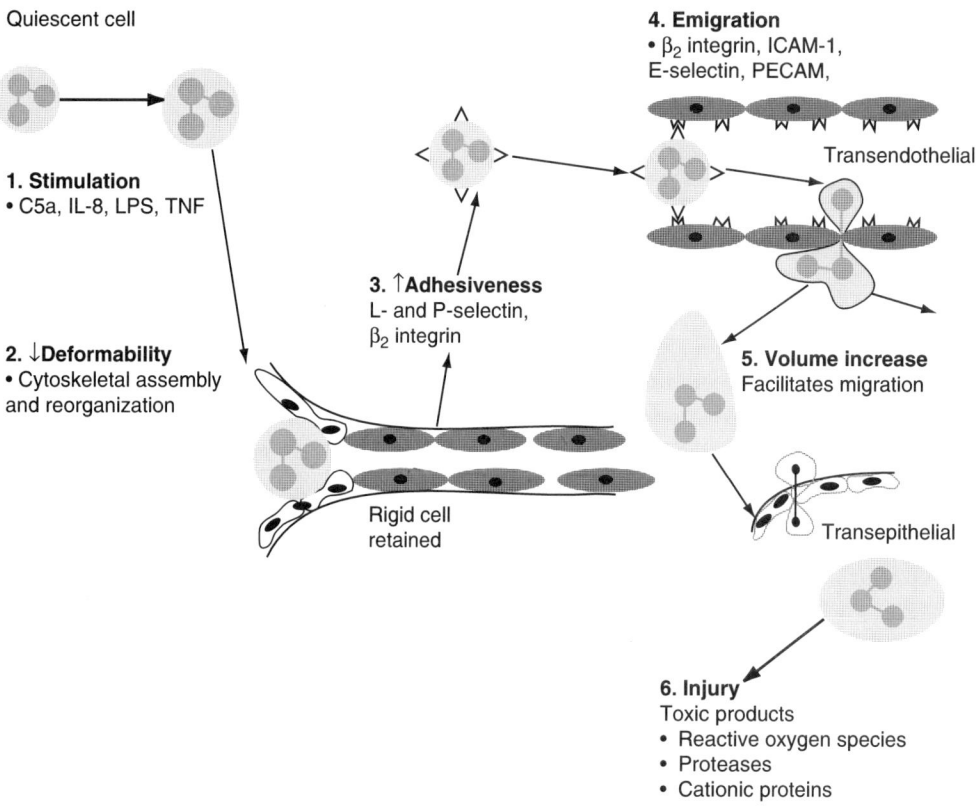

Figure 8.1 Mechanisms regulating neutrophil retention and emigration in the lung. Processes have been separated into six sequential steps for the purposes of clarity, but *in vivo* it is likely that these processes overlap and are difficult to isolate.

These data highlight an important difference between the pulmonary circulation and other circulatory beds, even though neutrophils can be shown to travel more slowly than erythrocytes in both. In the former, neutrophils may spend considerable periods of time in stationary contact with the local endothelium, a condition that may greatly predispose to adhesive and other interactions between the two. In systemic vascular beds, neutrophils are slowed relative to erythrocytes, but in contrast to the pulmonary circulation, this is accomplished by their rolling along the walls of post-capillary venules [4]. The factors that induce initial retention of neutrophils are also under different control mechanisms in the two circulations. The neutrophil has an average diameter of 8 μm, compared with a mean diameter of the pulmonary capillary of 5.5 μm. Thus, the neutrophil must deform in order to transit the lung. Neutrophils are fairly deformable at rest, but respond to chemoattractants so as to become considerably more stiff [5]. In addition, the size and stiffness of the other circulating leukocytes, monocytes and lymphocytes may also regulate the circulatory behavior of unstimulated cells [6].

The increase in stiffness consequent upon chemoattractant stimulation of neutrophils is accounted for largely by induction of cytoskeletal assembly and is accompanied by a redistribution of actin. The cells simultaneously express increased numbers of adhesion related glycoproteins, which may also contribute to the retention of these cells within the pulmonary microvasculature. Increased neutrophil adhesiveness has been demonstrated in response to C5a [7], tumor nucrosis factor (TNF) [8], interleukin (IL)-1 [9] and lipopolysaccharide (LPS) [10]. Neutrophils from patients with a deficiency of β_2 integrins do not adhere to the endothelium [11]. Only a few studies have directly assessed the role of adhesion molecules in neutrophil sequestration *in vivo*. These studies suggest that antibodies directed against the common β chain of the Mac-1, LFA-1, P150,95 family (CD11/CD18) can materially diminish neutrophil retention in skin [12] and gut [13], but appear to have less effect within the pulmonary microvasculature. Whether these data reflect an important role for the mechanical properties of the leukocyte, a different set of adhesion related molecules, or a fundamentally different endothelial surface in the lung compared to with systemic vascular beds, remains unclear but attempts to resolve this issue promise to yield a vigorous and constructive debate for several years.

A number of other features may modify neutrophil retention within the pulmonary microcirculation, in particular the expression of endothelial cell derived adhesion molecules. Treatment of endothelial cells with LPS [9], TNF [14], or IL-1 [15] results in enhanced adhesion due to upregulation of endothelial cell derived adhesion molecules. The relative importance of increased neutrophil versus endothelial adherence is not yet known in any *in vivo* system. However, the adherence of neutrophils occurs very rapidly [16,17], whereas the maximal endothelial response can take as long as 4–6 hours (see below). The endothelium is, however, capable of rapid responses due to generation of chemoattractants [18] and upregulation of readyformed adhesion molecules such as P-selectin [19]. Thus, the resulting adhesive interaction is regulated with respect to time,

intensity and cell specificity by both cell types.

Several different families of adhesion molecules have been identified, including the cellular adhesion molecule (CAM) members of the immunoglobulin superfamily (ICAM-1 [20], -2, and -3 (these latter two have not been implicated in neutrophil adherence), VCAM-1 [21] and PECAM-1 [22] and the members of the selectin family (E-selectin, P-selectin, L-selectin) and it is likely that more will be forthcoming. The identity of the cognate ligands on the neutrophil identified by these molecules is the subject of considerable controversy. ICAM-1 appears to interact with CD11a/CD18 (LFA-1) and CD11b/CD18 (Mac-1) on the surface of the neutrophil [23], while at least some selectins interact with sialated Lewis^x (sial-Le^x) [24,25] displayed on surface molecules. More recent studies indicate the ligands may be more complex [26].

Although the patterns of expression of adhesion molecules is complex, it is clear that they have significant effects on neutrophil sequestration, particularly after the initial deformability. Recent studies have begun to dissect the relative roles of these molecules in pulmonary inflammatory responses. In inflammation induced in rat lungs by immune complexes, CD11a (but not CD11b), L-selectin, and ICAM-1 appear important in regulating the accumulation of neutrophils from the vascular compartment. By contrast, CD11b and ICAM-1 appear important in regulating neutrophil appearance in the airway compartment, and in manifestations of lung injury, linked perhaps to induction of TNF expression [27].

It would appear that neutrophil sequestration *per se* in the pulmonary capillary bed is not necessarily associated with lung injury. For example, in a rabbit model of complement fragment induced lung injury there was no change in pulmonary permeability nor apparent tissue injury associated with neutrophil sequestration [28]. Furthermore, intratracheal instillation of CD11b blocks the injurious consequences of immune complexes whilst exerting no effect on neutrophil sequestration [27]. However, if initial retention occurs by mechanisms other than adherence, it remains possible that adherence is a critical prelude to injury. From *in vitro* studies it is known that activated neutrophils can cause endothelial damage, even in the absence of adherence, through the release of toxic mediators including oxidants and elastase [29]. However, in patients with leukocyte glycoprotein deficiency whose neutrophils neither adhere nor migrate localized inflammation/injury is not seen [11], suggesting that adherence is necessary.

REGULATION OF NEUTROPHIL MIGRATION

To reach the alveolus from the vascular space, cells must migrate through the vascular endothelium, basement membrane and alveolar epithelium. The route passes almost exclusively along the thick segment of the alveolar capillary membrane rather than the thin one [30], but the actual mechanism remains unclear. *In vitro* neutrophils migrate through endothelial monolayers without the addition of exogenous stimuli [31], a phenomenon not seen with fibroblast, smooth muscle or epithelial monolayers. This suggests that the endothelium may actually facilitate neutrophil migration, which is believed, based on ultrastructural examination, to occur between the endothelial cells [32]. The early notion that the endothelium participates in the migratory process has recently been given a molecular basis. The demonstration that ICAM-1 upregulation [33] on the endothelial cell, particularly in the context of coexpression of E-selectin [34], actively facilitates neutrophil migration across the endothelial cell and into the subendothelial spaces, indicates that upregulation may underlie certain migratory events *in vivo* and suggests new ways that migration may be regulated.

Once neutrophils are in the interstitium, migration may be regulated by external factors, such as the intensity of the chemoattractant gradient and cell motility. In the course of quantifying the inflammatory response to C5a in the lung, the volume of neutrophils in the lung has been measured using serial 0.5 μm sections and three dimensional reconstruction [35]. Neutrophils reconstructed within the vascular space, either in arterioles (158 μm^3), capillaries (128 μm^3) or venules (128 μm^3) were of similar volume, while those in the air space were markedly larger (266 μm^3). Neutrophils that had migrated into the abdominal wall (150 μm^3) were also significantly larger than those in the abdominal wall vasculature (100 μm^3). These increases in volume are much greater than the increase in volume ($\sim 15\%$) that neutrophils undergo when stimulated in suspension [36]. The much larger increase observed *in vivo* suggested that the process might have significance in the biology of the leukocyte and in the inflammatory process.

A major component of the volume response of neutrophils in suspension appears to be due to activation of the Na^+/H^+ antiport (NHE), a ubiquitous family of molecules that migrate as 110 kDa glycoproteins on sodium dodecyl sulfate (SDS) gels [37]. These transporters catalyze the electroneutral exchange of one Na^+ for one H^+. Amiloride and its analogs appear to bind without being transported, inhibiting exchange. There is an apparent allosteric modifier site for H^+ on the cytoplasmic portion that activates exchange when the cytoplasm is acidified. Under resting conditions, Na^+/H^+ exchange is nearly inactive and the induction of exchange requires activation. A major role of the exchanger appears to be in response to imposed shrinking. Activation of exchange leads to a one-for-one exchange of H^+ for Na^+ that increases cell volume because the proton disequilibrium is converted into a bicarbonate disequilibrium through action of Cl^-/HCO_3^- exchange (Figure 8.2). The net result is entry of osmotically active NaCl, followed by

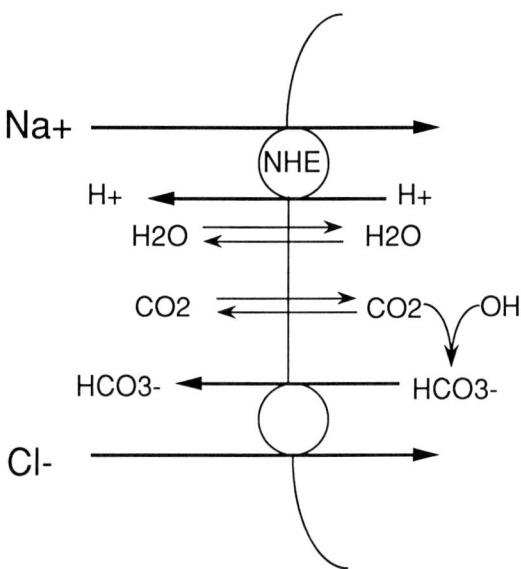

Figure 8.2 Mechanism by which Na^+/H^+ exchange (NHE) (top) coupled with Cl^-/HCO_3^- exchange (bottom) results in net movement of NaCl into the cell, followed by water entry. Interconversion of CO_2, H_2O, OH^-, and HCO_3^- are catalyzed by carbonic anhydrase in the cytoplasm.

water. Inhibitors of the antiport, such as amiloride and its analogs, therefore block both volume change and alkalinization.

The idea that activation of the antiport might be important in migration is supported by a positive correlation between the amount of intracellular alkalinization induced by formyl-met-leu-phe (FMLP) and the distance moved by a neutrophil in response to a chemotactic radiant [38]. Since amiloride and its analogs inhibit chemotaxis as well as cytoplasmic alkalinization [39], these experiments suggest important relationships between the Na^+/H^+ antiport, alkalinization and chemotaxis. If intracellular alkalinization is also considered to reflect the extent of sodium entry [40] (and hence the magnitude of the volume increase), such data suggest that the magnitude of the volume increase may regulate the extent of chemotaxis [41]. Similarly, intracellular pH has been shown to regulate or mod-

ulate the generation of superoxide and ion by human neutrophils [39].

Neutrophil granulocytes undergo substantial shape changes from the round, resting state to a complex polarized phenotype while migrating, which has made assessment of volume difficult. We measured cell volume changes in neutrophils migrating toward the chemotactic agent FMLP in collagen gels, using optical sectioning on a confocal microscope and three dimensional reconstruction. Migrating neutrophils displayed a significant volume increase of 35–60%. The cell swelling depended on sodium/proton antiport activity, which was abrogated by amiloride and dimethylamiloride, inhibitors of the antiport, and by substitution of sodium in the buffers by choline, which is not transported by the antiport. The volume increase appeared to facilitate neutrophil migration, as indicated by two lines of evidence. (1) Hypo-osmolar swelling enhanced, and hyperosmolar shrinking decreased, neutrophil migration toward FMLP in Boyden chambers. (2) Sodium/ proton antiport inhibitors decreased the extent of neutrophil migration in a fashion that was overcome in hypotonic buffers, which induced a volume increase similar to that seen in normal migrating cells. Hence, the volume increase associated with migration may be essential for optimal migration, suggesting that activation of the antiport is an important step in the signaling pathways used to initiate migration.

Several studies now link phosphorylation of the antiport to activation of protein kinase (PKC) by phorbol myristate acetate (PMA) [37] and/or inhibition of phosphatase 1 and 2A by okadaic acid [42]. However, none of these studies has been done in neutrophils, and most have involved non-physiologic circumstances. The finding that the antiport is activated by addition of okadaic acid, a purportedly specific phosphatase inhibitor, implies that one or more (currently unidentified) kinases are constitutively active in otherwise unstimulated cells. Since phosphatases 1 and 2A are generally regarded as typical P-Ser P-Thr phosphatases, the relevant kinase would be expected to be a serine/theronine kinase. Indeed, serine is the sole residue of the antiport phosphorylated by epidermal growth factor and thrombin in cultured cells [37]. Because the Na^+/H^+ antiport appears to be the target of multiple signaling pathways, including those activated by tyrosine kinase receptors and by G protein coupled phosphoinositide (PI) metabolism, this suggests convergence of the pathways on a common site.

REGULATION OF THE INJURIOUS POTENTIAL OF INFLAMMATORY CELLS

The migration of the neutrophil into the alveolus is not always associated with injury. Thus, neutrophil migration into the lungs of sheep induced by leukotriene (LT)B_4 was associated with no change in epithelial permeability [43]. What regulates the ability of the neutrophil to produce injury during, or perhaps after, its arrival in the alveolar compartment? Three major classes of injurious molecules are produced by inflammatory cells – oxygen metabolites, proteases and cations – but other toxic materials may eventually be identified. Amphipathic lipids may well be injurious, but have not received major emphasis, perhaps because they would also be toxic to the cell that produced them. This latter feature is of interest in that the inflammatory cell itself seems relatively resistant to its own toxic products – presumably an important feature in its primary role of host defence.

Toxic materials are secreted/released from inflammatory cells in a regulated fashion. Prior to the 1970s it was generally thought that inflammatory cells such as neutrophils released their contents during the process of lysis and destruction at the inflammatory site. While this certainly happens, particularly at points of infection with strains of bacteria that produce cytocidal toxins, it is now recognized that inflammatory cells actively secrete their contents, and like many other secretory processes this is inducible and under cellular control.

Neutrophil secretory products fall into three major categories: the contents of granules, lipid 'mediators' and oxygen metabolites. The azurophil granules contain acid hydrolases, elastase and many of the potentially toxic cations, and function in many regards like classical lysosomes. The neutrophil 'specific' granules, on the other hand, contain materials that tend to act at neutral pH and have been considered to serve as typical secretory granules [44]. Thus, discharge of the contents of these two organelles is under different control and probably occurs by different mechanisms [45,46]. Specific granules (and related storage structures) appear to discharge directly at the cell surface (exocytosis) and are released either to the outside or to the phagosome earlier than are the azurophil granules [47,48].

While it is well accepted that products contained within granules are secreted in a regulated fashion, it is less clear for other injurious products. Oxygen metabolites are thought to be produced at the cell surface itself, but may pass through anion channels (which are subject to regulation) in the membrane to gain access to the outside of the cell [49]. Lipid mediators have been assumed to diffuse passively, despite abundant evidence that many require protein carriers for transit through aqueous media. Recently, evidence points toward another level of regulation of movement of lipid mediators, such as platelet activating factor (PAF), across cell membranes. Bidirectional movement of PAF across both neutrophil and erythrocyte membranes is facilitated by the membrane becoming symmetrical [50,51]. Thus, release of lipid mediators that insert in the membrane may be enhanced by the membrane events that accompany stimulation, a glimpse into a much more complex view of the disposition of these molecules. This distinction between regulated secretion and passive lysis as a source of injurious materials is potentially important from a therapeutic perspective. Understanding the mechanisms involved in the secretory process would then allow the design of appropriate modulating agents.

PRIMING

Under some circumstances neutrophils can migrate into the lung without producing significant damage [28,52], although at other times great structural alteration ensues [53]. In an analogous fashion, neutrophil accumulation is sometimes considered to be the cause of disease (as in ARDS), and sometimes to be associated only with protection and to be followed by normal recovery of structure and functions (as in pneumonia). A potential explanation for these anomalies lies in the phenomenon of priming. Neutrophils (and most other inflammatory cells) can be raised to a heightened state of responsiveness by prior exposure to a stimulus which does not itself initiate the function in question. First shown for superoxide anion production [54] the prototypic priming agent was bacterial LPS. It is now appreciated that a wide variety of molecules can induce this altered responsivity, including PAF [55], TNF [56], granulocyte-macrophage colony stimulating factor (GM-CSF)[57], and agents typically viewed as triggering agents, such as IL-8 [58]. The cellular responses that are enhanced include secretion, adhesiveness and a number of synthetic functions. The nature of the secondary stimulus that actually induces the cell response (FMLP, C5a or immune complexes are often used experimentally) seems less important, suggesting that the primed cell responds in a stereotypical fashion to many triggering stimuli. It seems clear that complete neutrophil activation requires both steps (priming and stimulation), even if they both occur simultaneously and therefore cannot be independently detected.

An example of priming for cytotoxic effects is the destruction of cultured endothelial cells by neutrophils when stimulated with LPS and C5a together, but not by either agent alone [59]. In the context of a 'normal' inflammatory response, it is possible that neutrophils emigrate into the lung solely under the influence of chemotactic factors, but because they are not previously primed, secrete little of their contents, perhaps just enough to accomplish the emigration itself. Encountering bacteria and/or cytokines in the inflamed alveolus, the cells would undergo priming and the appropriate heightened responses required for removal of the infectious agents. If, however, neutrophils are primed before or during the emigration phase, injury to the tissues through which they migrate would ensue. Certainly, concurrent intravascular injections of LPS and chemoattractants were able to induce neutrophil dependent increases in pulmonary vascular leakage of albumin that were not evident with either stimulus alone [60]. In addition, interactions that less clearly involve stimulation, such as adherence [61], treatment with membrane perturbing agents and proteases [62], have all been demonstrated to enhance stimulation, particularly of oxidase.

ACTIVATION OF THE NADPH OXIDASE

Generation of superoxide anion (O_2^-) (Chapter 11) is the initial step in the synthesis of a variety of toxic oxidant products, including H_2O_2, OH, and hypochlorous acid involved in mediation of the injurious effects of neutrophils. Superoxide is generated by an NADPH oxidase, a multicomponent enzyme system whose assembly is regulated, at least in part, by both phosphorylation and the action of rac low molecular weight G proteins [63]. One observed effect of priming agents is to shorten the lag time between stimulation and production of O_2^-, whilst also increasing the initial rate and magnitude of the response [54]. While the molecular mechanisms of assembly of the oxidase are well understood, in part at least because of chronic granulomatous disease, those responsible for the enhanced responsiveness seen in primed cells remain uncertain.

STIMULATED EICOSANOID PRODUCTION

Arachidonic acid metabolites resulting from the action of 5-lipoxygenase, including LTB$_4$ and 5-hydroxyeicosotetraenoic acid (5-HETE), are released from neutrophils after stimulation [64–66]. These metabolites, particularly LTB$_4$, are potent neutrophil stimuli and may provide a paracrine loop to stimulate other leukocytes. As is the case with the oxidase, neutrophils stimulated directly with chemoattractants show a very limited capacity for synthesis of LTB$_4$. Once primed, however, neutrophil synthesis of LTB$_4$ increases quite significantly. Synthesis of LTB$_4$ requires arachidonic acid (AA) (whose release from phospholipids through the action of phospholipase may be regulated by microtubule associated protein (MAP) kinase, see below).

MECHANISMS OF PRIMING

The response of neutrophils to chemotactic stimuli reflects interaction with seven-transmembrane-spanning, G-protein linked receptors, of which the FMLP receptor is a prototype [67]. A variety of studies link ligand interaction with the FMLP receptor to activation of phospholipases [68], by mechanisms that are sensitive to pertussis toxin, and hence ascribed to involvement of G$_{i2}$[69]. Although the best described G$_i$ linked response is inhibition of adenylate cyclase [70], the a subunit of G$_i$ may activate ion channels [71] and induce mitogenesis [72]. Additionally, βγ subunits may regulate specific isoforms of phospholipase Cβ (PLCβ) [73]. Activation of PLCβ, which leads to generation of diacylglycerol, has been shown to activate PKC. Thus a variety of downstream events have been modeled by stimulation of

the cell with phorbol esters which directly activate PKC. Despite the undoubted relevance of these pathways to neutrophil activation, the events downstream of G$_{i2}$ remain obscure, and hence make unraveling mechanisms of priming difficult.

ROLE OF PKC IN PRIMING

A role for PKC in priming for O$_2^-$ can be adduced by the following: PMA, a potent activator of PKC, primes in low concentrations [74,75]. Elevations in diglyceride that may activate PKC appear to correlate with O$_2^-$ production, and some PKC inhibitors block priming by both PMA and TNF [76]. A series of persuasive reports by Bass and colleagues, however, have argued that the straightforward interpretation is oversimplified. Firstly, priming of neutrophils with diacylglycerols that activate PKC was not inhibited by a potent PKC antagonist, and the priming occurred at concentrations of alkylacylglycerol (AAG) that did not induce PKC translocation [77]. Secondly, priming for initiation of the respiratory burst [78] or for AA release [79] could be induced by ether acyl glycerides that were much less potent in activation of PKC. These studies suggest that at least some responses could be primed in a PKC independent fashion. However, it remains possible that particular PKC isoforms participate in a way not readily detectable. In addition, some functional responses, in particular prologation of the oxidase response, and activation of 5-hypoxygenase, were not primed by ether acyl glycerides, but were by AAGs. Furthermore, priming with PMA was associated with a reduction in PI breakdown, but an enhanced generation of diglycerides, indicating that the traditional PI-PLC is not the sole target of priming, and implicating production of diglyderides as an important component in the primed cell [75]. Others, however, have not been able to detect increased diglyceride levels after priming with TNF and stimulation with FMLP [80].

Another source of diglycerides in the neutrophil is phospholipase D, which generates, as one of its actions, phosphatidic acid. Although progress has been hampered by lack of a molecular description of this activity, it is clear from several reports that production of phosphatidic acid is enhanced in the stimulated cell after priming. This mechanism has been implicated in priming by TNF [80] and GM-CSF [81] and may directly stimulate the NADPH oxidase [82].

ROLE OF Ca²⁺ IN PRIMING

While chemoattractant stimuli induce a calcium transient, and calcium may be necessary for expression of the functions being primed, whether calcium is necessary for priming remains controversial. Thus, thapsigargin which induces a sustained elevation in Ca^{2+} can prime, but some priming stimuli induce no increase in intracellular Ca^{2+} [83]. Priming appears to occur in the absence of extracellular calcium, but some reports indicate that chelation of intracellular Ca^{2+} attenuates priming, while others do not [84]. It seems likely that some priming stimuli (such as PAF) require a certain level of Ca^{2+}, but may not necessarily involve the traditional stimulus induced transient.

Attempts to conceptualize these events into a coherent theory of priming have not so far been revealing. Recent increments in our understanding of pathways by which the neutrophil responds to stimulation, however, permit another approach. The recognition that the Ras-Raf MAP kinase pathway [85,86] is activated in neutrophils following stimulation by FMLP suggests clues to pathways activated by this and other chemoattractants.

PATHWAYS TO MAP KINASE (Figure 8.3)

Kinase pathways that include MAP kinases exist in cells of mammalian, amphibian and yeast ancestries, testifying to the remarkable evolutionary retention of this pathway [87].

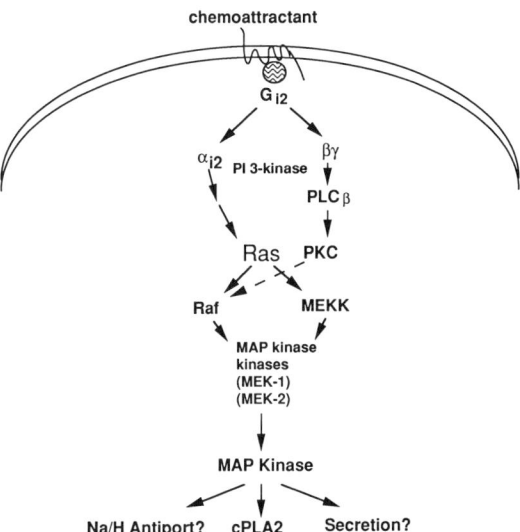

Figure 8.3 Signaling pathways used in response to chemoattractants in the neutrophil. The relative roles of the MAP kinase kinases Raf and MEKK remain unclear. Although MEK-1 and -2 are shown here, it is likely that other MEKs are awaiting discovery, and may serve to enforce specificity of pathways. Thus, while we indicate MAP kinase inducing a multiplicity of endpoints, it is again likely that other MAP kinases will be shown to be principally involved in these responses. The site at which priming acts is unknown.

MAP kinases are serine/threonine kinases phosphorylating and activating proteins such as Rsk90 [88], $cPLA_2$ [89] and cMyc [90]. Thus, analysis of the activation of MAP kinase and its related family members may provide clues to activation of $cPLA_2$ and AA release. MAP kinase activation requires phosphorylation on tyrosine and threonine residues [91], induced by a multifunctional MAP kinase kinase, or MEK (MAP ERK kinase), which itself is activated by phosphorylation [92]. Hence, elucidation of pathways leading to MEK activation may provide insight into upstream events.

Recent evidence suggests the existence of several pathways to activation of MEK, including a recently cloned MEKK [93], but the best delineated pathway uses the low molecular weight G-protein Ras to activate the kinase Raf which phosphorylates MEK in response to tyrosine kinase linked receptors [88]. In recent studies, both FMLP and C5a induced G_i dependent activation of Ras and Raf in the human neutrophil [94,95].

The recent flurry of reports implicating Raf as an important inhibitory target for cyclic AMP (cAMP) dependent kinase (PKA) [96–98] suggests that activation of PKA may reveal the importance of Raf activation. Thus, cell-permanent analogs of cAMP potently but transiently inhibited Raf activation by FMLP or C5a in neutrophils. Maneuvers that elevate intracellular cAMP attenuate actin assembly [94], chemotaxis [100], adherence [101], O_2^- secretion [102] and liberation of arachidonic acid [103]. This latter response is particularly noteworthy, as the cytosolic phospholipase A_2 is phosphorylated and activated by MAP kinase [89]. While not discounting the potential for other sites of action of cAMP and cAMP dependent protein kinase, these results suggest that inhibition of Raf activation interferes with neutrophil function, and that Raf may play a critical role in the transduction of such functions. Hence, the regulation of MAP kinase pathways in cells such as the neutrophil is predicted to play at least a modulatory role in specific differentiated functions, including chemotaxis and secretion.

INJURY ON A SURFACE

Once the primed and activated neutrophil is in contact with a surface, such as the vascular endothelium, the surface provides a localized site for cell secretion that may be shielded from the protective actions of plasma or tissue inhibitors. For example, the injury of endothelial cells by primed and stimulated neutrophils was unaffected by the presence of either plasma or α_1-antiprotease inhibitor, even though it was shown to be dependent on the expression of neutrophil elastase and the direct effect of purified elastase on the endothelial cells was clearly blocked by both. Three phenomena may explain this apparent discrepancy. Neutrophils apparently retain some of the elastase they 'secrete' on the plasma membrane [104] in a manner analogous to phosphatase as ectoenzymes after exocytosis of the granule [105]. This would result in application of the toxic enzyme at the point of surface stimulation of the cell and would concentrate it at that site. Secondly, local concentrations of injurious materials may be very high between the inflammatory cell and its target. Levels of H_2O_2 for example have been suggested to reach 10^{-2} mol/l [61]. Thirdly, the interaction between a stimulated inflammatory cell and its surface target seems to be tight enough to exclude protein molecules such as α_1-antiprotease [106]. Similar effects might be expected for neutrophils encountering connective tissue surfaces during migration across the interstitium. Finally, it has been appreciated for many years that neutrophils secrete more constituents when adherent [105], a phenomenon usually thought to be related to the normal phagolysosome fusion in a circumstance where the 'particle' to be phagocytosed is in fact the whole surface – a process called, colloquially, frustrated phagocytosis. The enhanced stimulation under these circumstances has been recently re-emphasized for neutrophils [61], where, under appropriate circumstances, stimuli that would not be triggers, such as GM and G-CSF, may serve as triggers of O_2^- secretion [107]. Thus, the mechanisms by which the primed cell in suspension responds with enhanced secretion are mimicked by a surface, likely representing interaction with specific receptors either on the cellular substatum or connective tissue. Elucidation of the mechanisms involved in these seemingly disparate responses is likely to greatly increase our understanding of the behavior of the neutrophil in pathophysiological processes.

ACKNOWLEDGEMENTS

The authors work was supported by grants (HL 40478 and HL30324) from the National Institutes of Health and from the MRC of Canada. The authors gratefully acknowledge the editorial assistance of Nina Eads.

REFERENCES

1. Lien, D.C., Wagner, W.W., Capen, R.L., *et al.* (1987) Physiologic neutrophil sequestration in the canine pulmonary circulation: evidence for localization in capillaries. *J. Appl. Physiol.*, **62**, 1236–43.

2. Lien, D.C., Worthen, G.S., Capen, R., *et al.* (1990) Neutrophil kinetics in the pulmonary microcirculation: effects of pressure and flow in the dependent lung. *Am. Rev. Respir. Dis.*, **141**, 953–9.

3. Lien, D.C., Worthen, G.S., Henson, P.M. and Bethel, R.A. (1992) Platelet-activating factor causes neutrophil accumulation and neutrophil-mediated increased vascular permeability in canine trachea. *Am. Rev. Respir. Dis.*, **145**, 693–700.

4. Schmid-Schonbein, G.W., Usami, S., Skalak, R. and Chien, S. (1980) Interaction of leukocytes and erythrocytes in capillary and post-capillary vessels. *Microvasc. Res.*, **19**, 45–70.

5. Worthen, G.S., Schwab, B., Elson, E.L. and Downey, G.P. (1989) Mechanics of stimulated neutrophils: cell stiffening induces retention in capillaries. *Science*, **245**, 183–5.

6. Downey, G.P., Chan, C.K., Lea, P. *et al.* (1992) Phorbol ester-induced actin assembly in neutrophils: role of protein kinase C. *J. Cell. Biol.*, **116**, 695–706.

7. Tonnesen, M.G., Anderson, D.C., Springer, T.A. *et al.* (1989) Adherence of neutrophils to cultured human microvascular endothelial cells: stimulation by chemotactic peptides and lipid mediator, and dependence on the Mac-1, LFA-1, p150,95 glycoprotein family. *J. Clin. Invest.*, **74**, 1581–92.

8. Kownatzki, E., Kapp, A. and Uhrich, S. (1988) Modulation of human neutrophil functions by recombinant human tumor necrosis factor and recombinant human lymphotoxin: promotion of adherence, inhibition of chemotactic migration and superoxide anion release from adherent cells. *Clin. Exp. Immunol.*, **74**, 143–8.

9. Pohlman, T.H., Stanness, K.A., Beatty, B.G. *et al.* (1986) An endothelial cell surface factor(s) induced *in vitro* by lipopolysaccharide, interleukin-8, and tumor necrosis factor increases neutrophil adherence by CDW18-dependent mechanism. *J. Immunol.*, **130**, 4548–53.

10. Worthen, G.S., Avdi, N., Vukajlovich, S. and Tobias, P.S. (1993) Neutrophil adherence induced by lipopolysaccharide *in vitro*: role of plasma component interaction with lipopolysaccharide. *J. Clin. Invest.*, **90**, 2526–35.

11. Anderson, D.C. and Springer, T.A. (1987) Leukocyte adhesion deficiency: an inherited defect in the Mac-1, LFA-1, and p150,95 glycoproteins. *Ann. Rev. Med.*, **38**, 175–94.

12. Doerschuk, C.M., Winn, R.K., Coxson, H.O. *et al.* (1990) CD18-dependent and independent mechanisms of nuetrophil emigration in the pulmonary and systemic microcirculation of rabbits. *J. Immunol.*, **144**, 2327–33.

13. Vedder, N.B., Winn, R.K., Rice, C.L. *et al.* (1988) A monoclonal antibody to the adherence-promoting leukocyte glycoprotein, CD18, reduces organ injury and improves survivial from hemorrhagic shock and resuscitation in rabbits. *J. Clin. Invest.*, **81**, 939–44.

14. Gamble, J.R., Harlan, J.M., Klebanoff, S.J. *et al.* (1985) Stimulation of the adherence of neutrophils to umbilical vein endothelium by human recombinant tumor necrosis factor. *Proc. Natl Acad. Sci. USA.*, **82**, 8667–74.

15. Bevilacqua, M.P., Pober, J.S., Wheeler, M.E. *et al.* (1985) Interleukin-1 acts on cultured human vascular endothelium to increase the adhesion of polymorphonuclear leukocytes, monocytes, and related leukocyte cell lines. *J. Clin. Invest.*, **76**, 2003–11.

16. Harlan, J.E., Hajduk, P.J., Yoon, H.S. and Fesik, S.W. (1994) Pleckstrin homology domains bind to phosphatidylinositol-4,5-bisphosphate. *Nature*, **371**, 168–70.

17. Tonnesen, M.G., Smedley, L. and Henson, P.M. (1984) Neutrophil-endothelial cell interactions: modulation of neutrophil adhesiveness induced by complement fragments C5a and C5a des arg and formyl-methionyl-leucyl-phenylalanine (FMLP) *in vitro*. *J. Clin. Invest.*, **74**, 1581–92.

18. Zimmermann, A., Keller, H.U. and Cottier, H. (1988) Heavy water (D_2O)-induced shape changes, movements and F-actin redistribu-

tion in human neutrophil granulocytes. *Eur. J. Cell. Biol.*, **47**, 320–6.

19. Geng, J.G., Bevilacqua, M.P., Moore, K.L. *et al.* (1990) Rapid neutrophil adhesion to activated endothelium mediated by GMP-140. *Nature*, **343**, 757–9.

20. Staunton, D.E., Marlin, S.D., Stratowa, C. *et al.* (1988) Primary structure of intercellular adhesion molecule 1 (ICAM-1) demonstrates interaction between members of the immunoglobulin and integrin supergene families. *Cell*, **52**, 925–33.

21. Osborn, L., Hession, C., Tizard, R. *et al.* (1989) Direct expression cloning of vascular adhesion molecule 1: a cytokine induced endothelial protein that binds to lymphocytes. *Cell*, **59**, 1203–11.

22. Newman, L.S. (1990) Dyspnea with diffuse interstitial infiltrates and hilar adenopathy, in *Pulmonary Grand Rounds*, (ed. M. Schwarz), B.C. Decker, Philadelphia, pp.44–52.

23. Smith, C.W., Macklin, S.D., Rothlein, R. *et al.* (1989) Cooperative interaction of LFA-1 and Mac-1 with intercellular adhesion molecule-1 in facilitating adherence and transendothelial migration of human neutrophils *in vitro. J. Clin. Invest.*, **83**, 2008–17.

24. Phillips, M.L., Nudelman, E., Gaeta, F.C.A. *et al.* (1990) ELAM-1 mediates cell adhesion by recognition of a carbohydrate ligand, sialle. *Science*, **250**, 1130–2.

25. Walz, G.A., Aruffo, A., Kolanus, W. *et al.* (1990) Recognition by ELAM-1 of the sial-le^x. *Science*, **250**, 1132–5.

26. Moore, K.L., Eaton, S.F., Lyons, D.E. *et al.* (1994) The P-selectin glycoprotein ligand from human neutrophils displays sialylated, fucosylated, O-linked poly-*n*-acetyl lactosamine. *J. Biol. Chem.*, **269**, 23318–27.

27. Mulligan, M.S., Vaporciyan, A.A., Warner, R.L. *et al.* (1995) Compartmentalized roles for leukocytic adhesion molecules in lung inflammatory injury. *J. Immunol.*, **154**, 1350–63.

28. Webster, R.O., Larsen, G.L., Mitchell, B.C. *et al.* (1982) Absence of inflammatory injury in rabbits challenged intravascularly with complement-derived chemotactic factors. *Am. Rev. Respir. Dis.*, **125**, 335–40.

29. Worthen, G.S., Henson, P.M., Henson, J.E. and Rees, A.J.. (1987) Mechanisms of vascular injury, in *Diseases of the Kidney*, 4th edn (eds R.W. Schrier and C.W. Gottschalk), Little Brown, Boston, pp. 2225–2252.

30. Parsons, P.E., Worthen, G.S. and Henson, P.M. (1991) Injury from inflammatory cells, in *Lung Injury* (eds R.G. Crystal and J.B. West), Raven Press, New York, pp. 221–31.

31. Beesley, J.E., Pearson, J.D, Carleton, J.S. *et al.* (1978) Interaction of leukocytes with vascular cells in culture. *J. Cell Sci.*, **33**, 85–101.

32. Marchesi, V.T. and Florey, H.W. (1960) Electron micrographic observations on the emigration of leukocytes. *Q. J. Exp. Physiol.*, **45**, 343–8.

33. Smith, C.W., Rothlein, R., Hughes, B.J. *et al.* (1988) Recognition of an endothelial determinant for CD18-dependent human neutrophil adherence and transendothelial migration. *J. Clin. Invest.*, **82**, 1746–56.

34. Luscinskas, F.W., Cybulsky, M.I., Kiely, J.M. *et al.* (1991) Cytokine-activated human endothelial monolayers support enhanced neutrophil transmigration via a mechanism involving both endothelial – leukocyte adhesion molecule-1 and intercellular adhesion molecule-1. *J. Immunol.*, **146**, 1617–25.

35. Worthen, G.S., Henson, P.M., Rosengren, S. *et al.* (1994) Neutrophils increase volume during migration *in vivo* and *in vitro. Am. J. Respir. Cell Mol. Biol.*, **10** 1–7.

36. Grinstein, S., Furuya, W. and Cragoe, E.J. Jr, (1986) Volume changes in activated human neutrophils: the role of Na$^+$/H$^+$ exchange. *J. Cell. Physiol.*, **128**, 33–40.

37. Sardet, C., Counillon, O., Franchi, A. and Pouyssegur, J. (1990) Growth factors induce phosphorylation of the Na$^+$/H$^+$ antiporter, glycoprotein of 110 kD. *Science*, **247**, 723–6.

38. Simchowitz, L. and Cragoe, E.J. Jr (1986) Regulation of human neutrophil chemotaxis by intracellular pH. *J. Biol. Chem.*, **261**, 6492–500.

39. Simchowitz, L. (1985) Intracellular pH modulates the generation of superoxide radicals by human neutrophils. *J. Clin. Invest.*, **76**, 1079.

40. Simchowitz, L. (1985) Chemotactic factor-induced activation of the Na$^+$/H$^+$ exchange in human neutrophils I. Sodium fluxes. *J. Biol. Chem.*, **260**, 13237–48.

41. Rosengren, S., Henson, P.M. and Worthen, G.S. (1994) Migration-associated volume changes in neutrophils facilitate the migratory process. *Am. J. Physiol.*, **267** C1623–32.

42. Bianchini, L., Woodside, M., Sardet, C. *et al.* (1991) Okadaic acid, a phosphatase inhibitor,

induces activation and phosphorylation of the Na^+/H^+ antiport. *J. Biol. Chem.,* **299**, 15406–13.

43. Staub, N.C., Schultz, E.L., Koike, K. and Albertine, K.H. (1985) Effect of neutrophil migration induced by leukotriene B_4 on protein permeability in sheep lung. *Fed. Proc.,* **44**, 30–5.

44. Gallin J.I. (1981) Abnormal phagocyte chemotaxis: pathophysiology, clinical manifestations, and management of patients. *Rev. Infect. Dis.,* **3**, 1196–220.

45. Lew, P.D., Monod, A., Waldvogel, F.A. *et al.* (1986) Quantitative analysis of the cytosolic free calcium dependency of exocytosis from three subcellular compartments in intact human neutrophils. *J. Cell Biol.,* **102**, 2197–204.

46. Wright, D.G. and Gallin, J.I. (1979) Secretory responses of human neutrophils: exocytosis of specific (secretory) granules by human neutrophils during adherence *in vitro* and during exudation *in vivo. J. Immunol.,* **123**, 284–94.

47. Bainton, D.F. (1973) Sequential degranulation of the two types of polymorphonuclear leukocyte granules during phagocytosis of microorganisms. *J. Cell Biol.,* **58**, 249–64.

48. Henson, P.M. (1971) The immunologic release of constituents from neutrophil leukocytes. II. Mechanisms of release during phagocytosis and adherence to nonphagocytosable surfaces. *J. Immunol.,* **107**, 1547–57.

49. Lynch, R.E. and Fridovich, I. (1978) Permeation of the erythrocyte stroma by superoxide radical. *J. Biol. Chem.,* **253**, 4697–9.

50. Bratton, D.L., Kailey, J.M., Clay, K.L. and Henson, P.M. (1991) A model for the extracellular release of PAF: the influence of plasma membrane phospholipid asymmetry. *Biochim. Biophys. Acta,* **1062**, 24–34.

51. Bratton, D.L. (1993) Release of platelet activating factor from activated neutrophils: transglutaminase-dependent enhancement of transbilayer movement across the plasma membrane. *J. Biol. Chem.,* **268**, 3364–73.

52. Meyrick, B., Hoffman, L.H. and Brigham, K.L. Chemotaxis of granulocytes across bovine pulmonary artery intimal explants without endothelial cell injury. *Tissue Cell,* **16**, 1–16.

53. Bachofen, M. and Weibel, E.R. (1982) Structural alterations of the lung parenchyma in the adult respiratory distress syndrome. *Clin. Chest Med.,* **3**, 35–56.

54. Guthrie, L.A., McPhail, L.C., Henson, P.M. and Johnston R.B. Jr (1984) The priming of neutrophils for enhanced release of oxygen metabolites by bacterial lipopolysaccharide: evidence for increased activity of the superoxide-producing enzyme. *J. Exp. Med.,* **160**, 1656–71.

55. Worthen, G.S., Seccombe, J.F., Guthrie, L.A. *et al.* (1988) Priming of neutrophils by lipopolysaccharide for enhanced production of platelet-activating factor: potential role in mediation of enhanced superoxide secretion. *J. Immunol.,* **140**, 3553–9.

56. Berkow, R.L., Wang, D., Larrick, J.W. *et al.* (1987) Enhancement of neutrophil superoxide production by preincubation with recombinant human tumor necrosis factor. *J. Immunol.,* **139**, 3783–91.

57. DiPersio, J.F., Billing, P., Williams, R. and Gasson, J.C. (1988) Human granulocyte-macrophage colony stimulating factor and other cytokines prime human neutrophils for enhanced arachidonic acid release and leukotriene B_4 synthesis. *J. Immunol.,* **140**, 4315–22.

58. Daniels, R.H., Finnen, M.J., Hill, M.E. and Lackie, J.M. (1992) Recombinant human monocyte IL-8 primes NADPH oxidase and phospholipase A_2 activation in human neutrophils. *Immunology,* **75**, 157–63.

59. Smedly, L.A., Tonnesen, M.G., Sandhaus, R.A. *et al.* (1986) Neutrophil-mediated injury to endothelial cells: enhancement by LPS and essential role of neutrophil elastase. *J. Clin. Invest.,* **77**, 1233–43.

60. Worthen, G.S., Haslett, C., Smedly, L.A. *et al.* (1986) Lung vascular injury induced by chemotactic factors: enhancement by bacterial endotoxins. *Fed. Proc.,* **45**, 7–12.

61. Nathan, C.F. (1987) Neutrophil activation on biological surfaces: massive secretion of hydrogen peroxide in response to products of macrophages and lymphocytes. *J. Clin. Invest.,* **80**, 1550–60.

62. Kusner, D.J., Aucott, J.N., Franceschi, D. *et al.* (1991) Protease priming of neutrophil superoxide production: effects on membrane lipid order and lateral mobility. *J. Biol. Chem.,* **266**, 16465–71.

63. Abo, A., Pick, E., Hall, A. *et al.* (1991) Activation of NADPH oxidase involves the small GTP-binding protein p21rac. *Nature,* **353**, 668–70.

64. McDonald, P., Pouliot, M. and Borgeat, P.

(1993) Enhancement by GM-CSF of agonist-induced 5-lipoxygenase activation in human neutrophils involves protein synthesis and gene transcription. *J. Lipid Med.*, **6**, 59–67.

65. Palmantier, R., Surette, M.E., Sanchez, A. *et al.* (1994) Priming for the synthesis of 5-lipoxygenase products in human blood *ex vivo* by human granulocyte-macrophage colony-stimulating factor and tumor necrosis factor-α. *Lab. Invest.*, **70**, 696–704.

66. Durstin, M., Durstin, S., Molski, T.F.P. *et al.* (1994) Cytoplasmic phospholipase A$_2$ translocates to membrane fraction in human neutrophils activated by stimuli that phosphorylate mitogen-activated protein kinase. *Proc. Natl Acad. Sci. USA*, **91**, 3142–6.

67. Thomas, K.M., Pyun, H.Y. and Navarro, J. (1990) Molecular cloning of the Met-Leu-Phe receptor from neutrophils. *J. Biol. Chem.*, **265**, 20061–4.

68. Cockcroft, S. and Stutchfield, J. (1989) The receptors for ATP and fMetLeuPhe are independently coupled to phospholipases C and A$_2$ via G-protein(s). Relationship between phospholipase C and A$_2$ activation and exocytosis in HL60 cells and human neutrophils. *Biochem. J.*, **263**, 715–23.

69. Bokoch, G.M. and Gilman, A.G. (1984) Inhibition of receptor-mediated release of arachidonic acid by pertussis toxin. *Cell*, **39**, 301–8.

70. Gilman, A.G. (1987) G proteins: transducers of receptor-generated signals. *Ann. Rev. Biochem.*, **56**, 615–49.

71. Yatani, A., Mattera, R., Codina, J. *et al.* (1988) The G protein-gated atrial K$^+$ channel is stimulated by three distinct Gi alpha-subunits. *Nature*, **336**, 680–2.

72. Seuwen, K., Kahan, C., Hartman, T. and Pouyssegur, J. (1990) Strong and persistent activation of inositol lipid breakdown induces early mitogenic events but not G$_0$ to S phase progression in hamster fibroblasts: comparison of thrombin and carbachol action in cells expressing M1 muscarinic acetylcholine receptors. *J. Biol. Chem.*, **265**, 22292–9.

73. Camps, M., Carozzi, A., Schnabel, P. *et al.* (1992) Isozyme-selective stimulation of phospholipase C-β2 by G protein βγ-subunits. *Nature*, **360**, 684–9.

74. McPhail, L.C. and Snyderman, R. (1983) Activation of the respiratory burst enzyme in human polymorphonuclear leukocytes by chemoattractants and other soluble stimuli:

evidence that the same oxidase is activated by different transductional mechanisms. *J. Clin. Invest.*, **72**, 192–200.

75. Tyagi, S.R., Tamura, M., Burnham, D.N. and Lambeth, J.D. (1988) Phorbol myristate acetate (PMA) augments chemoattractant-induced diglyceride generation in human neutrophils but inhibits phosphoinositide hydrolysis. *J. Biol. Chem.*, **263**, 13191–8.

76. Wilson, E., Olcott, M.C., Bell, R.M. *et al.* (1986) Inhibition of oxidative burst in human neutrophils by shingoid long-chain bases: role of protein kinase C in activation of the burst. *J. Biol. Chem.*, **261**, 616.

77. Bass, D.A., Gerard, C., Olbrantz, P. *et al.* (1987) Priming of the respiratory burst of neutrophils by diacylglycerol: independence from activation or translocation of protein kinase C. *J. Biol. Chem.*, **262**, 6643–9.

78. Bass, D.A., McPhail, L.C., Schmitt, J.D. *et al.* (1989) Selective priming of rate and duration of the respiratory burst of neutrophils by 1,2-diacyl and 1-0-alkyl-2-acyl diglycerides. *J. Biol. Chem.*, **264**, 19610–17.

79. Bauldry, S.A., Wykle, R.L. and Bass, D.A. (1988) Phospholipase A$_2$ activation in human neutrophils: differential actions of diacylglycerols and alkylacyglycerols in priming cells for stimulation by *N*-formyl-met-leu-phe. *J. Biol. Chem.*, **263**, 16787–95.

80. Bauldry, S.A., Bass, D.A., Cousart, S.L. and McCall, C.E. (1991) Tumor necrosis factor alpha priming of phospholipase D in human neutrophils: correlation between phosphatidic acid production and superoxide generation. *J. Biol. Chem.*, **266**, 4173–9.

81. Naccache, P.H., Hamelin, B., Gaudry, M. and Bourgoin, S. (1991) Priming of calcium mobilization in human neutrophils by granulocyte-macrophage colony-stimulating factor: evidence for an involvement of phospholipase D-derived phosphatidic acid. *Cell Signalling*, **3**, 635–44.

82. Agwu, D.E., McPhail, L.C., Sozzani, S. *et al.* (1991) Phosphatidic acid as a second messenger in human polymorphonuclear leukocytes: effects on activation of NADPH oxidase. *J. Clin. Invest.*, **88**, 531–9.

83. Garcia Rodriguez, C., Montero, M., Alvarez, J. *et al.* (1993) Dissociation of platelet-activating factor production and arachidonate release by the endomembrane Ca^{2+}-ATPase inhibitor thapsigargin: evidence for the involvement of

a Ca²⁺-dependent route of priming in the production of lipid mediators by human polymorphonuclear leukocytes. *J. Biol. Chem.*, **268**, 24751–7.

84. Gay, J.C., (1993) Mechanism and regulation of neutrophil priming by platelet-activating factor. *J. Cell. Physiol.*, **156**, 189–7.

85. Grinstein, S. and Furuya, W. (1992) Chemoattractant-induced tyrosine phosphorylation and activation of microtubule-associated protein kinase in human neutrophils. *J. Biol. Chem.*, **267**, 18122–5.

86. Thompson, H.L., Shiroo, M. and Saklatvala, J. (1993) The chemotactic factor N-formyl-methionyl-lencyl-phenylalanine activates microtubule-associated protein 2 (MAP) kinase and a MAP kinase kinase in polymophonuclear leukocytes. *Biochem. J.*, **290**, 483–8.

87. Pelech, S.L. (1993) Networking with protein kinase. *Curr. Biol.*, **3**, 513–5.

88. Wood, K.W., Sarnecki, C., Roberts, T.M. and Blenis, J. (1992) *ras* mediates nerve growth factor receptor modulation of three signal-transducing protein kinases: MAP kinase, *raf*-1, and RSK. *Cell.*, **68**, 1041–50.

89. Nemenoff, R.A., Winitz, S., Qian, N.X. *et al.* (1993) Phosphorylation and activation of a high molecular weight form of phospholipase A₂ by p42 microtubule-associated kinsae and protein kinase C. *J. Biol. Chem.*, **268**, 1960–4.

90. Seth, A., Alvarez, E., Gupta, S. and Davis R.J. (1991) A phosphorylation site located in the NH₂-terminal domain of c-Myc increases transaction of gene expression. *J. Biol. Chem.*, **266**, 23521–4.

91. Seger, R., Ahn, N.G., Boulton, T.G. *et al.* (1991) Microtubule-associated protein 2 kinases, ERK1 and ERK2, undergo autophosphorylation on both tyrosine and threonine residues: implications for their mechanism of activation. *Proc. Natl Acad. Sci. USA*, **88**, 7551–5.

92. Crews, C.M., Alessandrini, A. and Erikson, R.L. (1992) The primary structure of MEK, a protein kinase that phosphorylates the *ERK* gene product. *Science*, **258**, 478–80.

93. Lange-Carter, C.A., Pleiman, C.M., Gardner, A.M. *et al.* (1993) A divergence in the MAP kinase regulatory network defined by MEK kinase and *raf. Science*, **260**, 315–9.

94. Worthen, G.S., Avdi, N., Buhl, A.M. *et al.* (1994) FMLP activates ras and raf in human neutrophils: potential role in activation of MAP kinase. *J. Clin. Invest.*, **94**, 815–23.

95. Buhl, A.M., Avdi, N., Worthen, G.S. and Johnson, G.L. (1994) Mapping of the C5a receptor signal transduction in human neutrophils. *Proc. Natl Acad. Sci. USA*, **91**, 9190–4.

96. Wu, J., Dent, P., Jelinek, T. *et al.* (1993) Inhibition of the EGF-activated MAP kinase signalling pathway by adenosine 3', 5'-monophosphate. *Science*, **262**, 1065–9.

97. Cook, S.J. and McCormick, F. (1993) Inhibition by cAMP of ras-dependent activation of raf. *Science*, **262**, 1069–2.

98. Burgering, B.M.T., Pronk, G.J., van Weeren, P.C. *et al.* (1993) cAMP antagonizes p21ras-directed activation of extracellular signal-related kinase 2 and phosphorylation of mSos nucleotide exchange factor. *EMBO J*, **12**, 4211–20.

99. Downey, G.P., Elson, E.L., Schwab, B. III *et al.* (1991) Biophysical properties and microfilament assembly in neutrophils: modulation by cyclic AMP. *J. Cell Biol.*, **114**, 1179–90.

100. Rivkin, I, Rosenblatt, J. and Becker, E.L. (1975) The role of cAMP in in the chemotactic responsiveness and spontaneous motility of rabbit peritoneal neutrophils: the inhibition of neutrophil movement and elevation of cAMP level by catecholamines, prostaglandins, theophylline, and cholera toxin. *J. Immunol.*, **115**, 1126–34.

101. Chopra, J. and Webster, R.O. (1988) PGE1 inhibits neutrophil adherence and neutrophil-mediated injury to cultured endothelial cells. *Am. Rev. Respir. Dis.*, **138**, 915–20.

102. Fantone, J.C., Marasco, W.A., Elgas, L.J. and Ward, P.A. (1984) Stimulus specificity of prostaglandin inhibition of rabbit polymorphonuclear leukocyte lysosomal enzyme release and superoxide anion production. *Am. J. Pathol.*, **115**, 9–16.

103. Fonteh, A.N., Winkler, J.D., Torphy, T.J. *et al.* (1993) Influence of isoproterenol and phosphodiesterase inhibitors on platelet-activating factor biosynthesis in the human neutrophil. *J. Immunol.*, **151**, 330–50.

104. Fittschen, L.F., Sandhaus, R.A., Worthen, G.S. and Henson, P.M. (1988) Bacterial lipopolysaccharide enhanced chemoattractant-induced elastase secretion by human neutrophils. *J. Leukoc. Biol.*, **43** 547–56.

105. Henson, P.M., Tonnesen, M.G., Worthen, G.S.

and Parsons P.E. (1988) Pulmonary inflammation: mechanisms and effects of accummulation of inflammatory cells, in *Human Inflammatory Disease, Clinical Immunology. 1.* (eds C. Maronne, L.M. Lichtenstein, M. Kondorelli and A.S. Fauci), B.C. Decker, Toronto, pp. 69–76.

106. Campbell, E.J. and Campbell, M.A. (1988) Pericellular proteolysis by neutrophils in the presence of proteinase inhibitors: effects of substrate opsonization. *Cell Biol.*, **106**, 667–76.

107. Nathan, C.F. (1988) Respiratory burst in adherent human neutrophils: triggering by colony-stimulating factors CSF-GM and CSF-G. *Blood*, **73** 301–6.

S. Craig Stocks and Ian Dransfield

The extensive pulmonary vascularization and large number of marginated leukocytes of lung tissue allow for a rapid and wide spread cellular infiltrate in response to infection or other insult. Neutrophils are key effector cells in inflammatory responses, and once recruited they are capable of efficiently killing and degrading certain microorganisms (e.g. *streptococci*) using a battery of toxic metabolites and degradative enzymes [1,2]. However, excessive release of these histotoxic agents in healthy tissues may also inflict much unwanted tissue injury at sites of inflammation [3]. Thus, an inflammatory response that is too vigorous, or misdirected, may result in damage to host tissue. Such proinflammatory events are implicated in many diseases that are characterized by neutrophil accumulation and increased vascular permeability in the lung; including acute bacterial pneumonia, idiopathic pulmonary fibrosis and the syndrome of acute respiratory distress in adults (ARDS) [4,5].

One of the most prominent histological features of ARDS is the intense inflammatory cell infiltrate seen within the lung interstitium (Chapter 4). The predominantly neutrophilic nature of this infiltrate implicates the neutrophil as an important cell type in determining the pathogenesis of ARDS [6]. Analysis of bronchoalveolar lavage (BAL) obtained from patients with ARDS reveals increased numbers of neutrophils and their secretory products, including the proteases elastase and collagenase [7,8] (Chapter 16). It is therefore likely that neutrophil mediated lung injury and disruption of the capillary integrity makes a significant contribution to the observed leakage of protein-rich fluid exudate into the alveoli in established ARDS. Moreover, elevated levels of interleukin (IL)-8 and possibly other chemoattractants in BAL from ARDS patients rapidly following multiple trauma injury, suggests that an early event in ARDS is the establishment of a chemotactic gradient which leads to neutrophil recruitment [9,10].

In ARDS and at the initial phases of most other inflammatory diseases, early events are focused at the site of interaction between neutrophils and microvascular endothelial cells [11]. Intercellular adhesion processes are also critical in generating a microenvironment that promotes neutrophil mediated endothelial injury [12]. Neutrophil adhesion can be altered by many different host and bacterial derived products such that a spectrum of different adhesive states is possible, allowing adhesion to be matched to the severity of the provoking insult, whilst minimizing the risk of inappropriate adhesive interactions [13,14]. In addition to the molecular mechanisms which underlie neutrophil adhesion, the biophysical properties of the neutrophil and the unique hemodynamic properties of the lung microvasculature may also influence neutrophil emigration during inflammatory pro-

ARDS Acute Respiratory Distress in Adults. Edited by Timothy W. Evans and Christopher Haslett. Published in 1996 by Chapman & Hall, London. ISBN 0 412 56910 8

Table 9.1 Neutrophil adhesion receptors

Receptor family	Molecule	Leukocyte typing nomenclature
Selectins	L-selectin	Not determined
	E-selectin	Not determined
	P-selectin	CD62
Integrins	LFA-1	CD11a/CD18
	CR3/Mac-1	CD11b/CD18
	p150,95	CD11c/CD18
	VLA–6	CD49f/CD29
Immunoglobulins	ICAM-1	CD54
	ICAM-2	Not determined
	ICAM-3	CD50
	NCA	CD66/67
	LFA-3	CD58
Mucins	Leukosialin	CD43
Cartilage–link	Hermes/pgp-1	CD44
Carbohydrate	Lewis antigens	CD15, sCD15

cesses [15,16] (see also Mechanisms of leukocyte emigration, below).

Regulation of the repertoire and function of surface adhesion receptors allows dynamic two way communication between the neutrophil and its local microenvironment. Neutrophils are able to 'sense' and respond appropriately to local environmental stimuli through intracellular signals generated by binding to adhesive ligands. In this chapter we describe the molecular characteristics, binding specificities and functional regulation of the principal receptors mediating neutrophil adhesion to endothelial cells and the extracellular matrix (outlined in Table 9.1). In addition to the well characterized selectin [17], integrin [18] and immunoglobulin families [19], molecules such as CD43 (mucin family), CD44 (hyaluronate receptor) and carbohydrate moieties also play a key adhesive role. Recruitment of neutrophils to inflamed sites requires the coordinated regulation of activity of at least two receptor families (Figure 9.1) with initial rapid, low level interactions, termed 'rolling adhesion', mediated by molecules of the **selectin** family. Binding

via this mechanism serves to tether neutrophils to endothelium, permitting cellular activation events and as a prerequisite to leukocyte **integrin** dependent 'firm' adhesion and subsequent transmigration [20,21].

SELECTINS

Three members of the selectin family have so far been described. They are structurally related cell surface molecules with an N-terminal C-type (Ca^{2+} dependent) lectin domain followed by an epidermal growth factor-like domain and 2–9 short consensus repeat (SCR) motifs [22–25] (Figure 9.2). The nomenclature for selectins relates to the cell type on which the selectins were first described [26]. P-selectin was first identified as an activation marker of thrombin-stimulated **platelets**, but is also expressed on activated endothelium [27,28]. Similarly, E-selectin was identified as a surface glycoprotein present on activated **endothelium** [23] and L-selectin was first identified as a molecule having a role in lymphocyte homing,

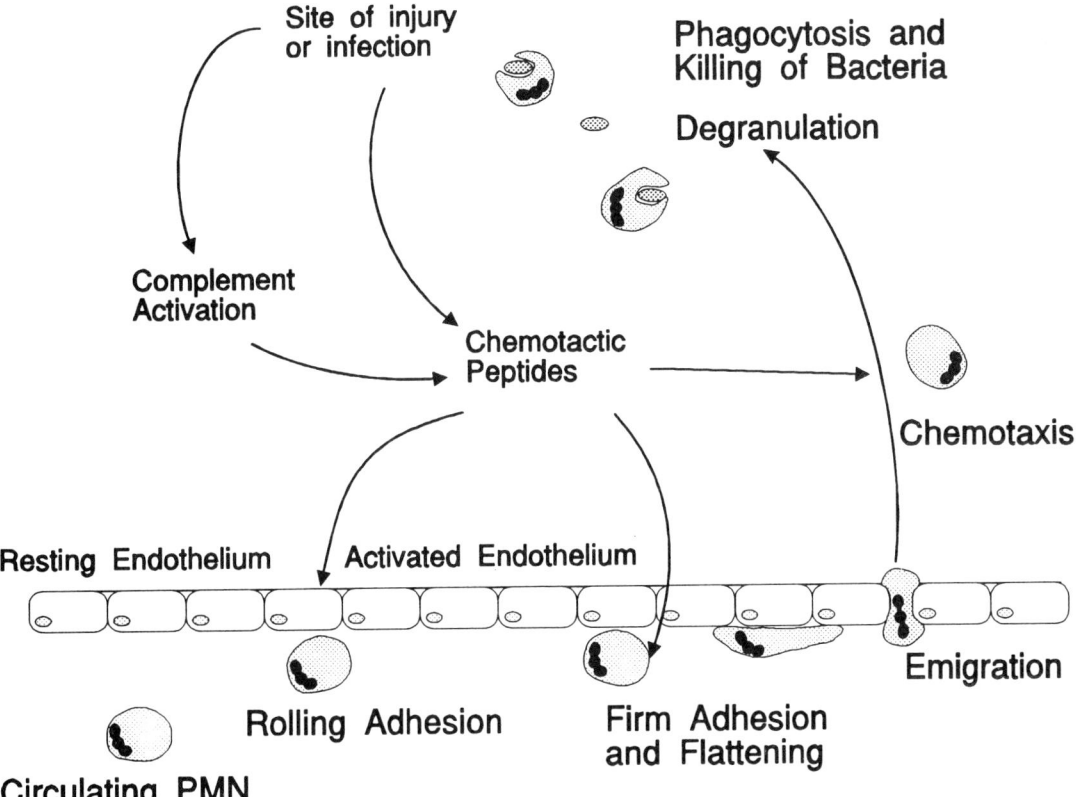

Figure 9.1 Events that occur during neutrophil adhesion and emigration to inflamed sites. Inflammatory events resulting in the release of chemotactic agents exert their effects upon both endothelium and circulating leukocytes (PMN). Endothelial cell activation facilitates 'rolling adhesion', whilst leukocyte activation initiates the process of firm adhesion and transmigration. After chemotactic migration to inflamed sites, triggering of effector cell function can result in further release of agents that serve to recruit leukocytes to inflammatory sites. Following removal of infectious agents and tissue repair during resolution of the inflammatory process, endothelium will return to the resting state and reduce further recruitment of leukocytes to these sites.

mediating the adhesion of lymphocytes to high endothelial venules [17,29,30].

The importance of selectins in neutrophil recruitment during inflammation is dramatically demonstrated by a rare disorder known as leukocyte adhesion deficiency 2 (LAD2). Patients lack fucosyl transferase activity, and so fail to express selectin ligands [31,32]. The clinical manifestations of LAD2 are recurrent bacterial infection (mainly pneumonia, periodontitis, otitis media and localized cellulitis), with the failure of pus formation in spite of high circulating leukocyte counts. *In vitro* tests on patients' neutrophils demonstrate an inability to engage in rolling adhesion, or to firmly adhere to cytokine activated endothelium, leading to failure of neutrophil recruitment. Although patients' neutrophils express normal levels of CD18 and have a normal phagocytic capacity, migration in response to chemoattractants is severely impaired. Demonstration that fucosylation of selectin ligands is essential for recognition *in vitro* was shown by transfection of a fucosyltransferase into nonbinding cell lines which then express ligands for selectins [33,34]. In addition to

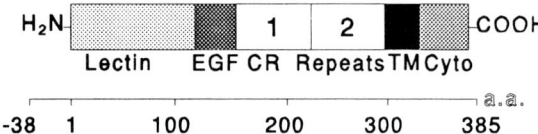

L-selectin

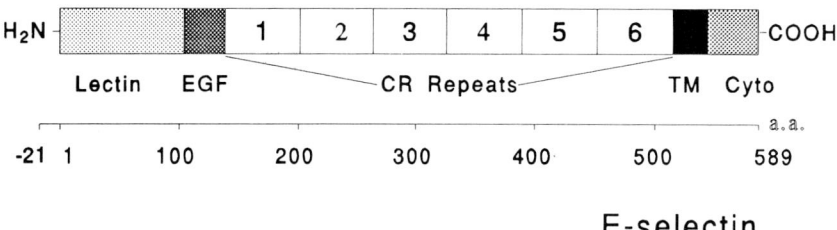

E-selectin

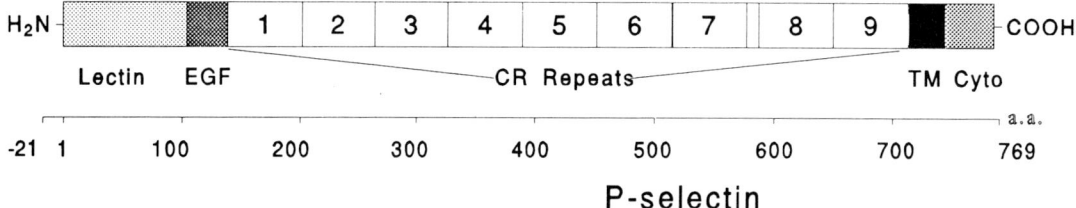

P-selectin

Figure 9.2 Selectin structure. Selectins are characterized by an N-terminal lectin-like domain that is thought to determine ligand binding specificity, followed by an epidermal growth factor (EGF)-like domain. Variable numbers of complement binding protein-like domains (CR) separate the EGF domain from the transmembrane sequences (TM). All three selectins are transmembrane proteins with a short cytoplasmic tail. The molecular weights of the selectins deduced by SDS gel electrophoresis are as follows: L-selectin – 90 kDa (neutrophils), 70–80 kDa (mononuclear cells); E-selectin – 100 kDa; P-selectin – 140 kDA.

defective inflammatory responses, patients with LAD2 also have severe mental retardation and short stature, indicating more widespread effects of this genetic defect.

SELECTIN LIGANDS

The binding of carbohydrate ligands in a Ca^{2+} dependent manner by selectins is conferred primarily by the lectin domain [35]. Extensive studies of the carbohydrate binding specificities of selectins has revealed similar, but dis-

tinct, binding characteristics (Figure 9.3). It is clear that the Lewis carbohydrate antigens Lewis[x] (Le[x]), Lewis[a] (Le[a]) and in particular their sialylated derivatives (sLe[x], sLe[a]) are recognized by both E- and P-selectin [33,36–44], and possibly also by L-selectin [45]. Unlike E-selectin, P-selectin recognizes a range of carbohydrate structures including nonsialylated Le[x] [46] and sulfoglucoronyl glycolipids, which are also recognized by L-selectin [47]. P-selectin has also been shown to bind to heterogeneous sulfated glycans

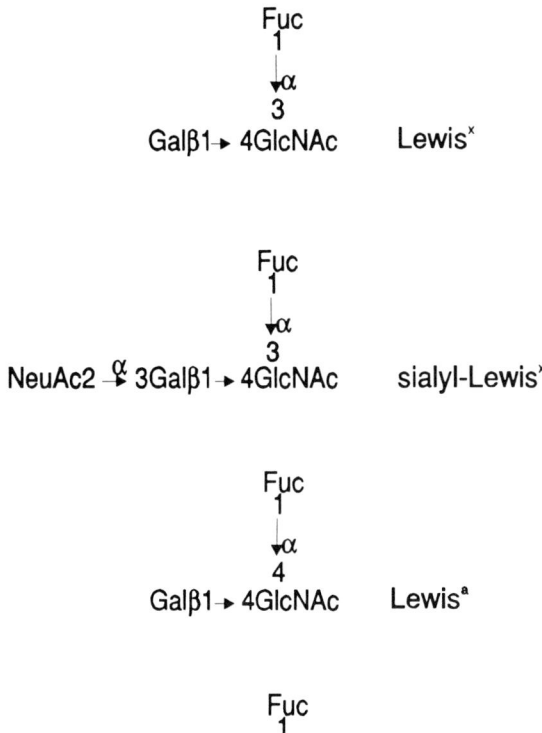

Figure 9.3 Carbohydrate structures recognized by selectins. The Lewis[x] and Lewis[a] carbohydrate moieties are key to selectin recognition. Carbohydrate residues are: Fuc, fucose; GlcNAc, *N*-acetylglucosamine; Gal, galactose; NeuAc, *N*-acetylneuraminic acid (sialic acid). Sialylation of the Lewis groups increases selectin binding.

[48], although this may serve a regulatory function rather than by direct competition for the ligand binding site [49].

Although Lewis groups are carried on glycolipids and glycoproteins, the neutrophil receptor for P-selectin is a glycoprotein [44] with O-linked carbohydrate groups [50]. P-selectin binding to a myeloid 120 kDa glycoprotein with O-linked sLe[x], has also been described [51]. A glycoprotein ligand for E-selectin has been identified on mouse myeloid cells, although a human homolog of this 150 kDa sialylated protein has not been identified [52]. L-selectin has been shown to recognize 50 and 90 kDa glycoproteins with O-linked, sulfated carbohydrate chains [53,54], and sulfated glycolipids [55], as well as Le[x] and Le[a] groups, with a preference for the nonsialylated forms [56]. The precise role of the different selectin ligands may alter when shear stress is reduced under conditions of low flow, e.g. vasodilatation, suggesting that selectins have a multirecognition capability to suit particular local conditions [57]. This finding implies an additional level of complexity in terms of interaction of selectin with ligand. Furthermore, it is likely that alternative ligands for the selectins have yet to be identified.

ROLE OF SELECTIN MEDIATED ADHESION

All three selectins mediate rolling adhesion, but each has a distinct role which probably contributes to the fine control of cellular recruitment during acute inflammation. P-selectin is of particular importance in the interaction between neutrophils and lung vascular endothelium. Studies *in vivo* show that cobra venom factor induced lung injury in rats is significantly ameliorated by administration of P-selectin monoclonal antibody (mAb) or the carbohydrate ligand groups recognized by P-selectin [58,59]. The effects observed on administration of synthetic sLe[x] oligosaccharides (but not a nonfucosylated analog) include a reduction in hemorrhage and extravascular leakage, as well as reduced neutrophil accumulation. It was suggested that low dosage (< 1μmol) administration of these oligosaccharides may have a therapeutic value in ARDS [58,59]. P-selectin mediated adhesion was found to account for the majority of 'spontaneous' rolling observed in canine mesenteric venules [60]. Inhibition observed after injection of neutralizing mAb was rapid (< 20 seconds) and persisted for up to 15 minutes, suggesting that the rate of P-selectin turnover within the plasma membrane may be rapid in order to replace

P-selectin shed from the cell surface [61,62]. The role of P-selectin adhesion in leukocyte recruitment *in vivo* was addressed using P-selectin deficient mice generated by specific gene targeting techniques [63]. Surprisingly, P-selectin deficient mice were healthy, even in the absence of a special pathogen-free environment. Further analysis revealed an elevated circulating neutrophil count and virtually no detectable rolling adhesion in mesenteric venules. Moreover, neutrophil recruitment in response to inflammatory stimuli administered intraperitoneally was delayed, but not totally blocked. The authors concluded that P-selectin adhesion has a key role in the early steps of leukocyte recruitment to sites of inflammation and that delayed recruitment observed in P-selectin deficient mice was probably a consequence of induction of E-selectin by inflammatory stimuli, thereby allowing neutrophil adhesion and subsequent recruitment [63].

Selectin mediated adhesion of neutrophils to activated platelets may be a significant contributory factor in atherosclerosis, thrombosis and ischemia. The severity of ischemia-reperfusion injury is reduced if neutrophil adhesion to endothelium/activated platelets is blocked; and anti-P-selectin antibody administered to a feline heart 10 minutes before reperfusion, following 80 minutes of ischemia, confers protective effects, reducing necrosis of myocardial tissue by 60% compared with controls [64]. The binding of neutrophils (and monocytes) to activated endothelium and platelets is also almost completely abolished by anti-P-selectin mAb [42,65–67] and P-selectin has been shown to mediate neutrophil rolling on immobilized activated platelets [68]. In addition to the well defined role for P-selectin in acute inflammatory responses, P-selectin may also have a role in continued leukocyte recruitment observed in chronic inflammation [69] and in thrombosis [70].

Partial inhibition of rolling by L-selectin mAb indicates that L-selectin is involved in neutrophil-endothelial adhesion, possibly binding to vascular selectins [68,71,72]. This suggestion is complicated by the finding that the carbohydrate ligands for the vascular selectins on neutrophils have been shown to be *O*-linked, but L-selectin has no sites for *O*-linked glycosylation. One possible explanation for these apparently discordant findings is that there is selective binding of particular ligands under different conditions (see above).

CONTROL OF SELECTIN MEDIATED ADHESION

One mechanism for the regulation of neutrophil adhesion is control of expression of selectins, or of their ligands. P-selectin is stored in platelet α granules and the Weibel–Palade bodies of endothelial cells and is rapidly translocated to the surface of these cells when they are activated [44,73–75]. Modulation of binding by sulphated glycans [49] or Ca^{2+} induced conformational changes in the lectin domain [74] of P-selectin have been proposed as mechanisms for control of ligand binding. Interestingly, rapid phosphorylation and subsequent dephosphorylation of platelet P-selectin occurs following platelet activation, although this was not shown to affect the avidity of P-selectin for ligand [76]. A soluble form of P-selectin lacking the transmembrane domain is present in small quantities in plasma [61], possibly serving an anti-inflammatory function by blocking integrin dependent adhesion of neutrophils to endothelial cells [46,77] and inhibiting neutrophil respiratory burst [78].

E-selectin is not expressed on resting endothelium but expression is inducible by lipopolysaccharide (LPS), tumor necrosis factor (TNF)α and IL-1. Induction requires *de novo* synthesis of the molecule [79,80], peaking 3–4 hours after stimulation and declining after about 9 hours [23,81,82]. Whereas the E- and P-selectins are expressed by vascular endothelium following activation, L-selectin is

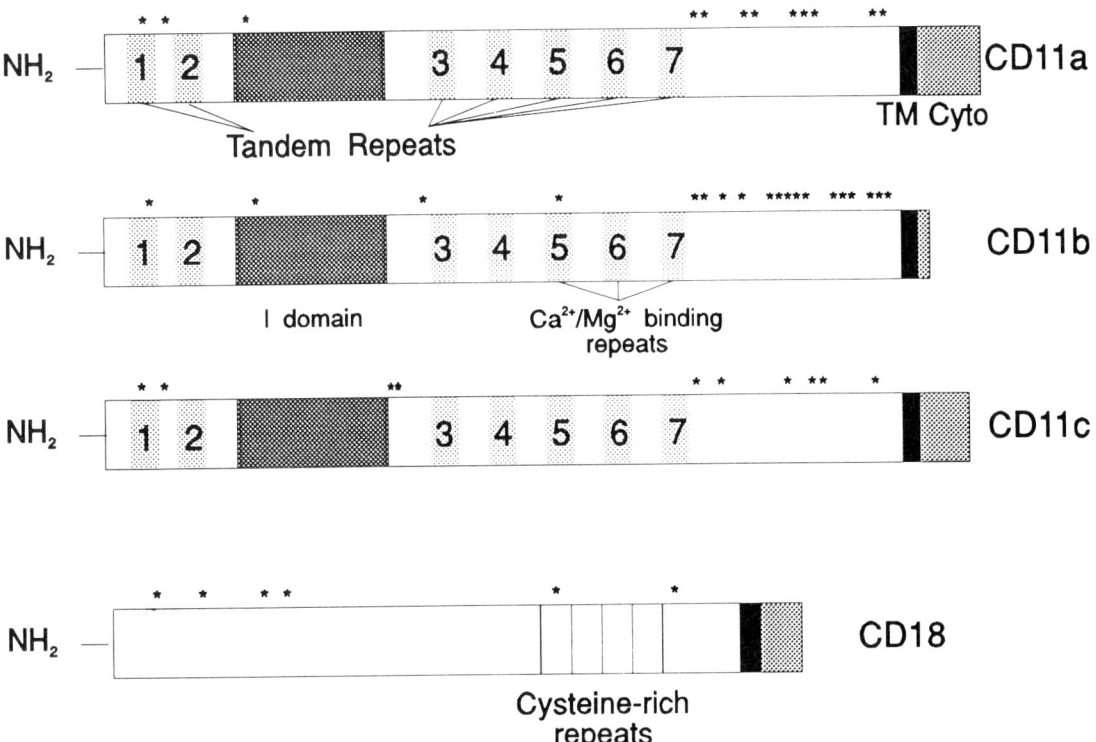

Figure 9.4 Leukocyte integrin subunit structure. Identified structures of the leukocyte integrin α subunits (approximately 1150 amino acids) are shown with N-terminus of each polypeptide to the left. Repeated domains (labeled 1–7) of approximately 60 amino acids, three of which (5, 6 and 7) contain sequences homologous to divalent cation binding domains. Inserted between domains 2 and 3 is a region of 180 amino acids (inserted or I domain) that shows homology to domains present in von Willebrand factor, cartilage matrix protein and the complement regulatory proteins factor B and H. TM represents the transmembrane spanning region, which is followed by a relatively short cytoplasmic domain (Cyto) (53 amino acids for CD11a, 19 amino acids for CD11b, and 29 amino acids for CD11c).

expressed constitutively on neutrophils. In contrast to the induction of expression observed for vascular selectins, L-selectin is rapidly shed from the surface of the cell by proteolysis following activation, indicating a role in the earliest stages of neutrophil responses to inflammatory stimuli [83]. Activation induced shedding of L-selectin correlates with downregulation of integrin independent adhesion following neutrophil activation [84]. A soluble form of L-selectin is also present in plasma and retains functional activity [85]. One intriguing possibility is that soluble selectin molecules may be bound to their natural ligands in inflammatory condi-

tions, serving to downregulate neutrophil adhesion. However, a corollary of this suggestion is that reduced levels of soluble selectins might have proinflammatory effects.

An additional level of regulation is that of selectin ligands on neutrophils. The selectin binding carbohydrate groups are expressed on a number of neutrophil glycoproteins, primarily nonspecific crossreacting antigen (NCA)-160 [86], but also L-selectin [72] and the β_2 integrins [87]. NCA-160, L-selectin, and the β_2 integrins have been implicated in recognition of the vascular selectins [72,88–90]. However, anti-NCA mAbs vary in their inhibitory potency [89], anti-β_2 mAb having no inhibitory effect [41,90] and neutrophils that do not express L-selectin are still able to bind E-selectin [91]. A number of neutrophil dependent mechanisms have been proposed for the regulation of selectin mediated neutrophil-endothelial interaction, including regulation of surface expression of the carbohydrate ligands and secretion of inhibitory factors such as sulfatides [48]. However, the role of the neutrophil ligands in control of the selectin mediated adhesion has received little study.

It is thought that initial neutrophil-endothelial contact, mediated by the neutrophil P- or E-selectin receptor, facilitates a critical interaction between endothelial cell associated platelet activating factor (PAF) and the PAF receptor on the neutrophil, which generates a signal resulting in activation of the leukocyte integrins [21,91–93]. Thus, binding of the neutrophils to vascular selectins acts as a trigger for further adhesion events (Figure 9.5), including activation dependent, integrin mediated adhesion necessary for subsequent transmigration. However, the finding that both CD18 dependent and CD18 independent neutrophil emigration pathways are used in response to different inflammatory stimuli in rabbits [94] suggests that the pathogen itself may influence the molecular mechanism by which neutrophils are recruited.

INTEGRINS

Integrins are receptors that serve as a link between cytoskeletal elements and extracellular matrix [95] and are potential regulators of cellular responses to micro environment. Integrin mediated adhesion requires the presence of extracellular divalent cations and is an active process dependent upon cellular metabolic activity. Integrin receptors are heterodimeric glycoproteins, comprising an α subunit noncovalently associated with a β subunit. There are now at least eight β subunits and 11 α subunits that have been cloned and sequenced [18] and the integrin family has been conveniently divided into subfamilies on the basis of subunit associations (Table 9.2).

Table 9.2 Integrin receptor subfamilies

β Subunit	α Subunit	Other name/ligand specificity
β_1	α_1	VLA-1 (collagens, laminin)
	α_2	VLA-2 (collagens, laminin)
	α_3	VLA-3 (fibronectin, laminin, collagen)
	α_4	VLA-4 (fibronectin, VCAM-1)
	α_5	VLA-5 (fibronectin)
	α_6	VLA-6 (laminin)
	α_7	Laminin receptor
	α_8	Not determined
β_2	α_L	LFA–1 ⎤
	α_M	CR3/Mac-1 ⎟ see Table 9.3
	α_X	p150,95 ⎦
β_3	α_{IIb}	IIb/IIa ⎤ multiple ligands
	α_V	Vitronectin receptor ⎦
β_4	α_6	Laminin receptor
β_5	α_V	Vitronectin receptor
β_6	α_V	Fibronectin receptor
β_7	α_4	Firbonectin/VCAM-1 receptor
β_8	α_V	Not determined

The β_2 integrin subfamily [96], LFA-1, CR3/Mac-1 and p150,95, or leukocyte integrins, are abundantly expressed on neutrophils and have a key role in neutrophil adhesive function. Neutrophil dysfunction in a relatively rare (< 70 patients worldwide) group of patients who suffer recurrent bacterial infections of soft tissues was found to be a consequence of a deficiency of β_2 integrins from patient leukocytes (leukocyte adhesion deficiency or LAD1; see below and reviewed in [97,98]). Other integrins expressed by neutrophils include the β_1 integrin $\alpha6\beta_1$ ('Very late activation antigen-6') that binds to the basement membrane component laminin [99] and a novel integrin immunologically related to β_3 integrin combined with an unidentified α subunit, which has been termed the 'leukocyte response integrin' in view of its ability to regulate other myeloid cell functions [100]. Antibodies defining integrins have been designated the following nomenclature: CD11a (LFA-1 α subunit), CD11b (CR3 α subunit), CD11c (p150,95 α subunit) and CD18 (β_2 subunit), CD29 (β_1 subunit), CD49f (VLA-6 α subunit).

LEUKOCYTE ADHESION DEFICIENCY

The clinical aspects of LAD are only briefly summarized here. Patients suffer from recurrent bacterial infections of soft tissues (e.g. gingivitis, pharyngitis) and infection of organs, such as the lung, may progress to sepsis and ultimately to death. Increased susceptibility to infection by pathogenic bacteria is not paralleled by increased incidence of viral infection and occurs despite persistent neutrophilia. The clinical symptoms of LAD are primarily the result of dysfunction of neutrophils due to defective expression of the leukocyte integrins [101–105]. Patients' neutrophils show a reduced ability to bind to and transmigrate on endothelial monolayers, accounting for the persistent neutrophilia and lack of polymorphonuclear cells (PMNs) in inflammatory infiltrates observed in this disease. The extent of the deficiency relates directly to the severity of the clinical manifestations, and patients with severe deficiency ($< 1\%$ normal levels of leukocyte integrin expression) rarely survive childhood, succuming to overwhelming infection. Since patients' leukocytes lack expression of all three leukocyte integrins, defects in the common β_2 subunit were suggested to be responsible for the disease [105]. Recently, recovery of leukocyte integrin expression in patients' cells transfected with the normal β_2 subunit cDNA has been demonstrated and thus this disease may possibly be a suitable candidate for gene therapy [106,107].

The α and β subunits of integrins are unrelated in terms of sequence, although both are transmembrane glycoproteins with large extracellular domains and a relatively short cytoplasmic tail (Figure 9.5). Correct folding and architecture of integrin β subunits probably depends on intrachain disulfides formed by highly conserved cysteine residues [108] and ligand binding and correct association of α and β subunits may involve a region approximately 100 amino acids from the N-terminus [109,110]. Since integrins that share the same β subunit are able to bind different ligands, the α subunit is thought to confer specificity. One functionally important region of the α subunits of some integrins, including the β_2 integrins, is termed the 'inserted' or 'I' domain (Figure 9.4). Mapping of the binding sites of many mAbs that inhibit function, and for one mAb that promotes leukocyte integrin function, map to this region [98,111,112]. The I domain lies within a series of seven tandem repeats of approximately 60 amino acids (Figure 9.4), three of which contain sequences that may also function as divalent cation binding units [113]. Since ligand binding by integrins requires divalent cations, it is thought that these regions are important for the process of ligand recognition. Recently, a novel divalent cation binding site has also been identified within the I domain [114].

Subtle modulation of leukocyte integrin

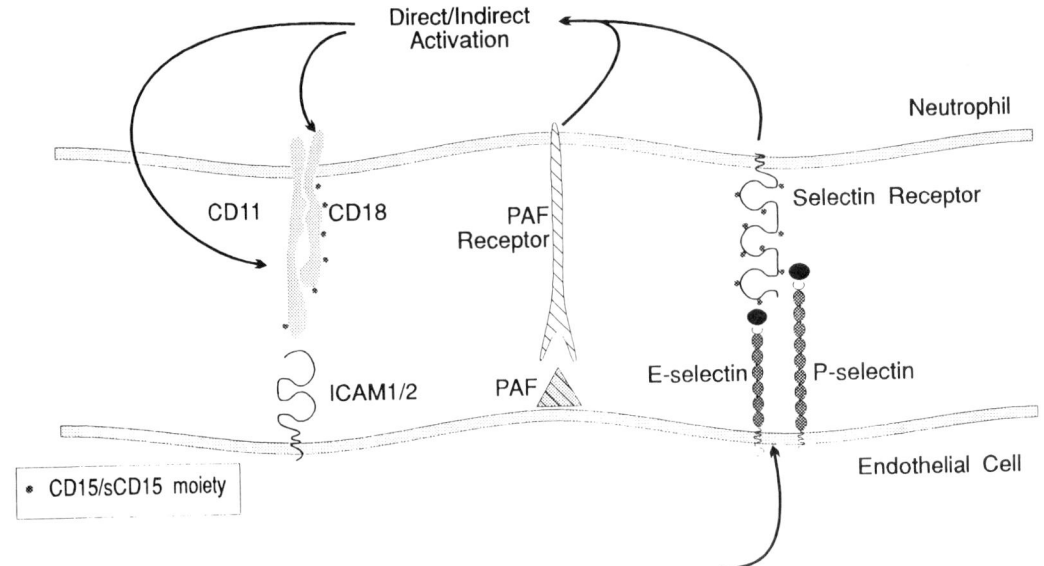

Figure 9.5 Possible sequence of events leading to β₂-integrin mediated binding to endothelium. Expression of selectins on endothelium is induced by inflammatory mediators initiating interaction with the neutrophil selectin receptor. Concomitant interaction of endothelial cell-associated PAF with the neutrophil PAF-receptor leads to activation of the leukocyte integrins, which are then able to bind ICAM-1/ICAM-2, resulting in neutrophil arrest. The precise mechanism for this activation is unclear but it may involve changes in integrin conformation and/or distribution.

functional activity may be achieved by differential carbohydrate modification. Differences in both the sulfation and the extent of sialylation of carbohydrate on leukocyte integrins have been reported [115,116]. The carbohydrate Le^x has also been found to be present on leukocyte integrins on neutrophils [117] and sLe^x presented by leukocyte integrins may act as a ligand for selectins [90]. Both α and β subunits of the leukocyte integrins can be phosphorylated *in vitro*, although only the β₂ subunit is phosphorylated in a regulated manner [118,119]. In view of the key role of the β₂ subunit cytoplasmic domain in the control of leukocyte integrin function [120], it may be that phosphorylation of cytoplasmic residues is associated with control of function.

LEUKOCYTE INTEGRIN LIGANDS

The molecules that are recognized by leukocyte integrins are diverse in terms of structure, including cell surface molecules, complement and clotting cascade proteins and LPS (Table 9.3). LFA-1 mediates a wide range of adhesion dependent functions of leukocytes, including adhesion to a number of cell types: endothelium, epithelium, keratinocytes and fibroblasts [121–123]. Three cellular counter receptors or ligands have been identified for LFA-1, termed intercellular adhesion molecule (ICAM)1, ICAM-2 and ICAM-3, all of which are related members of the immunoglobulin superfamily (see below).

Both CR3/Mac-1 and p150,95 mediate binding and phagocytosis of iC3b coated targets [124–127], although other ligands for CR3 include factor X and fibrinogen [128–130]. Chemoattractant stimulated neutrophils are able to bind to ICAM-1 on human umbilical vein endothelial cells (HUVEC) via CR3, an interaction confirmed using transfectants expressing ICAM-1 or CR3 and purified mol-

Table 9.3 Leukocyte integrins and their ligands

Name	Leukocyte typing nomenclature	Ligand(s)
LFA-1	CD11a/CD18	ICAM-1
		ICAM-2
		ICAM-3
CR3/Mac-1	CD11b/CD18	iC3b
		Fibrinogen
		Factor X
		ICAM-1
		LPS
p150,95	CD11c/CD18	iC3b
		Fibrinogen
		Endothelial ligand

ecules [131,132]. When compared to LFA-1–ICAM-1 binding, CR3–ICAM-1 binding is more sensitive to shear stress, indicating that the relative contributions of CR3 and LFA-1 may depend upon local environmental conditions. The ligand binding specificity of p150,95 has been less thoroughly studied than for LFA-1 and CR3. Binding of fibrinogen to TNF-stimulated neutrophils and of myeloid cells to endothelium is thought to involve p150,95 [133–135]. However, endothelial ligands for p150,95 are as yet unidentified.

REGULATION OF INTEGRIN FUNCTION

A broad spectrum of possible adhesive states is provided by a number of levels of control of leukocyte integrin mediated interactions. Regulation of ligand availability may be considered as a control mechanism that is independent of the cell type expressing leukocyte integrin receptors. On the other hand, regulation of receptor function allows leukocyte integrin bearing cells to remain unresponsive in the presence of abundant ligand or to hyperrespond to low levels of ligand. Dissociation between levels of surface expression and functional activity of leukocyte integrins suggests that they can be switched 'on' and 'off' in response to appropriate stimuli. Intracellular signals transmitted across the membrane result in altered leukocyte integrin responses, the strength and duration of which depend on the repertoire of signaling receptors engaged, permitting 'fine tuning' of adhesive interactions during an inflammatory response.

Altered expression or distribution of integrins or their ligands may control integrin mediated processes such as neutrophil recruitment. ICAM-1, in contrast to ICAM-2, is modulated by specific cytokines on a variety of cell types [123,136] and is present at sites of inflammation, suggesting that ICAM-1 serves as a stimulus specific adhesive ligand for recognition by leukocyte integrins. Cytoskeletal proteins such as talin and α-actinin have been demonstrated to be closely linked with integrins [137,138] possibly limiting lateral mobility of receptors and concentrating them at sites of interaction with ligand. Similarly, cytoskeletal association of integrin ligand, e.g. ICAM-1 [139], may also result in surface distribution changes. Multimeric complexes of leukocyte integrins or their ligands might permit more avid binding to surfaces bearing low density of ligand. Control of cytoskeletal associations may allow 'deadhesion' with resulting 'free' receptors diffusing away from the region of ligand binding.

In neutrophils, surface expression of CR3 and p150,95 is rapidly increased in response to inflammatory stimuli due to mobilization from intracellular pools [140–142]. Interestingly, upregulation of receptor expression and function seem to be separate events [143–145], newly mobilized receptors requiring a further activation signal, which may be particularly important for chemotaxis or transmigration [146]. There is now accumulating evidence that interaction of leukocyte integrins with ligand involves exposure of active sites which then confers functional activity [147]. Studies using a unique mAb, which binds to functionally active leukocyte integrins, have revealed that conformational alterations accompany integrin activation and are closely associated with functional regulation [148–151].

IMMUNOGLOBULIN SUPERFAMILY

Many receptors that mediate cellular recognition processes including adhesion are members of the immunoglobulin superfamily [19,152] The basic unit of immunoglobulin (Ig), termed an Ig domain, forms a modular framework which is particularly suited for recognition. The precise structure of this unit has been determined by crystallographic techniques and is formed by two parallel β sheets composed of either seven or eight parallel β strands. Variability of sequences between each of the β strands provides the potential for recognition of a diversity of molecular structures. The adhesion receptors expressed by neutrophils and endothelium that are members of this family are shown in Table 9.1. However, the key receptors that mediate neutrophil adhesion and recruitment in response to inflammatory stimuli are the neutrophil or NCAs, which display selectin ligands, and the intercellular adhesion molecules, ICAM-1 and ICAM-2, expressed by endothelium.

CEA FAMILY

The carcinoembryonic antigen (CEA), first described as an oncofetal antigen, and other closely related glycoproteins form an Ig subfamily with wide distribution in both normal and malignant tissues [153]. However, expression of CEA related antigens on leukocytes is restricted to polymorphonuclear cells. CEA related molecules, many of which mediate adhesion, have a single variable-like (lacking a disulfide bond), and a number of constant-like, Ig domains and a very high level of sequence homology with CEA. At least six CEA related antigens have been identified on neutrophils, including CD66 and CD67 antigens [154–156]. The 160 kDa neutrophil antigen (NCA-160) has been identified as the only neutrophil product of the BGP gene [157,158] and the 95 kDa antigen is probably a CGM 6 gene product [159].

Further complexity is introduced in that some CEA related glycoproteins, including CD67 (100 kDa) and the 95 kDa and 90 kDa antigens, are lipid anchored [156], whereas NCA-160 is a transmembrane protein. The method of membrane anchoring may have important functional implications in terms of association with cytoskeletal elements, generation of intracellular signals and possibly in regulation of receptor function. NCA-160 has been demonstrated to be phosphorylated cytoplasmically [160] and may also be a substrate for a neutrophil ectoprotein kinase [161], raising the possibility of multiple phosphorylation sites both inside and outside the cell. Interestingly, the YLYL motif, associated with signal transduction [162], is present in the cytoplasmic tail of one of the alternatively spliced variants of CGM1 and a similar domain is present in BGPa, which is identical to NCA-160 [163].

The role of NCA in adhesion has yet to be firmly established, although several CEA family members have been shown to mediate adhesion [164,165]. NCA-160 is heavily glycosylated (approximately 59% of the mature molecule is accounted for by carbohydrate), containing Le^x, Le^a and sLe^x which are recognized by selectins, and has been implicated in E-selectin binding [88]. The initiation of CD18 dependent adhesion responses by NCA mAb may indicate a role for NCA in triggering the events that lead to integrin activation [87]. Thus, neutrophil CEA related glycoproteins may be directly involved in neutrophil-endothelial adhesion events and indirectly in activation of independent adhesive interactions.

OTHER IMMUNOGLOBULIN FAMILY MOLECULES

Ligands for leukocyte integrins that are presented by endothelial cells are also members of the Ig superfamily. ICAM-1 comprises a single transmembrane polypeptide, with five unpaired Ig-like domains [166,167], which adopts a 'bent rod'-like structure, possibly with a hinge-like region between domains 2 and 3 [168]. Domain deletion and amino acid substitution experiments have localized the LFA-1 contact sites to residues in domains 1 and 2 of ICAM-1 [168,169] and CR3 contact sites to domain 3 [170]. The molecular weight of ICAM-1 is 90–115 kDa, but the core peptide is only 55 kDa, suggesting that ICAM-1 is heavily glycosylated. The ability of CR3 to bind ICAM-1 is altered by the extent of ICAM-1 glycosylation [132] and subtle differences in carbohydrate present on ICAM-1 may therefore affect the balance in the recruitment of lymphoid or myeloid cells that express LFA-1 or LFA-1/CR3 respectively. ICAM-2 is also a member of the Ig superfamily with two Ig-like domains [171]. When compared with ICAM-1, ICAM-2 is most homologous to those domains of ICAM-1 that are involved in LFA-1 binding, suggesting that both ICAM-1 and ICAM-2 may be recognized in a similar manner. Indeed, key residues implicated in LFA-1 binding are identical in both ICAM-1 and ICAM-2 [168,169].

A third adhesive ligand for LFA-1, termed ICAM-3, comprising five Ig-like domains has recently been identified [172–174]; it is identical to the molecule defined by CDw50 mAbs [175]. Unlike ICAM-1 or ICAM-2, ICAM-3 is abundantly expressed by neutro-phils, suggesting that it may be a major ligand mediating neutrophil interactions with LFA-1-bearing leukocytes. Such cellular adhesions may be necessary for regulation of inflammatory responses. Another neutrophil receptor of the Ig superfamily that may be important for neutrophil interactions with lymphocytes is LFA-3 which binds the T cell receptor associated molecule CD2 [176]. Adhesion receptors mediating neutrophil interaction with lymphocytes may serve to 'prime' neutrophil responses and may therefore have a critical role in control of neutrophil effector function [177].

Intracellular signals generated by occupancy of neutrophil matrix receptors also have the potential to alter neutrophil effector function [178,179]. Composition of the extracellular matrix may therefore exert control over neutrophil activation status and hence limit cellular injury and tissue damage. Non-integrin matrix receptors expressed by neutrophils include CD44 which binds hyaluronate [180], and fibronectin [181]. CD44 is a heavily glycosylated molecule with chondroitin sulphate present in addition to *N*- and *O*-linked carbohydrate and has sequence similarities with the cartilage link proteins that are involved in proteoglycan–hyaluronic acid binding [182]. Functional studies suggested that CD44 adhesion was important for binding of lymphocytes to high endothelial venules, possibly mediating tissue specific 'homing' of lymphocytes [183]. Although the widespread expression of the CD44 molecule seemed to argue against such a role, specificity may be conferred by functionally distinct variants generated by alternative splicing of the CD44 gene [184,185]. Furthermore, control of adhesion and migratory potential of cells may be determined in part by expression of CD44 variants, as tumor cells expressing certain splice variants of CD44 have increased metastatic potential [186].

Another highly glycosylated surface receptor that is thought to play a role in regulating adhesion of cells is CD43, or leukosialin. This receptor belongs to the mucin family of molecules and has 80–90 mucin-like carbohydrate groups attached extracellularly [187]. One possible function of CD43 (and other molecules which carry a net negative charge) may be to maintain cells in the circulation by exerting a net repulsion between interacting cell types [188]. In this regard it is interesting that activation of neutrophils results in proteolytic shedding of CD43 from the membrane, which may therefore facilitate adhesion [189]. CD43 is deficient in patients suffering from Wiskott–Aldrich syndrome and studies using patients' cells and recombinant proteins suggested that CD43 might serve as a receptor for ICAM-1, potentially further augmenting leukocyte integrin mediated adhesion to activated endothelium [190]. Induction of LFA-1-dependent homotypic aggregation of leukocytes as a result of cross-linking of CD43 using mAb also suggests that CD43 ligation may also serve as a signaling molecule and amplify integrin dependent leukocyte adhesion [191].

MECHANISMS OF LEUKOCYTE EMIGRATION

In the systemic circulation, leukocyte emigration occurs predominantly in the post-capillary venules, whereas in the lung it occurs through the capillary wall. Furthermore, the average diameter of the alveolar capillary is smaller than that of the neutrophil, and consequently it is thought that neutrophil deformability affects the retention time within the pulmonary circulation. Thus, 'rolling' adhesion, which may be an important factor in the arrest of neutrophils in the systemic circulation prior to transmigration events, may have a lesser role in recruitment of leukocytes into the alveolar space. However, P-selectin has a key role in neutrophil emigration processes in the lung [58,59], possibly altering the adhesion status of the neutrophil. Results from *in vivo* studies in animals using a monoclonal antibody to human CD18 also

suggest that for some pathogens neutrophil emigration into the lung may be CD18 independent [94,192]. However, the predominance of bacterial pneumonias observed in patients with LAD1(CD18 deficiency) clearly indicates that CD18 dependent emigration is critical for effective neutrophil recruitment. It is therefore likely that the mechanisms underlying neutrophil recruitment and emigration are complex.

SUMMARY

Neutrophils have been implicated as a key cell type in the development of ARDS. Interaction of neutrophils with endothelium is a prerequisite for neutrophil emigration, and neutrophil mediated cellular damage requires close apposition with endothelial surfaces. The diversity of structure and function of molecules mediating intercellular adhesion, selectins, integrins, immunoglobulin superfamily and other molecules (e.g. CD44 and CD43), allows exquisite regulation of these processes. However, additional levels of complexity within adhesion molecule families that are now beginning to be elucidated, particularly in the carbohydrate structures present on interacting cell types, provide further mechanisms for the fine control of adhesion that may be perturbed in disease states.

ACKNOWLEDGEMENTS

We would like to thank Rod Lawson for critical reading and helpful comments relating to this manuscript.

REFERENCES

1. Haslett, C., Savill, J.S. and Meagher, L. (1989) The neutrophil. *Curr. Opin. Immunol.*, **2**, 10–18.
2. Henson, P.M. and Johnston, R.B. (1987) Tissue injury in inflammation. Oxidants, proteinases and cationic proteins. *J. Clin. Invest.*, **79**, 669–74.
3. Weiss, S.J. (1989) Tissue destruction by neutrophils *N. Engl. J. Med.*, **320**, 365–76.

4. Malech, H.L. and Gallin, J.I. (1987) Neutrophils in human diseases. *N. Engl. J. Med.*, **317**, 687–94.

5. Worthen, G.S., Haslett, C., Rees, A.J. *et al.* (1987) Neutrophil-mediated pulmonary vascular injury. *Am. Rev. Respir. Dis.*, **136**, 19–28.

6. Rinaldo, J.E., and Rogers, R.M. (1982) Adult respiratory distress syndrome: changing concepts of lung injury and repair. *N. Engl. J. Med.*, **306**, 900–10.

7. Christner, P., Fein, A., Goldberg, S. *et al.* (1985) Collagenase in the lower respiratory tract of patients with the adult respiratory distress syndrome. *Am. Rev. Respir. Dis.*, **131**, 690–5.

8. Parsons, P.E., Fowler, A.A., Hyers, T.M. *et al.* (1985) Chemotactic activity in bronchoalveolar lavage fluid from patients with adult respiratory distress syndrome. *Am. Rev. Resp. Dis.*, **132**, 490–493.

9. Miller, E.J., Cohen, A.B., Nagao, S. *et al.* (1992) Elevated levels of NAP-1/interleukin-8 are present in the airspaces of patients with the adult respiratory distress syndrome and are associated with increased mortality. *Am. Rev. Respir. Dis.*, **146**, 427–32.

10. Donnelly, S.C., Strieter, R.M., Kunkel, S.L. *et al.* (1993) Interleukin-8 and development of adult respiratory distress syndrome in at-risk patient groups. *Lancet*, **341**, 643–7.

11. Osborn, L. (1990) Leukocyte adhesion to endothelium in inflammation. *Cell*, **62**, 3–6.

12. Smedley, L.A., Tonneson, M.G., Sandhous, R.A. *et al.* (1986) Neutrophil-mediated injury to endothelial cells. *J. Clin. Invest.*, **77**, 1233–43.

13. Young, S.K., Worthen, G.S., Haslett, C. *et al.* (1990) Interaction between chemoattractants and bacterial lipopolysaccharide in the induction and enhancement of neutrophil adhesion. *Am. J. Respir. Cell Mol. Biol.*, **2**, 523–32.

14. Worthen, G.S., Avdi, N., Vukajlovich, S. *et al.* (1992) Neutrophil adherence induced by lipopolysaccharide *in vitro*. *J. Clin. Invest.*, **90**, 2526–35.

15. MacNee, W. and Selby C., (1990) Neutrophil kinetics in the lung. *Clin. Sci.*, **79**, 97–107.

16. Downey, G.P., Doherty, D.E. and Schwab B. III, *et al.* (1990) Retention of leukocytes in capillaries; role of cell size and deformability. *J. Appl. Physiol.*, **69**, 1767–78.

17. Bevilacqua, M.P. and Nelson, R.M. (1993) Selectins. *J. Clin. Invest.*, **91**, 379–87.

18. Hynes, R.O. (1992) Integrins: versatility, modulation, and signaling in cell adhesion. *Cell*, **69**, 11–25.

19. Williams, A.F. and Barclay, A.N. (1988) The immunoglobulin superfamily-domains for cell surface recognition. *Ann. Rev. Immunol.*, **6**, 381–405.

20. Lawrence, M.B. and Springer, T.A. (1991) Leukocytes roll on a selectin at physiologic flow rates: distinction from and prerequisite for adhesion through integrins. *Cell*, **65**, 859–73.

21. Lorant, D.E., Patel, K.D., McIntyre, T.M. *et al.* (1991) Coexpression of GMP-140 and PAF by endothelium stimulated by histamine or thrombin: a juxtacrine system for adhesion and activation of neutrophils. *J. Cell Biol.*, **115**, 223–34.

22. Johnston, G.I., Cook, R.G. and McEver, R.P. (1989) Cloning of GMP-140, a granule membrane protein of platelets and endothelium: sequence similarity with proteins involved in cell adhesion and inflammation. *Cell*, **56**, 1033–4.

23. Bevilacqua, M.P., Pober, J.S., Mendrick, D.L. *et al.* (1987) Identification of an inducible endothelial-leucocyte adhesion molecule. *Proc. Natl Acad. Sci. USA*, **84**, 9238–42.

24. Hession, C., Osborn, L., Goff, D. *et al.* (1990) Endothelial leukocyte adhesion molecule 1: direct expression cloning and functional interactions. *Proc. Natl Acad. Sci. USA*, **87**, 1673–7.

25. Collins, T., Williams, A., Johnston, G.I. *et al.* (1991) Structure and chromosomal location of the gene for endothelial-leukocyte adhesion molecule 1. *J. Biol. Chem.*, **266**, 2466–73.

26. Bevilacqua, M., Butcher, E., Furie, B. *et al.* (1991) Selectins: a family of adhesion receptors. *Cell*, **67**, 233.

27. McEver, R.P. and Martin, M.N. (1984) A monoclonal antibody to a membrane glycoprotein binds only to activated platelets. *J. Biol. Chem.*, **259**, 9799–804.

28. Hsu-Lin, S.-C., Berman, C.L., Furie, B.C. *et al.* (1984) A platelet membrane protein expressed during platelet activation and secretion. *J. Biol. Chem.*, **259**, 9121–6.

29. Lasky, L.A., Singer, M.S., Yednock, T.A. *et al.* (1989) Cloning of a lymphocyte homing receptor reveals a lectin domain. *Cell*, **56**, 1045–55.

30. Siegelman, M.H. and Weissman, I.L. (1989) Human homologue of mouse lymph node homing receptor: evolutionary conservation

at tandem cell interaction domains. *Proc. Natl Acad. Sci. USA*, **86**, 5562–6.

31. Etzioni, A., Frydman, M., Pollack, S. *et al.* (1993) Brief report: recurrent severe infections caused by a novel leukocyte adhesion deficiency. *N. Engl. J. Med.*, **327**, 1789–92.

32. von Andrian, U.H., Berger, E.M., Ramezani, L. *et al.* (1993) *In vivo* behavior of neutrophils from two patients with distinct inherited leukocyte adhesion deficiency syndromes. *J. Clin. Invest.*, **91**, 2893–7.

33. Lowe, J.B., Stoolman, L.M., Nair, R.P. *et al.* (1990) ELAM-1-dependent cell adhesion to vascular endothelium determined by a transfected human fucosyltransferase cDNA. *Cell*, **63**, 475–84.

34. Goelz, S.E., Hession, C., Goff, D. *et al.* (1990) ELFT: a gene that directs the expression of the ELAM-1 ligand. *Cell*, **63**, 1349–56.

35. Hollenbaugh, D., Bajorath, J., Stenkamp, R. *et al.* (1993) Interaction of P-selectin (CD62) and its cellular ligand: analysis of critical residues. *Biochemistry*, **32**, 2960–6.

36. Phillips, M.L., Nudelman, E., Gaeta, F.C.A. *et al.* (1990) ELAM-1 mediates cell adhesion by recognition of a carbohydrate ligand, Sialyl-Le^x. *Science*, **250**, 1130–2.

37. Walz, G., Aruffo, A., Kolanus, W. *et al.* (1990) Recognition by ELAM-1 of the Sialyl-Le^x determinant on myeloid and tumor cells. *Science*, **250**, 1132–5.

38. Tiemeyer, M., Swiedler, S.J., Ishihara, M. *et al.* (1991) Carbohydrate ligands for endothelial-leukocyte adhesion molecule 1. *Proc. Natl Acad. Sci. USA*, **88**, 1138–42.

39. Tyrrell, D., James, P., Rao, N. *et al.* (1991) Structural requirements for the carbohydrate ligand of E-selectin. *Proc. Natl Acad. Sci. USA*, **88**, 10372–6.

40. Berg, E.L., Robinson, M.K., Mansson, O. *et al.* (1991) A carbohydrate domain common to both sialyl Le^a and sialyl Le^x is recognized by the endothelial cell leukocyte adhesion molecule ELAM-1. *J. Biol. Chem.*, **266**, 14869–72.

41. Larsen, E., Palabrica, T., Sajer, S. *et al.* (1990) PADGEM-dependent adhesion of platelets to monocytes and neutrophils is mediated by a lineage-specific carbohydrate, LNF III (CD15). *Cell*, **64**, 467–74.

42. Corral, L., Singer, M.S., Macher, B.A. *et al.* (1990) Requirement for sialic acid on neutrophils in a GMP-140 (PADGEM) mediated adhesive interaction with activated platelets. *Biochem. Biophys. Res. Commun.*, **172**, 1349–56.

43. Polley, M.J., Phillips, M.L., Wayner, E. *et al.* (1991) CD62 and endothelial cell-leukocyte adhesion molecule 1 (ELAM-1) recognize the same carbohydrate ligand, sialyl-Lewis x. *Proc. Natl Acad. Sci. USA*, **88**, 6224–8.

44. Moore, K.L., Varki, A. and McEver, R.P. (1991) GMP-140 binds to a glycoprotein receptor on human neutrophils: evidence for a lectin-like interaction. *J. Cell Biol.*, **112**, 491–9.

45. Foxall, C., Watson, S.R., Dowbenko, D. *et al.* (1992) The three members of the selectin receptor family recognize a common carbohydrate epitope, the sialyl Lewis^x oligosaccharide. *J. Cell Biol.*, **117**, 895–902.

46. Skinner, M.P., Lucas, C.M., Burns, G.F. *et al.* (1991) GMP-140 binding to neutrophils is inhibited by sulfated glycans. *J. Biol. Chem.*, **266**, 5371–4.

47. Needham, L.K. and Schnaar, R.L. (1993) The HNK-1 reactive sulfoglucuronyl glycolipids are ligands for L-selectin and P-selectin but not E-selectin. *Proc. Natl Acad. Sci. USA*, **90**, 1359–63.

48. Aruffo, A., Kolanus, W., Walz, G. *et al.* (1991) CD62/P-selectin recognition of myeloid and tumor cell sulfatides. *Cell*, **67**, 35–44.

49. Handa, K., Nudelman, E.D., Stroud, M.R. *et al.* (1991) Selectin GMP-140 (CD62; Padgem) binds to sialosyl-Le^a, and sialosyl-Le^x, and sulfated glycans modulate this binding. *Biochem. Biophys. Res. Commun.*, **181**, 1223–30.

50. Steininger, C.N., Eddy, C.A., Leimgruber, R.M. *et al.* (1992) The glycoprotease of *Pasteurella haemolytica* A1 eliminates binding of myeloid cells to P-selectin but not to E-selectin. *Biochem. Biophys. Res. Commun.*, **188**, 760–6.

51. Norgard, K.E., Han, H.J., Powell, L. *et al.* (1993) Enhanced interaction of L-selectin with the high endothelial venule ligand via selectively oxidized sialic acids. *Proc. Natl Acad. Sci. USA*, **90**, 1068–72.

52. Levinovitz, A., Muhlhoff, J., Isenmann, S. *et al.* (1993) Identification of a glycoprotein ligand for E-selectin on mouse myeloid cells. *J. Cell Biol.*, **121**, 449–59.

53. Imai, Y. and Rosen, S.D. (1993) Direct demonstration of heterogeneous, sulfated O-linked carbohydrate chains on an endothelail ligand for L-selectin. *Glycoconjugate J.*, **10**, 34–9.

54. Imai, Y., Singer, M.S., Fennie, C. *et al.* (1991) Identification of a carbohydrate-based endo-

thelial ligand for a lymphocyte homing receptor. *J. Cell Biol.*, **113**, 1213–21.

55. Suzuki, Y., Toda, Y., Tamatani, T. *et al.* (1993) Sulfated glycolipids are ligands for A lymphocyte homing receptor, L-selectin (LECAM-1), binding epitope in sulfated sugar chain. *Biochem. Biophys. Res. Commun.*, **190**, 426–34.

56. Green, P.J., Tamatani, T., Watanabe, T. *et al.* (1992) High affinity binding of the leucocyte adhesion molecule L-selectin to 3'-sulphated-Le^a and -Le^x oligosaccharides and the predominance of sulphate in this interaction demonstrated by binding studies with a series of lipid-linked oligosaccharides. *Biochem. Biophys. Res. Commun.*, **188**, 244–51.

57. Kojima, N., Handa, K., Newman, W. *et al.* (1992) Multi-recognition capability of E-selectin in a dynamic flow system, as evidenced by differential effects of sialidases and anti-carbohydrate antibodies on selectin-mediated cell adhesion at low vs. high wall shear stress: a preliminary note. *Biochem. Biophys. Res. Commun.*, **189**, 1686–94.

58. Mulligan, M.S., Polley, M.J., Bayer, R.J. *et al.* (1992) Neutrophil-dependent acute lung injury. Requirement for P-selectin (GMP-140). *J. Clin. Invest.*, **90**, 1600–7.

59. Mulligan, M.S., Paulson, J.C., De Frees, S. *et al.* (1993) Protective effects of oligosaccharides in P-selectin dependent lung injury. *Nature*, **364**, 149–51.

60. Dore, M., Korthuis, R.J., Granger, D.N. *et al.* (1993) P-selectin mediates spontaneous leukocyte rolling *in vivo*. *Blood*, **82**, 1308–16.

61. Dunlop, L.C., Skinner, M.P., Bendall, J.L. *et al.* (1992) Characterization of GMP-140 (P-selectin) as a circulating plasma protein. *J. Exp. Med.*, **175**, 1147–50.

62. Katayama, Y., Gottesman, S., Pumphrey, J. *et al.* (1988) The two-component, ATP-dependent Clp protease of *Escherichia coli*. Purification, cloning, and mutational analysis of the ATP-binding component. *J. Biol. Chem.*, **263**, 15226–36.

63. Mayadas, T.N., Johnson, R.C., Rayburn, H. *et al.* (1993) Leukocyte rolling and exravasation are severely compromised in P-selectin deficient mice. *Cell*, **74**, 541–54.

64. Weyrich, A.S., Ma, X., Lefer, D.J. *et al.* (1993) *In vivo* neutralization of P-selectin protects feline heart and endothelium in myocardial ischaemia and reperfusion injury. *J. Clin. Invest.*, **91**, 2620–9.

65. Hamburger, S.A. and McEver, R.P. (1990) GMP-140 mediates adhesion of stimulated platelets to neutrophils. *Blood*, **75**, 550–4.

66. Hakkert, B.C., Kuijpers, T.W., Leeuwenberg, J.F.M. *et al.* (1991) Neutrophil and monocyte adherence to and migration across monolayers of cytokine-activated endothelial cells: the contribution of CD18, ELAM-1, and VLA-4. *Blood*, **78**, 2721–6.

67. Larsen, E., Celi, A., Gilbert, G.E. *et al.* (1989) PADGEM protein: a receptor that mediates the interaction of activated platelets with neutrophils and monocytes. *Cell*, **59**, 305–12.

68. Buttrum, S.M., Hatton, R. and Nash, G.B. (1993) Selectin mediated rolling of neutrophils on immobilized platelets. *Blood*, **82**, 1165–74.

69. Grober, J.S., Bowen, B.L., Ebling, H. *et al.* (1993) Monocyte-endothelial adhesion in chronic rheumatoid arthritis. *J. Clin. Invest.* **91**, 2609–19.

70. Palabrica, T., Lobb, R., Furie, B.C. *et al.* (1993) Leukocyte accumulation promoting fibrin deposition is mediated *in vivo* by P-selectin on adherent platelets. *Nature*, **359**, 848–51.

71. Kishimoto, T.K., Warnock, R.A., Jutila, M.A. *et al.* (1991) Antibodies against human neutrophil LECAM-1 (LAM-1/Leu-8/DREG-56 antigen) and endothelial cell ELAM-1 inhibit a common CD18-indepedent adhesion pathway *in vitro*. *Blood*, **78**, 805–11.

72. Picker, L.J., Warnock, R.A., Burns, A.R. *et al.* (1991) The neutrophil selectin LECAM-1 presents carbohydrate ligands to vascular selectins ELAM-1 and GMP-140. *Cell*, **66**, 921–33.

73. McEver, R.P., Beckstead, J.H., Moore, K.L. *et al.* (1989) GMP-140, a platelet a-granule membrane protein, is also synthesized by vascular endothelial cells and is localized in Weibel-Palade bodies. *J. Clin. Invest.*, **84**, 92–9.

74. Geng, J.-G., Bevilacqua, M.P., Moore, K.L. *et al.* (1990) Rapid neutrophil adhesion to activated endothelium mediated by GMP-140. *Nature*, **343**, 757–60.

75. Patel, K.D., Zimmerman, G.A., Prescott, S.M. *et al.* (1991) Oxygen radicals induce human endothelial cells to express GMP-140 and bind neutrophils. *J. Cell Biol.*, **112**, 749–59.

76. Crovello, C.W., Furie, B.C. and Furie, B. (1993) Rapid phosphorylation and selctive dephosphorylation of P-selectin accompanies platelet activation. *J. Biol. Chem.*, **268**, 14590–3.

77. Gamble, J.R., Skinner, M.P., Berndt, M.C. *et al.*

(1990) Prevention of activated neutrophil adhesion to endothelium by soluble adhesion protein GMP-140. *Science*, **249**, 414–7.

78. Wong, C.S., Gamble, J.R., Skinner, M.P. *et al.* (1991) Adhesion protein GMP-140 inhibits superoxide anion release by human neutrophils. *Proc. Natl Acad. Sci. USA*, **88**, 2397–401.

79. Montgomery, K.F., Osborn, L., Hession, C. *et al.* (1991) Activation of endothelial-leukocyte adhesion molecule 1 (ELAM-1) gene transcription. *Proc. Natl Acad. Sci. USA*, **88**, 6523–7.

80. Suzuki, Y., Wang, W., Vu, T.H. *et al.* (1992) Effect of NADPH oxidase inhibition on endothelial cell ELAM-1 mRNA expression. *Biochem. Biophys. Res. Commun.*, **184**, 1339–43.

81. Klein, L.M., Lavker, L.M., Matis, W.L. *et al.* (1989) Degranulation of human mast cells induces an endothelial antigen central to leukocyte adhesion *Proc. Natl Acad. Sci. USA*, **86**, 8972–6.

82. Munro, M.J., Pober, J.S. and Cotran, R.S. (1991) Brief communication. Recruitment of neutrophils in the local endotoxin response: association with *de novo* endothelial expression of endothelial leukocyte adhesion molecule-1. *Lab. Invest.*, **64**, 295–9.

83. Kishimoto, T.K., Jutila, M.A., Berg, E.L. *et al.* (1989) Neutrophil Mac-1 and MEL-14 adhesion proteins inversely regulated by chemotactic factors. *Science*, **245**, 1238–41.

84. Dobrina, A., Carlos, T.M., Schwartz, B.R. *et al.* (1990) Phorbol ester causes down-regulation of CD11/CD18-independent neutrophil adherence to endothelium. *Immunology*, **69**, 429–34.

85. Schleiffenbaum, B., Spertini, O. and Tedder, T.F. (1992) Soluble L-selectin is present in human plasma at high levels and retains functional activity. *J. Cell Biol.*, **119**, 229–38.

86. Stocks, S.C. and Kerr, M.A. (1993) Neutrophil NCA-160 (CD66) is the major protein carrier of selectin binding carbohydrate groups Lewisx and sialyl-Lewisx. *Biochem. Biophys. Res. Commun.*, **195**, 478–83.

87. Asada, M., Furukawa, K., Kantor, C. *et al.* (1991) Structural study of the sugar chains of human leukocyte cell adhesion molecules CD11/CD18. *Biochemistry*, **30**, 1561–71.

88. Stocks, S.C. and Kerr M.A. (1992) Stimulation of neutrophil adhesion by antibodies recognizing CD15 (Lex) and CD15-expressing carcinoembryonic antigen-related glycoprotein NCA-160. *Biochem. J.*, **288**, 23–7.

89. Kuijpers, T.W., Hoogerwerf, M., van der Laan, L.J.W. *et al.* (1992) CD66 nonspecific cross-reacting antigens are involved in neutrophil adherence to cytokine-activated endothelial cells. *J. Cell Biol.*, **118**, 457–66.

90. Kotovuori, P., Tontti, E., Pigott, R. *et al.* (1993) The vascular E-selectin binds to the leukocyte integrins CD11/CD18. *Glycobiology*, **3**, 131–6.

91. Kuijpers, T.W., Hakkert, B.C., Hoogerwerf, M. *et al.* (1991) Role of endothelial leukocyte adhesion molecule-1 and platelet-activating factor in neutrophil adherence to IL-1 prestimulated endothelial cells. *J. Immunol.*, **147**, 1369–76.

92. Lorant, D.E., Topham, M.K., Whatley, R.E. *et al.* (1993) Inflammatory roles of P-selectin. *J. Clin. Invest.*, **92**, 559–70.

93. Lo, S.K., Lee, S., Ramos, R.A. *et al.* (1991) Endothelial leukocyte adhesion molecule-1 stimulates the adhesive activity of leukocyte integrin CR3 (CD11b/CD18, mac-1, amb2) on human neutrophils. *J. Exp. Med.*, **173**, 1493–1500.

94. Doerschuk, C.M., Winn, R.K., Coxson, H.O. *et al.* (1990) CD18-dependent and -independent mechanisms of neutrophil emigration in the pulmonary and systemic microcirculation of rabbits. *J. Immunol.*, **144**, 2327–33.

95. Tamkun, J.W., DeSimone, D.W., Fonda, D. *et al.* (1986) Structure of integrin, a glycoprotein involved in transmembrane linkage between fibronectin and actin. *Cell*, **46**, 271–82.

96. Hogg, N. (1989) The leukocyte integrins. *Immunol. Today*, **10**, 111–4.

97. Anderson, D.C. and Springer, T.A. (1987) Leukocyte adhesion deficiency; an inherited defect in the Mac-1, LFA-1 and p150, 95 glycoproteins. *Ann. Rev. Med.*, **38**, 175–94.

98. Arnaout, M.A. (1990) Leukocyte adhesion molecules deficiency: its structural basis, pathophysiology and implications for modulating the inflammatory response. *Immunol. Rev.*, **114**, 145–80.

99. Bohnsack, J.F. (1992) CD11/18-independent neutrophil adherence to laminin is mediated by the integrin VLA-6. *Blood*, **79**, 1545–52.

100. Gresham, H.D., Goodwin, J.L., Allen, P.M. *et al.* (1989) A novel member of the integrin receptor family mediates Arg-Gly-Asp-stimu-

lated neutrophil phagocytosis. *J. Cell Biol.*, **108**, 1935–43.

101. Anderson, D.C., Schmalsteig, F.C., Arnaout, M.A. *et al.* (1984) Abnormalities of poly-morphonuclear leukocyte function associated with a heritable deficiency of a high molecu-lar weight surface glycoprotein (gp138; com-mon relationship to diminished cell adherence. *J. Clin. Invest.*, **74**, 536–51.

102. Arnaout, M.A., Spits, H., Terhorst, C. *et al.* (1984) Deficiency of a leukocyte glycoprotein (LFA-1) in two patients with Mo1 deficiency. Effects of cell activation on Mo1/LFA-1 sur-face expression on normal and deficient leukocytes. *J. Clin. Invest.*, **74**, 1291–300.

103. Beatty, P.G., Harlen, J.M., Rosen, H. *et al.* (1984) Absence of a monoclonal antibody-defined protein complex in a boy with recur-rent bacterial infections. *Lancet*, **i**, 535–7.

104. Dana, N., Todd, R.F., Colten, H.R. *et al.* (1984) Deficiency of a monocyte-granulocyte surface glycoprotein (Mo1) in man. *J. Clin. Invest.*, **73**, 153–9.

105. Springer, T.A., Thompson, W.S., Miller, L.J. *et al.* (1984) Inherited deficiency of the Mac-1, LFA-1, p150,95 glycoprotein family and its molecular basis *J. Exp. Med.*, **160**, 1901–18.

106. Hibbs, M.L., Wardlaw, A.J., Stacker, S.A. *et al.* (1990) Transfection of cells from patients with leukocyte adhesion deficiency with an integ-rin beta subunit (CD18) restores lymphocyte function- associated antigen-1 expression and function. *J. Clin. Invest.*, **85**, 674–81.

107. Wilson, J.M., Ping, A.J., Krauss, J.C. *et al.* (1990) Correction of CD18-deficient lympho-cytes by retrovirus-mediated gene transfer. *Science*, **248**, 1413–6.

108. Kishimoto, T.K., O'Connor, K., Lee, A. *et al.* (1987) Cloning of the beta subunit of the leukocyte adhesion proteins: homology to an extracellular matrix receptor defines a novel supergene family. *Cell*, **48**, 681–90.

109. D'Souza, S.E., Ginsberg, M.H., Burke, T.A. *et al.* (1988) Localization of an Arg-Gly-Asp recognition site within an integrin adhesion receptor. *Science*, **242**, 91–3.

110. Smith, J.W. and Cheresh, D.A. (1988) The arg-gly-asp binding domain of the vitronectin receptor. *J. Biol. Chem.*, **263**, 18726–31.

111. Diamond, M.S., Garcia-Arguilar, J., Bickford, J.K. *et al.* (1993) The I domain is a major recognition site on the leukocyte integrin Mac-1 (CD11b/CD18) for four distinct adhe-sion ligands. *J. Cell Biol.*, **120**, 1031–43.

112. Landis, R.C., Bennett, R.I. and Hogg, N. (1993) A novel LFA-1 activation epitope maps to the I domain. *J. Cell Biol.*, **120**, 1519–27.

113. Edwards, J.G., Hameed, H. and Campbell, G. (1988) Induction of fibroblast spreading by Mn^{2+}: a possible role for unusual binding sites for divalent cations in receptors for pro-teins containing Arg-Gly-Asp. *J. Cell Sci.*, **89**, 507–13.

114. Michishita, M., Videm, V. and Arnaout, M.A. (1993) A novel divalent cation binding site in the A domain of the β_2 integrin CR3 (CD11b/CD18) is essential for ligand binding. *Cell*, **72**, 857–67.

115. Dahms, N.M. and Hart, G.W. (1985) Lympho-cyte function-associated antigen-1 (LFA-1) contains sulfated N-linked oligosaccharides. *J. Immunol.* **134**, 3978–86.

116. Takeda, A. (1987) Sialylation patterns of lym-phocyte function-associated antigen 1 (LFA-1) differ between T and B lymphocytes. *Eur. J. Immunol.*, **17**, 281–6.

117. Skubitz, K.M. and Snook, R.W. (1987) Mono-clonal antibodies that recognize lacto-*N*-fuco-pentaose III (CD15) react with the adhesion promoting glycoprotein family (LFA-1/HMAC-1/GP150, 95) and CR1 on human neutrophils. *J. Immunol.* **139**, 1631–9.

118. Chatila, T.A., Geha, R.F. and Arnaout, M.A. (1989) Constitutive and stimulus-induced phosphorylation of CD11/CD18 leukocyte adhesion molecule. *J. Cell Biol.*, **109**, 3435–44.

119. Merrill, J.T., Slade, S.G., Weissmann, G. *et al.* (1990) Two pathways of CD11b/CD18-medi-ated neutrophil aggregation with different involvement of protein kinase C-dependent phosphorylation. *J. Immunol.*, **145**, 2608–815.

120. Hibbs, M.L., Xu, H., Stacker, S.A. *et al.* (1991) Regulation of adhesion to ICAM-1 by the cytoplasmic domain of the LFA-1 integrin β subunit. *Science* **251**, 1611–3.

121. Haskard, D., Cavender, D., Beatty, P. *et al.* (1986) T lymphocyte adhesion to endothelial cells: mechanisms demonstrated by anti-LFA-1 monoclonal antibodies. *J. Immunol.*, **137**, 2901–6.

122. Dustin, M.L. and Springer, T.A. (1988) Lym-phocyte function-associated antigen-1 (LFA-1) interaction with intercellular adhesion mol-ecule-1 (ICAM-1) is one of at least three mech-

anisms for lymphocyte adhesion to cultured endothelial cells. *J. Cell Biol.* **107**, 321–31.

123. Dustin, M.L., Rothlein, R., Bhan, A.K. *et al.* (1986) Induction by IL-1 and interferon-gamma: tissue distribution, biochemistry and function of a natural adherence molecule (ICAM-1). *J. Immunol.*, **317**, 245–54.

124. Beller, D.I., Springer, T.A. and Schreiber, R.D. (1982) Anti-Mac-1 selectively inhibits the mouse and human type three complement receptor. *J. Exp. Med.*, **156**, 1000–9.

125. Wright, S.D., Rao, P.E., van Voorhis, W.C. *et al.* (1983) Identification of the C3bi receptor on human monocytes and macrophages by using monoclonal antibodies. *Proc. Natl Acad. Sci. USA*, **80**, 5699–703.

126. Micklem, R.J. and Sim, R.B. (1985) Isolation of complement fragment-iC3b-binding proteins by affinity chromatography. *Biochem. J.*, **231**, 233–6.

127. Myones, B.L., Dalzell, J.G., Hogg, N. *et al.* (1988) Neutrophil and monocyte cell surface p150, 95 has iC3b-receptor activity resembling CR3. *J. Clin. Invest.*, **82**, 640–51.

128. Altieri, D.C. and Edgington, T.S. (1988) The saturable high affinity association of factor X to ADP-stimulated monocytes defines a novel function of the Mac-1 receptor. *J. Biol. Chem.*, **263**, 7007–15.

129. Altieri, D.C., Bader, R., Mannucci, P.M. *et al.* (1988) Oligospecificity of the cellular adhesion receptor MAC-1 encompasses an inducible specificity for fibrinogen. *J. Cell Biol.*, **107**, 1893–1900.

130. Wright, S.D., Weitz, J.I., Huang, A.J. *et al.* (1988) Complement receptor type three (CD11b/CD18) of human polymorphonuclear leukocytes recognizes fibrinogen. *Proc. Natl Acad. Sci. USA*, **85**, 7734–8.

131. Smith, C.W., Marlin, S.D., Rothlein, R. *et al.* (1989) Cooperative interactions of LFA-1 and Mac-1 with intercellular adhesion molecule-1 in facilitating adherence and transendothelial migration of human neutrophils *in vitro*. *J. Clin. Invest.*, **83**, 2008–2017.

132. Diamond, M.S., Staunton, D.E., de Fougerolles, A.R. *et al.* (1990) ICAM-1 (CD54) a counter receptor for Mac-1 (CD11b/CD18). *J. Cell Biol*, **111**, 3129–39.

133. Loike, J.D., Sodeik, B., Cao, L. *et al.* (1991) CD11c/CD18 on neutrophils recognizes a domain at the N terminus of the A-α chain of fibrinogen. *Proc. Natl Acad. Sci. USA*, **88**, 1044–8.

134. Arnaout, M.A., Lanier, L.L. and Faller, D.V. (1988) Relative contribution of the leukocyte molecules Mo1, LFA-1, p150, 95 (LeuM5) in adhesion of granulocytes and monocytes to vascular endothelium is tissue- and stimulus-specific. *J. Cell. Physiol.*, **137**, 305–9.

135. Keizer, G.D., te Velde, A.A., Schwarting, R. *et al.* (1987) Role of p150, 95 in adhesion, migration, chemotaxis and phagocytosis of human monocytes. *Eur. J. Immunol.* **17**, 1317–22.

136. de Fougerolles, A.R., Stacker, S.A., Schwarting, R. *et al.* (1991) Characterization of ICAM-2 and evidence for a third counter-receptor for LFA-1. *J. Exp. Med.*, **174**, 253–67.

137. Otey, C.A., Pavalko, F.M. and Burridge, K. (1990) An interaction between alpha-actinin and the β1 integrin subunit *in vitro J. Cell Biol.*, **111**, 721–9.

138. Horwitz, A., Duggan, K., Burk, C. *et al.* (1986) Interaction of plasma membrane fibronectin receptor with talin – a transmembrane linkage *Nature*, **320**, 531–3.

139. Carpen, O., Pallai, P., Staunton, D.E. *et al.* (1992) Association of intercellular adhesion molecule-1 (ICAM-1) with actin-containing cytoskeleton and α-actinin. *J. Cell Biol.*, **118**, 1223–34.

140. Todd, R.F. III, Arnaout, M.A., Rosin, R.E. *et al.* (1984) Subcellular localization of the large subunit of Mo1 (Mo1α; formerly gp110), a surface glycoprotein associated with neutrophil adhesion. *J. Clin. Invest.*, **74**, 1280–90.

141. Bainton, D.F., Miller, L.J., Kishimoto, T.K. *et al.* (1987) Leukocyte adhesion receptors are stored in peroxidase negative granules of human neutrophils. *J. Exp. Med.*, **166**, 1641–53.

142. Sengelov, H., Kjeldsen, L., Diamond, M.S. *et al.* (1993) Subcellular localization and dynamics of Mac-1 (αmβ2) in human neutrophils. *J. Clin. Invest.*, **92**, 1467–76.

143. Buyon, J.P., Abramson, S.B., Philips, M.R. *et al.* (1988) Dissociation between increased surface expression of Gp165/95 and homotypic neutrophil aggregation. *J. Immunol.* **140**, 3156–60.

144. Vedder, N.B. and Harlen, J.M. (1988) Increased surface expression of CD11b/CD18 (Mac-1) is not required for stimulated neutrophil adherence to endothelium. *J. Clin. Invest.*, **81** 676–82.

145. Lo, S.K., Detmers, P.A., Levin, S.M. *et al.* (1989) Transient adhesion of neutrophils to endothelium. *J. Exp. Med.*, **169** 1779–93.

146. Hughes, B.J., Hollers, J.C., Crockett-Torabi, E. *et al.* (1992) Recruitment of CD11b/CD18 to the neutrophil surface and adherence-dependent cell locomotion. *J. Clin. Invest.* **90**, 1687–96.

147. Figdor, C.G., van Kooyk Y. and Keizer, G.D. (1990) On the mode of action of LFA-1. *Immunol. Today*, **11** 277–80.

148. Dransfield, I. and Hogg, N. (1989) Regulated expression of a Mg^{2+} binding epitope on leukocyte integrin alpha subunits. *EMBO J.*, **12**, 3759–65.

149. Dransfield, I., Cabanas, C., Craig, A. *et al.* (1992) Divalent cation regulation of the function of the leukocyte integrin LFA-1. *J. Cell Biol.*, **116**, 219–26.

150. Dransfield, I., Cabanas, C., Barrett, J. *et al.* (1992) Interaction of leukocyte integrins with ligand is necessary but not sufficient for function *J. Cell Biol.*, **116**, 1527–35.

151. Cabanas, C. and Hogg, N. (1993) Ligand intercellular adhesion molecule 1 has a necessary role in activation of integrin lymphocyte function-associated molecule 1. *Proc. Natl Acad. Sci. USA*, **90**, 5838–42.

152. Holness, C.L. and Simmons, D.L. (1994) Structural motifs for recognition and adhesion in members of the immunoglobulin superfamily. *J. Cell Sci.*, **107**, 2065–70.

153. Thomas, P., Toth, C.A., Saini, K.S. *et al.* (1990) The structure, metabolism and function of the carcinoembryonic antigen gene family. *Biochim.Biophys.Acta*, **1032**, 177–89.

154. Buchegger, F., Schreyer, M., Carrel, S. *et al.* (1984) Monoclonal antibodies identify a CEA crossreacting antigen of 95 kD (NCA-95) distinct in antigenicity and tissue distribution from the previously described NCA of 55 kD. *Int. J. Cancer*, **33**, 643–9.

155. Audette, M., Buchegger, F., Schreyer, M. *et al.* (1987) Monoclonal antibody against carcinoembryonic antigen (CEA) identifies two new forms of crossreacting antigens of molecular weight 90 000 and 160 000 in normal granulocytes. *Mol. Immunol.*, **24**, 1177–86.

156. Kuroki, M., Matsuo, Y. and Matsuoka, Y. (1990) Nonspecific cross-reacting antigen (NCA) expressed by human granulocytes: six species with different peptide sizes and membrane anchoring forms. *Biochem. Biophys. Res. Commun.*, **166**, 701–8.

157. Mahrenholz, A.M., Yeh, C.H., Shively, J.E. *et al.* (1993) Microsequence and mass spectral analysis of nonspecific cross-reacting antigen 160, a CD15 positive neutrophil membrane glycoprotein; demonstration of identity with biliary glycoprotein 1. *J. Biol. Chem.*, **268**, 13015–8.

158. Stoffel, A., Neumaier, M., Gaida, F.-J. *et al.* (1993) Monoclonal, anti-domain and anti-peptide antibodies assign the molecular weight 160 000 granulocyte membrane antigen of the CD66 cluster to a mRNA species encoded by the biliary glycoprotein gene, a member of the carcinoembryonic antigen gene family. *J. Immunol.*, **150**, 4978–84.

159. Berling, B., Kolbinger, F., Grunert, F. *et al.* (1990) Cloning of a carcinoembryonic antigen gene family member expressed in leukocytes of chronic myeloid leukemia patients and bone marrow. *Cancer Res.*, **50**, 6534–9.

160. Afar, D.E.H., Stanners, C.P. and Bell, J.C. (1992) Tyrosine phosphorylation of biliary glycoprotein, a cell adhesion molecule related to carcinoembryonic antigen. *Biochim. Biophys. Acta*, **1134**, 46–52.

161. Skubitz, K.M., Ducker, T.P. and Goueli, S.A. (1992) CD66 monoclonal antibodies recognize a phosphotyrosine containing protein bearing a carcinoembryonic antigen cross reacting antigen on the surface of human neutrophils. *J. Immunol.* **148**, 852–60.

162. Keegan, A.D. and Paul, W.E. (1992) Multichain imune recognition receptors: similarities in structure and signaling pathways. *Immunol. Today*, **13**, 63–8.

163. Nagel, G., Grunert, F., Kuijpers, T.W. *et al.* (1993) Genomic organization, splice variants and expression of CGM1, a CD66 related member of the carcinoembryonic antigen gene family. *Eur. J. Biochem.*, **214**, 27–35.

164. Oikawa, S., Inuzuka, C., Kuroki, M. *et al.* (1989) Cell adhesion activity of non-specific cross-reacting antigen (NCA) and carcinoembryonic antigen (CEA) expressed on CHO cell surface: homophilic and heterophilic adhesion. *Biochem. Biophys. Res. Commun.*, **164**, 39–45.

165. Oikawa, S., Kuroki, M., Matsuoka, Y. *et al.* (1992) Homotypic and heterotypic Ca^{++}-independent cell adhesion activities of biliary glycoprotein, a member of carcinoembryonic

antigen family, expressed on CHO cell surface. *Biochem. Biophys. Res. Commun.*, **186**, 881–7.

166. Simmons, D., Makgoba, M.W. and Seed, B. (1988) ICAM-1, an adhesion ligand of LFA-1, is homologous to the neural cell adhesion molecule NCAM. *Nature*, **331**, 624–7.

167. Staunton, D.E., Marlin, S.D., Stratowa, C. *et al.* (1988) Primary structure of ICAM-1 demonstrates interaction between members of the immunoglobulin and integrin supergene families. *Cell*, **52**, 925–33.

168. Staunton, D.E., Dustin, M.L., Erickson, H.P. *et al.* (1990) The arrangement of the immunoglobulin-like domains of ICAM-1 and the binding sites for LFA-1 and rhinovirus. *Cell*, **61**, 243–54.

169. Berendt, A.R., McDowall, A., Craig, A.G. *et al.* (1991) The binding site on ICAM-1 for *Plasmodium falciparum* infected erythrocytes overlaps but is distinct from the LFA-1 binding site. *Cell*, **68**, 71–81.

170. Diamond, M.S., Staunton, D.E., Marlin, S.D. *et al.* (1991) Binding of the integrin Mac-1 (CD11b/CD18) to the third immunoglobulin-like domain of ICAM-1 (CD54) and its regulation by glycosylation. *Cell*, **65**, 961–71.

171. Staunton, D.E., Dustin, M.L. and Springer, T.A. (1989) Functional cloning of ICAM-2, a cell adhesion ligand for LFA-1 homologous to ICAM-1. *Nature*, **339**, 61–4.

172. Fawcett, J., Holness, C.L.L., Needham, L.A. *et al.* (1992) Molecular cloning of ICAM-3, a third ligand for LFA-1, constitutively expressed on resting leukocytes. *Nature*, **360**, 481–4.

173. de Fougerolles, A., Klickstein, L.B. and Springer T.A. (1993) Cloning and expression of intercellular adhesion molecule 3 reveals strong homology to other immunoglobulin family counter-receptors for lymphocyte function-associated antigen 1. *J. Exp. Med.*, **177**, 1187–92.

174. Vazeux, R., Hoffman, P.A., Tomita, J.K. *et al.* (1992) Cloning and characterization of a new intercellular adhesion molecule ICAM-R. *Nature*, **360**, 485–8.

175. Juan, M., Vilella, R., Mila, J. *et al.* (1993) CDw50 and ICAM-3: two names for the same molecule. *Eur. J. Immunol.*, **23**, 1508–12.

176. Springer, T.A., Dustin, M.L., Kishimoto T.K. *et al.* (1987) The lymphocyte function-associated LFA-1, CD2, and LFA-3 molecules: cell adhesion receptors of the immune system. *Ann. Rev. Immunol.*, **5**, 223–52.

177. Zhang, J-H., Ferrante, A., Arrigo, A-P. *et al.* (1992) Neutrophil stimulation and priming by direct contact with activated human T lymphocytes. *J. Immunol.*, **148**, 177–81.

178. Nathan, C.F. (1987) Neutrophil activation on biological surfaces. *J. Clin. Invest.*, **80**, 1550–60.

179. Zhou, M. and Brown, E.J. (1993) CR3 (Mac 1, $\alpha M\beta_2$, CD11b/CD18) and FcγRIII cooperate in generation of a neutrophil respiratory burst: requirement for FcγRII and tyrosine phosphorylation. *J. Exp. Med.*, **178**, 1165–74.

180. Lesley, J., Hyman, R. and Kincade, P.W. (1993) CD44 and its interaction with extracullular matrix. *Adv. Immunol.*, **54**, 327–35.

181. Jalkanen, S. and Jalkanen, M. (1992) Lymphocyte CD44 binds the COOH terminal heparin binding domain of fibronectin. *J. Cell Biol.*, **116** 817–25.

182. Stamenkovic, I., Amiot, M., Pesando J.M. *et al.* (1989) A lymphocyte molecule implicated in lymph node homing is a member of the cartilage link protein family. *Cell*, **56**, 1057–62.

183. Goldstein, L.A., Zhou, D.F.H., Picker, L.J. *et al.* (1989) A human lymphocyte homing receptor, the Hermes antigen, is related to cartilage proteoglycan core and link proteins. *Cell*, **56**, 1063–72.

184. Dougherty, G.J., Lansdorp, P.M., Cooper, D.L. *et al.* (1991) Molecular cloning of CD44r1 and CD44r2 two novel isoforms of the human CD44 lymphocyte 'homing' receptor expressed by hemopoietic cells. *J. Exp. Med.*, **174**, 1–5.

185. Arch, R., Wirth, K., Hofmann, M. *et al.* (1992) Participation in normal immune responses of a metastasis-inducing splice variant of CD44. *Science* **257**, 682–5.

186. Gunthert, U., Hofmann, M., Rudy, W. *et al.* (1991) A new variant of glycoprotein CD44 confers metastatic potential to rat carcinoma cells. *Cell*, **65**, 13–24.

187. Hilkens, J., Ligtenberg, M.J.L., Vos, H.L. *et al.* (1992) Cell membrane-associated mucins and their adhesion-modualting capacity. *Trends Biochem. Sci.*, 17, 359–63.

188. Springer, T.A. (1990) Adhesion receptors of the immune system *Nature*, **346**, 425–34.

189. Rieu, P., Porteau, F., Bessou, G. *et al.* (1992) Human neutrophils release their major mem-

brane sialoprotein, leukosialin (CD43), during cell activation. *Eur. J. Immunol.,* **22**, 3021–6.

190. Rosenstein, Y., Park, J.K. Hahn, W.C. *et al.* (1991) CD43, a molecule defective in Wiscott–Aldrich syndrome, binds ICAM-1. *Nature,* **354**, 233–5.

191. deSmet, W., Walter, H. and van Hove, L. (1993) A new CD43 monoclonal antibody induces homotypic aggreagation of human leukocytes through a CD11a/CD18-dependent and -independent mechanism. *Immunology,* **79**, 46–54.

192. Vedder, N.B., Winn, R.K., Rice, C.L. *et al.* (1988) A monoclonal antibody to the adherence-promoting glycoprotein CD18 reduces organ injury and improves survival from haemorrhagic shock in rabbits. *J. Clin. Invest.,* **81**, 939–44.

PROTEINASES

10

Caroline A. Owen and Edward J. Campbell

There are several lines of evidence to indicate that proteinases play a critical role in both the pathogenesis and the resolution of the syndrome of acute respiratory distress in adults (ARDS). Firstly, through their capacity to injure endothelial cells, epithelial cells and interstitial structures, proteinases may play major roles in the initiation of lung injury and especially in the pathogenesis of abnormal capillary permeability. Secondly, polymorphonuclear neutrophils, (PMNs) which contain especially potent proteinases, are sequestered in large numbers in the microvasculature and air spaces of the lungs in patients with ARDS. Thirdly, abnormal proteinase activity has been well documented in ARDS. Finally, in the resolution/repair phase of ARDS, proteinases are necessary for clearing the proteinaceous debris that fills the alveolar spaces.

Essentially all of the enzymes discussed here have been cloned and sequenced, and a great deal is known about the biochemistry of their catalytic activity. However, throughout this chapter we emphasize that our knowledge of the individual roles of various proteinases in tissue injury and repair have not been fully elucidated. We will first review the biochemistry and cell biology of various proteinases that might be relevant to ARDS, then consider evidence for involvement of each in the pathogenesis and resolution of the syndrome. Finally, the prospects for inhibition of

proteinases as a potential therapeutic strategy in ARDS are reviewed.

CLASSIFICATION SCHEMES

Proteinases, or endopeptidases, are capable of cleaving peptide bonds in the central regions of polypeptides. To facilitate understanding of the potential roles of proteinases in lung disease, it is useful to group them by structure, activity and source. Thus, proteinases can be classified by [1] the chemical nature of their active site; [2] the predominant type of substrate(s) they prefer; or [3] the predominant cell type(s) from which they originate. A fourth grouping, that of the pH at which they have greatest activity (Table 10.1), will not be considered separately.

BIOCHEMISTRY OF THE ACTIVE SITE

Four distinct classes of proteinases can be identified by the amino acid groups and biochemical mechanisms responsible for their catalytic activities. These include serine proteinases, metalloproteinases, aspartic proteinases and cysteine proteinases. As can be seen from Table 10.1, serine and metalloproteinases are most active at neutral pH and, it is therefore apparent that they could play a major role in degradation of extracellular structural proteins. By contrast, the aspartic and cysteine proteinases have acidic pH optima; their main role is in intracellular pro-

ARDS Acute Respiratory Distress in Adults. Edited by Timothy W. Evans and Christopher Haslett. Published in 1996 by Chapman & Hall, London. ISBN 0 412 56910 8

Table 10.1 Classification of proteinases according to catalytic mechanism

Mechanism	Active Site	pH Optimum	Examples	Location
Serine proteinases	'Catalytic triad' Asp, His, **Ser**	Neutral (pH 7–9)	Human leukocyte elastase, cathepsin G, proteinase 3	PMNs, monocytes, eosinophils, basophils
			Plasminogen activators	Synthesized and secreted (leukocytes, endothelial cells) Cell surface of leukocytes
			Thrombin and plasmin	Plasma
			Tryptase	Granules of mast cells and basophils
Metalloproteinases	Zn^{2+} coordinated to amino acids	Neutral (pH 7–9)	See Table 10.2	See Table 10.2
Cysteine proteinases	**Cys**, His	Acidic (pH 3–6)[a]	Cathepsin S Cathepsin L Cathepsin B	Lysosomes of most cells
Aspartic proteinases	Asp (2 residues)	Acidic (pH 2–5)	Cathepsin D	Lysosomes of most cells

[a] At pH 7, cathepsin S retains 25% of its catalytic activity.

tein digestion, which occurs within the acidic environment of lysosomes. However, the latter classes of proteinases may also play a role in the degradation of extracellular matrix macromolecules if they are released in high enough concentrations and/or in a microenvironment that allows the local maintenance of an acid pH, such as the area subjacent to activated phagocytes [1,2].

A mechanism based classification is useful not only for understanding the biochemistry of the enzymes but also for understanding the spectrum of activity of proteinase inhibitors, most of which are targeted against enzymes having a specific catalytic mechanism.

Serine proteinases

Serine proteinases have a catalytically essential serine residue at their active site, and are the largest class of mammalian proteinases. Mammalian serine proteinases have the sequence Asp-Ser-Gly at their reactive center, and their activity depends upon a 'catalytic triad' consisting of residues Asp^{102}, His^{57}, and Ser^{195} (chymotrypsin numbering). These amino acid residues are widely separated in the primary sequence but are brought together at the active site of the enzymes in their tertiary structure [3].

The extensive structural homologies among serine proteinases has led to the hypothesis that they have all diverged from a primitive digestive enzyme through the process of gene duplication and mutation. This class of proteinases includes many of the proteins involved in the cascades of coagulation, fibrinolysis and complement activation, as well as the digestive enzymes trypsin and chymotrypsin. The importance of serine proteinases in physiologic and pathologic processes is underscored by the fact that inhibitors of these enzymes comprise about 10% of all plasma proteins.

Most serine proteinases are synthesized as inactive precursors (zymogens) that require limited proteolysis to activate them. Notable exceptions to this rule are leukocyte serine proteinases, including human leukocyte elastase, cathepsin G and proteinase 3, which are stored in an active form within specialized granules.

Selected examples of leukocyte serine proteinases that are particularly relevant to ARDS are given in the paragraphs below.

Human leukocyte elastase (HLE)

HLE is glycoprotein consisting of a single polypeptide chain of 218 amino acid residues and contains two asparagine-linked carbohydrate side chains [4]. It is highly cationic, with a strongly basic isoelectric point (pH 10–11). Several isoforms of HLE can be isolated from neutrophils that differ in their carbohydrate structure and are of uncertain importance [5]. HLE preferentially cleaves bonds that are C-terminal to small, hydrophobic residues (particularly bonds having valine at the P1 position).

During the host inflammatory response, HLE is released from activated living cells and/or from dying cells. It may contribute to tissue damage by its direct cytotoxic effects on cells (see below) and by catalyzing the hydrolysis of matrix macromolecules. A wide variety of important matrix components are susceptible to attack by this HLE including: (1) elastin [6]; (2) fibronectin [7]; (3) type III collagen, a major supporting component of lung connective tissue and blood vessels [8]; (4) type IV collagen, an important structural component of epithelial and endothelial basement membranes [9]; (5) type VI collagen microfibrils, which form important links between the major components of the extracellular matrix [10]; and (6) proteoglycans [11]. In addition, HLE has been shown to hydrolyze several plasma proteins, including immunoglobulins, clotting factors and complement components [12,13]. Activation or inactivation of these plasma cascades may lead to important local and systemic consequences. HLE has also induced lymphocyte activation and platelet aggregation [12].

Proteinase 3

Proteinase 3 is a cationic serine proteinase that consists of a 228 residue polypeptide chain with 54% homology to HLE [14]. It is a glycoprotein with two potential N-linked glycosylation sites. Like HLE, proteinase 3 prefers to cleave peptide bonds with small aliphatic amino acids (alanine, serine and valine) at the P1 site [15].

Proteinase 3 degrades a variety of substrates *in vitro*, including mature elastin, fibronectin, laminin, vitronectin and collagen type IV, but shows little or no activity against interstitial collagens types I and III [15].

Cathepsin G

Cathepsin G is an even more cationic serine proteinase that shares 37% sequence homology with HLE. It consists of a 235 residue polypeptide chain that has the potential for only one asparagine-linked carbohydrate residue at Asp^{64} [16]. It has a chymotrypsin-like catalytic activity, in that it preferentially cleaves peptide bonds that are C-terminal to bulky aliphatic or aromatic residues (particularly bonds having phenylalanine at the P1 position).

The natural substrates for cathepsin G are less certain than are those for HLE and proteinase 3. However, it is known that cathepsin G enhances the activity of HLE against elastin [17], and that it is a converting enzyme for angiotensin I [18]. Moreover, it has bactericidal activities [19] and also promotes platelet activation and aggregation [20].

Metalloproteinases

This class of proteinases contains enzymes that are dependent on Zn^{2+} for their activity. X-ray crystallography of human fibroblast-type collagenase has revealed that the zinc ion is at the bottom of the catalytic cleft and is ligated to three histidine residues (each 2.1 Å (0.21 nm) distant) in a highly conserved consensus sequence [21]. Several excellent reviews of this class of enzymes have been published in recent years [22–25].

The metalloproteinase genes are normally silent. Expression is inducible under certain physiologic situations, such as embryonic development and wound healing. If regulation goes awry, a variety of destructive diseases may result. The gene regulation for these enzymes is generally under strict transcriptional control by a variety of growth factors and cytokines. The enzymes are rapidly secreted as proenzymes following translation. Exceptions to this rule are neutrophil collagenase and neutrophil gelatinase, which are stored in secondary granules.

Matrix metalloproteinase proenzymes can be activated by organomercurials, chaotropic agents or limited proteolysis. The 'cysteine switch' model holds that a conserved cysteine residue in these enzymes is coordinated to the zinc atom at the active site of the proenzyme forms, thereby excluding water from the reactive center. Any of a variety of disturbances, including proteolysis and conformational change in the proenzymes, can break the cysteine–zinc contact and activate the enzyme [26]. The mechanism of activation *in vivo* is unknown, but recent data support the possibility that cell surface bound enzymes activate at least some metalloproteinases [27].

To date, 11 human metalloproteinases have been identified by cDNA cloning and sequencing (Table 10.2). The nomenclature of metalloproteinases tends to be confusing, as the enzymes have often been named before the full spectrum of their catalytic activities were known; thus, multiple names are commonly used to describe single enzymes. The predicted amino acid sequences of human metalloproteinases indicate a high degree of conservation ($\sim$ 40–50%); moreover, domains within these sequences have been identified that have specific functions (Figure 10.1). All of the enzymes have an N-terminal propeptide domain that confers the capacity for secretion in zymogen form, and a catalytic domain near the middle of the linear sequence of the molecule that contains the Zn^{2+} binding region. Most metalloproteinases also have a C-terminal domain that is structurally similar to several extracellular matrix proteins. For example, a vitronectin-like domain is found in all metalloproteinases except matrilysin. The gelatinases have additional domains that are inserted into the catalytic domain; both gelatinases have a domain that is homologous to the collagen binding region of fibronectin, a feature that is likely to be responsible for their substantial capacity to degrade gelatin. Gelatinase B has an additional collagen-like domain, the function of which is not known. The membrane-type matrix metalloproteinase has a distinctive transmembrane domain, which leads to cell surface localization [27].

Collectively, the metalloproteinases have the capacity to degrade all of the components of the extracellular matrix. They are known to be important both in normal remodeling of connective tissues and in tissue injury. The interstitial collagenases are the most substrate specific of this class of enzymes. Their catalytic activity is quite specific for cleavage of several native helical collagens, including types I, II, III and X, at a single locus; however, they have also been reported to cleave and inactivate serine proteinase inhibitors [28–31]. The gelatinases and stromelysins have much broader proteolytic activities when compared to interstitial collagenases. The gelatinases further degrade collagens that have been denatured by interstitial collagenases and also degrade types IV, V, VII and X collagen and elastin. Membrane-type matrix metalloproteinase specifically activates progelatinase A at the cell surface [27]. Stromelysins act synergistically with both the interstitial collagenases and gelatinases to degrade collagen, and also degrade proteoglycans and many components of the extracellular matrix, including laminin and

Table 10.2 Matrix metalloproteinases (MMPs)

Common name	MMP No.	Preferred substrates	Cell(s) of origin
Fibroblast-type collagenase	MMP-1	Collagens I, II, III, VII, VIII, X Entactin, serpins	Fibroblasts, endothelial cells, mesothelial cells, keratinocytes
PMN collagenase	MMP-5	Collagens (as above)	PMNs Eosinophils
Collagenase-3	MMP-13	Collagen I (and II, III?)	Breast carcinoma (and other?) cells
72 kDA gelatinase (A) (72 kDA type IV/V collagenase)	MMP-2	Gelatins Collagens IV, V, VII, X, XI Elastin	Fibroblasts Mononuclear phagocytes
92 kDA gelatinase (B) (92 kDA type IV/V collagenase)	MMP-9	Fibronectin Entactin	Endothelial cells Mesothelial cells
Stomelysin-1	MMP-3	Proteoglycans	Fibroblasts
Stomelysin-2	MMP-10	Laminin, fibronectin	Mononuclear phagocytes
Stomelysin-3[a]	MMP-11	Collagens IV, V, IX, X Procollagenase, (elastin)	Endothelial cells
Matrilysin (PUMP)[b]	MMP-7	Proteoglycans, elastin Fibronectin, laminin, entactin Collagen IV, gelatins, procollagenase	Monocyte-derived macrophages Tumor cells
Human macrophage elastase	MMP-12	Elastin, collagen IV Fibronectin, laminin, entactin	Macrophages (Other cells?)
Membrane-type matrix metalloproteinase	MMP-14	Pro-gelatinase A (activates)	Cell membranes of tumor (and other?) cells

[a] Has sequence homology to other metalloproteinases, but no known catalytic activities.
[b] PUMP = punctuated metalloproteinase.

fibronectin. Matrilysin has broad substrate specificity that includes elastin and proteoglycans [32,33]. In addition, matrilysin has very potent activity against basement membrane components. Human macrophage elastase has only recently been cloned and sequenced. This enzyme has clearly been shown to be expressed by alveolar macrophages [34]; however, its expression by other cell types has not yet been investigated. Human macrophage elastase has potent elastolytic activity. It also has the capacity to degrade basement membrane components, and is at least as potent as matrilysin against components of basement membranes, including fibronectin, laminin, entactin and type IV collagen [35].

Cysteine proteinases

Mammalian cysteine proteinases have a common catalytic mechanism, a two domain globular structure, and a similar size (about 23–27 kDa). There is a striking conservation of Cys^{25} and His^{150} (papain numbering), both of which are directly involved in catalysis. An intact active-site cysteine is critical for catalytic activity.

Mammalian lysosomal proteinases (cathepsins B, H, L and S) are members of the papain superfamily of cysteine proteinases. All are synthesized as higher molecular weight glycoprotein proenzymes that are processed by limited proteolysis to the active,

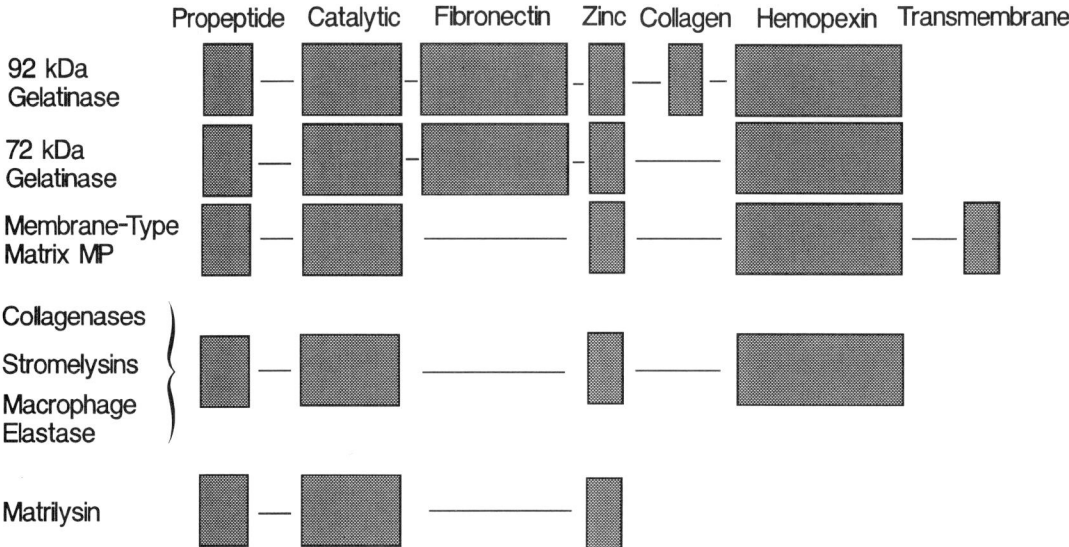

Figure 10.1 Domain structure of matrix metalloproteinases. The amino-terminal portions of the enzymes are to the left. The metalloproteinases are assemblages of homologous domains that vary from enzyme to enzyme, as indicated by the blocks. The presence or absence of the various domains largely determines the size of the enzymes. Each enzyme is translated with an amino-terminal signal peptide that is not shown. The length of each block is roughly proportional to its domain size.

usually double chain, forms found in lyso-somes. They share with papain an affinity for hydrophobic amino acid side chains. Cysteine proteinases typically have no catalytic activity above pH 6, and often are inactivated by exposure to neutral pH. The major role ascribed to these enzymes has been in intra-cellular protein digestion and destruction of endocytosed proteins. Cathepsin S, however, has an extended pH range, retaining ~25% of its catalytic activity at neutral pH [36]. Thus, in contrast to the other cysteine proteinases, cathepsin S may be poised to play an import-ant role in extracellular protein degradation.

Physiologically important proteins that can be degraded by cathepsin B and L include proteoglycans, and the N-terminal peptides of collagen that contain the crosslinks within and between the molecules; cathepsin L is tenfold more active against the latter sub-strate. Cathepsins L and S also have the capacity to degrade elastin [36–38].

Aspartic proteinases

Two aspartic acid residues, each surrounded by a conserved sequence, are integral to the catalytic activity of these proteinases. The car-bonyl groups of the aspartic acid residues are separated by 2.9 Å (0.29 nm), and are con-nected to one another through extensive hydrogen bonds. A solvent water molecule is held between them. The structure of these enzymes is bilobar, with a large catalytic cleft containing the active-site aspartic acid resi-dues separating the two domains [39].

Mammalian aspartic proteinases are mem-bers of a multigene family that includes pep-sin and renin, and share ~5% sequence identity [39,40]. The proenzyme forms of these proteinases have an N-terminal propep-tide of up to 50 amino acid residues.

The most prominent lysosomal proteinase acting at acid pH is cathepsin D. It is found in the lysosomes of most cells, including fibro-blasts, but its activity is highest in phagocytic cells, such as macrophages, where it is increased further by cellular activation. At sites of inflammation, cathepsin D is secreted by macrophages into the extracellular space. Although cathepsin D has no activity at or above pH 7, it is possible that at sites of inflammation the pericellular pH may be sufficiently low to allow cathepsin D to degrade matrix macromolecules [1]; this process may be facilitated by the lack of inhibitors of cathepsin D in mammalian tissues. The aspartic proteinases tend to have an extended substrate specificity, and except for renin have a broad peptide bond specificity. Extracellular matrix components that are susceptible to cathepsin D include proteoglycans and a few peptide bonds in native collagens.

TYPES OF SUBSTRATES PREFERRED

When considering proteinases in the context of tissue injury and repair, it is useful to classify them according to their substrate specificity. We will consider three groups of enzymes classified in this way: elastases, collagenases and plasminogen activators.

Elastases

Elastin is an intensely hydrophobic and very inert macromolecule that has a critical structural and mechanical role in the lungs. Elastases are defined as enzymes that have the capacity to degrade insoluble, mature (cross linked) elastin into soluble peptides. There are several elastases that are associated with inflammatory cells.

The serine proteinases HLE, proteinase 3 and cathepsin G have varying degrees of elastolytic activity. HLE, the most intensively studied of the PMN enzymes, has potent elastolytic activity. Proteinase 3 also degrades elastin; its elastolytic activity at acid pH is greater than that of HLE, but is it less active at neutral pH [41]. The role of cathepsin G in extracellular degradation of elastin is less

clear. In contrast to HLE, minimal cathepsin G is released following exposure of PMN to agents that promote lysosomal degranulation, and cathepsin G is very weakly elastolytic *in vitro*. However, cathepsin G has been shown to increase the elastolytic activity of HLE [17].

Several metalloproteinases have the capacity to solubilize elastin. Human macrophage elastase and matrilysin have potent elastolytic activity [33,34]. The 72 kDa and 92 kDa gelatinases also exhibit activity against elastin *in vitro* [33,42].

The cysteine proteinases cathepsin L [38] and cathepsin S [36] are strongly elastolytic *in vitro*. The extended pH range of cathepsin S [36] suggests the possibility that it may have an unusual role among cysteine proteinases in the degradation of extracellular proteins.

Collagenases

Collagen molecules are composed of three polypeptide chains arranged in a rigid triple helical conformation. This structure tends to render the molecules resistant to proteolytic attack by all enzymes other than specific collagenases. Interstitial collagenases are enzymes that catalyze both the initial and rate limiting step in collagen degradation by cleaving the collagen helix under physiologic conditions [43–45].

Interstitial collagens (types I–III) are major structural components of the extracellular space. The classical interstitial collagenase (MMP-1) is the most thoroughly studied. It is secreted by fibroblasts, mesothelial cells and mononuclear phagocytes. This enzyme, along with the structurally similar neutrophil collagenase, cleaves interstitial collagens by a common mechanism, catalyzing the scission of all three constituent collagen polypeptide chains at a single locus three quarters of the distance from the amino-terminal end of the molecule. This reaction produces two fragments that spontaneously denature at physiologic temperature into randomly coiled gelatinous peptides that are susceptible to digestion by a variety of other proteinases.

Other collagenases are involved in degradation of type IV (basement membrane) collagen; these include matrilysin, 72 kDa and 92 kDa gelatinases, stromelysin and human macrophage elastase. The 72 kDa and 92 kDa gelatinases cleave type IV collagen in its helical domain, whereas human macrophage elastase and stromelysin cleave the molecule in its non-helical domain [35,46,47]. Pericellular collagen (type V) is cleaved by 72 kDa and 92 kDa gelatinases and matrilysin [32]. Collagen type IX, a fibril associated collagen that connects fibrils to other matrix elements, is degraded by stromelysin. HLE is capable of cleaving collagen type III [48], type IV [9,49] and type VI [10]. However, the rate of catalytic cleavage of type III collagen by HLE is less than 2% of that exhibited by the interstitial collagenases [50].

Plasminogen activators

Plasminogen activators are serine proteinases that convert plasminogen, which is abundant in most body fluids, to plasmin, a serine proteinase that can degrade fibrin. Degradation (or lack of degradation) of the provisional fibrin matrix at sites of inflammation may be critical determinants of the outcome of an inflammatory process. In addition, plasmin participates in the degradation of other matrix and basement glycoproteins such as fibronectin, laminin, proteoglycans and possibly type V collagen [51,52]. Finally, plasmin activates procollagenases to active collagenases that are required for the degradation of helical collagen molecules [53]. Thus, by working in concert, the cascade of activated enzymes derived from plasminogen activator can degrade many of the components of extracellular matrix.

There are two principal plasminogen activators: urokinase-type plasminogen activator (u-PA) and tissue-type plasminogen activator (t-PA). Plasminogen activators are distributed on many cell types (see below). As detailed below, plasminogen activators have been implicated in many cellular responses involving tissue degradation and cellular migration, as well as in inflammation [54,55].

CELLULAR SOURCES OF PROTEINASES

Proteinases that are relevant to lung tissue injury and repair originate from a variety of cell types, including both inflammatory and resident cells. In many cells, synthesis and/or release of proteolytic enzymes is strikingly altered by mediators that are released at sites of inflammation. It is also noteworthy that many examples exist of cells that contain or concurrently synthesize both enzymes and inhibitors of those enzymes, such as: (1) serine proteinases and α_1-antitrypsin/human elastase inhibitors in PMNs [56] and monocytes [57]; (2) metalloproteinases and tissue inhibitor of metalloproteinases in various cell types [58–60]; and (3) cysteine proteinases and cystatin in macrophages [61]. It is likely that concomitantly released proteinase inhibitors serve to confine catalytic activity of enzymes to the zone immediately surrounding the cell.

Polymorphonuclear neutrophils

PMNs are replete with a number of proteolytic enzymes that are of pathogenetic importance in ARDS. At least six neutral proteinases have been identified within neutrophils including: (1) serine proteinases (HLE, cathepsin G, proteinase 3 and plasminogen activator); and (2) metalloproteinases (neutrophil collagenase and gelatinase). Together these enzymes can degrade most, if not all, of the constituents of the extracellular matrix.

The proteinases found in PMNs are generally stored within two distinct types of cytoplasmic granules that are formed at different stages in myelopoietic development. The azurophil (primary) granules are produced at the promyelocyte stage of development and contain HLE, cathepsin G and proteinase 3, while the specific (secondary) granules are formed at the myelocyte stage and contain the PMN collagenase. A third small vesicular organelle, the C particle [62], contains gelatinase and plasminogen activator.

HLE and cathepsin G are the most extensively studied neutral proteinases of PMNs. PMNs contain approximately 1 μg each of HLE and cathepsin G per 10^6 cells [63]. Within minutes of an appropriate stimulus these enzymes can be released from the azurophil granules into the extracellular space. It is clear that mature PMNs do not contain mRNA for HLE, cathepsin G or proteinase 3 and do not have the capacity to synthesize them *de novo* [64–66]; rather, synthesis of these proteinases is complete at the promyelocyte stage of development of PMNs. Because of the limited synthetic capabilities of mature PMNs, synthesis of most of their other proteinases is thought to be completed in bone marrow precursors as well. By contrast, plasminogen activator is synthesized *de novo* by circulating PMNs. The production of this proteinase can thus be modulated by factors that regulate protein synthesis.

Mononuclear phagocytes

Mononuclear phagocytes express an array of proteolytic enzymes that are under developmental control and are also highly regulated by physiologic and pharmacologic stimuli. Circulating monocytes tend to contain intracellular serine proteinases but have only a limited capacity to produce metalloproteinases and cysteine proteinases. By contrast, macrophages produce predominantly metalloproteinases (Table 10.2). The general pattern is that monocytes contain rapidly mobilized, active serine proteinases, while macrophages rely upon regulated synthesis and secretion of enzymes such as metalloproteinases that are synthesized on demand and secreted in zymogen form [67].

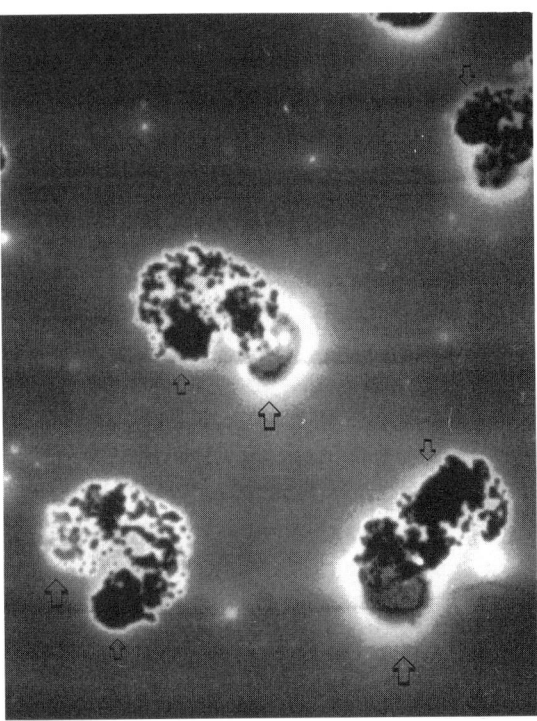

Figure 10.2 Proteolytic activity of PMNs occurring despite the presence of a proteinase inhibitor. (×100.) The light background in the micrograph is immunofluorescent staining of fibronectin, which had been coated onto the surface of a glass slide. Human PMNs were added in the presence of an excess of α_1-antitrypsin then incubated for 45 minutes. Note that the 'lawn' of fibronectin is intact throughout much of the micrograph because the α_1-antitrypsin has protected it from being degraded by the proteinases released by the neutrophils. In the dark areas, the fibronectin has been degraded by HLE derived from the cells. Each of these areas corresponds to the path of a single neutrophil on the surface. The cells initially attached at the sites marked by the small arrows, then migrated a distance of 5–7 cell diameters. Their final positions are marked by the large arrows. At the sites of initial attachment, and subjacent to the cells along the paths of their migration, fibronectin was degraded in very sharply localized zones despite the presence of the inhibitor. Some mechanisms that might allow this proteolysis to occur are depicted in Figure 10.3. (Reproduced with permission from Campbell, E.J. and Campbell, M.A. (1988) *J. Cell Biol*, **106**, 667–76.)

Monocytes

Circulating human monocytes contain the serine proteinases HLE, cathepsin G and proteinase 3. HLE and cathepsin G are known to reside in peroxidase-positive cytoplasmic granules that resemble the azurophil granules of neutrophils [63,68], and proteinase 3 is presumed to be contained within the same granules. Like PMNs, monocytes do not contain measurable amounts of mRNA for HLE, cathepsin G or proteinase 3 [64–66], indicating that their synthesis of these enzymes has been completed prior to release of mature cells from the bone marrow.

Monocytes rapidly release their granules containing proteinases when appropriately stimulated [63]. Additional complexity is added by observations that monocytes can also take up HLE that has been released by neutrophils, because HLE has been shown to bind to monocyte surface receptors, and is rapidly internalized into the phagolysosomes [69–71].

Monocytes have only a limited capacity to secrete metalloproteinases. Exposure to the lectin concanavalin A induces monocytes to release interstitial collagenase; however, the amounts are less than 5% of those secreted by macrophages [59]. Monocytes also secrete gelatinase B and tissue inhibitor of metalloproteinases (TIMP), but again in substantially smaller amounts than those secreted by macrophages, and their release is not subject to significant regulation by extracellular signals.

Heterogeneity of human monocytes

Human monocytes are greatly heterogeneous with regard to a variety of cellular characteristics and activities. We have recently identified two distinct, naturally occurring subsets of circulating monocytes that differ strikingly in their expression of serine and metalloproteinases: proinflammatory (P) and immune-modulatory (I) monocytes [72,73]. P monocytes constitute 20–30% of circulating monocytes and express a striking neutrophil-like phenotype characterized by: (1) responsiveness to chemotactic signals; (2) adherence to extracellular matrix macromolecules through high level expression of β_1 and β_2 integrins; (3) high phagocytic activity; (4) high capacity to generate reactive oxygen species; and (5) inability to present antigen to lymphocytes. In contrast, I monocytes have a low proinflammatory potential, but express high level, cell surface HLA-DR antigen, indicating that their main role is to modulate specific immune responses.

Work from our laboratory indicates that expression of the serine proteinases, HLE and cathepsin G, is restricted to P monocytes [73]. These cells contain $\sim$ 200 ng of each enzyme per 10^6 cells, or about 20% of the amount contained within PMNs. P monocytes have the capacity to produce extensive HLE mediated proteolysis of fibronectin, even in the presence of high concentrations of proteinase inhibitors [73]. These data are all consistent with the possibility that only a restricted population of monocytes is recruited to sites of inflammation. Moreover, these cells are rich in serine proteinases, and when they mature in the tissues they have the capacity to produce high levels of metalloproteinases. Thus, proteinases released by P monocytes could play an important pathogenetic role in lung injury in ARDS and other diseases associated with tissue inflammation.

Macrophages

As monocytes mature into macrophages, serine proteinases and metalloproteinases are progressively lost [74]; however, macrophages are not necessarily devoid of serine proteinases. Macrophages, like monocytes, express specific cell surface receptors for HLE and cathepsin G and can thus internalize that which has been released into the extracellular space by other inflammatory cells, such as PMNs and monocytes [69,70,75]. In addition, macrophages phagocytose and remove apoptotic neutrophils (and their contents) within tissues [76]. Internalized HLE can be released slowly by mononuclear phagocytes, a process that can be accelerated by hypoxic injury to the cells [77].

Macrophages also express u-PA. Interestingly, the activity of this enzyme appears to be critical for macrophage expression of elastolytic activity *in vitro*, probably by exposing matrix elastin to the activity of other macrophage derived proteinases [78]. Moreover, u-PA and its cell surface receptor appear to have important roles in the adherence and locomotion of mononuclear phagocytes [79,80] that are independent of their roles in extracellular proteolysis.

Maturation of monocytes into macrophages is also associated with increased expression of a variety of metalloproteinases [74]. Macrophages have the capacity for regulated secretion of several metalloproteinases, including interstitial collagenase, stromelysins 1 and 2, gelatinase B, and human macrophage elastase, in addition to the counter-regulatory TIMP. Matrilysin synthesis is unclear at present because monocyte derived macrophages, but not alveolar macrophages, have been found to have regulated synthesis of this enzyme [81]. Expression of metalloproteinases by macrophages can be regulated by physiologic and pharmacologic stimuli.

In general, the secretion of all metalloenzymes is upregulated by bacterial endotoxin, and to a lesser extent by phorbol esters; gelatinase B is regulated much less strikingly than the remainder of the metalloproteinases. Stimuli upregulate metalloproteinase secretion by increasing macrophage production of prostaglandin E_2 and intracellular cAMP [82], although some data indicate that the mechanisms may differ from enzyme to enzyme [83]. Metalloproteinase expression by macrophages can also be downregulated by agents that suppress eicosanoid synthesis such as interferon γ, interleukin 4 and dexamethasone [82,84].

Macrophages also express two elastinolytic cysteine proteinases, cathepsins L and S [36–38]. Cathepsin S appears poised to play a role in extracellular proteolytic events because it has activity at neutral pH [36]. However, macrophages have the capacity to create acidic microenvironments in the immediate pericellular space [1], in part through activity of a proton pump in the cell membrane [2].

Other inflammatory cells

Other leukocytes have been shown to contain proteinases that are thought to play a role in ARDS. Human eosinophils contain a collagenase stored within cytoplasmic granules which can specifically cleave human collagen types I and III, the two major connective tissue components of human lung parenchyma [85]. More recently, eosinophils have been shown to contain an elastase that is physically and immunologically identical to HLE within both types of dense cytoplasmic granules [86].

Human basophils and mast cells also contain serine proteinases that play a role in degradation of the extracellular matrix. Mast cells and basophils contain HLE within their cytoplasmic granules in amounts that represent 3–20% of those found within human PMNs [87]. Mast cells express proteinase 3 on their cell surface [88]. Mast cells also contain tryptase, a 134 kDa trypsin-like serine proteinase, which is stored within their granules and constitutes more than 25% of the dry weight of these cells [89]. Trace amounts of this enzyme are also found within the granules of basophils. Human mast cell tryptase can directly degrade type VI collagen microfibrils which link the major elements of the extracellular matrix [10]. Tryptase also activates the zymogen form of stromelysin which, in turn, activates latent interstitial collagenase [90,91]. Once activated, stromelysin can degrade fibronectin, laminin, type IV and IX collagen, gelatin and proteoglycans. Activation of stromelysin by tryptase can thus be an important step in the initiation of matrix degradation.

Resident cells

Resident cells such as endothelial cells, fibroblasts, mesothelial cells and alveolar epithelial cells express proteinases.

Endothelial cells express proteinases of both the serine and metalloproteinase subclasses. Serine proteinases expressed by endothelial cells include plasminogen activators and proteinase 3. Human endothelial cells produce both t-PA and u-PA forms of plasminogen activator activity, but t-PA production and secretion is elevated most frequently [92]. The t-PA form functions predominantly in endothelial cell mediated fibrinolysis, whereas the u-PA form is thought to be more involved in tissue remodeling. Recent observations have indicated that tumor necrosis factor (TNF)α and TNFβ upregulate the synthesis and secretion of u-PA by endothelial cells, thereby increasing their capacity to degrade and invade the subendothelial extracellular matrix [92] (Chapter 7). Proteinase 3 is expressed on the cell surface of human endothelial cells, and exposure to TNFα, interleukin 1α/β, and interferon γ induces translocation of preformed proteinase 3 from intracellular stores to the cell surface [93]. Metalloproteinases produced by endothelial cells include interstitial collagenase [31], gelatinases [94] and stromelysins [95,96].

Fibroblasts and mesothelial cells are sources of metalloproteinases. Fibroblasts express interstitial collagenase, gelatinase A and stromelysin [22, 97], and fibroblast secretion of metalloproteinases is regulated by a variety of cytokines, growth factors and pharmacologic agents [97]. Mesothelial cells express interstitial collagenase, 72 kDa and 92 kDa gelatinases and TIMP, and their expression is modified by the state of cellular differentiation [60].

Type II alveolar epithelial cells, which repopulate the epithelial lining layer following acute lung injury, synthesize and secrete u-PA, and thus play an important role in the repair process [98]. Type II alveolar epithelial cells and Clara cells secrete antileukoproteinase and elafin [99,100], two important inhibitors of HLE in the lower respiratory tract, indicating that these cells may play a role in the defense of the peripheral lung against HLE secreted by leukocytes during the acute exudative phase of ARDS.

Cell biology of extracellular protein degradation

In contrast to the wealth of information about the structure and biochemistry of proteinases and inhibitors, remarkably little exists about the mechanisms by which inflammatory cells use and control their proteolytic enzymes to degrade extracellular proteins *in vivo*. It is known from a variety of studies that inhibitors confine the proteolytic activity of inflammatory cells to the immediate pericellular microenvironment, but that they cannot inhibit degradation of proteins that are in direct contact with the cells. Our understanding of the cell biology of this confined proteolytic activity has lagged far behind our knowledge of the structure and biochemistry of the enzymes and inhibitors themselves. Controlled (or **confined**) activity of these enzymes in the extracellular space permits an effective inflammatory response to injury, infection or other insults. By contrast, uncontrolled proteolysis during inflammation can result in disabling tissue injury, such as ARDS.

The plasma and interstitial space are replete with proteinase inhibitors [101] that serve to confine and terminate proteolytic events. During tissue inflammation there is increased synthesis of plasma proteinase inhibitors by the liver [102]; moreover, the increased vascular permeability that is associated with inflammation results in increased transudation of these inhibitors into sites of

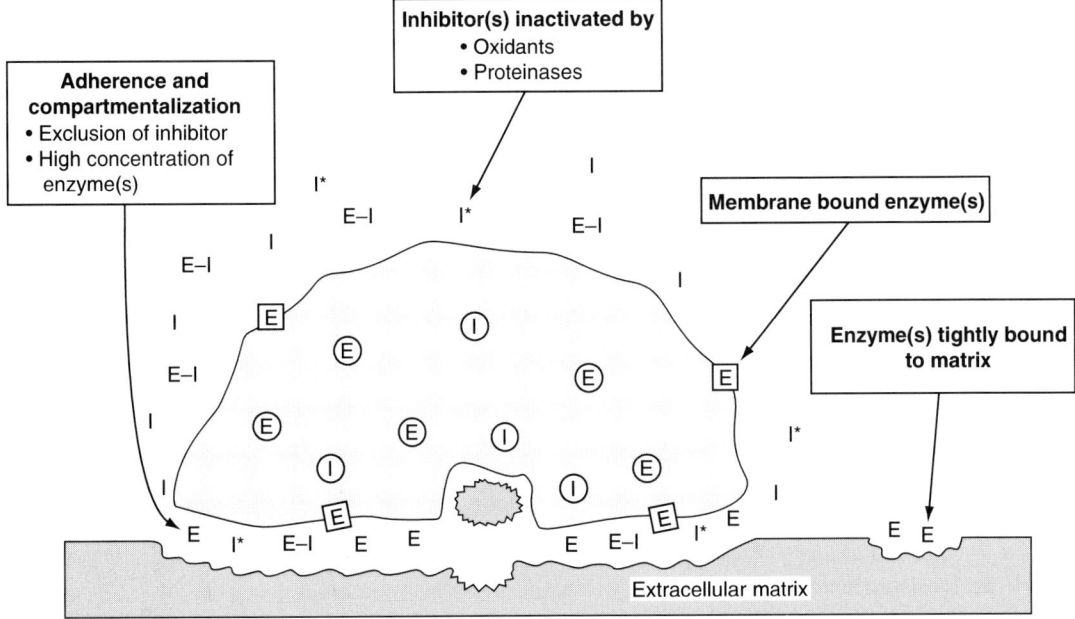

Figure 10.3 Interaction of an inflammatory cell with extracellular matrix, showing mechanisms that might permit matrix degradation despite the presence of proteinase inhibitors. E = proteolytic enzyme(s); I = proteinase inhibitor(s); E-I = inhibited enzyme; I* = inactivated inhibitor. Enzyme released freely into the extracellular space is subject to inhibition (E-I), but enzyme released into zones of close contact between the cell and the matrix is more likely to retain activity. The high concentrations of enzyme that exist near the site of release from the cell may transiently overwhelm local inhibitor concentrations. Membrane bound enzyme may be resistant to inhibitors. Diffusion of inhibitors into zones of tight adherence between the cells and subajacent proteins may be impaired. Some inhibitor in the extracellular space may be inactivated. (Reproduced with permission from Campbell E.J., Senior, R.M. and Welgus, H.G. (1987) *Chest*, **92**, 161–7.)

tissue inflammation. Mechanisms that allow such degradation of extracellular proteins *in vivo* must circumvent the effects of proteinase inhibitors in the extracellular milieu. A number of such mechanisms have been proposed (Figure 10.3). For the specific case of proteolytic activity of PMNs, evidence exists to support all of the mechanisms shown in Figure 10.3.

Compartmentalization

Our laboratory [63,103–106] and others [107–114] have demonstrated that inflammatory cells degrade extracellular substrates despite the presence of inhibitors *in vitro*

(Figure 10.2). Our early studies [63,105,106] and work from other laboratories [114–118] indicated that proteolysis occurs most effectively (and in some systems exclusively) when the cells are in direct contact with the substrate. Moreover, we [63,105] and others [114] have found that proteinase inhibitors **confine** proteolytic activity to the pericellular microenvironment, but **cannot inhibit degradation of proteins at or near the cell surface**.

Compartmentalization of proteinases and their inhibitors can exist in the interstitial space as a result of close apposition of inflammatory cells to matrix proteins, thereby forming a microenvironment that: (1) excludes

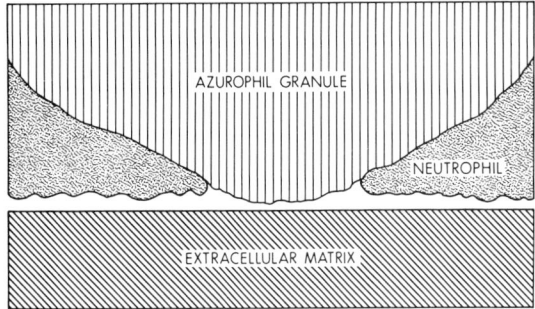

Figure 10.4 A neutrophil that has attached to a cell surface. In zones in which neutrophils are tightly adherent, the separation between the cell and the underlying surface is very small. An azurophil granule, containing both serine proteinases and myeloperoxidase, is shown being released. Note that the granule has a diameter of approximately 0.3 μm. The high concentration of enzymes within the granule can be expected, at least transiently, to overwhelm local proteinase inhibitors within the extracellular fluid separating the cell from the surface. Moreover, the cell is capable of preventing free diffusion of additional inhibitors into the zone of its contact with the surface. (Reproduced with permission from Fishman, *Update: Pulmonary Disease and Disorders*, 2nd edn, published by McGraw-Hill, 1992).

high molecular weight inhibitors such as α_1-proteinase inhibitor [105] and α_2-macroglobulin [119] from penetrating into zones of contact between cells and the substrate; and/or (2) contains high concentrations of enzymes relative to inhibitors, due to discharge of granule contents into the subcellular cleft (Figure 10.4).

As an example of the high concentrations of proteinases that can exist in the pericellular microenvironment *in vivo*, we have calculated that the concentration of HLE within an azurophil granule is in the millimolar range [120]. Since that concentration is two orders of magnitude higher than the concentration of α_1-antitrypsin in plasma, release of an azurophil granule into the extracellular space **must** be accompanied by at least a transient burst of proteolytic activity. Catalytic activity will persist until diffusion of the granule contents

away from the site allows the ratio of enzyme concentration to inhibitor concentration to fall to $< 1{:}1$.

Reduced effectiveness of inhibitors

Inactivation of inhibitors in the pericellular environment may promote local proteolysis. Both oxidants and metalloproteinases have been shown to inactivate α_1-antitrypsin [28–31,108] and other proteinase inhibitors [28,31,121–123]. Moreover, PMNs and mononuclear phagocytes release oxidants locally at the site of their contact with a surface [124]. Such events could provide a microenvironment surrounding the cell in which proteolysis is facilitated by inactivation of proteinase inhibitors.

Membrane bound enzymes

Cell surface binding may be a mechanism by which proteolytic activity is localized to specific microenvironments, allowing local degradation of extracellular matrix while minimizing injury to adjacent structures [125]. Recent unpublished studies from our laboratory have demonstrated that PMNs also express HLE and cathepsin G on their cell surface in a catalytically active form. Cell surface expression of HLE and cathepsin G is minimal on unstimulated PMNs; however, exposure of PMNs to phorbol ester stimulates a 30-fold increase in cell surface expression of these enzymes. Priming of PMNs with lipopolysaccharide (LPS) or TNFα followed by stimulation with chemoattractants also induces striking upregulation of cell surface expression of HLE and cathepsin G by PMNs. In marked contrast to enzymes that are released into the extracellular space, cell surface HLE is remarkably resistant to inhibition by naturally occurring proteinase inhibitors.

Other laboratories have shown that proteinase 3 is present on the cell surface of PMNs [88] and that priming and activation of

PMNs results in increased translocation of proteinase 3 to the cell surface [126,127]. The catalytic activity and susceptibility to inhibition of cell surface bound proteinase 3 have not been studied. It is noteworthy that HLE, cathepsin G and proteinase 3 are also expressed on the cell surface of human monocytes [88,128,129].

Catalytically-active u-PA of fibroblasts [130] and mononuclear phagocytes [118,131,132] is expressed on the cell surface. Moreover, membrane bound uPA: (1) has a distribution that is strikingly restricted to focal contacts of fibroblasts [130,133]; (2) has a 40% lower association rate constant for the plasminogen activator inhibitors PAI-1 and PAI-2 than the soluble form [134]; and (3) converts membrane bound plasminogen to plasmin that is resistant to α_2-antiplasmin (an inhibitor that is quite effective against free plasmin [118]). The u-PA receptor of U937 cells recognizes an amino-terminal growth factor-like sequence, a region that is remote from the active site and not required for catalytic activity [135]. Normal human alveolar macrophages appear to share this u-PA receptor [136], that preferentially binds catalytically-active enzyme and protects it from inhibition by PAI-2. Finally, plasminogen activation by single chain u-PA is accelerated 16-fold following binding of the enzyme to U937 cells [137]. Thus, it has been hypothesized that cell surface bound u-PA and plasmin appear ideally suited to facilitate cell migration through fibrin clots and tissue barriers.

Matrix metalloproteinases and cathepsin B have been found in a catalytically-active form on cell surfaces; moreover, cell surface binding is a proposed mechanism for activation of latent metalloproteinases [125].

Together, these observations indicate that persistently active proteinases on the surface of inflammatory cells facilitate their egress from the vasculature, penetration of tissue barriers and local degradation of matrix macromolecules at sites of inflammation.

Tight binding of enzyme(s) to substrate(s)

In vitro studies have demonstrated that naturally occurring inhibitors have reduced effectiveness against catalytic activity of HLE following its binding to elastin [138,139]. Moreover, studies in which HLE has been found in association with interstitial elastin in human emphysematous lungs suggest the intriguing possibility that this elastin bound HLE retains catalytic activity *in vivo*. As another example, binding of HLE or plasmin to fibrin markedly reduces the susceptibility of these enzymes to inhibition [140].

ROLE OF PROTEINASES IN THE PATHOGENESIS OF ARDS

INJURY TO LUNG ARCHITECTURE

Diffuse damage to the lung alveolar-capillary barrier is the initial pathologic feature of ARDS. Proteinases have the capacity to injure all three components of this barrier (endothelium, interstitium and epithelium), thereby contributing to the development of inflammatory edema and refractory hypoxemia (Figure 10.5). In particular, cationic proteinases released from activated phagocytes such as HLE and cathepsin G, as well as thrombin, a plasma serine proteinase, have been shown to injure both cellular components of this barrier.

HLE, cathepsin G and thrombin can alter the properties of the alveolar-capillary barrier. Exposure of cultured endothelial and epithelial monolayers to cathepsin G or thrombin leads to progressive retraction of cells with the development of intercellular gaps [141–143], and increased transendothelial albumin influx [141,143,144]. In addition, exposure of epithelial monolayers to zymosan activated neutrophils induces increased epithelial permeability [145]. This process can be inhibited by α_1-proteinase inhibitor, a major inhibitor of HLE and cathepsin G.

HLE and cathepsin G can induce endothelial cell detachment [146] and frank lysis of

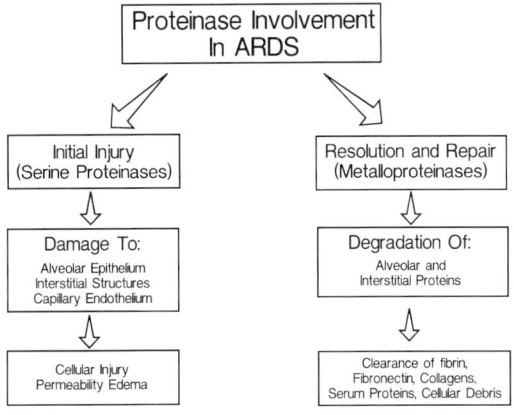

Figure 10.5 Potential roles of proteinases in the pathogenesis and resolution of ARDS. Serine proteinases, predominantly derived from PMNs, can cause injury to all of the components of the alveolar-capillary barrier, with resulting cellular injury and alveolar flooding with protein-rich exudate. In later stages of ARDS, proteinases are required to degrade the abnormal proteins that result from alveolar and interstitial flooding and ingrowth of fibroblasts into the alveolar spaces. Proteolytic activity must also be involved in the clearance of cellular debris. It is likely that this activity is largely attributable to metalloproteinases derived from resident cells and mononuclear phagocytes, although endocytosed proteins and debris could be degraded by cysteine and aspartic proteinases.

cultured endothelial [147] cells *in vitro*. In addition, primed and stimulated neutrophils can induce detachment of alveolar epithelial cells [148] and lysis of cultured endothelial cells by mechanisms that are mimicked by the isolated enzyme [147] and blocked by inhibitors of HLE [147,148]. Moreover, infusion of HLE, cathepsin G or thrombin into the lungs of experimental animals leads to increased vascular permeability [141,146], sequestration of neutrophils within the pulmonary vasculature and progressive pulmonary failure [149].

The mechanism(s) by which HLE and cathepsin G induce increased permeability of the alveolar-capillary barrier of the lung is not clear, but there is evidence that it may be related, in part, to their high positive charge at physiologic pH rather than their enzymatic activities because: (1) heat inactivation of cathepsin G only partially protects endothelial cells from increased permeability [141]; and (2) other highly positively charged molecules, including polylysine and protamine, are toxic to cells both *in vitro* and *in vivo* [143,150–153] and can also increase vascular permeability [152,153]. Thus, is it likely that HLE and cathepsin G act via their cationic nature, either directly or by promoting increased binding to cell surfaces.

Destruction of the extracellular matrix components of the endothelial and epithelial basement membranes, and interstitial space in ARDS is well documented [154]. Proteinases contained within neutrophils and mononuclear phagocytes (see below) have the capacity to degrade many if not all of the constituents of the extracellular matrix, including fibronectin, collagen types I – IV, elastin, laminin, entactin and proteoglycans [67,106,155–159]. Destruction of these structural proteins is likely to facilitate the movement of fluid, proteins and inflammatory cells into the alveolar space, leading to impairment of gas exchange. In addition, proteolytically released fragments of elastin and collagen have chemotactic activity for inflammatory cells *in vitro*. Thus, proteolysis of matrix components may perpetuate the accumulation of inflammatory cells in the lungs of patients with ARDS, and amplify tissue injury.

ABNORMAL PROTEINASE ACTIVITY IN ARDS

Evidence of abnormal proteinase activity has been found in patients with ARDS. Investigation of patients with established ARDS has shown large numbers of neutrophils sequestered in the lung microvasculature [149, 160–162] and bronchoalveolar lavage (BAL) fluid [163–166]. In addition, there is a direct correlation between lung neutrophil number and: (1) the severity of abnormalities in gas exchange; and (2) lung protein permeability [164].

Patients with ARDS have increased circulating levels of lactoferrin [167] and lysozyme [168], which are proteins stored within the granules of phagocytes. These observations indicate that there is activation, degranulation and release of proteinases by phagocytes in patients with ARDS.

High levels of HLE have been detected in plasma [169], tracheal aspirate [170] and BAL [163,171,172] samples from the majority of patients with established ARDS, whereas HLE is found infrequently and at low levels in healthy subjects or patients with chronic pulmonary diseases [163,169]. Several studies have demonstrated that the high elastase levels in BAL fluid are associated with reduced levels of functional α_1-antitrypsin and there is evidence that this is due to oxidative inactivation of this proteinase inhibitor [163,171].

Patients with ARDS have high serum concentrations of 7S collagen, an N-terminal peptide which is cleaved by HLE from type IV collagen, an important basement membrane component [173,174]. Moreover, the serum concentration of 7S collagen is strongly correlated with disease severity and survival. These observations indicate that disruption of the endothelial basement membrane is an important pathogenetic event in ARDS.

High levels of other phagocyte derived proteinases that can injure the extracellular matrix in the lung parenchyma, such as types I and III collagenase activity [164,166], have also been reported in patients with established ARDS.

There are striking abnormalities in the activities of proteolytic enzymes that are involved in the both coagulation and fibrinolytic pathways in ARDS. Specifically, there is evidence that patients with ARDS have enhanced activation of the coagulation pathway with concomitant depressed fibrinolysis [175]. The development of this procoagulant and antifibrinolytic state may contribute to the formation and persistence of hyaline membranes, and subsequently to intra-alveolar fibrosis, which are both characteristic pathologic features of ARDS. Augmented activity of both the intrinsic [176] and extrinsic [175,177] coagulation pathways have been demonstrated in BAL fluid from patients with ARDS; most of the procoagulant activity in the latter pathway is due to increased levels of tissue factor complexed with factor VII [175]. The normal pathway of bronchoalveolar fibrinolysis is markedly depressed even during the early exudative phase of ARDS [175,178]. Patients with ARDS have normal levels of immunoreactive u-PA and plasminogen in BAL fluid, but an almost complete loss of urokinase activity [175,178]. The decreased enzymatic activity is due, in part, to the presence of an excess of PAI-1 and, in part, to excess antiplasmins, such as α_2-antiplasmin, in BAL fluid that are capable of inhibiting any plasmin formed [175,178]. The sources of the excess PAI-1 and antiplasmins have not yet been elucidated.

PROTEINASES IN RESOLUTION OF ARDS

Proteinases are almost certainly involved in the resolution/repair phase that follows the initial injury in ARDS (Figure 10.5). Sequential pathological studies of lung tissue in ARDS have revealed diffuse damage to the alveolar-capillary barrier that is accompanied by an intra-alveolar exudate rich in platelets, fibrin, fibronectin and other plasma proteins. Prominent deposition of fibrin and fibronectin along alveolar ducts leads to the formation of hyaline membranes. These sites of early fibrin deposition correlate with the subsequent location of fibrosis in ARDS; fibrin and fibronectin are important substrates for fibroblasts and the growth of fibroblasts into these deposits is followed by the deposition of collagen types I and III and fibronectin [179–181].

In survivors of ARDS, an extensive remodeling process occurs leading to the eventual return of nearly normal lung anatomy and physiologic function in these individuals [182–184]. Restoration of lung architecture to normal during the resolution phase of ARDS requires the removal of these deposited proteins. This process is likely to require the activities of a number of proteolytic enzymes from various sources.

Removal of fibrin requires the formation of plasmin from plasminogen which is catalyzed by plasminogen activators. The bulk of plasminogen activator activity in BAL fluid is soluble u-PA. Neutrophils, mononuclear phagocytes and alveolar type II epithelial cells synthesize and secrete u-PA; moreover, mononuclear phagocytes express cell associated u-PA which is resistant to inhibition by inhibitors of PA. However, the relative contributions of these cellular sources of uPA in the clearance of fibrin from the lungs in ARDS has yet to be determined.

Removal of fibronectin, collagen and proteinaceous debris that fills the alveolar spaces is likely to involve elastases, collagenases, gelatinases, plasminogen activators and cathepsins from plasma and inflammatory cells, such as neutrophils, mononuclear phagocytes, platelets and fibroblasts. The cellular sources of these proteinases, and the signaling events that control them, are largely unknown. However, *in situ* hybridization studies may help to resolve these questions in the coming years. Such studies may lead to interventions that promote healing of the injured lung in ARDS.

PROSPECTS FOR REDUCING LUNG INJURY

Proteinase inhibition is a reasonable strategy for ameliorating the initial lung injury in ARDS. As detailed above, a single proteolytic enzyme (HLE) accounts for most of the extracellular proteolytic activity of neutrophils and could represent a final common pathway for serious lung tissue injury during acute inflammation, regardless of the initial inciting cause of lung inflammation. Some promising results have been obtained with inhibition of leukocyte elastase in animal models of acute lung injury. For example, the abnormalities in lung lymph flow, lung lymph protein clearance and lung mechanics in response to endotoxin in sheep is ameliorated by inhibiting leukocyte elastase [185]. In another study, a synthetic HLE inhibitor (ICI 200,355) blunted rat leukocyte elastase activity in lung tissue in a model of thrombin induced pulmonary edema [186]. In the latter model, a protective effect of the elastase inhibitor was demonstrated by reductions in lung weight and lung water content.

The pharmaceutical industry has shown considerable interest in developing inhibitors of HLE. Patients with ARDS will be logical target populations for successfully developed HLE inhibitors because of the serious morbidity, mortality and economic costs associated with this syndrome. The results of such intervention in humans are difficult to predict, and the design of clinical trials (particularly development of inclusion and exclusion criteria for entry) will be daunting challenges. However, HLE inhibition appears to offer at least a reasonable chance of substantially reducing the initial lung injury, particularly if therapy is begun very early or is given to patients in high risk groups **before** they develop symptoms and signs of ARDS.

ACKNOWLEDGEMENTS

Supported in part by United States Public Health Service Grant HL46440, The Council For Tobacco Research, USA, Inc., and the Department of Veterans Affairs. E.J.C. is a Clinical Investigator of the Department of Veterans Affairs. C.A.O. is supported by a Research Training Fellowship Grant from the American Lung Association.

REFERENCES

1. Etherington, D.J., Mason, R.W., Taylor, M.A.J. and Wardale, R.J. (1984) Production of a monospecific antiserum to cathepsin L: the

histochemical location of enzyme in rabbit fibroblasts. *Biosci. Rep.*, **4**, 121–7.

2. Blair, H.C., Teitelbaum, S.L., Ghiselli, R. and Gluck, S. (1989) Osteoclastic bone resorption by a polarized vacuolar proton pump. *Science*, **245**, 855–7.

3. Neurath, H. (1984) Evolution of proteolytic enzymes. *Science*, **224**, 350–7.

4. Sinha, S., Watorek, W., Karr, S. *et al.* (1987) Primary structure of human neutrophil elastase. *Proc. Natl Acad. Sci. USA*, **84**, 2228–32.

5. Watorek, W., van Halbeek, H. and Travis, J. (1993) The isoforms of human neutrophil elastase and cathepsin G differ in their carbohydrate side chain structures. *Biol. Chem. Hoppe-Seyler*, **374**, 385–93.

6. Janoff, A. and Scherer, J. (1968) Mediators of inflammation in leukocyte lysosomes: IX. Elastinolytic activity in granules of human polymorphonuclear leukocytes. *J. Exp. Med.*, **128**, 1137–51.

7. McDonald, J.A. and Kelley, D.G. (1980) Degradation of fibronectin by human leucocyte elastase: release of biologically active fragments. *J. Biol. Chem.*, **255**, 8848–58.

8. Mainardi, C.L., Hasty, D.L. Seyer, J.M. and Kang, A.H. (1988) Specific cleavage of human type III collagen by human polymorphonuclear leukocyte elastase. *J. Biol. Chem.*, **255**, 12006–10.

9. Mainardi, C.L., Dixit, S.N. and Kang, A.H. (1980) Degradation of type IV (basement membrane) collagen by a proteinase isolated from human polymorphonuclear leukocyte granules. *J. Biol. Chem.*, **255**, 5435–41.

10. Kielty, C.M., Lees, M., Shuttleworth, C.A. and Woolley, D. (1993) Catabolism of intact type VI collagen microfibrils: susceptibility to degradation by serine proteinases. *Biochem. Biophys. Res. Commun.*, **191**, 1230–6.

11. Keiser, H., Greenwald, R.A., Feinstein, G. and Janoff A. (1976) Degradation of cartilage proteoglycan by human leukocyte granule neutral proteases – a model of joint injury. II. Degradation of isolated bovine nasal cartilage proteoglycan. *J. Clin. Invest.*, **57**, 625–32.

12. Janoff, A. (1985) State of the art. Elastases and emphysema. Current assessment of the protease-antiprotease hypothesis. *Am. Rev. Respir. Dis.*, **132**, 417–33.

13. Havemann, K. and Gramse M. (1984) Physiology and pathophysiology of neutral protein-ases of human granulocytes. *Adv. Exp. Med. Biol.*, **167**, 1–21.

14. Campanelli, D., Melchior, M., Fu, Y. *et al.* (1990) Cloning of cDNA for proteinase 3: a serine protease, antibiotic, and autoantigen from human neutrophils. *J. Exp. Med.*, **172**, 1709–15.

15. Rao, N.V., Wehner, N.G., Marshall, B.C. *et al.* (1994) Characterization of proteinase-3 (PR-3), a neutrophil serine proteinase. *J. Biol. Chem.*, **266**, 9540–8.

16. Salvesen, G., Farley, D., Shuman, J. *et al.* (1987) Molecular cloning of human cathepsin G: structural similarity to mast cell and cytotoxic T lymphocyte proteinases. *Biochemistry*, **26**: 2289–93.

17. Boudier, C., Holle, C. and Bieth, J.G. (1981) Stimulation of the elastolytic activity of leukocyte elastase by leukocyte cathepsin G. *J. Biol. Chem.*, **256**, 10256–8.

18. Snyder, R.A., Kaempfer, C.E. and Wintroub BU. (1985) Chemistry of a human monocyte-derived cell line (U937): identification of the angiotensin I-converting activity as leukocyte cathepsin G. *Blood*, **65**, 176–82.

19. Elsbach, P. and Weiss, J. (1992) Oxygen-independent antimicrobial systems of phagocytes, in *Inflammation. Basic Principles and Clinical Correlates*. 2nd edn, (eds J.I. Gallin, I.M. Goldstein and R. Snyderman), Raven Press, New York, pp. 603–36.

20. Selak, M.A., Chignard, M. and Smith, J.B. (1988) Cathepsin G is a strong platelet agonist released by neutrophils. *Biochem. J.*, **251**, 293–9.

21. Lovejoy, B., Cleasby, A., Hassell, A.M. *et al.* (1994) Structure of the catalytic domain of fibroblast collagenase complexed with an inhibitor. *Science*, **263**, 375–7.

22. Murphy, G. and Docherty, A.J.P. (1992) The matrix metalloproteinases and their inhibitors. *Am. J. Respir. Cell Mol. Biol.*, **7**, 120–5.

23. Woessner, J.F. Jr. (1991) Matrix metalloproteinases and their inhibitors in connective tissue remodeling. *FASEB J.*, **5**, 2145–54.

24. Jiang, W. and Bond, J.S. (1992) Families of metalloendopeptidases and their relationships. *FEBS Lett.*, **312**, 110–4.

25. Matrisian, L.M. (1992) The matrix-degrading metalloproteinases. *Bioessays*, **14**, 455–63.

26. Springman, E.B., Angleton, E.L., Birkedal-Hansen, H. and Van Wart H.E. (1990) Multiple modes of activation of latent human

fibroblast collagenase: evidence for the role of a Cys[73] active-site zinc complex in latency and a 'cysteine switch' mechanism for activation. *Proc. Natl Acad. Sci. USA.*, **87**, 364–8.

27. Sato, H., Takino, T., Okada, Y. *et al.* (1994) A matrix metalloproteinase expressed on the surface of invasive tumour cells. *Nature*, **370**, 61–5.

28. Reddy, V.Y. Pizzo, S.V. and Weiss, S.J. (1989) Functional inactivation and structural disruption of human alpha 2-macroglobulin by neutrophils and eosinophils. *J. Biol. Chem.*, **264**, 13801–9.

29. Desrochers, P.E. and Weiss, S.J. (1988) Proteolytic inactivation of alpha-1-proteinase inhibitor by a neutrophil metalloproteinase. *J. Clin. Invest.*, **81**, 1646–50.

30. Vissers, M.C.M., George, P.M., Bathurst, I.C. *et al.* (1988) Cleavage and inactivation of alpha$_1$-antitrypsin by metalloproteinases released from neutrophils. *J. Clin. Invest.*, **82**, 706–11.

31. Desrochers, P.E. Jeffrey, J.J. and Weiss, S.J. (1991) Interstitial collagenase (matrix metalloproteinase-1) expresses serpinase activity. *J. Clin. Invest.*, **87**, 2258–65.

32. Quantin, B., Murphy, G. and Breathnach, R. (1989) Pump-1 cDNA codes for a protein with characteristics similar to those of classical collagenase family members. *Biochemistry*, **28**, 5327–34.

33. Murphy, G., Cockett, M.I., Ward, R.V. and Docherty, A.J.P. (1991) Matrix metalloproteinase degradation of elastin, type IV collagen, and proteoglycan. A quantitative comparison of the activities of 95 kDa and 72 kDa gelatinases, stromelysins-1 and -2 and punctated metalloproteinase (PUMP). *Biochem. J.*, **277**, 277–9.

34. Shapiro, S.D., Kobayashi, D.K. and Ley T.J. (1993) Cloning and characterization of a unique elastolytic metalloproteinase produced by human alveolar macrophages. *J. Biol. Chem.*, **268**, 23824–9.

35. Gronski, T.J., Kobayashi, D.K. and Shapiro, S.D. (1994) Expression and purification of recombinant human macrophage metalloelastase: a potent basement membrane degrading enzyme. *Am. J. Respir. Crit. Care Med.*, **149**, A370 (abstract).

36. Shi, G.-P., Munger, J.S., Meara, J.P. *et al.* (1992) Molecular cloning and expression of human alveolar macrophage cathepsin S, an elastinolytic cysteine protease. *J. Biol. Chem.*, **267**, 7258–62.

37. Chapman, H.A. Jr, Reilly, J.J. Jr, Yee, R. and Mason B. (1987) Synthesis and expression of an elastolytic enzyme, cathepsin L, by human alveolar macrophages. *Am. Rev. Respir. Dis.*, **135**, 292A (abstract).

38. Mason, R.W., Johnson, D.A., Barrett, A.J. and Chapman, H.A. Jr (1986) Elastinolytic activity of human cathepsin L. *Biochem. J.*, **233**, 925–7.

39. Szecsi, P.B. (1992) The aspartic proteases. *Scand. J. Clin. Lab. Invest.*, **52** (suppl. 210), 5–22.

40. Barrett, A.J. (1980) The many forms and functions of cellular proteinases. *Fed. Proc.*, **39**, 9–14.

41. Kao, R.C., Wehner, N.G., Skubitz, K.M. *et al.* (1988) Proteinase 3. A distinct human polymorphonuclear leukocyte proteinase that produces emphysema in hamsters. *J. Clin. Invest.*, **82**, 1963–73.

42. Senior, R.M., Griffin, G.L., Fliszar, C.J. *et al.* (1991) Human 92- and 72-kilodalton type IV collagenases are elastases. *J. Biol. Chem.*, **266**, 7870–5.

43. Welgus, H.G., Jeffrey, J.J. and Eisen, A.Z. (1981) The collagen substrate specificity of human skin fibroblast collagenase. *J. Biol. Chem.*, **256**, 9511–5.

44. Gross, J. and Nagai, Y. (1965) Specific degradation of the collagen molecule by tadpole collagenolytic enzyme. *Proc. Natl Acad. Sci. USA*, **54**, 1197–204.

45. Welgus, H.G., Jeffrey, J.J., Stricklin, G.P. and Eisen A.Z. (1982) The gelatinolytic activity of human skin fibroblast collagenase. *J. Biol. Chem.*, **257**, 11534–9.

46. Chin, J.R., Murphy, G. and Werb, Z. (1985) Stromelysin, a connective tissue-degrading metalloendopeptidase secreted by stimulated rabbit synovial fibroblasts in parallel with collagenase. *J. Biol. Chem.*, **260**, 12367–76.

47. Whitham, S.E., Murphy, G., Angel, P. *et al.* (1986) Comparison of human stromelysin and collagenase by cloning and sequence analysis. *Biochem. J.*, **240**, 913–6.

48. Gadek, J.E., Fells, G.A., Wright, D.G. and Crystal, R.G. (1980) Human neutrophil elastase functions as a type III collagen 'collagenase'. *Biochem. Biophys. Res. Commun.*, **95**, 1815–22.

49. Pipoly, D.J. and Crouch, E.C. (1987) Degrada-

tion of native type IV procollagen by human neutrophil elastase. Implications for leukocyte-mediated degradation of basement membranes. *Biochemistry*, **26**, 5748–54.

50. Welgus, H.G., Burgeson, R.E., Wootton, J.A.M. *et al.* (1985) Degradation of monomeric and fibrillar type III collagens by human skin collagenase: kinetic constants using different animal substrates. *J. Biol. Chem.*, **260**, 1052–9.

51. Salonen, E.-M., Zitting, A. and Vaheri, A. (1984) Laminin interacts with plasminogen and its tissue-type activator. *FEBS Lett.*, **172**, 29–32.

52. Dano, K., Andreasen, P.A., Grondahl-Hansen, J. *et al.* (1985) Plasminogen activators, tissue degradation, and cancer. *Adv. Cancer Res.*, **44**, 139–266.

53. Saksela, O. and Rifkin, D.B. (1988) Cell-associated plasminogen activation: regulation and physiological functions. *Ann. Rev. Cell Biol.*, **4**, 93–126.

54. Kirchheimer, J.C. and Remold, H.G. (1989) Endogenous receptor-bound urokinase mediates tissue invasion of human monocytes. *J. Immunol.*, **143**, 2634–9.

55. Stossel, T.P. (1993) On the crawling of animal cells. *Science*, **260**, 1086–94.

56. Mason, D.Y., Cramer, E.M., Massé, J.-M. *et al.* (1991) Alpha$_1$-antitrypsin is present within the primary granules of human polymorphonuclear leukocytes. *Am. J. Pathol.*, **139**, 623–8.

57. Perlmutter, D.H., Kay, R.M., Cole, F.S. *et al.* (1985) The cellular defect in alpha-1 proteinase inhibitor (alpha-1-PI) deficiency is expressed in human monocytes and in *Xenopus* oocytes injected with human liver mRNA. *Proc. Natl Acad. Sci. USA*, **82**, 6918–21.

58. Stricklin, G.P. and Welgus, H.G. (1983) Human skin fibroblast collagenase inhibitor: purification and biochemical characterization. *J. Biol. Chem.*, **258**, 12252–8.

59. Campbell, E.J., Cury, J.D., Lazarus, C.J. and Welgus, H.G. (1987) Monocyte procollagenase and tissue inhibitor of metalloproteinases: identification, characterization, and regulation of secretion. *J. Biol. Chem.*, **262**, 15862–8.

60. Marshall, B.C., Santana, A., Xu Q.-P., *et al.* (1993) Metalloproteinases and tissue inhibitor of metalloproteinases in mesothelial cells. *J. Clin. Invest.*, **91**, 1792–9.

61. Chapman, H.A. Jr, Reilly, J.J. Jr, Yee, R. and Grubb A. (1990) Identification of cystatin C, a cysteine proteinase inhibitor, as a major secretory product of human alveolar macrophages *in vitro*. *Am. Rev. Respir. Dis.*, **141**, 698–705.

62. Dewald, B., Bretz, U. and Baggiolini, M. (1982) Release of gelatinase from a novel secretory compartment of human neutrophils. *J. Clin. Invest.*, **70**, 518–25.

63. Campbell, E.J., Silverman, E.K. and Campbell, M.A. (1989) Elastase and cathepsin G of human monocytes. Quantification of cellular content, release in response to stimuli, and heterogeneity in elastase-mediated proteolytic activity. *J. Immunol.*, **143**, 2961–8.

64. Takahashi, H., Nukiwa, T., Basset, P. and Crystal, R.G. (1988) Myelomonocytic cell lineage expression of the neutrophil elastase gene. *J. Biol. Chem.*, **263**, 2543–7.

65. Hanson, R.B., Connolly, N.L., Burnett, D. *et al.* (1990) Developmental regulation of the human cathepsin G gene in myelomonocytic cells. *J. Biol. Chem.*, **265**, 1524–30.

66. Sturrock, A.B., Franklin, K.F., Rao, G. *et al.* (1992) Structure, chromosomal assignment, and expression of the gene for proteinase-3. The Wegener's granulomatosis autoantigen. *J. Biol. Chem.*, **267**, 21193–9.

67. Shapiro, S.D., Campbell, E.J., Senior, R.M. and Welgus, H.G. (1991) Proteinases secreted by human mononuclear phagocytes. *J. Rheumatol.*, **27**, 95–8.

68. Kargi, H.A., Campbell, E.J. and Kuhn, C. III (1990) Elastase and cathepsin G of human monocytes. Heterogeneity and subcellular localization to peroxidase-positive granules. *J. Histochem. Cytochem.*, **38**, 1179–86.

69. Campbell, E.J. (1982) Human leukocyte elastase, cathepsin G, and lactoferrin: a family of neutrophil granule glycoproteins which bind to an alveolar macrophage receptor. *Proc. Natl Acad. Sci. USA*, **79**, 6941–5.

70. Campbell, E.J., White, R.R., Senior, R.M. *et al.* (1979) Receptor-mediated binding and internalization of leukocyte elastase by alveolar macrophages *in vitro*. *J. Clin. Invest.*, **64**, 824–33.

71. Campbell, E.J. and Wald, M.S. (1983) Fate of human neutrophil elastase following receptor-mediated endocytosis by human alveolar macrophages: implications for connective tissue injury. *J. Lab. Clin. Med.*, **101**, 527–36.

72. Owen, C.A., Campbell, M.A., Boukedes, S.S. and Campbell, E.J. (1994) Monocytes recruited to sites of inflammation express a

distinctive pro-inflammatory (P) phenotype. *Am. J. Physiol.*, **267**, L786–96.

73. Owen, C.A., Campbell, M.A., Boukedes, S.S. *et al.* (1994) A discrete subpopulation of human monocytes expresses a neutrophil-like proinflammatory (P) phenotype. *Am. J. Physiol.*, **267**, L775–85.

74. Campbell, E.J., Cury, J.D., Shapiro, S.D. *et al.* (1991) Neutral proteinases of human mononuclear phagocytes. Cellular differentiation markedly alters cell phenotype for serine proteinases, metalloproteinases, and TIMP. *J. Immunol.*, **146**, 1286–93.

75. White, R.R., Janoff, A., Gordon, R. and Campbell, E.J. (1982) Evidence for *in vivo* internalization of human leukocyte elastase by human alveolar macrophages. *Am. Rev. Respir. Dis.*, **125**, 779–81.

76. Savill, J.S., Henson, P.M. and Haslett, C. (1989) Phagocytosis of aged human neutrophils by macrophages is mediated by a novel 'charge-sensitive' recognition mechanism. *J. Clin. Invest.*, **84**, 1518–27.

77. Campbell, E.J. and Wald, M.S. (1983) Hypoxic injury to human alveolar macrophages accelerates release of previously bound neutrophil elastase: implications for lung connective tissue injury including pulmonary emphysema. *Am. Rev. Respir. Dis.*, **127**, 631–5.

78. Chapman, H.A. Jr, Reilly, J.J. Jr and Kobzik, L. (1988) Role of plasminogen activator in degradation of extracellular matrix protein by live human alveolar macrophages. *Am. Rev. Respir. Dis.*, **137**, 412–9.

79. Waltz, D.A., Sailor, L.Z. and Chapman, H.A. (1993) Cytokines induce urokinase-dependent adhesion of human myeloid cells. A regulatory role for plasminogen activator inhibitors. *J. Clin. Invest.*, **91**, 1541–52.

80. Gyetko, M.R., Todd, R.F. III, Wilkinson, C.C. and Sitrin R.G. (1994) The urokinase receptor is required for human monocyte chemotaxis *in vitro*. *J. Clin. Invest.*, **93**, 1380–7.

81. Busiek, D.F., Ross, F.P., McDonnell, S. *et al.* (1992) The matrix metalloprotease matrilysin (PUMP) is expressed in developing human mononuclear phagocytes. *J. Biol. Chem.*, **267**, 9087–92.

82. Wahl, L.M. and Corcoran, M.L. (1993) Regulation of monocyte/macrophage metalloproteinase production by cytokines. *J. Periodontol.*, **64**, 467–73.

83. Saarialho-Kere, U.K., Welgus, H.G. and Parks, W.C. (1993) Distinct mechanisms regulate interstitial collagenase and 92-kDa gelatinase expression in human monocytic-like cells exposed to bacterial endotoxin. *J. Biol. Chem.*, **268**, 1–8.

84. Shapiro, S.D., Campbell, E.J., Kobayashi, D.K. and Welgus H.G. (1990) Immune modulation of metalloproteinase production in human macrophages. Selective suppression of interstitial collagenase and stromelysin biosynthesis by interferon-gamma. *J. Clin. Invest.*, **86**, 1204–10.

85. Davis, W.B., Fells, G.A., Sun, X.-H. *et al.* (1984) Eosinophil-mediated injury to lung parenchymal cells and interstitial matrix. A possible role for eosinophils in chronic inflammatory disorders of the lower respiratory tract. *J. Clin. Invest.*, **74**, 269–78.

86. Lungarella, G., Menegazzi, R., Gardi, C. *et al.* (1992) Identification of elastase in human eosinophils: immunolocalization, isolation, and partial characterization. *Arch. Biochem. Biophys.*, **292**, 128–35.

87. Meier, H.L., Schulman, E.S., Heck, L.W. *et al.* (1989) Release of elastase from purified human lung mast cells and basophils. *Inflammation*, **13**, 295–308.

88. Braun, M.G., Csernok, E., Gross, W.L. and Muller-Hermelink, H.K. (1991) Proteinase 3, the target antigen of anticytoplasmic antibodies circulating in Wegener's granulomatosis. Immunolocalization in normal and pathologic tissues. *Am. J. Pathol.*, **139**, 831–8.

89. Schwartz, L.B., Lewis, R.A., Seldin, D. and Austin, K.F. (1981) Acid hydrolases and tryptase from secretory granules of dispersed human lung mast cells. *J. Immunol.*, **126**, 1290–6.

90. Gruber, B.L., Schwartz, L.B., Ramamurthy, N.S. *et al.* (1988) Activation of latent rheumatoid synovial collagenase by human mast cell tryptase. *J. Immunol.*, **140**, 3936–42.

91. Gruber, B.L., Marchese, M.J., Suzuki, K. *et al.* (1989) Synovial procollagenase activation by human mast cell tryptase dependence upon matrix metalloproteinase 3 activation. *J. Clin. Invest.*, **84**, 1657–62.

92. Niedbala, M.J. (1993) Cytokine regulation of endothelial cell extracellular proteolysis. *Agents Actions*, **42**, 179–93.

93. Mayet, W.J., Csernok, E., Szymkowiak, C. *et al.* (1993) Human endothelial cells express proteinase 3, the target antigen of anti-

cytoplasmic antibodies in Wegener's granulomatosis. *Blood*, **82**, 1221–9.

94. Desrivieres, S., Lu, H., Peyri, N. *et al.* (1993) Activation of the 92 kDa type IV collagenase by tissue kallikrein. *J. Cell. Physiol.*, **157**, 587–93.

95. Herron, G.S., Banda, M.J., Clark, E.J. *et al.* (1986) Secretion of metalloproteinases by stimulated capillary endothelial cells. II. Expression of collagenase and stromelysin activities is regulated by endogenous inhibitors. *J. Biol. Chem.*, **261**, 2814–8.

96. Herron, G.S., Werb, Z., Dwyer, K. and Banda, M.J. (1986) Secretion of metalloproteinases by stimulated capillary endothelial cells. I. Production of procollagenase and prostromelysin exceeds expression of proteolytic activity. *J. Biol. Chem.*, **261**, 2810–3.

97. Birkedal-Hansen, H., Moore, WGI, Bodden, M.K. *et al.* (1993) Matrix metalloproteinases: A review. *Crit. Rev. Oral Biol. Med.*, **4**, 197–250.

98. Marshall, B.C., Sageser, D.S., Rao, N.V. *et al.* (1990) Alveolar epithelial cell plasminogen activator. Characterization and regulation. *J. Biol. Chem.*, **265**, 8198–204.

99. Sallenave, J.-M., Silva, A., Marsden, M.E. and Ryle, A.P. (1993) Secretion of mucus proteinase inhibitor and elafin by Clara cell and type II pneumocyte cell lines. *Am. J. Respir. Cell Mol. Biol.*, **8**, 126–33.

100. De Water, R., Willems, L.N.A., Van Muijen, G.N.P. *et al.* (1986) Ultrastructural localization of bronchial antileukoprotease in central and peripheral human airways by a gold-labeling technique using monoclonal antibodies. *Am. Rev. Respir. Dis.*, **133**, 882–90.

101. Travis, J. and Salvesen, G.S. (1983) Human plasma proteinase inhibitors. *Annu. Rev. Biochem.*, **52**, 655–709.

102. Carrell, R.W. (1986) Alpha$_1$-antitrypsin: molecular pathology, leukocytes, and tissue damage. *J. Clin. Invest.*, **78**, 1427–31.

103. Campbell, E.J., Senior, R.M., McDonald, J.A. and Cox, D.L. (1982) Proteolysis by neutrophils. Relative importance of cell–substrate contact and oxidative inactivation of proteinase inhibitors *in vitro*. *J. Clin. Invest.*, **70**, 845–52.

104. Campbell, E.J. and Campbell, M.A. (1987) Proteolysis by neutrophils while in contact with substrate: incomplete protection of substrate by proteinase inhibitors, in *Pulmonary Emphysema and Proteolysis*, Vol. II (eds (C.

Mittman and J.C. Taylor), Academic Press, New York, pp. 235–44.

105. Campbell, E.J. and Campbell, M.A. (1988) Pericellular proteolysis by neutrophils in the presence of proteinase inhibitors: effects of substrate opsonization. *J. Cell Biol.*, **106**, 667–76.

106. Senior, R.M., Connolly, N.L., Cury, J.D. *et al.* (1989) Elastin degradation by human alveolar macrophages: a prominent role of metalloproteinase activity. *Am. Rev. Respir. Dis.*, **139**, 1251–6.

107. Johnson, K.J. and Varani, J. (1981) Substrate hydrolysis by immune complex-activated neutrophils: effect of physical presentation of complexes and protease inhibitors. *J. Immunol.*, **127**, 1875–9.

108. Weiss, S.J. and Regiani, S. (1984) Neutrophils degrade subendothelial matrices in the presence of alpha-1-proteinase inhibitor: cooperative use of lysosomal proteinases and oxygen metabolites. *J. Clin. Invest.*, **73**, 1297–303.

109. Ossanna, P.J., Test, S.T., Matheson, N.R. *et al.* (1986) Oxidative regulation of neutrophil elastase-alpha-1-proteinase inhibitor interactions. *J. Clin. Invest.*, **77**, 1939–51.

110. Weiss, S.J., Curnutte, J.T. and Regiani, S. (1986) Neutrophil-mediated solubilization of the subendothelial matrix: oxidative and non-oxidative mechanisms of proteolysis used by normal and chronic granulomatous disease phagocytes. *J. Immunol.*, **136**, 636–41.

111. Sibille, Y., Lwebuga-Mukasa, J.S., Palomski, L. *et al.* (1986) An *in vitro* model for polymorphonuclear-leukocyte-induced injury to an extracellular matrix: relative contribution of oxidants and elastase to fibronectin release from amniotic membranes. *Am. Rev. Respir. Dis.*, **134**, 134–40.

112. Weitz, J.I., Huang, A.J., Landman, S.L. *et al.* (1988) Elastase-mediated fibrinogenolysis by chemoattractant-stimulated neutrophils occurs in the presence of physiologic concentrations of antiproteinases. *J. Exp. Med.*, **166**, 1838–50.

113. Schalkwijk, J., Van den Berg, W.B. Van de Putte, L.B.A. and Joosten, L.A.B. (1987) Elastase secreted by activated polymorphonuclear leucocytes causes chondrocyte damage and matrix degradation in intact articular cartilage: escape from inactivation by alpha-

1-proteinase inhibitor. *Br. J. Exp. Pathol.*, **68**, 81–8.

114. Rice, W.G. and Weiss, S.J. (1990) Regulation of proteolysis at the neutrophil–substate interface by secretory leukoprotease inhibitor. *Science*, **249**, 178–81.

115. Chapman, H.A. Jr and Stone, O.L. (1984) Comparison of live human neutrophil and alveolar macrophage elastolytic activity *in vitro*. Relative resistance of macrophage elastolytic activity to serum and alveolar proteinase inhibitors. *J. Clin. Invest.*, **74**, 1693–700.

116. Chapman, H.A. Jr and Stone, O.L. (1984) Co-operation between plasmin and elastase in elastin degradation by intact murine macrophages. *Biochem. J.*, **222**, 721–8.

117. Chapman, H.A. Jr, Stone, O.L. and Vavrin, Z. (1984) Degradation of fibrin and elastin by intact human alveolar macrophages *in vitro*. Characterization of plasminogen activator and its role in matrix degradation. *J. Clin. Invest.*, **73**, 806–15.

118. Plow, E.F., Freaney, D.E., Plescia, J. and Miles, L.A., (1986) The plasminogen system and cell surfaces: evidence for plasminogen and urokinase receptors on the same cell type. *J. Cell Biol.*, **103**, 2411–20.

119. Wright, S.D. and Silverstein, S.C. (1984) Phagocytosing macrophages exclude proteins from zones of contact with targets. *Nature*, **309**, 359–61.

120. Campbell, E.J. (1986) Preventive therapy of emphysema: lessons from the elastase model. *Am. Rev. Respir. Dis.*, **134**, 435–7.

121. Desrochers, P.E., Mookhtiar, K., Van Wart, H.E. *et al.* (1992) Proteolytic inactivation of alpha 1-proteinase inhibitor and alpha 1-antichymotrypsin by oxidatively activated human neutrophil metalloproteinases. *J. Biol. Chem.*, **267**, 5005–12.

122. Reddy, V.Y., Desrochers, P.E., Pizzo, S.V. *et al.* (1994) Oxidative dissociation of human alpha 2-macroglobulin tetramers into dysfunctional dimers. *J. Biol. Chem.*, **269**, 4683–91.

123. Kramps, J.A., Van Twisk, C., Appelhans, H. *et al.* (1990) Proteinase inhibitory activities of antileukoprotease are represented by its second COOH-terminal domain. *Biochim. Biophys. Acta*, **1038**, 178–85.

124. Vissers, M.C.M., Day, W.A. and Winterbourn, C.C. (1985) Neutrophils adherent to a non-phagocytosable surface (glomerular basement membrane) produce oxidants only at the site of attachment. *Blood*, **66**, 161–6.

125. Chen, W.-T. (1992) Membrane proteases: roles in tissue remodeling and tumour invasion. *Curr. Opin. Cell Biol.*, **24947**, 26992–8526.

126. Csernok, E., Ernst, M., Schmitt, W. *et al.* (1994) Activated neutrophils express proteinase 3 on their plasma membrane *in vitro* and *in vivo*. *Clin. Exp. Immunol.*, **95**, 244–50.

127. Gross, W.L., Csernok, E. and Flesch, B.K. (1993) 'Classic' anti-neutrophil cytoplasmic autoantibodies (cANCA), 'Wegener's auto-antigen' and their immunopathogenic role in Wegener's granulomatosis. *J. Autoimmun.*, **6**, 171–84.

128. Lavie, G., Zucker-Franklin, D. and Franklin, E.C. (1980) Elastase-type proteases on the surface of human blood monocytes: possible role in amyloid formation. *J. Immunol.*, **125**, 175–80.

129. Zucker-Franklin, D., Lavie, G. and Franklin, E.C. (1981) Demonstration of membrane-bound proteolytic activity on the surface of mononuclear leukocytes. *J. Histochem. Cytochem.*, **29**, 451–6.

130. Pollanen, J., Hedman, K., Nielsen, L.S. *et al.* (1988) Ultrastructural localization of plasma membrane-associated urokinase-type plasminogen activator at focal contacts. *J. Cell Biol.*, **106**, 87–95.

131. Chapman, H.A. Jr, Vavrin, Z. and Hibbs, J.B. (1982) Macrophage fibrinolytic activity: identification of two pathways of plasmin formation by intact cells and of a plasminogen activator inhibitor. *Cell*, **28**, 653–62.

132. Nielsen, L.S., Kellerman, G.M., Behrendt, N. *et al.* (1988) A 55 000–60 000 Mr receptor protein for urokinase-type plasminogen activator. Identification in human tumor cell lines and partial purification. *J. Biol. Chem.*, **263**, 2358–63.

133. Pollanen, J., Saksela, O., Salonen, E. *et al.* (1987) Distinct localizations of urokinase-type plasminogen activator and its type 1 inhibitor under cultured human fibroblasts and sarcoma cells. *J. Cell Biol.*, **104**, 1085–96.

134. Ellis, V., Wun, T.-C., Behrendt, N. *et al.* (1990) Inhibition of receptor-bound urokinase by plasminogen-activator inhibitors. *J. Biol. Chem.*, **265**, 9904–8.

135. Picone, R., Kajtaniak, E.L., Nielsen, L.S. *et al.* (1989) Regulation of urokinase receptors in monocytelike U937 cells by phorbol ester

phorbol myristate acetate. *J. Cell Biol.*, **108**, 693–702.

136. Chapman, H.A. Jr, Bertozzi, P., Sailor, L.Z. and Nusrat, A.R. (1990) Alveolar macrophage urokinase receptors localize enzyme activity to the cell surface. *Am. J. Physiol.*, **3**, L432–8.

137. Ellis, V., Scully, M.F. and Kakkar, V.V. (1989) Plasminogen activation initiated by single-chain urokinase type plasminogen activator. Potentiation by U937 monocytes. *J. Biol. Chem.* **264**, 2185–8.

138. Morrison, H.M., Welgus, H.G., Stockley, R.A. *et al.* (1990) Inhibition of human leukocyte elastase bound to elastin: relative ineffectiveness and two mechanisms of inhibitory activity. *Am. J. Respir. Cell Mol. Biol.*, **2**, 263–9.

139. Bruch, M. and Bieth, J.G. (1986) Influence of elastin on the inhibition of leucocyte elastase by alpha₁-proteinase inhibitor and bronchial inhibitor. Potent inhibition of elastin-bound elastase by bronchial inhibitor. *Biochem. J.*, **238**, 269–73.

140. Kolev, K., Lerant, I., Tenekejiev, K. and Machovich, R. (1994) Regulation of fibrinolytic activity of neutrophil leukocyte elastase, plasmin, and miniplasmin by plasma protease inhibitors. *J. Biol. Chem.*, **269**, 17030–4.

141. Peterson, M.W. (1989) Neutrophil cathepsin G increases transendothelial albumin flux. *J. Lab. Clin. Med.*, **113**, 297–308.

142. Laposata, M., Dovnarsky, D.K. and Shin, H.S. (1983) Thrombin-induced gap formation in confluent endothelial cell monolayers *in vitro*. *Blood*, **62**, 549–56.

143. Rochat, T.R., Casale, J.M., Hunninghake, G.W. and Peterson, M.W. (1988) Neutrophil cathepsin G increases permeability of cultured type II pneumocytes. *Am. J. Physiol.*, **24**, C603–11.

144. Garcia, J.G.N., Siflinger-Birnboim, A., Bizios, R. *et al.* (1986) Thrombin-induced increase in albumin permeability across the endothelium. *J. Cell. Physiol.*, **128**, 96–104.

145. Sugahara, K., Cott, G.R., Parsons, P.E. *et al.* (1986) Epithelial permeability produced by phagocytosing neutrophils *in vitro*. *Am. Rev. Respir. Dis.*, **133**, 875–61.

146. Harlan, J.M. (1985) Leukocyte-endothelial interactions. *Blood*, **65**, 513–25.

147. Smedly, L.A., Tonnesen, M.G., Sandhaus, R.A. *et al.* (1986) Neutrophil-mediated injury to endothelial cells. Enhancement by endotoxin and essential role of neutrophil elastase. *J. Clin. Invest.*, **77**, 1233–43.

148. Brown, D.M., Brown, G.M., MacNee, W. and Donaldson, K. (1992) Activated human peripheral blood neutrophils produce epithelial injury and fibronectin breakdown *in vitro*. *Inflammation*, **16**, 21–30.

149. Stokke, T., Burchardi, H., Hensel, I. and Horl, W.H. (1985) Experimental studies on the adult respiratory distress syndrome: effects of induced DIC; granulocytes and elastase in mini pigs. *Eur. J. Clin. Invest.*, **15**, 415–21.

150. Seiler, M.W., Rennke, H.G., Venkatachalam, M.B. and Cotran, R.S. (1977) Pathogenesis of polycation-induced alterations ('fusion') of glomerular epithelium. *Lab. Invest.*, **36**, 48–61.

151. Peterson, M.W., Clark, R., Stone, P. and Shasby, D.M. (1985) Neutrophil cationic protein increases endothelial albumin transport. *Am. Rev. Respir. Dis.*, **131**, A421 (abstract).

152. Vehaskari, V.M., Chang, C.T.-C., Stevens, J.K. and Robson A.M. (1984) The effects of polycations on vascular permeability in the rat. A proposed role for charge sites. *J. Clin. Invest.*, **73**, 1053–61.

153. Nagy, Z., Peters, H. and Huttner, G. (1983) Charge-related alterations of the cerebral endothelium. *Lab. Invest.*, **49**, 662–71.

154. Demling, R.H. (1988) The role of mediators in human ARDS *J. Crit. Care.*, **3**, 56–72.

155. Crouch, E., Moxley, M.A. and Longmore, W. (1987) Synthesis of collagenous proteins by pulmonary type II epithelial cells. *Am. Rev. Respir. Dis.*, **135**, 1118–23.

156. Pipoly, D. and Crouch, E. (1986) Degradation of basement membrane collagen by human leukocyte elastase and hydrogen peroxide. *Am. Rev. Respir. Dis.*, **133**, A258.

157. Senior, R.M. and Campbell, E.J. (1983) Neutral proteinases from human inflammatory cells: a critical review of their role in extracellular matrix degradation. *Clin. Lab. Med.*, **3**, 645–66.

158. Campbell, E.J., Senior, R.M. and Welgus, H.G. (1987) Extracellular matrix injury during lung inflammation. *Chest*, **92**, 161–7.

159. Sires, U.I., Griffin, G.L., Broekelmann, T.J. *et al.* Degradation of entactin by matrix metalloproteinases. Susceptibility to matrilysin and identification of cleavage sites. *J. Biol. Chem.*, **268**, 2069–74.

160. Crapo, J.D., Barry, B.E., Gehr, P. *et al.* (1982) Cell number and cell characteristics of the normal human lung. *Am. Rev. Respir. Dis.* **125**, 332–7

161. Rinaldo, J.E. and Rogers, R.M. (1982) Adult respiratory distress syndrome. Changing concepts of lung injury and repair. *N. Engl. J. Med.*, **306**, 900–9.

162. Warshawaki, R.J., Sibbald, W.J., Driedger, A.A. and Cheung, H. (1986) Abnormal neutrophil–pulmonary interaction in the adult respiratory distress syndrome. Qualitative and quantitative assessment of pulmonary neutrophil kinetics in humans with the *in vivo* indium-111 neutrophil scintigraphy. *Am. Rev. Respir. Dis.*, **122**, 797–804.

163. Lee, C., Fein, A., Lippmann, M. *et al.* (1981) Elastolytic activity in pulmonary lavage fluid from patients with adult respiratory-distress syndrome. *N. Engl. J. Med.*, **304**, 192–6.

164. Weiland, J., Davis, W.B., Holter, *et al.* (1986) Lung neutrophils in the adult respiratory distress syndrome. *Am. Rev. Respir. Dis.*, **133**, 218–25.

165. Fowler, A.A., Hyers, T.M., Fisher, B.J. *et al.* (1987) The adult respiratory distress syndrome. Cell populations and soluble mediators in the air spaces of patients at high risk. *Am. Rev. Respir. Dis.*, **136**, 1225–31.

166. Christner, P., Fein, A., Goldberg, S. *et al.* (1985) Collagenase in the lower respiratory-tract of patients with adult respiratory-distress syndrome. *Am. Rev. Respir. Dis.*, **131**, 690–5.

167. Hallgren, R., Borg, T., Venge, P. and Modig, J. (1984) Signs of neutrophil and eosinophil activation in adult respiratory distress syndrome. *Crit. Care Med.*, **12**, 14–8.

168. Baldwin, S.R., Simon, R.H., Grum, C.M. *et al.* (1986) Oxidant activity in expired breath of patients with adult respiratory distress syndrome. *Lancet*, **i**, 11–4.

169. Zheutlin, L.M., Thonar, J.-M.A., Jacobs, E.R. *et al.* (1986) Plasma elastase levels in the adult respiratory distress syndrome. *J. Crit. Care*, **1**, 39–44.

170. Speer, C.P., Ruess, D., Harms, K. *et al.* (1993) Neutrophil elastase and acute pulmonary damage in neonates with severe respiratory distress syndrome. *Pediatrics*, **91**, 794–9.

171. Cochrane, C.G., Spragg, R.G., Revak, S.D. *et al.* (1983) The presence of neutrophil elastse and evidence of oxidation activity in broncho-alveolar lavage fluid of patients with adult respiratory distress syndrome. *Am. Rev. Respir. Dis.*, **127**, S25–7.

172. McGuire, W.W., Spragg, R.G., Cohen, A.B. and Cochrane, C.G. (1982) Studies on the pathogenesis of the adult respiratory distress syndrome. *J. Clin. Invest.*, **69**, 543–53.

173. Kawamura, M., Yamasawa, F., Ishizaka, A. *et al.* (1994) Serum concentration of 7S collagen and prognosis in patients with the adult respiratory distress syndrome. *Thorax*, **49**, 144–6.

174. Kondoh, Y., Taniguchi, H., Taki, F. *et al.* (1992) 7S collagen in bronchoalveolar lavage fluid of patients with adult respiratory distress syndrome. *Chest*, **101**, 1091–4.

175. Idell, S., James, J.K., Levin, E.G. *et al.* (1989) Local abnormalities in coagulation and fibrinolytic pathways predispose to alveolar fibrin deposition in the adult respiratory distress syndrome. *J. Clin. Invest.*, **84**, 695–705.

176. Idell, S., Kucich, U., Fein. A. *et al.* (1985) Neutrophil elastase-releasing factors in bronchoalveolar lavage from patients with adult respiratory distress syndrome. *Am. Rev. Respir. Dis.*, **132**, 1098–105.

177. Idell, S., Gonzalez, K., Bradford, H. *et al.* (1987) Procoagulant activity in bronchoalveolar lavage in the adult respiratory distress syndrome. *Am. Rev. Respir. Dis.*, **136**, 1466–74.

178. Bertozzi, P., Astedt, B., Zenzius, L. *et al.* (1990) Depressed bronchoalveolar urokinase activity in patients with adult respiratory distress syndrome. *N. Engl. J. Med.*, **322**, 890–7.

179. Pratt, P. (1978) Pathology of adult respiratory distress syndrome, in *The Lung: Structure Function, and Disease* (eds W.M. Thurlbeck and M.R. Abell), Williams & Wilkins, Baltimore, pp. 45–7.

180. Bassett, F., Ferrans, V.J. Soler, P., *et al.* (1986) Intraluminal fibrosis in interstitial lung disorders. *Am. J. Pathol.*, **122**, 443–61.

181. Zapol, W.M., Trelstad, R.L., Coffey, J.W. *et al.* (1979) Pulmonary fibrosis in severe acute respiratory failure. *Am. Rev. Respir. Dis.*, **119**, 547–54.

182. Elliot, C.G., Morris, A.H. and Cengiz M. (1981) Pulmonary function and exercise gas exchange in survivors of adult respiratory distress syndrome. *Am. Rev. Respir. Dis.*, **123**, 492–5.

183. Alberts, W.M., Priest, G.R. and Moser, K.M. (1983) The outlook for survivors of ARDS. *Chest*, **84**, 272–4.

184. Peters, J.I., Bell, R.C., Prihoda, T.J. *et al.* (1989) Clinical determinants of abnormalities in pulmonary functions in survivors of the adult respiratory distress syndrome. *Am. Rev. Respir. Dis.*, **139**, 1163–8.

185. Gossage, J.R., Kuratomi, Y., Davidson, J.M. *et al.* (1993) Neutrophil elastase inhibitors, SC-37698 and SC-39026, reduce endotoxin-induced lung dysfunction in awake sheep. *Am. Rev. Respir. Dis.*, **147**, 1371–9.

186. Ahn, C.M., Sandler, H., Glass, M. and Saldeen, T. (1993) Effect of a synthetic leukocyte elastase inhibitor on thrombin-induced pulmonary edema in the rat. *Exp. Lung Res.*, **19**, 125–35.

11

REACTIVE OXYGEN SPECIES, ANTIOXIDANT PROTECTION AND LUNG INJURY

John M.C. Gutteridge and Gregory J. Quinlan

ARDS AND OXIDANT STRESS

The syndrome of acute respiratory distress in adults (ARDS) is characterized by refractory hypoxemia secondary to nonhydrostatic pulmonary edema and is associated with a wide variety of precipitating factors, often not directly involving the lung [1,2]. Thus, ARDS can result from such diverse clinical conditions as sepsis, gastric aspiration, polytrauma, pancreatitis, hemorrhagic shock, severe burns, oxygen toxicity and cardiopulmonary bypass [2]. In spite of the increasing complexity and scientific basis of medical support, ARDS still carries a mortality rate of around 50%, little changed from when it was first described [3].

The precise mechanisms that lead to acute lung injury are at present unknown, but recent evidence suggests that patients with ARDS are exposed to a severe oxidative burden from a variety of sources. In support of this concept, myeloperoxidase and oxidized α_1-antiproteinase have been found in bronchoalveolar lavage (BAL) fluids [4,5] and hydrogen peroxide (H_2O_2) can be detected in the expired breath [6,7] of patients with ARDS. Furthermore, ascorbic acid and α-tocopherol have been found to be depleted in body fluids [8,9], plasma proteins are exces- sively damaged [10] and products of peroxidized lipids have been detected in BAL fluids and plasma retrieved from patients with severe lung injury [8,9].

When patients die within the first three days of the onset of ARDS, their primary illness is usually thought to be responsible, but late deaths are more commonly attributable to infection. Patients in whom the lung is the primary site of infection appear to have the worst prognosis, often responding poorly to antibiotic therapy [11]. When ARDS is triggered by sepsis, bacterial lipopolysaccharides are thought to elicit the expression of a number of cytokines, activating the complement and coagulation cascades. These changes have important effects upon several cellular systems, including circulating and resident phagocytic cells in the lung [12,13]. Activation of neutrophils, sequestered within the lung, causes the release of reactive oxygen species such as superoxide, hydrogen peroxide and hypochlorous acid, as well as other damaging agents including eicosanoids and proteases [14].

When suitable transition metal complexes are present, O_2^-, H_2O_2 and lipid peroxides (LOOH) can form highly reactive species such as hydroxyl radicals ($^\bullet$OH), ferryl ions

ARDS Acute Respiratory Distress in Adults. Edited by Timothy W. Evans and Christopher Haslett. Published in 1996 by Chapman & Hall, London. ISBN 0 412 56910 8

(FeO^{2+}), alkoxyl ($LO^{\bullet}$) and peroxyl ($LO_2^{\bullet}$) radicals, all of which are capable of damaging biological molecules. Iron is by far the most abundant transition metal in the body, and therefore the most likely participant in electron transfers leading to the formation of aggressive oxidants [15]. In order to protect against iron driven radical reactions, iron is maintained in 'safe' protein transport and storage forms, which limit its reactivity in free radical reactions [15,17]. In addition to iron sequestration in extracellular fluids, the body utilizes protective enzymes to catalyze the oxidation of ferrous ions to the less reactive ferric state (ferroxidases). The most important ferroxidase in human plasma is the copper-containing protein ceruloplasmin, termed ferroxidase 1 [18].

In addition to neutrophil activation, the unavoidable requirement of ARDS patients for high inspired oxygen concentrations (F_{IO_2}) also contributes to oxidative stress. Oxidant stress may be defined as an imbalance between the generation of oxygen derived species and the level of antioxidant protection within a system. Normally these are approximately in balance, but when the balance is tipped in favor of the oxygen derived species cellular biochemistry is disturbed and a state of 'oxidative stress' exists, which can lead to molecular damage. Cells can respond to oxidative stress in several ways, such as recognizing and removing damaged molecules, increasing the levels of some antioxidants or redistributing transition metals within the body. Because of the biological complexity of oxidative stress and the antioxidant response we have introduced the reader to the basic biochemistry of oxygen reduction to reactive intermediates, and the body's protection against them with antioxidants. In the next section we discuss in some detail the major reactive forms of oxygen and their interaction with transition metals, particularly iron, to produce biologically damaging species.

OXYGEN ACTIVATION BY PHAGOCYTIC CELLS

Most of the phagocytic cells in the human bloodstream are neutrophils (polymorphonuclear cells). When human tissue is injured, an acute inflammatory response develops. The arterioles in and around the injured area relax, so that the capillary network becomes engorged with blood. The permeability of the blood vessel walls increases so that protein-rich fluid leaks out, causing edema.

Neutrophils enter the inflamed tissue by crossing the vessel wall. Their migration appears to be produced by a number of compounds, known as chemotactic factors, such as products of complement activation and lipid oxidation. Lungs also contain larger phagocytic cells called alveolar macrophages. When a phagocytic cell contacts opsonized bacteria (or particles) the bacteria are engulfed and killed within the phagocytic vacuole.

At the onset of phagocytosis there is a marked increase in oxygen uptake known as the 'oxidative burst' ('respiratory burst' is a term also used, although the phenomenon has nothing to do with cell respiration). During this process the free radical superoxide (O_2^-) is produced by an NADPH dependent enzyme complex associated with the plasma membrane [19]. In addition, neutrophils contain an enzyme, myeloperoxidase, which is used along with superoxide and hydrogen peroxide to help kill engulfed microorganisms. In the presence of hydrogen peroxide and chloride ions (Cl^-), myeloperoxidase forms hypochlorous acid (HOCl), a powerful oxidant. Hypocholorous acid may also form hydroxyl radicals by reaction with superoxide or ferrous ions [20,21].

HYPEROXIA AND OXYGEN ACTIVATION

When oxygen enters the lungs it dissolves in the lipid and aqueous phases of lung tissue and diffuses across alveolar membranes into the capillaries, where it is picked up by red blood cell hemoglobin.

It is well established that when oxygen is supplied to the lungs at concentrations greater than those present in air (21%) at normal atmospheric pressure (normobaric), tissue injury occurs. For example, when adult rats are exposed to greater than 95% oxygen they die within 60–72 hours. In 1954 Gerschman and colleagues first proposed that oxygen toxicity was caused by the formation of free radicals [22] which led to tissue damage. This was later demonstrated in hyperoxic rat lungs where the pulmonary production of oxygen radicals came mainly from mitochondria [23]. Hyperoxia also appears to amplify the susceptibility of lung cells to neutrophil mediated oxidant damage [24].

FREE RADICALS, REACTIVE OXYGEN SPECIES AND TRANSITION METALS IN BIOLOGICAL SYSTEMS

CHEMISTRY OF OXYGEN

The element oxygen (O) exists in air as a molecule (O_2) known as dioxygen or molecular oxygen. It was first isolated and characterized between 1772 and 1774 by the individual skills of the great European scientists Priestley, Lavoisier and Scheele. Dioxygen, hereafter referred to as oxygen, appeared in significant amounts on the surface of the Earth some 2.5×10^9 years ago, and geological evidence suggests that this was due to the photosynthetic activity of micro-organisms (blue-green algae). As they split water to obtain their essential requirement for hydrogen, blue-greens released tons of oxygen into the atmosphere, creating the worst case of environmental pollution ever recorded on this planet. The slow and steady rise in atmospheric oxygen concentration was accompanied by the formation of the ozone layer in the stratosphere. Both oxygen and the ozone layer acted as critical filters against the intense solar ultraviolet light reaching the surface of the Earth. Ascending in altitude from the Earth's atmosphere into outer space relatively heavy molecules such as O_2, N_2, H_2O give way to lighter molecules atoms and ions such as $H^{\bullet}$, H^+, $^{\bullet}OH$ and electrons, which are dominant above 800 km. The universe consists predominantly of hydrogen (H) and helium (He), with the Earth as a unique centre of oxidation in an otherwise reducing universe.

The percentage of oxygen in dry air is now around 21%, making it, after nitrogen (78%), the second most abundant element in the atmosphere. However, this amount of oxygen in the air is negligible when compared with that present as part of the water molecule in oceans, lakes and rivers, and that present as part of mineral reservoirs in the Earth's crust, where it is by far the most abundant element. When the Earth's atmosphere changed from a highly reducing state to the oxygen-rich state that we know today, anaerobic life forms ceased to exist or retreated to places where oxygen was excluded. The slow change from anaerobic to aerobic life necessitated the evolution of specialized antioxidants to protect against the toxic properties of oxygen. Aerobic life uses oxygen to oxidize (burn) carbon- and hydrogen-rich substrates (foods) to obtain the chemical energy and heat essential for life. Unfortunately, when we oxidize molecules with oxygen, the oxygen molecule itself becomes reduced and forms intermediates; two of which are free radicals (equations 1–4).

$$O_2 + e + H^+ \longrightarrow HO_2^{\bullet}$$
$$\text{(hydroperoxyl radical)} \tag{1}$$

$$HO_2^{\bullet} \xrightarrow{pH\,7.4} H^+ + O_2^- \text{ (superoxide radical)}$$
$$O_2^- + 2H^+ + e \longrightarrow H_2O_2$$
$$\text{(hydrogen peroxide)} \tag{2}$$

$$H_2O_2 + e \longrightarrow OH^- + {}^{\bullet}OH$$
$$\text{(hydroxyl radical);} \tag{3}$$

$${}^{\bullet}OH + e + H^+ \longrightarrow H_2O \tag{4}$$

Under normal conditions oxygen is a stable, odorless, tasteless and colorless gas of limited solubility in water – three volumes of gas dissolving in 100 volumes of water. This limited solubility is vital to aquatic life and essential for normal respiratory functions in man. The air dissolved in water contains a higher percentage of oxygen (34%, because nitrogen has a solubility around 2 volumes per 100 volumes) than does dry air (21%). Oxygen is considerably more soluble in organic solvents than it is in water. For example, the fat solvent chloroform ($CHCl_3$) at 10°C can dissolve up to 219.5 ml of oxygen per liter at one atmosphere, whereas under the same conditions water dissolves only 38.2 ml of oxygen. These differences in solubility are important when considering the availability of oxygen for chemical reactions inside biological membranes, which consist predominantly of lipids.

When compared with the other elements, oxygen has the third highest affinity for electrons and should be considerably more reactive than it is observed to be. The reason why its reactivity is masked involves the electronic structure of oxygen, and only when this is overcome can the 'true' reactivity of oxygen be expressed.

Oxidation = removal of electrons
Reduction = addition of electrons
Redox processes = electron exchange between reducing and oxidizing agents.

Chemical molecules of interest to biologists and chemists differ in their tendency to accept or donate electrons, and the voltage required to oppose this tendency in aqueous solution under defined conditions is known as the 'redox potential'.

When oxygen is reduced by the stepwise addition of electrons (equations 1–4), two free radicals ($HO_2^\bullet$, $^\bullet OH$) are formed, together with H_2O_2, which is not a free radical. At a physiological pH value of 7.4 the hydroperoxyl radical ($HO_2^\bullet$) with a pKa of 4.8 (the pH value at which equal concentrations of both

acid ($HO_2^\bullet$) and base (O_2^-) are present) dissociates to give the superoxide anion radical (O_2^-):

$$HO_2^\bullet \longrightarrow H^+ + O_2^- \qquad (5)$$

It is now considered unnecessary to show the unpaired electron (bold dot $\bullet$) on the superoxide anion radical ($O_2^{\bullet-}$) because it is less of a radical than molecular oxygen (which has two unpaired electrons but is never shown as $O_2^{\bullet\bullet}$). At this point, before going on to discuss free radicals, we need a simple definition of a free radical.

A free radical may be defined as any chemical species, capable of independent existence, that contains one or more unpaired electrons.

This definition is a broad biological one [25] which does not specify exactly where the unpaired electron is. It is preferred because it allows us to classify most of the transition metal ions as free radicals, and so better understand the close inter-relationship between oxygen and reactive metal ions.

OXYGEN AND ITS REDUCTION INTERMEDIATES

The superoxide anion

Superoxide (O_2^-) is a radical anion formed when one electron enters one of the π^*2p orbitals of oxygen. The chemistry of superoxide differs greatly depending on its solution environment. In aqueous solution O_2^- is a weak oxidizing agent able to oxidize molecules such as ascorbic acid and thiols. However, O_2^- is a much stronger reducing agent, and is able to reduce several iron complexes such as cytochrome c and ferric-ethylene diaminetetra-acetic acid (EDTA). Superoxide rapidly disappears in aqueous solution due to its dismutation reaction in which hydrogen peroxide and oxygen are formed:

$$O_2^- + O_2^- + 2H^+ \longrightarrow H_2O_2 + O_2 \qquad (6)$$

superoxide dismutase (SOD), discovered by McCord and Fridovich in 1968, greatly accelerates the above reaction [26]. Several different forms of the enzyme are known to exist in plant, microbial and mammalian cells, differing in structure and transition metal ions at their active centers but catalyzing exactly the same chemical reaction, shown in equation 6 [27]. The protonated form of O_2^-, the hydroperoxyl radical ($HO_2^\bullet$), is both a more powerful oxidant and reductant than O_2^-, but little $HO_2^\bullet$ will be present at a physiological pH (7.4).

Hydrogen peroxide

Any system producing superoxide will, as a result of the dismutation reaction, also produce H_2O_2. Many enzymes such as urate oxidase, glucose oxidase and D-amino acid oxidase produce H_2O_2 directly by the transfer of two electrons to oxygen. H_2O_2 is a weak oxidant and a weak reducing agent that is relatively stable in the absence of transition metal ions. The molecule has an uncharged covalent structure. It readily mixes with water, and is treated as a water molecule by the body, rapidly diffusing across cell membranes. The redox properties of H_2O_2 and its ability to form highly reactive free radicals in the presence of transition metal ions have necessitated the evolution of body defenses against it. Unwanted H_2O_2 is removed from cells by the action of enzymes such as catalase, glutathione peroxidase (selenium containing) and certain other peroxidases:

$$Catalase + 2H_2O_2 \longrightarrow O_2 + 2H_2O \qquad (7)$$

$$Peroxidase + H_2O_2 \longrightarrow$$
$$cofactor\ oxidation + H_2O + cofactor \qquad (8)$$

Hydroxyl radicals

The hydroxyl radical ($^\bullet OH$) is a major product arising from the high energy ionization of water (radiolysis):

$$H_2O \longrightarrow {}^\bullet OH + H^\bullet$$
$$+ e_{aq}^- + H_2O_2 + H_3O^+ \qquad (9)$$

Most of our definitive knowledge about the hydroxyl radical comes from studies by radiation chemists who, by convention, show the unpaired electron on the hydrogen atom, i.e. $OH^\bullet$. This is incorrect because the unpaired electron is on the oxygen atom. The $^\bullet OH$ radical is an extremely aggressive oxidant that can attack most biological molecules at an almost diffusion controlled rate. Three types of chemical reactions commonly occur with the $^\bullet OH$ radical:

1. hydrogen abstraction
2. aromatic hydroxylation
3. electron transfer.

Use is often made of these reactions for detecting biological damage caused by $^\bullet OH$ radicals.

Singlet oxygen

Singlet oxygen ($^1\Delta g\ O_2$) is not a free radical as it does not contain an unpaired electron. Nevertheless, it is a highly reactive form of oxygen in which the spin restriction of oxygen (two unpaired electrons with parallel spins) is removed, thereby increasing its oxidizing ability. In addition to $^1\Delta g\ O_2$, another form of singlet oxygen exists ($^1\Sigma g^+ O_2$). However, this state is extremely energetic and rapidly decays to the $^1\Delta g$ form in biological systems. Formation of singlet oxygen is extremely important when considering photochemical reactions.

Ozone

The pale blue gas ozone (O_3) provides an important protective shield (global antioxidant) in the stratosphere against solar radiation. At ground level, however, ozone is a toxic and unwanted pollutant. Ozone is produced in polluted urban air and by intensive light sources used in scientific equipment and some photocopying machines. It is extremely damaging to the lung, readily oxidizing proteins, DNA and lipids.

Oxides of nitrogen

Nitric oxide (NO) and nitrogen dioxide (NO_2) contain odd numbers of electrons, and are therefore free radicals, whereas nitrous oxide (N_2O) does not. Nitrogen dioxide is a dense brown poisonous gas, and a powerful oxidizing agent. Nitric oxide, on the other hand, is a colourless gas and a weak reducing agent, it was first recognized as a distinct gas by Joseph Priestley in 1772, who prepared an iron complex of it. Recently, biological interest in nitric oxide has centered around the observation that the vascular endothelium and other cells in the body produce small amounts of the gas from the amino acid L-arginine (reviewed in [28]). At present, nitric oxide is indistinguishable from the vasodilator, endothelium derived relaxing factor (EDRF). Nitric oxide has been shown to have protective effects, including the inhibition of lipid peroxidation [29]. Inhaled nitric oxide has been shown to inhibit neutrophil mediated oxygen radical dependent leak in isolated rat lungs [30] (Chapter 29). Nitric oxide can also react with another endogenous free radical, superoxide, to produce a reactive intermediate peroxynitrite ($ONOO^-$) [31,32]. Peroxynitrite is a powerful oxidant, able to damage many biological molecules, and is thought to decompose to release some hydroxyl radicals independent of metal catalysis [33] (equation 10). The chemistry of peroxynitrite has been recently reviewed [34]. Nitrous oxide is a colorless gas, with a sweetish odor and taste, that is used as an anesthetic ('laughing gas').

$$ONOO^- + H^+ \longrightarrow {}^\bullet OH + NO_2 \qquad (10)$$

TRANSITION METAL IONS AND FREE RADICAL FORMATION

When the Earth's atmosphere changed to an aerobic state, iron (the fourth most abundant element, present in the reduced ferrous (FeII) state) oxidized to the insoluble ferric state (FeIII). Poor solubility placed considerable restrictions upon its availability to early life forms, such as micro-organisms, that required iron as a catalyst for aerobic processes. To overcome the limited bioavailability of iron, micro-organisms adapted by synthesizing iron chelators (siderophores) that were able to chelate, solubilize and capture ferric ions, and internalize them by receptor recognition to provide the iron required. Today, microbial siderophores, such as desferrioxamine, are among some of the most effective iron chelators used to treat iron overload diseases. Hereafter, a close relationship evolved between oxygen and iron, and together with copper these metals form the major catalysts for aerobic metabolism often found at the active center of oxidases, oxygenases, antioxidants, electron transport and oxygen transport proteins.

Interaction of iron and oxygen to form reactive intermediates

During the 1890s the Cambridge chemist H.J.H. Fenton described a reaction between iron salts and hydrogen peroxide that caused oxidative damage to the organic molecule tartaric acid [35]. This reaction is known as the 'Fenton reaction' and is widely represented as follows:

$$Fe^{2+} + H_2O_2 \longrightarrow Fe^{3+} + OH^- + {}^\bullet OH \qquad (11)$$
$$Fe^{3+} + H_2O_2 \longrightarrow Fe^{2+} + HO_2^\bullet + H^+ \qquad (12)$$

overall reaction

$$\text{iron salt} + 2H_2O_2 \longrightarrow 2H_2O + O_2 \qquad (13)$$

Reactions 11 and 12 are gross oversimplifications of the chemistry involved, particularly when such reactions are considered in biological systems.

At physiological pH values (7.4), ferrous ions (FeII), in the presence of oxygen and phosphate ions (PO_4^{2-}), exist only transiently before auto-oxidizing to the ferric state (FeIII). In the process of changing from the ferrous to the ferric state an electron is transferred from iron to oxygen to make superoxide as, follows:

$$Fe^{2+} + O_2 \rightleftharpoons Fe^{2+}O_2 \longleftrightarrow Fe^{3+}O_2^-$$
$$\rightleftharpoons Fe^{3+} + O_2^- \qquad (14)$$

The intermediates $Fe^{2+}O_2$ and $Fe^{3+}O_2^-$ are known as the perferryl ion.

Discovery of the SOD enzymes [26] changed biological thinking concerning oxygen radicals, previously considered the domain of radiation chemists. It is not surprising, therefore, that many theoretical aspects of radiation chemistry were transferred into biological Fenton chemistry without careful consideration of the full implications. One such example is the protection afforded by 'hydroxyl radical scavengers'. Hydroxyl radical scavengers are usually low molecular mass chemicals with known second order rate constants for reaction with the hydroxyl radical that are determined by competition kinetics using techniques such as pulse radiolysis [36].

The homolysis (radiolysis) of water produces a variety of products, a major species being the hydroxyl radical ($^\bullet OH$):

$$H_2O \longrightarrow e^-_{aq} + H^\bullet + H_3O^+$$
$$+ \ ^\bullet OH + H_2O_2 \qquad (9)$$

$$H^\bullet + O_2 \longrightarrow H^+ + O_2^- \qquad (15)$$

$$e^-_{aq} + O_2 \longrightarrow O_2^- \qquad (16)$$

The hydroxyl radical produced by X-or γ irradiation of water is formed free in solution, and can react with any added chemical at a rate calculated in moles per second (mol/s) as its second order rate constant. Most of the 'scavengers' used in radiation chemistry react at high rates with $^\bullet OH$ ($1 - 6 \times 10^9$ mol/s). The ability to protect a selected detector molecule from damage by $^\bullet OH$ will be a function of concentration present and the second order rate constant. Do these considerations still hold true for $^\bullet OH$ radicals formed in Fenton chemistry?

The answer is 'no' because biological Fenton chemistry is dependent upon iron ions, which in the ferric form are insoluble and unreactive at physiological pH. Biological systems overcome the problem of iron solubility by binding iron ions to a ligand. If the bound iron still remains redox active, any $^\bullet OH$ radicals generated by its participation in Fenton chemistry will be site directed to the ligand holding the iron. Iron therefore determines which biological molecules will receive $^\bullet OH$ radical damage, and this tends to overrule predictions for scavengers based on rate constants and concentrations present.

The administration of hydroxyl radical scavengers to animals or humans is therefore unlikely to achieve simple competitive scavenging because, in most cases, insufficient scavenger will enter cells to compete with fast site specific chemistry. Many hydroxyl radical scavengers will, of course, have a multitude of pharmacological properties in their own right, which may explain why some remarkable responses have been reported. Even in simple test tube 'Fenton' experiments we do not see hydroxyl radical scavengers behaving as predicted from their concentrations and second order rate constants. To explain these discrepancies, others have suggested that the oxidizing species formed during Fenton chemistry is not the $^\bullet OH$ radical but an oxo-iron species, such as the ferryl ion (FeO^{2+}) [37,38], in which iron has an oxidation number of IV. So far, the ferryl ion has not been chemically or spectroscopically identified outside a heme ring and, although it is expected to have considerable oxidizing power, its 'footprints' of attack on scavengers, or more complex biological molecules such as DNA, do not support the view that it is an absolute alternative to the $^\bullet OH$ radical (reviewed in [15]).

It seems more likely that the ferryl ion is often formed as an intermediate in Fenton chemistry, leading to $^\bullet OH$:

$$Fe^{2+} + H_2O_2 \longrightarrow FeO^{2+} \longrightarrow {}^{\bullet}OH \qquad (17)$$

and that its reaction with detector molecules or added scavengers will depend upon the experimental conditions used.

How does Fenton chemistry occur in vivo?

Superoxide is produced continuously in the body during aerobic metabolism, and by the dismutation reaction will form H_2O_2 both in the presence or absence of the SOD enzymes. When O_2^- and H_2O_2 are produced in quantities that exceed the ability of protective enzymes, such as SOD catalase and glutathione peroxidase, to remove them, they can facilitate the release of iron from iron-containing proteins. Redox active iron + O_2^- + H_2O_2 make hydroxyl radicals, thus the excessive production of O_2^- can provide all the necessary ingredients for Fenton chemistry to take place (reviewed in [39]).

If SODs only make H_2O_2 why do we need them?

Superoxide dismutase deficient bacterial mutants have confirmed that SOD is essential for aerobic life. The poor reactivity of O_2^- has led to the identification of only a few examples, in plant and microbial systems, which suggest a direct toxic effect of O_2^-. Yet we know that the generation of O_2^- in biological systems can lead to extensive molecular damage, and protection can be afforded by SOD. The only plausible explanation we have at present, is that the SODs protect by preventing the O_2^- dependent reduction of redox active iron complexes (i.e. SODs are anti-reductants). Our knowledge of the redox active iron complexes present in biological systems is still, however, sadly lacking [40].

As previously mentioned, superoxide can react with another endogenous free radical, NO, to form peroxynitrite. Superoxide dismutase prevents this reaction and the subsequent formation of damaging ONOO$^-$ and

$^{\bullet}$OH, as well as prolonging the biological activity of NO.

Iron containing proteins as free radical catalysts

Several claims have been made that iron storage, transport and functional proteins are Fenton catalysts (reviewed in [41]). Under normal physiological conditions, however, this is extremely unlikely. Iron correctly loaded into transferrin, lactoferrin and into the core of ferritin do not facilitate Fenton chemistry. A small amount of labile iron associated with ferritin, but not at its ferric core, is often available (depending on the preparation of the sample) to participate in Fenton chemistry. Similarly, iron in the plasma of patients with hemochromatosis, and in the synovial fluid of patients with rheumatoid arthritis, appears to be more labile under conditions of pH, or oxidant stress, than that present in normal control patients [42]. This iron can be detected by using the ability of bleomycin to degrade DNA in the presence of the iron that it chelates from the biological sample. Heme proteins have been observed to stimulate Fenton chemistry because that iron leaves the heme protein and not the $^{\bullet}$OH radical [43]. Incubation of heme proteins with H_2O_2 causes the release of chelatable iron that is available for Fenton chemistry [43].

Copper as a biological free radical catalyst

Copper is a trace element in the Earth's crust, and some 60 times less abundant than iron in the human body. Copper salts are usually more reactive than iron in oxygen radical reactions, but bioavailability and avid protein binding often mask this increased reactivity. Absorption of dietary copper takes place in the stomach, or upper small intestine, from whence it is transported to the liver as an albumin complex – human albumin having one high affinity binding site for copper. The liver incorporates most of the copper into the plasma protein ceruloplasmin, said to show sequence homology with lactoferrin and coagulation factor V. Ceruloplasmin has a molecular mass of around 130 000, and contains some six or seven copper ions per mole of protein. Its biological function has been considered mainly as an acute phase protein. Proteins showing an increase in plasma concentration after trauma or in the acute phase of an inflammatory response are often called acute phase reactants. The acute phase proteins have been defined as those plasma proteins which increase in concentration by 25% or more in the first 7 days following tissue damage. Acute phase proteins are synthesized by the liver and induced by cytokines derived from the inflammatory focus. The purpose of the acute phase response appears to be the activation of a protective screen against further tissue injury caused by the release of proteolytic enzymes and biological pro-oxidants from damaged cells. Ceruloplasmin's ferroxidase activity has been proposed as such a protective defense [44,45] against oxidative damage.

Ceruloplasmin does not donate or specifically bind copper ions while in the circulation; however, it is able to enter cells and release copper for the synthesis of copper-containing proteins, undergoing proteolytic degradation in the process. Total plasma copper levels are essentially a measure of ceruloplasmin, although many established texts report that up to 10% of plasma copper is labile and bound to amino acids. Using a molecular recognition assay similar to that of the bleomycin assay but specific for copper (based on 1, 10-phenanthroline), we have been unable to detect labile copper in freshly taken normal human plasma [46]. Whenever plasma is stored or mishandled, however, labile copper readily appears due to rapid proteolytic degradation of ceruloplasmin. Copper released from ceruloplasmin in this way causes the peroxidation of plasma lipoproteins. The resulting oxidized lipid–protein–copper complex has a ferroxidase

activity (ferroxidase II) similar to that of ceruloplasmin (ferroxidase I) but not inhibited by azide. The potential for artifacts when studying plasma copper biochemistry are enormous (reviewed in [47]).

When copper ions are nonspecifically attached to amino acids and proteins they can usually redox cycle to generate oxygen radicals. However, many of these radicals may not be seen by an added 'detector' molecule because the reaction is so highly site specific, to the copper binding molecule.

CHANGES IN PLASMA IRON CHEMISTRY

IRON DISTRIBUTION IN THE BODY

The body of an average adult human male contains some 4.5 g iron, absorbs about 1 mg iron per day, and when in iron balance excretes the same amount. Only slight disturbances to the delicate balance between iron intake and iron loss can push the body into conditions of iron overload or iron deficiency. It has been estimated that in the world today some 500 million people are iron deficient and several millions are iron overloaded. No specific mechanisms exist for iron excretion, loss occurring by the turnover of intestinal epithelial cells, in sweat, feces, urine and by menstrual bleeding in women.

Most of the body's iron (some two thirds) is found in the oxygen carrying protein hemoglobin, with smaller amounts present in myoglobin, various enzymes, the iron transport proteins transferrin and lactoferrin, and the iron storage proteins ferritin and hemosiderin. Transferrin binds, with high affinity ($Ka = 10^{28}$), two moles of iron per mole of protein and is normally only one third loaded with iron, retaining a considerable metal binding capacity. Metals other than iron, such as aluminum, can bind to transferrin and enter cells via the transferrin receptor. Lactoferrin shares many similarities with transferrin, but is immunologically distinct and can hold on to bound iron down to pH values of 4.0.

The iron storage protein ferritin consists of a protein shell surrounding a core of ferric ions, and when fully loaded contains some 4500 iron ions per mole of protein. Iron enters ferritin in the reduced ferrous state and is laid down in the core by a process of oxidation involving the 'ferroxidase' activity of the protein, and the growth of ferric oxide crystal. For iron to leave the core it has to be reductively mobilized back to the ferrous state, either by the entry of a reductant to the ferritin core or by long range electron transfer through the coat of ferritin. Hemosiderin is an insoluble iron – protein complex that probably arises as a lysosomal degradation product of ferritin, although similar conversions can be made by subjecting ferritin to free radical oxidations (48).

Most of our dietary intake of iron is in the form of nonheme ferric ion. This requires reduction and solubilization before absorption from the intestine can occur. Gastric hydrochloric acid and ascorbate (vitamin C) facilitate absorption in this way. Dietary heme iron is mostly derived from red meat products, and can be directly absorbed by the intestine. Only a small, and carefully controlled, fraction of the total iron ingested is absorbed and allowed to enter the circulation bound to transferrin. Cells requiring iron for essential aerobic processes have transferrin receptors which allow uptake of iron into the cell. Once inside the cell reductive release of iron from transferrin occurs, allowing the apotransferrin molecule (devoid of iron) to return to the circulation to continue iron transport functions.

TRANSFERRIN CHANGES

Transferrin is a β-globulin, with a relative molecular mass of around 76 000, which has the essential function of binding and transporting mononuclear iron in the body. It is often loosely referred to as an 'acute phase protein' but, like albumin, often shows a decrease following trauma.

Recent studies in patients with ARDS have shown that transferrin levels are low in plasma but high in BAL fluids when compared with normal healthy control subjects (Tables 11.1 and 11.8). When patients with ARDS who show evidence of multiorgan failure are compared with those who do not, the multiorgan failure group show evidence of impaired liver function (mean bilirubin value 121 ± 43 µmol/l), transient iron overload, and significantly lower transferrin levels (0.82 ± 0.13 g/l) (Table 11.1).

PLASMA IRON AND TRANSFERRIN IRON SATURATION

The iron transport protein transferrin is normally only one third loaded with iron and

Table 11.1 Plasma transferrin values reported in patients with ARDS

Patient group studied (n)	Transferrin (g/l)	Transferrin as % of total proteins	References
Normal healthy controls (10)	2.91±0.12	3.48±0.23	49
Normal healthy controls (19)	2.63±0.17[a]	3.51±0.10	50
ARDS: no evidence of multiorgan failure (10) sequential sampling; 99 samples (group A)	1.76±0.13	2.91±0.12	49
ARDS: multiorgan failure with transient iron overload (5) sequential sampling; 13 samples (group B)	0.82±0.13	1.62±0.25	51
ARDS: random sampling of patients (14)	1.14±0.13	2.5±0.20	50

[a] Calculated from the authors' data using a Mr for transferrin of 76 500.

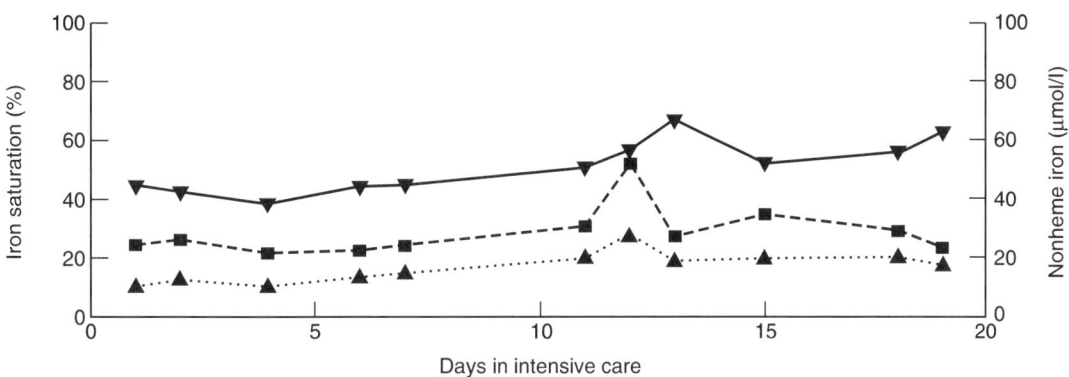

Figure 11.1 Changes in plasma iron chemistry of a patient with ARDS during intensive care. (▼) Total iron-binding capacity (μmol/1); (▲ total nonheme iron; (■) % saturation of transferrin.

retains a considerable iron binding capacity (see next section). When the iron binding capacity of transferrin is saturated, low molecular mass iron can be detected in the plasma using the bleomycin assay (52). Bleomycin detectable iron has been demonstrated in the plasma of patients with iron overload conditions, such as idiopathic hemochromatosis (53), leukemic patients on chemotherapy (54), in the plasma of neonates (55, 56) and in cardiopulmonary bypass patients (57). Two groups of patients with ARDS have been investigated for abnormalities in their plasma iron: group A patients had no evidence of multiorgan failure; group B patients showed transient iron overload with the presence of bleomycin detectable iron in at least one of their plasma samples (51). All patients in the second group had evidence of impaired liver function, and often multiorgan failure. Group A patients showed an increased percentage iron saturation of their transferrin (Table 11.1) compared with normal healthy controls, but none had bleomycin detectable iron present, as would be expected from their high plasma iron binding capacities.

Of considerable importance when interpreting chemical data in plasma from patients with ARDS are the large day to day variations that occur. These are illustrated in Figure 11.1, which shows daily changes in plasma iron

concentration and the percentage saturation of transferrin of a patient during intensive care. Biochemical studies on patients with ARDS using single time point sampling could introduce large errors, and may account for some of the inconsistencies reported in the literature.

The patients from group B with liver damage had bleomycin detectable iron (1.20 ± 0.60 μmol/l) in six of 13 samples analyzed, suggesting that transient iron overload had occurred. This finding was confirmed by the high percentage saturation of the low levels of transferrin present. Survival within this group was low (20%) compared with group A (60%). A pilot study to determine the presence or absence of bleomycin chelatable iron in BAL fluid taken from patients with lung injury has been carried out in our laboratory, and this indicates that low micromolar concentrations of chelatable iron are often present in some fluids.

Nontransferrin bound low molecular mass iron is a pro-oxidant form of iron that imposes additional oxidative stress on biological systems. The finding [51] that such iron can transiently appear in the plasma of some patients with ARDS already under considerable oxidative stress is of considerable interest for future antioxidant intervention therapies with chelator regimens.

ANTIOXIDANT DEFICIENCIES

INTRODUCTION TO BIOLOGICAL ANTIOXIDANTS

The term 'antioxidant' is frequently used in the biomedical literature, but rarely is it defined, with a strong implication that it refers to chemicals with chain breaking properties such as vitamin E (α-tocopherol) and vitamin C (ascorbic acid). The authors [25] take a much broader view than this and define an antioxidant as:

> Any substance, when present at low concentrations compared with those of the oxidizable substrate, that significantly delays, or inhibits, oxidation of that substrate.

Antioxidants can act at several different stages in an oxidative sequence, and we can illustrate this by considering lipid peroxidation in cell membranes or food products. Antioxidants can act by:

1. removing O_2 or decreasing local O_2 concentrations;
2. removing catalytic metal ions;
3. removing key reactive oxygen species (ROS) such as O_2^- and H_2O_2;
4. scavenging initiating radicals such as $^\bullet OH$, $RO^\bullet$, $RO_2^\bullet$;
5. breaking the chain of an initiated sequence;
6. quenching or scavenging singlet oxygen.

Antioxidants inhibiting lipid peroxidation by mechanisms (1), (2), (4) and (6) can be called 'preventative' antioxidants. Those acting by mechanism (3) are also preventative but as they are enzymes (e.g. catalase, SOD and glutathione peroxidase) they are not consumed by the reaction. Chain breaking antioxidants (5), singlet oxygen quenchers (6) and metal chelators (2) will be consumed while carrying out their protective functions. Many antioxidants have more than one mechanism of action. Propylgallate, for example, a partially water soluble phenolic antioxidant used by the food industry, is a chain breaking

antioxidant, a powerful scavenger of $^\bullet OH$ radicals and an iron binding agent.

It has been known for a long time that when two different antioxidants are present at the same time they can protect against oxidation far better than each can individually. This phenomenon is known as 'antioxidant synergism'.

PROTECTION OF CELLS AGAINST OXIDATIVE DAMAGE

Cells have a formidable armamentarium of defenses against oxidative damage, many of which may not readily be recognized as antioxidants.

Antioxidant protection can operate at several different levels within cells, for example by:

1. preventing radical formation;
2. intercepting formed radicals;
3. repairing oxidative damage;
4. increasing elimination of damaged molecules;
5. nonrepair recognition of excessively damaged molecules in order to prevent mutations occurring;
6. gene regulated oxidative stress proteins.

Oxygen metabolism occurs within cells, and it is here we expect to find antioxidants evolved to deal speedily and specifically with reduced intermediates of oxygen (Table 11.2). Enzymes such as the SODs rapidly promote the dismutation of superoxide into hydrogen peroxide and oxygen at a rate considerably faster than it occurs uncatalyzed:

$$2O_2^- + 2H^+ \xrightarrow{\text{SOD}} H_2O_2 + O_2 \tag{6}$$

Hydrogen peroxide, a product of the dismutation reaction, can be destroyed by two different enzymes, namely catalase (equation 7) and glutathione peroxidase (GSHPx selenium containing enzyme) (equation 8).

$$2H_2O_2 \xrightarrow{\text{catalase}} O_2 + 2H_2O \tag{7}$$

$$H_2O_2 \xrightarrow[\text{GSHPx}]{\text{GSH}} GSSG + 2H_2O \tag{8}$$

Table 11.2 Intracellular antioxidants

Antioxidant	Function/activity
Superoxide dismutases (Cu,Zn,Mn)	Removes O_2^- (catalytically)
Catalase (contains 4 NADPH molecules) (Fe)	Removes H_2O_2 when present in high concentrations
Gluthatione peroxidase (Se)	Removes H_2O_2 when present at low steady state levels. Can remove organic hydroperoxides
Prevention of O_2^-, H_2O_2, $\cdot$OH formation by cytochrome oxidase (Cu)	No release of active oxygens during the reduction of O_2 to H_2O

Table 11.3 Membrane antioxidants

Antioxidant	Function/activity
Vitamin E	Lipid soluble, chain breaking antioxidant
β-Carotene	Lipid soluble radical scavenger and singlet oxygen quencher
Co-enzyme Q	May act as an antioxidant in addition to its major role in energy metabolism
Membrane structural organization	Phospholipid: cholesterol. Types of phospholipids and fatty acids important for memnbrane integrity

During normal aerobic metabolism these enzymes function in concert within the cell to eliminate toxic reduction intermediates of oxygen, thereby allowing a small, low molecular mass iron to safely exist for DNA synthesis and the manufacture of iron containing proteins.

Prevention of radical formation inside cells is an obvious mechanism that must have evolved to restrict oxygen toxicity. A good example of this is cytochrome oxidase, the terminal oxidase of the mitochondrial electron transport chain, which does not release reactive oxygen intermediates from its active center while functioning catalytically.

PROTECTION OF MEMBRANES AGAINST OXIDATIVE DAMAGE

Within the hydrophobic lipid interior of membranes different types of lipophilic radicals are formed from those seen in the intracellular aqueous milieu. Lipophilic radicals require different types of antioxidants for their removal (Table 11.3). Vitamin E (α-tocopherol), a fat soluble vitamin, is a poor antioxidant outside a membrane bilayer but is extremely effective when incorporated into the membrane. If vitamin E is extracted from its association with plasma lipoproteins and tested *in vitro* for its ability to scavenge peroxyl radicals ($RO_2^{\bullet}$), it appears as the most important lipophilic chain breaking antioxidant of human plasma. However, caution should be exercised when asking what the 'most important' biological antioxidant is, because the answer will vary and depend on which pro-oxidant was used to drive radical production. The body appears to have several mechanism to 'spare' vitamin E consumption. It can regenerate oxidized forms using enzymes, as well as use nonenzymic reduction with molecules such as vitamin C.

An important part of membrane stability and protection is the way in which the membrane is assembled from its lipid components. Structural organization requires that the 'correct' ratios of phospholipids to cholesterol are present, and that the 'correct' types of phospholipids and their fatty acids are attached (reviewed in [39]).

PROTECTION IN EXTRACELLULAR FLUIDS AGAINST OXIDATIVE DAMAGE

Body extracellular fluids contain little, or no, catalase activity, and extremely low levels of SOD. Glutathione peroxidases, in both selenium containing and nonselenium containing forms, are present in plasma but there is little glutathione (GSH) in plasma (< 1 µmol) to satisfy an enzyme with a Km for GSH in the millimolar range. 'Extracellular' superoxide dismutases (EC-SODs) have recently been identified and shown to contain copper and attached carbohydrate groups (glycosylated) [58]. The EC-SOD enzymes bind to heparin *in vitro*, which has led to the proposal that they may occupy heparin binding sites on the endothelial cell surface and thereby form a first line of cellular defense [58]. By allowing the limited survival of O_2^- and H_2O_2 in extracellular fluids the body can utilize these molecules, and others such as nitric oxide (NO), as useful messenger, signal or trigger molecules [59,60]. A key feature of such a proposal is that O_2^- and H_2O_2 do not meet with reactive iron or copper, and that extracellular antioxidant protection has evolved to keep iron and copper in poorly reactive or nonreactive forms [47,59,61].

The iron transport protein transferrin is normally one third loaded with iron and keeps the concentration of 'free' iron in plasma at effectively nil. Iron bound to transferrin will not participate in radical reactions, and the available iron binding capacity gives it a powerful antioxidant property towards iron stimulated radical reactions [61]. Similar considerations apply to lactoferrin [61] which, like transferrin, can bind two moles of iron per mole of protein, but hold on to its iron down to pH values as low as 4.0. Hemoglobin, myoglobin and heme compounds can accelerate lipid peroxidation by at least two different mechanisms: the heme ring can react with peroxides to form active oxo-iron species, such as perferryl (iron oxidation state V) and ferryl (IV) [62]; and a molar excess of

peroxide can cause fragmentation of the cyclic tetrapyrrol rings, releasing chelatable iron [43]. Plasma also contains proteins such as haptoglobins and hemopexin specifically to bind and conserve hemoglobin and heme iron respectively. Binding to these proteins greatly diminishes the ability of heme proteins to accelerate lipid peroxidation [63,64].

The major copper-containing protein of human plasma is ceruloplasmin, unique for its intense azure coloration. Apart from its known acute phase reactant properties, its biological functions have remained an enigma. Proposals that it plays a major role in iron metabolism as a ferroxidase enzyme (catalyzing the oxidation of ferrous ions to the ferric state for binding to transferrin) has not been widely accepted (reviewed in [47]). However, the authors and their colleagues [44,45,47] have pointed out that the protein's ferroxidase activity makes a major contribution to extracellular antioxidant protection against iron driven lipid peroxidation and Fenton chemistry. Ceruloplasmin (Cu^{2+}-Cp) rapidly removes ferrous ions from solution and simultaneously reduces oxygen to water (equations 18 and 19), with the transfer of four electrons at the enzyme's active center:

$$Fe^{2+} + Cu^{2+}\text{-}Cp \longrightarrow Cu^+\text{-}Cp + Fe^{3+} \quad (18)$$

$$4\,Cu^+\text{-}Cp + O_2 + 4\,H^+ \longrightarrow 4\,Cu^{2+}\text{-}Cp \\ + 2H_2O \quad (19)$$

This is another example of antioxidant protection by nonrelease of reactive forms of oxygen into the aqueous milieu, as would occur if the oxidation of ferrous ions were not catalyzed by ceruloplasmin [47]. Ceruloplasmin has been shown to react stoichiometrically with both O_2^- and H_2O_2 [65,66], although it does not have catalytic SOD and peroxidase activities, as often claimed.

Plasma contains a variety of redox activity low molecular mass molecules, and many of these have been ascribed primary antioxidant roles [67,68]. Thus, using iron independent generation of peroxyl radicals from an azo

Table 11.4 Extracellular antioxidants

Antioxidant	Function/activity
Transferrin	Binds ferric ions (2 per mole of protein)
Lactoferrin	Binds ferric ions at lower pH (2 per mole of protein)
Haptoglobins	Binds hemoglobin
Hemopexin	Binds heme
Albumin	Binds copper, heme, and scavenges HOCl
Ceruloplasmin	Ferroxidase activity – stoichiometric O_2^- scavenging binds copper ions (nonspecific), utilizes H_2O_2 for reoxidation of coppers
EC-SOD	Removes O_2^- catalytically
EC-GSHpase	Removes H_2O_2 and hydroperoxides catalytically; little GSH available in plasma (1–2 µmol/l)
Protein thiols/GSH	Total thiols around 500 µmol/l
Bilirubin	Scavenges peroxyl radicals (< 0.09 µmol/l)
Mucus	Scavenges ·OH radicals
Urate	Radical scavenger and metal binder (0.08 µmol/l)
Glucose	·OH radical scavenger (4–6 mmol/l)
Ascorbic acid	·OH radical scavenger (0.03 µmol/l)

Lipoprotein antioxidants
  Vitamin E
  β-Carotene
  Retinyl stearate
  Lycopene	

Red blood cells	Diffusion of H_2O_2 into the cell and passage of O_2^- through the anion channel (RBCs contain catalase and SOD)

Values in parentheses are normal plasma concentration.

initiator, these authors have found vitamin E, uric acid, bilirubin and ascorbic acid to be important plasma antioxidants. Plasma contains numerous lipid particles, the lipoproteins, which carry lipids such as phospholipids, cholesterol esters, cholesterol and triglycerides around the body. The major lipoproteins are low density lipoproteins (LDL), high density lipoproteins (HDL), very low density lipoproteins (VLDL) and chylomicrons. Classification has historically been based on physical properties, such as charge, density or particle size. The lipid portion of isolated lipoproteins is prone to oxidize when the natural antioxidants that are associated with it, such as vitamin E, α-carotene, lycopene and retinyl stearate, are consumed [69]. There are suggestions that a similar process occurs *in vivo* and contributes to the development of atheromatous plaque (reviewed in [70]).

When serum or plasma samples are stored or mishandled, proteolytic enzymes present in plasma degrade ceruloplasmin, releasing copper-containing fragments that cause the peroxidation of lipoproteins [71]. The copper–peroxidized lipoprotein complex possesses a ferroxidase-like activity (ferroxidase II) similar to that of ceruloplasmin except that it is not inhibited by azide [72]. Normal, freshly taken human plasma does not, however, contain ferroxidase II activity.

Table 11.4 shows iron- and copper-inactivating protein as well as low molecular mass scavengers for oxygen radicals which can be described as plasma antioxidants.

PLASMA ANTIOXIDANT CHANGES IN ARDS

In the preceding discussions of this section we defined and classified plasma antioxidants by their biological sites of action and their specialized functions. Here we discuss antioxidant changes that have been reported to occur in the plasma of patients with ARDS.

Iron binding antioxidant activities

Compared with normal healthy control subjects, patients with ARDS (without multiorgan failure) show decreased levels of plasma iron binding antioxidant activity (Table 11.5). Decreased protection was seen in three different assay systems generating different radical species [49]. The decreased ability of ARDS plasma to protect against iron

stimulated oxygen radical formation correlates with the percentage iron saturation of the transferrin (Table 11.6). Large day to day variations in the iron saturation of transferrin were observed, suggesting episodes of iron release during treatment (Figure 11.1). A small group of patients with ARDS, showing impaired liver function as part of their wider multiorgan failure, had low molecular mass iron present in their plasma (p. 177) and a high iron saturation of their transferrin. In these patients antioxidant protection was greatly reduced, or even lost (Table 11.5).

Table 11.5 Plasma iron binding antioxidant changes in patients with ARDS: radicals formed and detector molecules damaged

Patient group (n)	Lipid radicals Phospholipids (% inhibition)	Hydroxyl radicals Deoxyribose (% inhibition)	Oxo-iron species DNA (% inhibition)	References
Normal healthy controls (12)	86.4±1.14	96.0±0.57	61.3±1.53	49
ARDS (10): without multiorgan failure; sequential study, 99 samples	65.6±3.83	87.1±2.93	46.5±2.94	49
ARDS (5): multiorgan failure and transient iron-overload; sequential study, 13 samples	27	–	2.61(S)	51

S = Stimulation of radical damage.

Table 11.6 Plasma iron and transferrin iron saturation values reported in patients with ARDS

Patients studied (n)	Total nonheme iron (μmol/l)	% Saturation of transferrin	Chelatable low Mr iron (μmol/l)	Unsaturated iron-binding capacity (UIBC) (μmol/l)	References
Normal controls (10)	15.7±6.05	25.6±8.8	0	61.2	49
ARDS (10): without multiorgan failure; sequential sampling, 99 samples	14.9±2.13	33.9±3.8	0	30.3	49
ARDS (5): with transient iron-overload and multiorgan failure; sequential sampling, 13 samples	18.6±4.30	71.0±6.89	1.20±0.60	7.4	51
ARDS (14): random sampling of patients	11.9[a]	41%[a]	Not tested	17.1±7.1 (6)	50

[a] Values calculated from published data of these authors, which reported UIBC, and transferrin levels (50). Normal control values were as published or calculated from the authors' data, i.e. total nonheme iron 30.7 μmol/l, % saturation of transferrin 45% and UIBC 38.1±6.9 (50) (7 patients).

Iron oxidizing antioxidant activities

Ceruloplasmin is the main copper-containing protein of human plasma. It has an iron oxidizing activity (ferroxidase) which is considered an important biological primary antioxidant function for the protein (p. 181). As an acute phase protein, concentrations of ceruloplasmin will increase in the plasma following tissue trauma. In animal models serum ceruloplasmin has also been observed to increase after exposure to hyperoxia by a mechanism independent of the acute phase response [73].

In two recent studies plasma ceruloplasmin levels were reported as raised [49] and as normal [50] when compared with healthy controls. The latter finding is surprising in view of the known response of ceruloplasmin to trauma and hyperoxia. The iron oxidizing antioxidant activity of ARDS plasma in the first study was, however, similar to that of normal control plasma, in spite of the measured higher ceruloplasmin protein levels present (Table 11.7). The reason for this remains unclear but may suggest that some of the ceruloplasmin present in plasma is not fully functional as a ferroxidase [49]. Ceruloplasmin is particularly susceptible to proteolytic damage and increased proteolytic activity in ARDS plasma or lung tissue, where it is also synthesized [74], may contribute to the apparent loss of activity. Typical changes in plasma ceruloplasmin levels in a patient with ARDS, and its relationship to iron oxidizing antioxidant activity, are shown in Figure 11.2.

Scavenging antioxidant activities

Numerous nonspecific low molecular mass molecules present in plasma have been ascribed biological antioxidant properties. These include glucose, uric acid, bilirubin, ascorbic acid, vitamin E and thiols (reviewed in [49]). In addition, plasma also contains low concentrations of specific high molecular mass scavengers, such as EC-SOD, EC-glutathione peroxidase and catalase (p. 180).

Plasma thiols

Plasma from normal healthy controls contains around 500 μmol/l of thiols mainly associated with the sulphydryl groups of plasma proteins. Plasma thiol values are lower in ARDS patients (around 300 μmol/l) [10] and even lower than this when expressed for nonsurviving members of the ARDS group [10]. Interestingly, nonsurvivors have higher levels of plasma proteins compared with the surviving ARDS group. When plasma from ARDS patients is tested in an antioxidant assay system, which measures only radical scavenging (iron binding and iron oxidizing activities have been removed) it shows lower activity than normal controls [49].

The lung is a primary target for oxidant injury and damage to lung tissue leads to loss of sulfydryl groups of both protein and non-

Table 11.7 Plasma iron oxidizing antioxidant changes in patients with ARDS: Radicals formed and detector molecules damaged

Patient group (n)	Lipid radicals Phospholipids (% inhibition)	Hydroxyl radicals Deoxyribose (% inhibition)	Oxo-iron species DNA (% inhibition)	References
Normal healthy controls (12) Ceruloplasmin 0.26±0.03 g/l	64.0±2.9	73.8±1.3	27.9±1.4	49
ARDS (10): without multiorgan failure; sequential study, 99 samples Ceruloplasmin 0.38±0.04 g/l	64.0±3.1	69.5±2.6	19.7±2.8	49

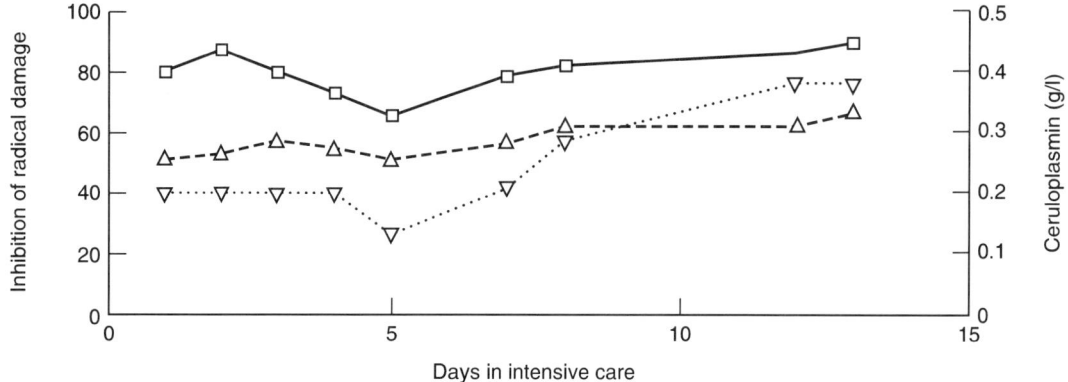

Figure 11.2 Changes in plasma iron oxidizing antioxidant properties. ($\triangle$) Protection against organic oxygen radicals (% inhibition); ($\square$) protection against inorganic oxygen radicals (% inhibition); (∇) ceruloplasmin levels (g/l).

protein molecules (reviewed in [75]). Thiol groups are particularly susceptible to oxidation and can be destroyed by biological oxidants such as hydrogen peroxide, peroxynitrite, iron salts, and peroxyl and hydroxyl radicals. Patients with ARDS have depleted levels of plasma, and red blood cell, GSH (nonprotein thiol) [76]. The antioxidant properties of the drug N-acetylcysteine [77], together with the observed depletion of thiols in ARDS patients, have led to clinical trials designed to replace or protect vital thiol groups with this drug. Clinical trials so far, however, have not demonstrated that thiol supplementation is of great benefit to patients with ARDS [78] but it may yet be shown that subgroups within the ARDS population would benefit from thiol supplementation, whereas others would not.

Ascorbate acid (vitamin C)

Using fresh single plasma samples randomly selected from eight patients with ARDS, Cross *et al.* [8] found extremely low levels of ascorbate, ranging from < 1 to 5 μmol/l, compared with 49 ± 1 μmol/l in normal healthy controls. The authors interpreted these findings as evidence of increased oxidative stress *in vivo* and suggested that the

low plasma ascorbate levels reflect increased neutrophil activity.

α-Tocopherol (vitamin E)

α-Tocopherol is carried in plasma by lipoproteins; for example, in LDL there are around six molecules of α-tocopherol for each LDL particle. α-Tocopherol is a fat soluble antioxidant (p. 180) that offers little protection to the surrounding aqueous milieu [79]. In three separate studies, plasma α-tocopherol levels have been reported to be low in patients with ARDS, with values of 7.73 ± 0.54 mg/l (*n* = 12) [9], 10.4 ± 3.5 mg/l (*n* = 25) [80] and 4.0 mg/l (*n* = 6) [81], compared with normal healthy control values of 11.46 ± 0.55 mg/l (*n* = 7), 14.9 ± 2.5 mg/l (*n* = 16) and 11.2 mg/l (*n* = 7) respectively. In a follow up study, Cross *et al.* [8] concluded that α-tocopherol was not significantly lower in patients with ARDS when standardized to the total plasma cholesterol present. Further studies are required to resolve these reported differences.

Extracellular antioxidant enzymes

Hydrogen peroxide levels are increased in breath condensates of patients with ARDS receiving mechanical ventilation [6,7], supporting the proposal that neutrophils play a major role in the oxidant stress seen in this syndrome. However, only low or undetectable amounts of H_2O_2 are found in plasma extracts from patients with ARDS [80]. When H_2O_2 destroying enzymes, such as catalase and glutathione peroxidases, were measured in the serum of septic patients with ARDS and appropriate controls, the ARDS group had higher catalase activity [82], which may explain the undetectable levels of H_2O_2 in ARDS plasma. Interestingly, there was no evidence to support red blood cell hemolysis as the origin of the increased serum catalase. Extending these studies to include serum manganese-containing superoxide dismutase (Mn-SOD), these researchers assessed enzyme levels and other protein makers as predictors for patients with sepsis who were most likely to develop ARDS [83]. Of 26 patients with sepsis, six who developed ARDS had higher serum levels of MnSOD and catalase activity [83].

BAL FLUID ANTIOXIDANT CHANGES

Lung epithelial lining fluid (LELF) is a thin layer of plasma ultrafiltrate, and locally secreted molecules, that covers the lower respiratory tract epithelium and forms the first barrier to oxidant stress from ambient air. LELF contains a variety of plasma proteins, several of which have been ascribed important antioxidant roles in the plasma. In addition, LELF contains several nonprotein antioxidants, such as ascorbic acid, α-tocopherol and GSH. LELF is collected by lavage and so becomes BAL fluid (BALF) by undergoing a substantial dilution. BALF can, however, be corrected back to LELF by use of the urea dilution technique [84]:

$$\text{LELF (ml)} = \frac{[\text{urea}]\ \text{BALF}}{[\text{urea}]\ \text{serum}} \times \text{volume BALF.}$$

Data reported on BAL fluids will depend upon the volume of saline used to aspirate LELF, the recovery of fluid achieved, and the degree to which the fluid is concentrated before analysis. Results from different laboratories are therefore difficult to compare (Table 11.8).

Iron binding antioxidant activities

LELF fluid from normal subjects contains microgram quantities of transferrin, which has a substantial iron binding capacity because it inhibits iron stimulated lipid peroxidation, a property that can be reversed by presaturating LELF with an iron salt [85]. Analysis of BAL fluids from patients with ARDS reveals higher total protein concentrations, and higher levels of transferrin (Table 11.8), making the fluid an even more potent inhibitor of iron stimulated lipid peroxidation [86]. It has been suggested that the high permeability pulmonary edema of ARDS, although disadvantageous to gas exchange, may be beneficial for antioxidant protection of the lung [86].

Iron oxidizing antioxidant activities

On a molar basis LELF fluid contains 20-fold less ceruloplasmin than transferrin, and appears to offer little ferroxidase dependent antioxidant protection against lipid peroxidation [85]. However, when BAL fluids from patients with ARDS are assayed for ferroxidase antioxidant activity in a similar free radical generating system, they show considerable protection [86] consistent with their increased concentrations of ceruloplasmin (Table 11.8). In addition to its well defined ferroxidase antioxidant activity, ceruloplasmin has been reported to protect against the oxidative inactivation of α-protease [88] and to reduce the adhesion of neutrophils to endothelial cells [87].

Table 11.8 Lung epithelial lung lining fluid (LELF) and bronchoalveolar lavage fluid (BALF) protein values in ARDS and controls

Patient group (n)	Total protein (µg/ml)	Albumin (µg/ml)	Transferrin (µg/ml)	Ceruloplasmin (µg/ml)	References
Normal controls (18) Non-smokers LELF[a]	9 000±1,000	4600±600	324.2±42.1	22.2±2.6	85
Normal controls: BALF 100 ml wash concentrated to 1.5–2.5 ml	77.3±7.0 (12)	–	2.78±0.30 (4)	0.26±0.02 (4)	86
Normal controls (38): BALF 250 ml wash concentrated to 17.5 ml	1 000±100	–	30.6±8.0	0.26	50
ARDS (11); BALF 100 ml wash concentrated to 1.5–2.5 ml	2 536.8±408.2	–	77.8±15.3	36.5±5.6	87
ARDS (23); BALF 250 ml wash concentrated to 12.5 ml	20 000±3,000	–	413.1±84.0	120±26.0	50

[a] LELF volumes were calculated by use of the urea dilution technique (84).

Scavenging antioxidant protection

Lung epithelial lining fluid contains high concentrations of GSH compared with plasma from the same individual [89]. Most of the GSH (96%) is in the reduced form, and some 140-fold higher than that present in plasma. Normal human plasma GSH values reported in the literature are somewhat variable, probably due to the labile nature of the molecule and the nonspecific methods used to measure it. However, it is likely that normal human plasma contains around 1–2 µmol/l. Reduced GSH can act as a scavenging antioxidant by reacting with hydroxyl radicals (9×10^9/mol/s), and as a substrate for the hydrogen peroxide removing enzyme glutathione peroxidase. However, GSH can also slowly react with superoxide radicals ($< 7.7 \times 10^5$/mol/s) in a sequence that can lead to singlet oxygen formation. Other pro-oxidant reactions can also occur with GSH, due to its ability to reduce ferric ions and to form thiyl radicals. Indeed, the pro-oxidant properties of plasma from normal patients and those with ARDS, shown in one of our assay systems [49], can be ascribed to protein-SH groups.

Patients with ARDS have decreased levels of GSH in LELF (21.7 µmol/l ± 7.8) compared with normal controls (91.8 µmol/l ± 14.5) [90], consistent with increased oxidant activity associated with activated neutrophils.

EVIDENCE OF OXIDATIVE MOLECULAR DAMAGE

MOLECULAR DAMAGE TO BIOLOGICAL MOLECULES MEDIATED BY OXYGEN

Oxygen damage to living cells was originally attributed to the oxygen molecule itself. However, although isolated examples of this do exist in biology it was soon realized that the rates of enzyme inactivation by oxygen were too slow to account for the extreme toxicity seen in plant and animal systems.

Gershman, Gilbert and colleagues [22] first proposed that the damaging effects of oxygen were caused by oxygen radicals. Their theory was latter expanded and extended, following the discovery of the SODs, by McCord and Fridovich [26] into the 'superoxide theory of oxygen toxicity'. This theory proposes that superoxide is a major biological toxin, and that the SOD enzymes provide a key biological defense against oxygen toxicity. Twenty-five years on, the theory still holds true although there are still some intriguing puzzles to solve. As previously discussed, much of our early biological knowledge of radicals came from radiation studies which led to the proposal that hydrogen peroxide reacted directly with superoxide to yield hydroxyl radicals. It soon became obvious that this reaction could not occur in biological systems and that a catalyst was required, much along the lines (involving iron) proposed by Haber and Weiss in 1932. The 'Haber–Weiss reaction', shown below (equations 20, 6 and 11), can also be described as a 'superoxide driven Fenton reaction'.

$$O_2^- + Fe^{3+} \longleftrightarrow Fe^{2+} + O_2 \qquad (20)$$

$$2O_2^- + 2H^+ \longrightarrow H_2O_2 + O_2 \qquad (6)$$

$$Fe^{2+} + H_2O_2 \longrightarrow Fe^{3+} + OH^- + {}^\bullet OH \qquad (11)$$

LIPID CHANGES

Twelve patients with ARDS and pulmonary or extrapulmonary sepsis were monitored for changes in their plasma fatty acids using the technique of gas chromatography [9]. These studies were conducted over a 24 hour period and showed significant decreases in the percentage of essential fatty acids present (linoleic and arachidonic acid), and an increase in the ratio of oleic acid to linoleic acid. Studies in our laboratory over longer periods of time, using the technique of gas chromatography mass spectrometry, have shown similar marked changes in plasma fatty acid patterns in patients with ARDS. Major decreases in linoleic acid are associated with increases in oleic acid and palmitoleic acid [91] and a loss of protein thiol groups suggestive of oxidative damage. However, the reverse ratio can also ensue (Figure 11.3). Most of the patient with ARDS in our intensive care unit during

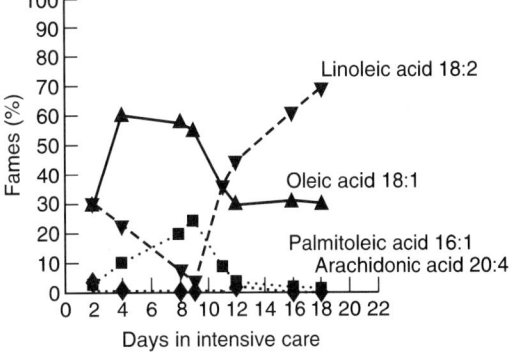

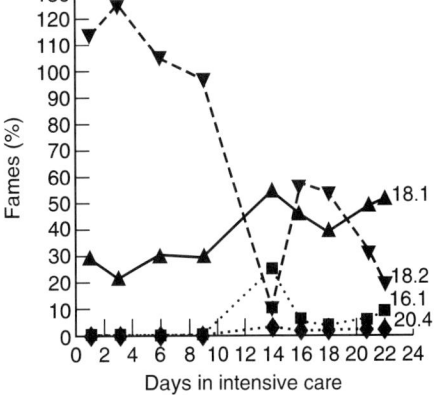

Figure 11.3 Percentage changes in plasma fatty acids of two typical ARDS patients during intensive care. (▽) 18:2, (△) 18:1, (□) 16:1, (◇) 20:4. FAMES = fatty acid methyl esters measured by gas chromatography – mass spectrometry.

this study were given parenteral nutrition, often including a lipid supplement.

Linoleic acid can be converted to arachidonic acid, which is a substrate for prostaglandin synthesis, and some loss of linoleic acid observed in our study may be attributable to such enzymic peroxidation.

Levels of plasma esterified cholesterol are considerably lower in patients with ARDS than those seen in normal healthy controls, and this is also reflected in the cholesterol ester to free cholesterol ratio [8], suggesting abnormalities in cholesterol metabolism also exists in patients with ARDS. These authors suggested that patients with ARDS are suffering from a deficiency of plasma lecithin–cholesterol acyltransferase activity [8].

Unsaturated fatty acid oxidation products in plasma and BAL fluids

The free radical peroxidation of polyunsaturated lipids has long been associated with tissue damage. Peroxidation products of lipids can be detected in most disease states, often giving rise to the false assumption that lipid peroxidation is a cause of many diseases [92]. In most cases, however, lipid peroxidation is an inevitable consequence of tissue damage [92].

Animal models of lung injury induced by a variety of techniques, such as complement activation [93], oleic acid [94], endotoxin [95] and *Escherichia coli* peritonitis [96], have demonstrated evidence of lipid peroxidation based on techniques such as conjugated dienes and thiobarbituric acid reactivity (TBAR).

There is, however, surprisingly little information concerning peroxidative changes in ARDS patients. Mechanically ventilated patients in intensive care were studied by Iakeda and colleagues [97] and shown to have increased levels of TBAR, which were ascribed to the presence of plasma lipid peroxides, and decreased levels of vitamin E compared with preoperative control patients. Similar increases in plasma lipid hydroperoxides were found in sepsis patients, many pulmonary, using a specific and sensitive assay for peroxides [98]. Cross and colleagues [8], using a highly sensitive assay for lipid hydroperoxides (detection limit 0.3μ mol/l), found no lipid peroxides in freshly taken plasma from patients with ARDS, but did find nanomolar concentrations in LELF. Others, however, using nonspecific assays, such as the TBAR test, have reported increased plasma levels in patients with ARDS [9]. Sequential plasma studies on patients with ARDS in our own laboratory

have shown no evidence for increased formation of TBARs, diene conjugates and fluorescent adducts characteristic of polyunsaturated fatty acid peroxidation. We do, however, find an increased formation of plasma 4-hydroxynonenal (0.412 ± 0.023 nmol/l compared with 0.205 ± 0.018 nmol/l in healthy controls) which parallels the loss of linoleic acid [99]. 4-Hydroxynonenal has been shown to be a potent chemoattractant and to possess a wide range of biological activities, such as the ability to inactivate β adrenoceptors (time and concentration dependent) in rat lung membranes [100].

PROTEIN OXIDATION

Proteins are important targets for free radical attack. Amino acids within the protein structure can be modified by free radicals in a variety of ways, altering the chemical and physical properties of the molecule. For example, aromatic amino acids, such as phenylalanine and tyrosine can be hydroxylated, thiol group-containing amino acids such as cysteine can be oxidized to disulfides, and methionine to methionine sulfoxide. In addition, many amino acids can be oxidized to yield thiobarbituric acid reactive products [101] and carbonyl functions (reviewed in [102]).

Studies in our laboratory monitoring sequential changes in plasma protein thiol and carbonyl groups in patients with ARDS have shown two distinct patterns, one for survivors and one for nonsurvivors [10]. An example of these changes is shown in Figure 11.4. As can be seen, survivors showed decreased plasma thiol levels with increasing carbonyl values. As they recovered, their thiols increased, often reaching normal levels, as carbonyls fell. Nonsurvivors, however, show low thiols and high carbonyl values which rarely change during their stay in intensive care. Values obtained in eight patients with ARDS are summarized in Table 11.9.

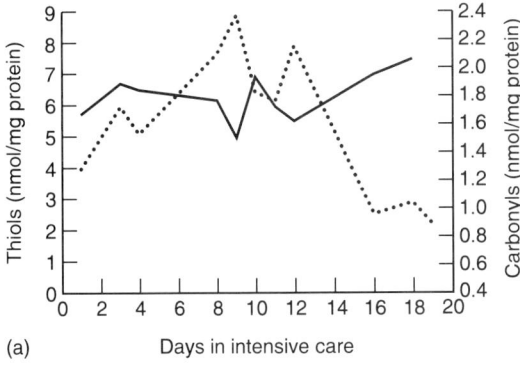

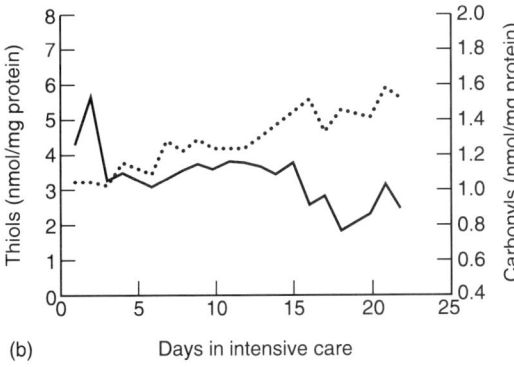

Figure 11.4 Changes in (·····) plasma thiols (nmol/mg protein) and (——) carbonyls (nmol/mg protein) in (a) a nonsurviving and (b) a surviving patient with ARDS.

Oxidative damage to specific proteins

The enzyme xanthine dehydrogenase can be converted to its oxidase form by oxidative modification and by limited proteolysis. Once formed, xanthine oxidase can oxidize a wide range of substrates, including xanthine, hypoxanthine, acetaldehyde and a variety of other biological aldehydes, with the coupled reduction of molecular oxygen to superoxide and hydrogen peroxide. Xanthine oxidase activity has been reported to be increased in the plasma of six of 15 patients with ARDS when compared with intensive care unit control patients [103]. Several groups have dem-

onstrated, using animal models, that xanthine oxidase derived from endothelial cells contributes to lung injury through several mechanisms including oxidant formation [104–106], which also leads to increased cytokine expression [107].

Methionine sulfoxide formation from methionine has been used as a marker of oxidant damage to proteins [108]. Behr and colleagues [108] measured methionine sulfoxide in BAL fluids taken from patients with diffuse fibrosing alveolitis and found significant increases compared with appropriate controls. Interestingly, there was a positive correlation between methionine sulfoxide formation and the number of neutrophils present. Similar studies in patients with chronic bronchitis have also revealed increased levels of methionine sulfoxide in BAL fluid [109]. Methionine residues of the elastase inhibiting protein, α-antiproteinase, appear to be critical targets for damage. When these residues are oxidized the protein is unable to inhibit elastase, allowing increased proteolytic damage [110]. Aromatic hydroxylation of tyrosine in the *ortho* position (*o*-tyrosine) provides a marker of hydroxyl radical attack on proteins [111] and increased formation of *o*-tyrosine has been detected in the plasma of patients with ARDS [112]. Peroxynitrite formation has been implicated in the pathology of ARDS, based on the detection of the 3-nitrotyrosine in lung tissue from patients with acute lung injury [113].

DNA DAMAGE

DNA is a critical molecule for oxidative damage leading to base modifications and strand breaks. Pulmonary artery and aortic endothelial cells exposed to 50 μmol H_2O_2 have been shown to undergo DNA damage [114]. This occurred whether the cells were directly incubated with H_2O_2 or glucose oxidase or xanthine oxidase. Inhibitor studies clearly identified the penultimate reactive species as H_2O_2, presumably acting through Fenton-

Table 11.9 Plasma protein values in surviving and nonsurviving patients with ARDS

Patient code	Number of samples	Total protein (mg/ml)	Total thiols (nmol/mg protein)	Carbonyls (nmol/mg protein)	Total autofluorescence (RFI units)
A	9	49.9±2.1	6.26±0.67	1.649±0.14	64.63±5.30
B	12	57.4±2.63	6.40±0.24	1.610±0.14	51.96±2.22
C	9	57.3±3.8	6.07±0.32	1.350±0.08	42.60±2.70
D	11	74.3±2.59	3.68±0.24	1.135±0.07	57.60±3.12
E	15	85.7±1.45	3.10±0.15	1.077±0.04	60.50±2.50
F	15	67.4±1.47	4.04±0.29	1.460±0.04	50.60±3.67
G	14	71.2±2.10	3.57±0.13	1.750±0.06	–
H	19	92.4±1.60	3.39±0.17	1.270±0.04	–
ARDS survivors (*n* = 3)		53.9±2.15	6.24±0.09	1.536±0.09	53.1±6.39
ARDS nonsurvivors (*n* = 5,[a]3)		78.2±4.68	3.56±0.16	1.338±0.12	[a]56.2±2.55
ARDS total (*n* = 8,[a]6)		69.5±5.17	4.56±0.50	1.413±0.09	[a]54.6±3.22
Normal controls (*n* = 12)		83.6±1.82	6.55±0.52	0.940±0.04	64.4±2.94
Non-ARDS ICU controls (*n* = 10)		60.5±3.0	5.5±0.27	1.24±0.090	–

RFI = relative flourescence intensity units.
[a] Number of patient samples available for analysis.
Source: Quinlan *et al.* [10].
Patients A,B and C survived ARDS; patients D,E,F,G and H did not.
Values shown are for patients with ARDS the mean ±SEM of venous and arterial plasma samples assayed in duplicate.

type chemistry with a transition metal ion closely associated with DNA. Similar strand breaks were also observed in lymphocytes under the same reaction conditions. The oxidant oxone has also been shown to cause single strand breaks in DNA of rat lung macrophages [115] collected from lavage fluid, as well as human fibroblasts in the presence of arachidonic acid. The involvement of arachidonic acid suggests that lipid peroxidation may also be a requirement to mediate DNA damage under these conditions.

SUMMARY AND CONCLUSIONS

ARDS is an acute lung injury syndrome in which patients are experiencing severe oxidative stress from the disease process as well as from treatment with high F_{IO_2} regimens. So far, however, there is no strong evidence to support the view that oxidative stress causes the disease. Antioxidants have, so far, had a poor record in modifying human diseases in

which free radicals are thought to play a damaging role. It seems likely, therefore, that until the molecular mechanisms of oxidant injury are better understood and effective antioxidant delivery systems developed, presently available antioxidants will only make a minor contribution to the clinical management of the syndrome.

REFERENCES

1. Wardle, E.N. (1984) Shock lungs; the post traumatic respiratory syndrome. *Quarterly Journal of Medicine*, **53**, 317–29.
2. Macnaughton, P.D. and Evans, T.W. (1992) Adult respiratory distress syndrome. *Lancet*, **339**, 469–72.
3. Ashbaugh, D.G., Bigelow, D.B., Petty, T.L. and Levine, B.E. (1967) Acute respiratory distress syndrome in adults. *Lancet*, **ii**, 319–23.
4. Cochrane, C.G., Spragg, R.C. and Revak, S.D. (1983) The presence of neutrophil elastase and evidence of oxidation activity in bronchoalveolar lavage fluid of patients with adult respiratory distress syndrome. *American Review of Respiratory Disease*, **127**, 525–7.

5. Weiland, J.E., Davis, W.B. and Holter, J.F. (1986) Lung neutrophils in the adult respiratory distress syndrome: clinical and pathophysiological significance. *American Review of Respiratory Disease*, **14**, 218–25.

6. Baldwin, S.R., Grum, C.M., Boxer, L.A. *et al.* (1986) Oxidant activity in expired breath of patients with adult respiratory distress syndrome. *Lancet*, **i**, 11–4.

7. Sznajder, J.I., Fraiman, A., Hall, J.B. *et al.* (1989) Increased hydrogen peroxide in the expired breath of patients with acute hypoxemic respiratory failure. *Chest*, **96**, 606–12.

8. Cross, C.E., Forte, T., Stocker, R. *et al.* (1990) Oxidative stress and abnormal cholesterol metabolism in patients with adult respiratory distress syndrome. *Journal of Laboratory and Clinical Medicine*, **115**, 391–404.

9. Richard, C. Lemonnier, F. Thibault, M *et al.* (1990) Vitamin E deficiency and lipoperoxidation during adult respiratory distress syndrome. *Critical Care Medicine*, **18**, 4–9.

10. Quinlan, G.J., Evans, T.W. and Gutteridge, JMC (1994) Oxidative damage to plasma proteins in adult respiratory distress syndrome. *Free Radical Research*, **20**, 289–298.

11. Seidenfeld, J.J., Pohl, D.F., Bell, R.C. *et al.* (1986) Incidence site and outcome of infections in patients with the adult respiratory distress syndrome. *American Review of Respiratory Disease*, **134**, 12–6.

12. Kinkel, S.L., Standiford, T. Kasahara, K *et al.* (1991) Interleukin-8 (IL-8): the major neutrophil chemotactic factor in the lung. *Experimental Lung Research*, **17**, 17–23.

13. Fantone, J.C., Feltner, D.E. and Brieland, J.K. (1987) Phagocytic cell-derived inflammatory mediators and lung disease. *Chest*, **91**, 428–34.

14. Tate, R.M. and Repine, J.E. (1983) Neutrophils and the adult respiratory distress syndrome. *American Review of Respiratory Disease*, **125** 552–9.

15. Gutteridge, J.M.C and Halliwell, B (1989) Iron toxicity and oxygen radicals, in *Iron Chelating Therapy* (ed. C. Hershko), Baillière Tindall, London, pp. 195–256.

16. Aust, S.D., Morehourse, L.A. and Thomas, C.E. (1985) Role of metals in oxygen radical reactions. *Journal of Free Radical Biology and Medicine*, **1**, 3–25.

17. Halliwell, B. and Gutteridge, J.M.C. (1992) Biologically relevant metal ion-dependent hydroxyl radical generation. An update. *FEBS Letters*, **307**, 108–12.

18. Osaki, S. Johnson, D.A. and Frieden, E (1966) The possible significance of the ferrous oxidase activity of ceruloplasmin in normal human plasma. *Journal of Biological Chemistry*, **241**, 2746–51.

19. Babior, B.M. (1978) Oxygen-dependent microbial killing by phagocytes. *New England Journal of Medicine*, **298**, 721–5.

20. Candeias, L.P., Patel, K.B., Stratford, M.R.L. *et al.* (1993) Free hydroxyl radicals are formed on reaction between the neutrophil-derived species superoxide anion and hypochlorous acid. *FEBS Letters*, **333**, 151–3.

21. Candeias, L.P., Stratford, M.R.L. and Wardman, P. (1994) Formation of hydroxyl radicals on reaction of hypochlorous acid with ferrocyanite. A model iron (II) complex. *Free Radical Research*, **20**, 241–9.

22. Gerschman, R., Gilbert, D.L., Nye, S. *et al.* (1954) Oxygen poisoning and X-irradiation: a mechanism in common. *Science*, **199**, 623–6.

23. Feeman, B.A. and Crapo, J.D. (1981). Hyperoxia increases oxygen radical production in rat lungs and lung mitochondria. *Journal of Biological Chemistry*, **256**, 10986–92.

24. Suttorp, N. and Simon, L.M. (1982) Lung cell oxidant injury. Enhancement of polymorphonuclear leukocyte-mediated cytotoxicity in lung cells exposed to sustained *in vitro* hyperoxia. *Journal of Clinical Investigation*, **70**, 342–50.

25. Halliwell, B. and Gutteridge, J.M.C. (1989) *Free Radicals in Biology and Medicine* 2nd edn, Oxford University Press, Oxford.

26. McCord, J.M. and Fridovich, I. (1969) Superoxide dismutase and enzymic function for erythrocuprein (hemocuprein). *Journal of Biological Chemistry*, **224**, 6049–55.

27. Fridovich, I. (1983) Superoxide radical: an endogenous toxicant. *Annual Reviews of Pharmacology and Toxicology*, **23**, 239–57.

28. Moncada, S. and Higgs, E.A. (1991) Endogenous nitric oxide: physiology, pathology and clinical relevance. *European Journal of Clinical Investigation*, **21**, 361–74.

29. Rubbo H., Radi R., Trujillo M. *et al.* (1994) Nitric oxide regulation of superoxide and peroxynitrite-dependent lipid peroxidation. *Journal of Biological Chemistry*, **269**, 26066–75.

30. Guidot D.M., Repine M.J., Brooks M. *et al.* (1995) Inhaled nitric oxide prevents neutro-

phil-mediated, oxygen radical-dependent leak in isolated rat lungs. *Americal Journal of Physiology,* **269**, L2–50.

31. Beckman, J.S., Beckman, T.W., Chen, J. *et al.* (1990) Apparent hydroxyl radical production by peroxynitrite: implications for endothelial injury from nitric oxide and superoxide. *Proceedings of the National Academy of Sciences of the USA,* **87**, 1620–4.

32. Saran, M., Michel, C. and Bors, W. (1990) Reaction of NO with O_2. Implications for the action of endothelium-derived relaxing factor (EDRF). *Free Radical Research Communications,* **10**, 221–6.

33. Radi, R., Beckman, J.S., Bush, K.M. *et al.* (1991) Peroxynitrite oxidation of sulfhydryls. The cytotoxic potential of superoxide and nitric oxide. *Journal of Biological Chemistry,* **266**, 4244–50.

34. Pryor W.A. and Squadrito G.L. (1995) The chemistry of peroxynitrite: a product from the reaction of nitric oxide with superoxide. *American Journal of Physiology,* **268**, L699–722.

35. Fenton, H.J.H. (1894) Oxidation of tartaric acid in presence of iron. *Journal of the Chemical Society,* **65**, 899–909.

36. Anbar, M. and Neta, P. (1967) A compilation of specific bimolecular rate constants for the reactions of hydrated electrons, hydrogen atoms and hydroxyl radicals with inorganic and organic compounds in aqueous solution. *International Journal of Applied Radiation and Isotopes,* **18**, 493–523.

37. Rush, J.D. and Koppenol, W.H. (1986) Oxidising intermediates in the reaction of ferrous EDTA with hydrogen peroxide. *Journal of Biological Chemistry,* **261**, 6730–6733.

38. Sutton, H.E., Vile, G.F. and Winterbourn, C.C. (1987) Radical driven Fenton reactions. Evidence from paraquat radical studies for production of tetravalent iron in the presence and absence of ethylenediamine tetracetic acid. *Archives of Biochemistry and Biophysics,* **256**, 462–71.

39. Gutteridge, J.M.C., Westmarck, T. and Halliwell, B. (1985) Oxygen radical damage in biological systems, in *Free Radicals, Aging and Degenerative Diseases* (eds J.E. Johnson Jr, R. Walford *et al.*), Alan R. Liss, New York, pp. 99–139.

40. Gutteridge, J.M.C. (1991) Reduction of low molecular mass iron by reducing molecules present in plasma, and the protective action of caeruloplasmin. *Journal of Trace Elements and Electrolytes in Health and Disease* **5**, 279–81.

41. Halliwell, B. and Gutteridge, J.M.C. (1990) Role of free radicals and catalytic metal ions in human disease: an overview. *Methods in Enzymology,* **186**, 1–85.

42. Gutteridge, J.M.C. (1988) Bleomycin-iron in biological fluids. What does the assay measure? in *Free Radicals: Methodology and Concepts* (eds C. Rice-Evans and B. Halliwell), Richelieu Press, London, pp. 429–46.

43. Gutteridge, J.M.C. (1986) Iron promoters of the Fenton reaction and lipid peroxidation can be released from haemoglobin by peroxides. *FEBS Letters,* **201**, 291–5.

44. Gutteridge, J.M.C. (1978) Caeruloplasmin: a plasma protein, enzyme and antioxidant. *Annals of Clinical Biochemistry,* **15**, 293–6.

45. Gutteridge, J.M.C. (1983) Antioxidant properties of caeruloplasmin towards iron and copper dependent oxygen radical formation. *FEBS Letters,* **157**, 37–40.

46. Gutteridge, J.M.C. (1984) Copper-phenanthroline induced site-specific oxygen radical damage to DNA. Detection of loosely bound trace copper in biological fluids. *Biochemical Journal,* **218**, 983–5.

47. Gutteridge, J.M.C. and Stocks, J. (1981) Caeruloplasmin: physiological and pathological perspectives. *Critical Reviews in Clinical Laboratory Sciences,* **14**, 257–329.

48. O'Connell, M.J., Baum, H. and Peters, T.J. (1986) Hemosiderin-like properties of free-radical-modified ferritin. *Biochemical Journal,* **240**, 297–300.

49. Gutteridge, J.M.C., Quinlan, G.J., Mumby, S. *et al.* (1994), Primary plasma in adult respiratory distress syndrome patients: changes in iron-oxidising, iron-binding and free radical scavenging proteins. *Journal of Laboratory and Clinical Investigation,* **124**, 263–73.

50. Kresek-Staples, J.A., Kew, R.R. and Webster, R.O. (1992) Ceruloplasmin and transferrin levels are altered in serum and bronchoalveolar lavage fluid of patients with the adult respiratory distress syndrome. *American Review of Respiratory Disease,* **145**, 1009–15.

51. Gutteridge, J.M.C., Quinlan, G.T. and Evans, T.W. (1994) Transient iron-overload with bleomycin-detectable iron in the plasma of patients with adult respiratory distress syndrome. *Thorax,* **49**, 707–10.

52. Gutteridge, J.M.C. and Hon, Y. (1986) Iron complexes and their reactivity in the bleomycin assay for radical-promoting loosely-bound iron. *Free Radical Research Communications*, **2**, 143–51.

53. Gutteridge, J.M.C., Rowley, D.A., Griffiths, E. *et al.* (1985) Low-molecular weight iron complexes and oxygen radical reactions in idiopathic haemochromatosis. *Clinical Science*, **68**, 463–7.

54. Halliwell, B., Aruoma, O.I., Mufti, G. *et al.* (1988) Bleomycin-detectable iron in serum from leukaemic patients before and after chemotherapy: therapeutic implications for treatment with oxidant-generating drugs. *FEBS Letters*, **241**, 202–4.

55. Evans, P.J., Evans, R., Kovar, I.Z. *et al.* (1992) Bleomycin-detectable iron in the plasma of premature and full-term neonates. *FEBS Letters*, **303**, 210–2.

56. Lindeman, J.H., Houdkamp, E., Lentjes, E.G. *et al.* (1992) Limited protection against iron-induced lipid peroxidation by cord blood plasma. *Free Radical Research Communications*, **16**, 285–94.

57. Pepper, J.R., Mumby, S. and Gutteridge, J.M.C. (1994) Transient iron-overload with bleomycin-detectable iron present during cardiopulmonary bypass surgery. *Free Radical Research*, **21**, 53–58.

58. Marklund, S.L., Holme, E. and Hellner, L. (1982) Superoxide dismutase in extracellular fluids. *Clinica Chimica Acta*, **126**, 41–51.

59. Halliwell, B. and Gutteridge, J.M.C. (1986) Oxygen free radicals in relation to biology and medicine: some problems and concepts. *Archives of Biochemistry and Biophysics*, **246**, 501–14.

60. Saran, M. and Bors, W. (1989) Oxygen radicals in extracellular fluids. *Biochemical Society Transactions*, **10**, 72–3.

61. Gutteridge, J.M.C., Paterson, S.K., Segal, A.W. *et al.* (1981) Inhibition of lipid peroxidation by the iron-binding protein lactoferrin. *Biochemical Journal*, **199**, 259–61.

62. Rice-Evans, C.A., Diplock, A.T. and Symons, M.C.R. (1991) *Techniques in Free Radical Research*, Elsevier, Amsterdam.

63. Gutteridge, J.M.C. (1987) The antioxidant activity of haptoglobin towards haemoglobin stimulated lipid peroxidation. *Biochimica et Biophysica Acta*, **917**, 219–23.

64. Gutteridge, J.M.C. and Smith, A. (1988) Antioxidant protection by haemopexin of haemoglobin stimulated lipid peroxidation. *Biochemical Journal*, **256**, 861–5.

65. Bannister, J.V., Bannister, W.H., Hill, H.A.O. *et al.* (1980) Does caeruloplasmin dismute superoxide? No. *FEBS Letters*, **118**, 127–9.

66. Calabrese, L. and Carboraro, M. (1986) An e.p.r. study of the non-equivalence of the copper sites of caeruloplasmin. *Biochemical Journal*, **238**, 291–5.

67. Frei, B., Stocker, R. and Ames, B.N. (1988) Antioxidant defenses and lipid peroxidation in human blood plasma. *Proceedings of the National Academy of Sciences of the USA*, **85**, 9748–52.

68. Wayner, D.D., Burton, G.W., Ingold, K.U. *et al.* (1985) Quantitative measurement of the total, peroxyl radical-trapping antioxidant capability of human blood plasma by controlled peroxidation: the important contribution made by plasma proteins. *FEBS Letters*, **187**, 33–7.

69. Esterbauer, H., Gebicki, J., Puhl, H. *et al.* (1992) The role of lipid peroxidation and antioxidants in oxidative modification of LDL. *Free Radical Research Communications*, **13**, 341–90.

70. Steinberg, D. (1993) Modified forms of low-density lipoprotein and atherosclerosis. *Journal of Internal Medicine*, **233**, 227–32.

71. Gutteridge, J.M.C., Winyard, P., Brailsford, S. *et al.* (1985) The behaviour of caeruloplasmin in stored human extracellular fluids in relation to ferroxidase II activity, lipid peroxidation and phenanthroline detectable copper. *Biochemical Journal*, **230**, 517–23.

72. Williams, D.M., Christensen, D.D., Lee, G.R. *et al.* (1974) Serum azide-resistant ferroxidase activity. *Biochimica et Biophysica Acta*, **350**, 129–34.

73. Moak, S.A. and Greenwald, R.A. (1984) Enhancement of rat serum ceruloplasmin levels by exposure to hyperoxia. *Proceedings of the Society for Experimental Biology and Medicine*, **177**, 97–103.

74. Fleming, R.E., Whitman, I.P. and Gitlin, J.D. (1991) Induction of ceruloplasmin gene expression in rat lung during inflammation and hyperoxia. *American Journal of Physiology*, **260**, L68–74.

75. Paterson, C.E. and Rhoades, R.A. (1988) Protective role of sulfhydryl reagents in oxidant

lung injury. *Experimental Lung Research*, **14**, 1005–19.

76. Bernard, G.R., Swindell, B.B., Meredith, M.J. *et al.* (1989) Glutathione (GSH) repletion by *N*-acetylcysteine (NAC) in patients with the adult respiratory distress syndrome (ARDS). *American Review of Respiratory Disease*, **139**, A221.

77. Aruoma, O.I. Halliwell, B., Hoey, B.M. *et al.* (1989) The antioxidant action of *N*-acetylcysteine: its reaction with hydrogen peroxide, hydroxyl radicals, superoxide and hypochlorous acid. *Free Radical Biology and Medicine*, **6**, 593–7.

78. Jepson, S., Herlevsen, P., Knudesen, P. *et al.* (1992) Antioxidant treatment with *N*-acetylcysteine during adult respiratory distress syndrome: a prospective, randomized, placebo-controlled study. *Critical Care Medicine*, **20**, 918–23.

79. Gutteridge, J.M.C. (1978) The membrane effects of vitamin E, cholesterol and their acetates an peroxidative susceptibility. *Research Communications in Chemical Pathology and Pharmacology*, **22**, 563–71.

80. Frei, B., Yamamoto, Y., Niclas, D. *et al.* (1988) Analysis of oxidants and antioxidants in human plasma of healthy subjects and of patients with adult respiratory distress syndrome, in *Free Radicals, Methodology and Concepts* (eds C. Rice-Evans and B. Halliwell), Richelieu Press, London, pp. 349–68.

81. Bertrand, Y., Pincemail, J., Hanique, G. *et al.* (1989) Differences in tocopherol – lipid ratios in ARDS and non-ARDS patients. *Intensive Care Medicine*, **15**, 87–93.

82. Leff, J.A., Parson, P.E., Day, C.E. *et al.* (1992) Increased serum catalase activity in septic patients with the adult respiratory distress syndrome. *American Review of Respiratory Disease*, **146**, 985–9.

83. Leff, J.A., Parson, P.E., Day, C.E. *et al.* (1993) Serum antioxidants as predictors of adult respiratory distress syndrome in patients with sepsis. *Lancet*, **341**, 777–80.

84. Rennard, S.I., Basset, G., Lecossier, D. *et al.* (1986) Estimation of the volume of epithelial lining fluid recovered by lavage using urea as marker of dilution. *Journal of Applied Physiology*, **60**, 532–8.

85. Pacht, E.R. and Davis, B. (1988) Role of transferrin and ceruloplasmin in antioxidant activity of lung epithelial lining fluid. *Journal of Applied Physiology*, **64**, 2092–9.

86. Lykens, M.G. Davis, B.W. and Pacht, E.R. (1992) Antioxidant activity of bronchoalveolar lavage fluid in the adult respiratory distress syndrome. *American Journal of Physiology*, **262**, L169–75.

87. Broadley, C. and Hoover, R.L. (1989) Ceruloplasmin reduces the adhesion and scavenges superoxide during the interaction of activated polymorphonuclear leukocytes with endothelial cells. *American Journal of Pathology*, **138**, 647–55.

88. Taylor, J.C. and Oey, L. (1982) Ceruloplasmin: plasma inhibitor of the oxidative inactivation of alpha-protease inhibitor. *American Review of Respiratory Disease*, **126**, 476–82.

89. Cantin, A.M., North, S.L., Hubbard, R.C. *et al.* (1987) Normal alveolar epithelial lining fluid contains high levels of glutathione. *Journal of Applied Physiology*, **63**, 152–7.

90. Pacht, E.R., Timerman, A.P., Lykens, M.G. *et al.* (1991) Deficiency of alveolar fluid glutathione in patients with sepsis and the adult respiratory distress syndrome. *Chest*, **100**, 1397–403.

91. Quinlan, G.J., Evans, T.W. and Gutteridge, J.M.C. (1994) Linoleic acid and protein thiol changes suggestive of oxidative damage in the plasma of patients with adult respiratory distress syndrome. *Free Radical Research*, **20**, 299–306.

92. Halliwell, B. and Gutteridge, J.M.C. (1984) Lipid peroxidation, oxygen radicals, cell damage and antioxidant therapy. *Lancet*, **i**, 1396–7.

93. Ward, P.A., Till, G.O., Hatherill, J.R. *et al.* (1985) Systemic complement activation, lung injury, and products of lipid peroxidation. *Journal of Clinical Investigation*, **76**, 517–27.

94. Spragg, R.G., Abraham, J.L. and Loomis, W.H. (1982) Pulmonary platelet deposition accompanying acute oleic-acid-induced pulmonary injury. *American Review of Respiratory Disease*, **126**, 553–7.

95. Demling, R.H., Lalonde, C., Jin, L.J. *et al.* (1986) Endotoxemia causes increased lung tissue lipid peroxidation in anaesthetized sheep. *Journal of Applied Physiology*, **60**, 2094–100.

96. Ishizaka, A., Stephens, K.E., Tazelaar, H.D. *et al.* (1988) Pulmonary edema after *Escherichia coli* peritonitis correlates with thiobarbituric-acid-reactive material in bronchoalveolar lav-

age fluid. *American Review of Respiratory Disease*, **137**, 783–9.

97. Iakeda, K., Shimada, Y., Masaru, A. *et al.* (1984) Plasma lipid peroxides and alpha-tocopherol in critically ill patients. *Critical Care Medicine*, **12**, 957–9.

98. Keen, R.R., Stella, L.A., Flanigan, D.P. *et al.* (1991) Differential detection of plasma hydroperoxides in sepsis. *Critical Care Medicine*, **19**, 1114–9.

99. Quinlan, G.J., Evans, T.W. and Gutteridge, J.M.C. (1994) 4-Hydroxy-2-nonenal levels in the plasma of patients with adult respiratory distress syndrome as linoleic acid appears to fall. *Free Radical Research*, **21**, 95–106.

100. Leurs, R., Rademaker, B., Kramer, K. *et al.* (1986) The effects of 4-hydroxyl-2-3-*trans* nonenal on α-adrenoceptors of rat lung membranes. *Chemical and Biological Interactions*, **59**, 211–8.

101. Gutteridge, J.M.C. (1981) Thiobarbituric acid-reactivity following iron-dependent free radical damage to aminoacids and carbohydrates.

102. Stadtman, E.R. (1990) Metal ion-catalysed oxidation of proteins: biochemical mechanisms and biological consequences. *Free Radicals in Biology and Medicine*, **9**, 315–25.

103. Grum, C.M., Ragsdale, R.A., Ketai, L.H. *et al.* (1987) Plasma xanthine oxidase activity in patients with adult respiratory distress syndrome. *Journal of Critical Care*, **2**, 22–6.

104. Rodell, T.C., Heronis, J.C., Ohnemus, C.L. *et al.* (1987) Xanthine oxidase mediates elastase-induced injury to isolated lungs and endothelium. *Journal of Applied Physiology*, **63**, 2159–63.

105. Phan, S.H., Gannon, D.E., Varani, J. *et al.* (1989) Xanthine oxidase activity in rat pulmonary artery endothelial cells and its alteration by activated neutrophils. *American Journal of Pathology*, **134**, 1201–11.

106. Till, G.O., Friedl, H.P. and Ward, P.A. (1991) Lung injury and complement activation: role of neutrophils and xanthine oxidase. *Free Radical Biology and Medicine*, **10**, 379–86.

107. Schwartz M.D., Repine J.E., and Abraham E. (1995) Xanthine oxidase-derived oxygen radicals increase lung cytokine expression in mice subjected to hemorrhagic shock. *American Journal of Respiratory Cell and Molecular Biology*, **12**, 434–40.

108. Behr, J., Maier, K, Krombach, F. *et al.* (1991) Pathogenic significance of reactive oxygen species in diffuse fibrosing alveolitis. *American Review of Respiratory Disease*, **144**, 146–50.

109. Maier, K.L., Leuschel, L. and Costabel, V. (1992) Increased oxidised methionine residues in BAL fluid proteins in acute or chronic bronchitis. *European Respiratory Journal*, **5**, 651–8.

110. Carp, H., Miller, F. Hoidal, J.R. *et al.* (1982) Potential mechanism of emphysema: α1-proteinase inhibitor recovered from lungs of cigarette smokers contains oxidised methionine and has decreased elastase inhibitory capacity. *Proceedings of the National Academy of Sciences of the USA*, **79**, 2041–5.

111. Karam, L.R. and Simic, M.G. (1990) Formation of ortho-tyrosine by radiation and organic solvents in chicken tissue. *Journal of Biological Chemistry*, **265**, 11581–5.

112. Quinlan, G.J., Evans, T.W. and Gutteridge, JMC (1994) Ortho-tyrosine levels in the plasma proteins of patients with adult respiratory distress syndrome are increased: implications for hydroxyl radical damage. *American Journal of Respiratory and Critical Care Medicine*, **149**, A428.

113. Kooy N.W., Royall J.A., Yao Z. *et al.* (1995) Evidence for *in vivo* peroxynitrite production in human acute lung injury. *American Journal of Respiratory Critical Care Medicine*, **151**, 1250–4.

114. Spragg, R.C. (1991) DNA strand break formation following exposure of bovine pulmonary artery and aortic endothelial cells to reactive oxygen products. *American Journal of Respiratory Cell and Molecular Biology*, **4**, 4–10.

115. Hanley, N.M., Kozumbo, W.J., Costa, D.L. *et al.* (1993) Induction of DNA single strand breaks in lung cells by ozone exposure *in vivo* and *in vitro*. *American Review of Respiratory Disease*, **147**, A670.

Elizabeth L. Aronsen and John M. Shannon

Since the mid-1970s, increasing attention has been paid to the biological responses of alveolar epithelial type II cells following acute lung injury and their contribution to the syndrome of acute respiratory distress in adults (ARDS) [1]. Research has been greatly aided by techniques developed to isolate and culture type II cells in an environment separated from the complex milieu of the whole lung. In addition, application of molecular biological techniques to the study of these cells has rapidly expanded our understanding of the type II cell's role in the structure and function of the alveolus, which will improve our knowledge of the mechanism by which a diverse group of risk factors can lead to the common final endpoint which is called ARDS, and may result in the development of specific therapies and interventions by which it can be treated [2,3].

This chapter reviews current knowledge of alveolar type II cell biology, particularly relating to acute lung injury from a variety of causes. An overview will outline the pathology of the type II cell in the normal and injured alveolus. Subsequent sections will review type II cell functions: (1) in ion transport, (2) in surfactant synthesis and secretion, and (3) as the type I cell progenitor in repair of the injured alveolar epithelium. We attempt to relate observations at the alveolar epithelial cellular level to events occurring in the clinical syndrome.

Specifically, ARDS can be divided into three major clinicopathological phases (Chapters 4 and 16):

1. an acute exudative phase in which ion transport and surfactant abnormalities may predominate;
2. a proliferative phase in which cytokines and growth factors are likely to play an important role;
3. a resolution phase that involves type II cell differentiation into type I cells with restoration of normal alveolar architecture and function.

A fourth phase, mentioned briefly in this chapter, is the fibrotic phase, with failure of normal alveolar restoration, that occurs in patients with recurrent lung insults [4]. Death can occur during any of these clinical/pathological phases. Each phase will be reviewed with specific reference to type II cell biology.

PATHOLOGY

In the normal adult human lung, type II cells comprise approximately 15% of the total lung cell population. These cuboidal cells are found in the corners of the alveolus and are polarized, with their microvilli projecting into the alveolar lumen and the basement membrane adjacent to the basement membrane of capillary endothelial cells and interstitial fibroblasts. By electron microscopy characteristic lamellar bodies, the organelles of surfactant storage, can be identified. Besides

ARDS Acute Respiratory Distress in Adults. Edited by Timothy W. Evans and Christopher Haslett. Published in 1996 by Chapman & Hall, London. ISBN 0 412 56910 8

surfactant synthesis and secretion, type II cells function in vectorial solute transport and are the progenitor cells of alveolar type I cells [5]. As type II cells proliferate and differentiate into type I cells, they attenuate their metabolic machinery (mitochondria, endoplasmic reticulum, Golgi), lose their storage granules (lysosomal bodies, multivesicular bodies, lamellar bodies) and become flattened. Although representing less than 10% of the total lung cell number, type I cells cover more than 90% of the apical alveolar surface. The very thin type I cell surface is the site of alveolar gas exchange. Morphometry estimates reveal that potential oxygen delivery through this barrier is proportional to the oxygen requirements of the animal [6].

An important concept is that while there are many causes of ARDS, the response of the lung to injury is limited, resulting in a similar pathologic picture irrespective of etiology [7–12]. In histological sections taken from patients who have developed ARDS and died during the acute exudative phase (Chapter 4), the earliest lesion appears to be interstitial edema [11]. There is a twofold increase in septal width and a two- to threefold increase in the volume of the alveolar epithelial cells [5]. Intercellular tight junctions show a decrease in the number of junctional strands and an irregularity in distribution [12] as type I epithelial cells swell. There are areas of focal alveolar collapse and flooding. The pulmonary edema fluid is composed of proteinaceous material, inflammatory cells, cell debris, blood and surfactant remnants. Amorphous, fibrinous hyaline membranes line the alveolar septae, particularly near the distal terminal bronchioles where they form rings at the entrances to the alveolar spaces. Soon after, gross alveolar epithelial cell damage is visible. The swollen type I cells necrose, leaving intercellular gaps and a denuded, but often intact, basement membrane with overlying hyaline membranes. The type I alveolar epithelial cell is highly vulnerable to injury for at least two reasons. Firstly, there is a very large

surface to volume ratio of the cell, thus leaving a large surface area exposed to injurious agents. Secondly, compared to other lung cell types, particularly the progenitor type II cell, the type I cell has relatively few intracellular organelles associated with energy production or the synthesis of macromolecules that might be associated with cellular defense against injury. By inference from cell culture results, type I cells have a significant decrease in catalase, glutathione reductase, and glutathione peroxidase activities compared with type II cells [14] (chapter 11). By contrast, type II cells have a high endogenous content of antioxidant enzymes such as manganese superoxide dismutase [15] that may protect them from the injury seen in type I cells.

Hyperplastic and hypertrophic type II cells characterize the proliferative phase of ARDS. Normal type II cell turnover *in vivo* is about 4–5 weeks, but following acute lung injury there is a dramatic increase in type II cell labeling index of up to 23% [16]. These cells can be demonstrated to be metabolically active in the synthesis of type IV collagen matrix and surfactant protein A [17]. In the proliferative phase of ARDS there are two competing phenomena: type II cell proliferation with restoration of the normal alveolar architecture, and the fibroproliferative response with organization of the intra-alveolar space exudate. If type II cell restoration prevails, clinical and pathologic resolution occurs. If the fibroproliferative response dominates, the fibrotic phase (also termed sclerosing alveolitis) results.

In the resolution phase of ARDS, type II cells differentiate into type I cells and restore the normal alveolar epithelial barrier. Type II cells that do not differentiate into type I cells synthesize and secrete surfactant to line the alveolus. Epithelial polarity is re-established with the return of vectorial solute transport (Chapter 20). There is restoration of the normal alveolar architecture histologically, with corresponding clinical improvement in gas exchange, increased pulmonary compliance, decreased physiological shunt and clearing of the chest radiograph.

Although the pathological lesion of acute lung injury is diffuse alveolar damage, it is important to recognize that different areas of the lung parenchyma are variably affected, resulting in a patchy injury and response [18]. This patchy response has also been suggested clinically by regions of uneven nitrogen washout seen acutely in trauma patients [19] (Chapter 15). One mechanism may be that irregularly distributed corner alveolar capillaries become obstructed with cellular-fibrin debris, regional hypoxia occurs and nearby epithelial cells are more severely injured. Regional alveolar capillary plugging has been demonstrated in rabbits injured by intravenous administration of ethchlorvynol [20]. Enhanced coagulation and suppressed fibrinolysis activity have been demonstrated in bronchoalveolar lavage (BAL) fluid from patients with ARDS [21,22]. Since alveolar injury results in surfactant abnormalities and decreased alveolar compliance, mechanical ventilation, itself a necessary therapy for ARDS, may result in the more compliant normal alveolus becoming overdistended (Chapter 23).

ARDS-like lesions can be produced experimentally in a number of ways:

- Mechanical
    serial lung lavage [23]
- Chemical
    high F_{IO_2} [24]
    hydrochloric acid [25]
    endotoxin [R. Deterding and R. Mason, personal communication]
    oleic acid [26]
    ethchlorvynol [20]
    N-nitroso-N-methylurethane (NNNMU) [27,28]
- Radiation [29]
- Infectious
    viral [30]
    bacterial [31].

These are only a few of the methods that have been used to induce acute lung injury. In animals given NNNMU subcutaneously, the alveolar epithelium is preferentially injured with relative sparing of the endothelium [27]. Lung compliance decreases as epithelial cell necrosis occurs and is restored with epithelial regeneration. No experimental animal model exactly duplicates the conditions and response of ARDS in humans. Furthermore, the mechanisms of injury can probably involve either a direct or indirect toxic effect on the alveolar epithelial cell, since risk factors for the syndrome include both inhalation and intravenous (systemic) routes of injury.

Intense investigations are in progress to find the causative factor(s) in the propagation of lung injury in ARDS. One hypothesis is that the influx of inflammatory cells, particularly neutrophils, is injurious to the alveolar epithelial cells, either by direct toxic effects or indirectly by the secretion of products detrimental to the bystanding alveolus. Parsons and colleagues [32] demonstrated neutrophil chemotactic activity present in BAL from 14 of 16 patients with ARDS but no activity in normal controls (Chapter 6). Patients with ARDS have alveolar macrophages that release more interleukin (IL)-1 than normal subjects [33]. Eosinophil cationic protein and myeloperoxidase, markers of eosinophil and neutrophil activation, respectively, are increased in the BAL of patients with ARDS [34,35]. C5a and C3, products of complement activation and neutrophil chemoattractants, are elevated in the BAL of patients with ARDS [36]. These patients have higher levels of BAL neutrophil elastase [37,38]. Although neutrophils have been intensely studied as the agents which propagate acute lung injury, they are not absolutely required to produce ARDS, which may develop in neutropenic patients [39,40] (Chapter 5).

There is evidence of oxygen free radicals (OFRs) in acute lung injury [41] (Chapter 11). These can inactivate proteinase inhibitors such as α_1-protease inhibitor, which are then more susceptible to digestion by proteolytic cleavage by other enzymes such as neutrophil elastase. In addition, OFRs inhibit type II cell surfactant synthesis *in vitro* [42]. Xanthine oxidase instilled intratracheally into guinea pigs results in decreased BAL surfactant and decreased lung compliance [43]. *Streptococcus pneumoniae* strains deficient in pneumolysin produce hydrogen peroxide in concentrations that are directly toxic to rat alveolar epithelial cells [44]. BAL glutathione, an important antioxidant, is reduced in patients with ARDS [45]. Guinea pig type II cells cultured under normoxic conditions have significant amounts of glutathione. When exposed to hyperoxic conditions, cell injury is significantly correlated with the amounts of reduced glutathione and inversely correlated with the amounts of total intracellular glutathione; inhibition of new glutathione synthesis is associated with increased susceptibility to hyperoxic injury [19].

The type II cell may have a role in the defense against oxygen toxicity and the generation of OFRs by inflammatory cells. For example, surfactant protein (SP)-A preincubation significantly decreases alveolar macrophage superoxide production [46]. Exposure to hyperoxia produces a twofold stimulus in SP-A and SP-B mRNA synthesis by type II cells [47]. Tumor necrosis factor (TNF)α is abundant in type II cells at all stages of ARDS [48]. Cytokines such as TNF and IL-1 protect against hyperoxic lung injury [24], possibly via an increase in alveolar cell antioxidant enzymes such as manganese superoxide dismutase [49] (Chapter 7).

ION TRANSPORT AND THE ALVEOLAR EPITHELIAL BARRIER

The polarized alveolar epithelial type II cell functions in active transepithelial solute transport of sodium from the alveolar space to the interstitium, allowing resorption of alveolar fluid. In addition, tight junctions between type II cells and neighboring type I cells form the basis for an alveolar epithelial barrier that is 15 times tighter than the adjacent endothelial barrier and thus provides the major defense against noncardiogenic pulmonary leak that is characteristic of ARDS (Chapter 20).

Several methods have been employed to demonstrate and measure alveolar barrier dysfunction in humans [50–52]. In general, there is agreement that there is an increase in permeability of the air–capillary barrier in acute lung injury, whether measured as a function of extravascular lung water or in terms of solute or serum protein leakage into the alveolar space [34]. Radiolabeled aerosol clearance is also increased in patients at risk for and with ARDS [50,53,54], demonstrating that the increased barrier permeability is not due to an increase in vectoral transport by the alveolar epithelial cells. In a study of 34 mechanically ventilated patients, clinical improvement in gas exchange and radiographic abnormalities were associated with restoration of active ion transport accompanied by alveolar fluid resorption and an increase in alveolar protein concentration [55].

There is a significant increase in extravascular lung water as early as 1 hour after intravenous oleic acid injection into rats, preceding the influx of inflammatory cells in the BAL at 4 hours, suggesting that the initial mechanism of increased barrier permeability is not due to mediator release from neutrophils [56]. Neutrophil depletion prior to injury does decrease the permeability changes, suggesting that these cells may have some effect on the type II cell's ability to restore the alveolar barrier.

In patients with increased capillary permeability, protein leakage results in BAL protein contents 12–35 times that of normal controls [57,58]. Most studies agree that there is loss of size selectivity of the alveolar epithelium, as large molecular weight proteins such as albumin, IgM, and α_2-macrogobulin can be recovered in BAL from affected patients. The loss of size selectivity could be secondary to loss of epithelial intercellullar junctional integrity or to epithelial cell death with resultant basement membrane denudation. The degree of injury probably affects the degree of protein leakage and size selectivity. Jenkins and colleagues found that the increase in BAL total protein content in septic animals was primarily due to low molecular weight plasma proteins, suggesting a relative preservation of the size selectivity of the alveolar-capillary barrier in this model of acute lung injury [31]; alveolar protein leak was completely blocked by pretreatment with ibuprofen. Byrne and colleagues [59] also demonstrated that ibuprofen could block protein leak as well as maintain arterial oxygen content and lung compliance in a sepsis model of acute lung injury. Nonsteroidal anti-inflammatory agents such as ibuprofen inhibit prostaglandin synthetase, suggesting that arachidonic acid metabolites may be important in the pathogenesis of ARDS, particularly in disrupting the alveolar epithelial barrier function of type I and type II cells. Related to this concept is the demonstration of elevated BAL leukotriene D_4, but not B_4 or C_4 or prostaglandin E_2, in patients with ARDS compared with controls [60]. Adult type II cells produce prostaglandins *in vitro* [61]. Prostaglandins in turn affect fibroblast proliferation, collagen synthesis, and collagenase secretion. These observations also suggest a possible therapeutic intervention in the early, exudative phase of ARDS and perhaps in the later proliferative phase. However, these agents could also exert detrimental effects through other mechanisms. It is important to note that aspirin, whose mechanism of action is similar to that of the nonsteroidal anti-inflammatory agents such as ibuprofen, has, with overdose, itself been reported to induce ARDS [62].

An interesting autosomal recessive clinical disorder, lysinuric protein intolerance, is characterized by a basolateral epithelial diamino acid transport defect. These patients are predisposed to ARDS and the concentration of diamino acids in the BAL of asymptomatic patients is increased [63], suggesting that epithelial transport functions of type II cells may be very important in the cellular mechanisms of ARDS.

SURFACTANT FUNCTION (CHAPTER 16)

Type II alveolar epithelial cells synthesize surfactant in microsomes and store it in lamellar bodies. Surfactant is normally composed of a complex of phospholipids, proteins and neutral lipids. Proteins comprise approximately 4% by weight of surfactant obtained in normal BAL fluid. There have been four major surfactant apoproteins identified, including SP-A, SP-B, SP-C and SP-D [for review see [64]. cDNAs for these proteins have been cloned and sequenced for several species and their secondary structure is largely known. SP-A is a glycosylated protein with a collagen-rich region that forms large oligomers under native conditions. Its molecular weight under reducing conditions ranges from 26 to 36 kDa, depending on the degree of post-translational modifications. In the normal lung, surfactant synthesis and reuptake is an active, temperature dependent process highly regulated by type II cells. The activity of these cells in this function depends on feedback loops that monitor the amount of surfactant present in the surrounding milieu. Regulation of surfactant synthesis and reuptake is a major function of SP-A, which acts via a receptor on the type II cell plasma membrane. SP-B and SP-C are small (reduced molecular weights of 8 kDa and 4 kDa, respectively) proteolipids that are very hydrophobic and whose major function is to optimize the biophysical properties of alveolar surfactant in reducing surface tension. SP-D is more recently described and its functions are largely unknown, although its lectin properties make it an attractive candidate for local defense against invading microbes [65].

Phospholipids comprise the greatest proportion of surfactant, 90% by weight. The most abundant surfactant phospholipid by far is the disaturated form of phosphatidyl-choline (PC), dipalmitoyl-phosphatidyl-choline (DPPC). Type II cells utilize the cytidine diphosphate (CDP)-choline pathway for *de novo* synthesis of PC. Lesser quantities of phosphatidylglycerol (PG), phosphatidyle-thanolamine (PE), phosphatidylinositol (PI), sphingomyelin (SM) and others are also present. Normally, there is less than 1% lyso-phosphatidylcholine present in BAL [42]. Neutral lipids comprise approximately 6% of total surfactant by weight. The majority of this is cholesterol.

There are several factors known to regulate type II cell surfactant secretion *in vivo* or *in vitro* (for review see [66], including β-adrenergic and cholinergic agonists [67,68], vasopressin [69], hyperventilation [70,71], changes in pH [72], diglycerides, lipid media-tors [73], phorbol esters, calcium ionophores, arachidonic acid metabolites [74], adenosine, ATP, cAMP [75] and even cell shape and extracellular matrix (ECM) interactions [76–78]. ATP and cAMP also stimulate SP-A synthesis which in turn, through a receptor-mediated mechanism, inhibits type II cell surfactant secretion [79]. Stilbene disulfonates also inhibit *in vitro* type II cell surfactant secretion [80].

There are at least six mechanisms proposed [81,82] by which surfactant abnormalities in acute lung injury can result in ARDS:

1. inadequate surfactant synthesis leading to a surfactant lining layer insufficient to maintain alveolar patency;
2. altered surfactant composition resulting in decreased or altered surfactant function;
3. abnormal surfactant metabolism;
4. inhibition of surfactant synthesis and/or function by serum proteins exuded into the alveolar space;
5. direct surfactant biochemical toxicity or structural alteration by proteases or free oxygen radicals;
6. compartmentalization of surfactant into

intra-alveolar hyaline membranes render-ing it unavailable to function.

In the alveolar microenvironment all of these mechanisms may play some role in acute lung injury.

INADEQUATE SURFACTANT SYNTHESIS

There is some disagreement as to the total BAL phospholipid content in patients with ARDS. Some have found an increase in total phospholipid [83], while others demonstrated no change [84,85], and still others found a decrease [86]. In rats with experimental peri-tonitis, type II cells have a marked decrease in their ability to synthesize surfactant phospho-lipids, as measured by their reduced uptake of choline and fatty acids [87]. Ambroxol, an experimental agent that acts as a secreta-gogue, increases surfactant choline but not fatty acid incorporation in rabbits with perito-nitis and produces no marked histologic dif-ference in these animals as compared with uninjured controls [88].

ALTERED SURFACTANT COMPOSITION

After describing ARDS, Petty and colleagues went on to demonstrate that the syndrome was associated with fundamental abnormal-ities in surfactant composition and properties [89]. They were able to isolate three lipid–protein aggregates from the lungs of patients with ARDS rather than one major aggregate from normal lavage. *Ex vivo*, the abnormal surfactant was much more compressible, sug-gesting a mechanism for alveolar instability in the syndrome. Autopsied lungs from these patients demonstrated a significant loss of volume and reduced compliance similar to clinical premortem findings. More recently, investigations have focused on BAL content in ARDS patients [90].

Many studies indicate alterations in BAL surfactant composition in humans (reviewed in [81,82,91–93]). In general, BAL phospholipid composition in patients with ARDS is altered so that the relative amounts of phosphatidylcholine (especially DPPC) and phosphatidylglycerol decrease, while phosphatidylinositol, phosphatidylethanolamine, and sphingomyelin increase. Similar alterations in surfactant composition have been reported in a variety of animal models [28,94,95]. The observation that lysophosphatidylcholine increases as well [28] is intriguing because this compound indirectly inhibits surfactant function (see below). One study [96] also demonstrated a 20-fold increase in BAL glycolipids in ARDS patients, a potentially important observation because glycolipids decrease surfactant activity *in vitro*. SP-D binds glucosylceramide, a glycolipid found in BAL [97], suggesting a mechanism for glycolipid regulation. Pison and colleagues demonstrated a decrease in BAL SP-A in 19 patients with multiple trauma and correlated this decrease with the severity of lung injury [98]. Gregory *et al.* [86] showed that SP-A is decreased in both patients at risk for, or with ARDS.

ABNORMAL SURFACTANT METABOLISM

In NNNMU-treated animals, Lewis and colleagues [28] demonstrated a decrease in the BAL large aggregate surfactant and an increase in DPPC in lamellar bodies. This was followed by increased DPPC secretion and an increase in BAL inactive small aggregate surfactant. The small aggregate fraction is believed to be a surfactant form that has been metabolized prior to reuptake and recycling by type II cells. Others have also found an increase in the less active small aggregate fraction in BAL from ARDS patients [84]. A chronic form of ARDS induced experimentally in mice by radiation treatment is associated with an increase in BAL total phospholipid and protein content, an increase in the high density large aggregate surfactant

subtype, and a decrease in the nonactive low density small aggregate surfactant subtype [29], the latter apparently due to a protein inhibitor of the conversion from high to low density surfactant present in the alveolar fluid [99]. These studies taken together indicate that type II cells may have very different acute and chronic responses to lung injury.

There is also evidence that the surfactant proteins and phospholipids may have altered patterns of metabolism during hyperoxic injury [100]. In this hamster model, SP-A, -B and -C declined, while DPPC increased, during exposure to hyperoxia.

Mechanical stimulation (stretch) of the alveolus stimulates surfactant secretion as well. Conversely, one might suppose that conditions of less stretch (e.g. shallow breathing) might have the opposite effect; that is, the aggregation of surfactant into less functional forms, with increased surface tension and atelectasis [101].

INHIBITION OF SURFACTANT SYNTHESIS AND/OR FUNCTION BY PLASMA PROTEINS

Plasma proteins inhibit the active, temperature-dependent surfactant synthesis and endocytosis by type II cells [102] *in vitro*. Fibrinogen degradation products and laminin also inhibit surfactant surface tension activity (103). Fibrinogen and its degradation products are found in the vast majority of patients with ARDS [92]. In oleic acid-treated rabbits there is a rapid decrease in compliance and lung volume, associated with a marked increase in cell-free BAL protein content but no significant change in phospholipid content or composition [57]. The alteration in BAL protein content is associated with a significant decrease in surface activity. Thus, plasma proteins in the alveolus can have profound effects on surfactant synthesis and function, suggesting this is an important mechanism of lung dysfunction in ARDS.

DIRECT SURFACTANT STRUCTURAL ALTERATION

One degradation product of surfactant PC and DPPC is lysophosphatidylcholine (LPC), formed by plasma phospholipase A_2 (PLA) digestion. PLA activity is increased in patients with septic shock [104], especially in those with ARDS. Intravenous administration of PLA into rats results in intra-alveolar pulmonary edema that can be blocked by pretreatment with indomethacin [105]. In rabbits injured by oleic acid, Casals and colleagues [94] found that although BAL PLA activity was decreased after acute lung injury, whole lung microsomal PLA activity was increased. They also reported an increase in BAL LPC in these animals at 2.5 hours after injury. LPC increases fibrinogen inhibition of surfactant function *in vitro* [106]. Type II cells, as well as Clara cells, synthesize uteroglobin, a PLA inhibitory and anti-inflammatory protein [107]. These data, taken together, demonstrate not only direct surfactant structural alteration but suggest that the alveolar epithelium may have mechanisms to counteract these alterations.

SURFACTANT COMPARTMENTALIZATION

There is currently no direct evidence for compartmentalization of surfactant into intra-alveolar hyaline membranes rendering it unavailable as a mechanism of abnormal surfactant function in acute lung injury. However, as hyaline membranes are a significant finding in ARDS lesions, and as their physico-chemical properties are such that they might be expected to neutralize surfactant function *in vitro* and *in vivo*, we include this possibility here for completeness.

SURFACTANT REPLACEMENT THERAPY

Recognition of surfactant abnormalities and the successful use of exogenous surfactant in the therapy of neonatal respiratory distress syndrome has led to similar interest in the use of surfactant replacement as therapy for ARDS [43,91,108–112]. A number of investigations have studied the effects of exogenous surfactant in healthy and injured animal models.

In guinea pigs, lung injury induced by repeated lung lavage could be reversed by surfactant replacement. The treated animals had significant improvement in gas exchange as well as histologically demonstrated improvement in alveolar air expansion [23]. Surfactant replacement in rabbits injured by intratracheal instillation of hydrochloric acid restored normal recoil, but these authors found no effect on gas exchange as measured by arterial blood gases [25]. Gas exchange was significantly improved in acute lung injury produced in rats by Sendai virus infection after intratracheal surfactant administration [113]. Possible explanations for these apparent discrepancies in the effects on gas exchange include the mechanism of lung injury, or the time, dose or specific differences in the composition of surfactant administered. Exogenous surfactant administered to healthy rabbits appears to stimulate both synthesis and secretion of endogenous surfactant [114] by type II cells. It does not appear to normalize either the decrease in DPPC nor the decrease in small aggregates (i.e. normalize the altered surfactant metabolism) in NNNMU-injured rabbits [115].

Surfactant therapy must be approached with caution. Human surfactant is immunogenic, as can be shown by demonstrating circulating immune complexes in ARDS patients [116]. Mice inoculated intraperitoneally with hybridomas producing antibodies to surfactant apoproteins develop acute respiratory failure with histologic lesions similar to those seen in ARDS [117].

Intratracheal administration of antibodies which recognize SP-A actually improved gas exchange in rats depleted of surfactant by repeated lung lavage [118]. SP-A accelerates generation of thromboplastin and inhibits fibrinolysis, inhibits surfactant release and facilitates surfactant reuptake. This suggests that there are very complex interactions among the various surfactant components that must be carefully considered while instituting clinical trials of surfactant therapy.

PROLIFERATION AND REPAIR

Several processes contribute to lung remodeling after acute lung injury; these include alveolar interstitial thickening, intra-alveolar connective tissue matrix deposition, alveolar collapse and alveolar contraction [119]. Appropriate remodeling and resolution of injury is likely to result from a highly synchronized spatiotemporal expression of autocrine and paracrine factors. Failure of these checks and balances could result in an overabundant fibroproliferative response in the alveolar space and propagation of chronic scarring [120, 121]. In the proliferative phase of diffuse alveolar damage, there is rapid proliferation of fibroblasts in the interstitium and obliteration of the air spaces [122]. Fibroblasts deposit type III collagen and EDIIIa-containing fibronectin which can, in turn, serve as receptors for cell adhesion molecules of the integrin type. Cell adhesion molecules are found on all types of interstitial and alveolar cells, thus cellular proliferation and migration may depend on ECM signals from specific types of collagen or fibronectin.

Remodeling of the ECM by fibroblasts and type II epithelial cells probably involves a balance between collagen deposition and degradation. Christner and colleagues [123] measured BAL collagenase activity in ARDS patients and found evidence of both type I and type III collagenase activity in the majority of these subjects. Similar activity was not detectable in their controls. Interestingly, in one patient they were able to follow sequentially, type III collagenase activity peaked before type I activity. In the normal lung, type IV collagen is deposited by type II epithelial cells and found in a uniform distribution along the basement membrane [124]. Type III collagen, produced by fibroblasts, is found at alveolar entrance rings, in the alveolar septae and within the interstitium. Importantly, in acute lung injury, type III and type I collagens have increased deposition in the interstitium, alveolar septae and alveolar spaces, with type III collagen deposition preceding type I collagen deposition. It appears that in ARDS a remodeling of the alveolar structure occurs, and that this takes place in an ordered fashion and depends on the balance between type II cells, fibroblasts, probably other lung cell types, and the extracellular matrix. Alveolar type II cell–fibroblast interactions may play an important role in repair. Through gaps in the basement membrane, close contacts are established and fibroblast type I collagen secretion is stimulated by a factor released by type II cells; fibroblasts reciprocally stimulate SP-A mRNA synthesis by type II cells [125].

A number of soluble factors have been demonstrated to stimulate type II cell DNA synthesis *in vitro*:

- epidermal growth factor (EGF) [126]
- hepatocyte growth factor/scatter factor (HGF/SF)
- keratinocyte growth factor (KGF)
- acidic fibroblast growth factor (aFGF)
- insulin [127]
- cholera toxin [128]
- serum
- BAL fluid [129]
- pituitary extract [130]
- gastrin releasing peptide (GRP) [130].

While HGF is probably produced by alveolar macrophages in the microenvironment, HGF receptor mRNA can be demonstrated in isolated type II cells [131]. Both KGF and KGF receptor mRNA are found early in lung development and in adult lung (J. Shannon, unpublished observations). Insulin-like growth factors IGF-1 and IGF-2 stimulate fibroblast but not type II cell proliferation [130]. There has been a great deal of interest in the use of various cytokines to stimulate type II cell specific proliferation in injury

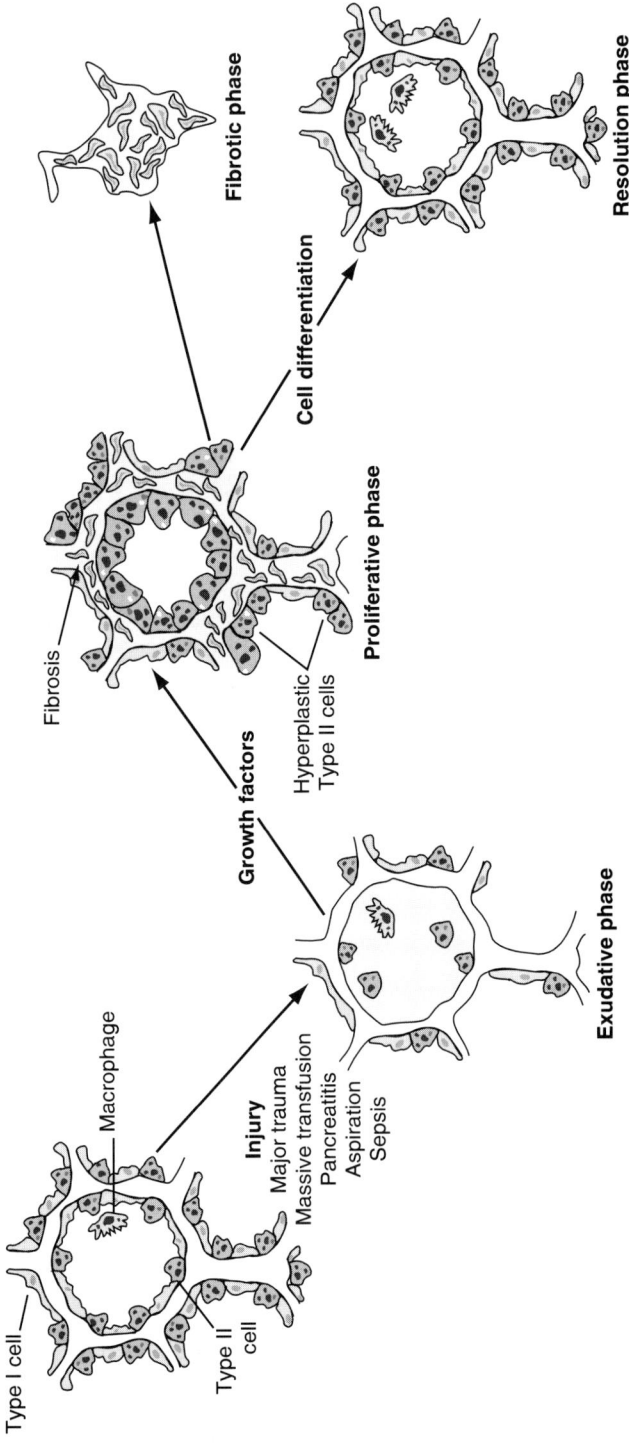

Figure 12.1 Lung injury and repair in ARDS. Following various systemic or inhalational insults, the alveolus characteristically undergoes four major clinicopathological phases. These are (1) the exudative phase, distinguished by interstitial edema, type I epithelial cell death, and alveolar flooding; (2) the proliferative phase, charaterized by increases in growth factor and cytokine expression as well as both type II epithelial cell and fibroblast proliferation; and (3) the resolution phase during which type II cells differentiate into type I cells and migrate via cell–cell and cell–extracellular matrix adhesion molecule regulation to restore normal alveolar architecture and function. The fourth, fibrotic, phase results from repeated insults and/or excessive fibroblast compared to epithelial cell proliferation. (Courtesy of Leigh Landskronen.)

models as well. It is likely that in the near future clinical trials will begin.

The concept that the ECM is more than simply an inert framework is now firmly established. The normal ECM is a complex of collagens, glycosaminoglycans, proteoglycans and cell adhesion molecules (such as laminin and fibronectin) that are involved in cell–ECM adhesive interactions. Through transmembrane signal transduction and tyrosine kinase activation, cell adhesion molecules appear to trigger cellular proliferation and differentiation [132]. During development, inflammation and repair, integrin-type fibronectin–fibrinogen receptors are upregulated [133]. Isolated type II cells cultured on a fibronectin substratum develop a significantly higher transepithelial resistance as compared with those cultured on collagen, indicating that ECM has a significant effect on the formation of tight junctions and a polarized epithelium [134]. Neutrophil products, such as metalloproteases, elastase and cathepsin G, solubilize ECM *in vitro* [135] and likely affect the balance as well.

Other families of adhesion molecules are found in the alveolus as well. The immunoglobulin type adhesion molecule ICAM-1 is normally expressed primarily on type I cells, especially near junctions. In acute lung injury induced by hyperoxia, ICAM-1 is found more dispersed on the surface of the type I cells and its expression is markedly induced on type II epithelial cells [136]. ICAM-1 is not detectable on freshly isolated type II cells but is upregulated when these cells are cultured on substrata that promote spreading [137]. The counterreceptors for this molecule include LFA-1 and Mac-1, which are found on leukocytes, and may contribute to transmigration across the alveolar epithelium and pulmonary sequestration of inflammatory cells during acute lung injury.

Transmembrane glycoprotein cell adhesion molecules of the cadherin type mediate homotypic intercellular adhesion. Although epithelial (E)-cadherin appears to be the major cadherin in the normal adult lung, isolated type II cells contain mRNA for both E-cadherin and another cadherin, placental (P)-cadherin (E. Aronsen, unpublished observations). It is not known whether P-cadherin may be important in type II cell proliferation or differentiation into type I cells although P-cadherin expression in fetal lung development makes this an attractive hypothesis. It is obvious that disruption of homotypic intercellular adhesion can be a mechanism leading to the alveolar leak syndrome seen early in acute lung injury and that re-establishment of normal cell–cell contacts is critical to restoring the integrity of the alveolar epithelium.

CONCLUSION

ARDS is a devastating illness with high mortality (Chapter 2). Many of the clinical manifestations can be understood in the context of type II cell biology (Figure 12.1). Understanding how the type II cell responds in both its proliferative and differentiated capacities may result in specific therapeutic interventions.

REFERENCES

1. Ashbaugh, D.G., Bigelow, C.B., Petty, T.L. and Levine, B.E. (1967) Acute respiratory distress in adults. *Lancet*, **ii**, 319–23.
2. Goldstein, G. and Luce, J.M. (1990) Pharmacologic treatment of the adult respiratory distress syndrome. *Clin. Chest Med.*, **11**, 773–87.
3. Jacobs, E.R. and Bone, R.C. (1986) Therapeutic implications of acute lung injury. *Crit. Care Clin.*, **2**, 615–28.
4. Tomashefski, J.F. Jr (1990) Pulmonary pathology of the adult respiratory distress syndrome. *Clin. Chest Med.*, **11**, 593–619.
5. Adamson, I.Y.R. and Bowden, D.H. (1974) The type 2 cell as progenitor of alveolar epithelial regeneration. *Lab. Invest.*, **30**, 35–42.
6. Weibel, E.R. (1983) How does the lung affect gas exchange? *Chest*, **83**, 657–65.
7. Albertine, K.H. (1985) Ultrastructural abnormalities in increased-permeability pulmonary edema. *Clin. Chest Med.*, **6**, 345–69.

8. Blennerhassett, J.B. (1985) Shock lung and diffuse alveolar damage: pathological and pathogenetic considerations. *Pathology*, **17**, 239–47.

9. Hasleton, P.S. (1983) Adult respiratory distrss syndrome – a review. *Histopathology*, **7**, 307–32.

10. Joka, T., Obertacke, U., Atay, Z. *et al.* (1989) Cytological changes in alveolar cells with ARDS. *Prog. Clin. Biol. Res.*, **308**, 51–5.

11. Riede, U.N., Mittermayer, C., Friedburg, H. *et al.* (1979) Morphologic development of human shock lung. *Pathol. Res. Pract.*, **165**, 269–86.

12. Riede, U.N. and Shah, I. (1984) Diagnostic morphometry of the adult respiratory distress syndrome. *Pathol. Res. Pract.*, **179**, 204–6.

13. Barrios, R., Inoue, S. and Hogg, J.C. (1977) Intercellular junctions in 'shock lung'. A freeze-fracture study. *Lab. Invest.*, **36**, 628–35.

14. Kinnula, V.L., Chang, L., Everitt, J.I. and Crapo, J.D. (1992) Oxidants and antioxidants in alveolar epithelial type II cells: *in situ*, freshly isolated, and cultured cells. *Am. J. Physiol.*, **262**, 69–77.

15. Clyde, B.L., Chang, L.Y., Auten, R.L. *et al.* (1993) Distribution of manganese superoxide dismutase mRNA in normal and hyperoxic rat lung. *Am. J. Respir. Cell Mol. Biol.*, **8**, 530–7.

16. Smith, L.J. and Brody, J.S. (1981) Influence of methylprednisolone on mouse alveolar type 2 cell response to acute lung injury. *Am. Rev. Respir. Dis.*, **123**, 459–64.

17. Sugiyama, K.L. and Kawai, T. (1993) Diffuse alveolar damage and acute interstitial pneumonitis: histochemical evaluation with lectins and monoclonal antibodies against surfactant apoprotein and collagen type IV. *Mod. Pathol.*, **6**, 242–8.

18. Yazdy, A.M., Tomashefski, J.F. Jr, Yagan, R. and Kleinerman J. (1989) Regional alveolar damage (RAD): a localized counterpart of diffuse alveolar damage. *Am. J. Clin. Pathol.*, **92**, 10–15.

19. Aerts, C., Wallaert, B. and Voisin C. (1992) *In vitro* effects of hyperoxia on alveolar type II pneumocytes: inhibition of glutathione synthesis increases hyperoxic cell injury. *Exp. Lung Res.*, **18**, 845–61.

20. Gil, J. and McNiff, J.M. (1982) Early tissue damage in ethchlorvynol-induced alveolar edema in rabbit lung. *Am. Rev. Respir. Dis.*, **126**, 701–7.

21. Idell, S., James, K.K., Levin, E.G. *et al.* (1989) Local abnormalities in coagulation and fibrinolytic pathways predispose to alveolar fibrin deposition in the adult respiratory distress syndrome. *J. Clin. Invest.*, **84**, 695–705.

22. Seeger, W., Hubel, J., Klapettek, K. *et al.* (1991) Procoagulant activity in bronchoalveolar lavage of severely traumatized patients – relation to the development of acute respiratory distress. *Thromb. Res.* **61**, 53–64.

23. Berggren, P., Lachmann, B., Curstedt, T. *et al.* (1986) Gas exchange and lung morphology after surfactant replacement in experimental adult respiratory distress syndrome induced by repeated lung lavage. *Acta Anaesthesiol. Scand.*, **30**, 321–8.

24. White, C.W., Ghezzi, P. and Dinarello, C.A. *et al.* Recombinant tumor necrosis factor/cachectin and interleukin 1 pretreatment decreases lung oxidized glutathione accumulation, lung injury, and mortality in rats exposed to hyperoxia. *J. Clin. Invest.*, **79**, 1868–73.

25. Lamm, W.J. and Albert, R.K. (1990) Surfactant replacement improves lung recoil in rabbit lungs after acid aspiration. *Am. Rev. Respir. Dis.*, **142** 1279–83.

26. Schuster, D.P. (1994) ARDS: clinical lessons from the oleic acid model of acute lung injury. *Am. J. Respir. Crit. Care Med.*, **149**, 245–60.

27. Barrett, C.R. Jr, Bell, A.L. Jr and Ryan, S.F. (1979) Alveolar epithelial injury causing respiratory distress in dogs: physiologic and electron-microscopic correlations. *Chest*, **75**, 705–11.

28. Lewis, J.F., Ikegami, M. and Jobe, A.H. (1990) Altered surfactant function and metabolism in rabbits with acute lung injury. *J. Appl. Physiol.*, **69**, 2303–10.

29. Gross, N.J. (1991) Surfactant subtypes in experimental lung damage: radiation pneumonitis. *Am. J. Physiol.*, **260**, L302–10.

30. van Daal, G.J., Eijking, E.P. and So, K.L. *et al.* (1992) Acute respiratory failure during pneumonia induced by Sendai virus. *Adv. Exp. Med. Biol.*, **316**, 319–26.

31. Jenkins, J., Carey, P., Byrne, K. *et al.* (1991) Sepsis-induced lung injury and the effects of ibuprofen pretreatment. Analysis of early alveolar events via repetitive bronchoalveolar lavage. *Am. Rev. Respir. Dis.*, **143**, 155–61.

32. Parsons, P.E., Fowler, A.A., Hyers, T.M. and Henson, P.M. (1985) Chemotactic activity in bronchoalveolar lavage fluid from patients with adult respiratory distress syndrome. *Am. Rev. Respir. Dis.*, **132**, 490–3.

33. Jacobs, R.F., Tabor, D.R., Burks, A.W. and Campbell, G.D. (1989) Elevated interleukin-1 release by human alveolar macrophages during the adult respiratory distress syndrome. *Am. Rev. Respir. Dis.*, **140**, 1686–92.

34. Hallgren, R., Samuelsson, T. and Modig, J. (1987) Complement activation and increased alveolar-capillary permeability after major surgery and in adult respiratory distress syndrome. *Crit. Care Med.*, **15**, 189–93.

35. Hallgren, R., Samuelsson, T., Venge, P. and Modig, J. (1987) Eosinophil activation in the lung is related to lung damage in adult respiratory distress syndrome. *Am. Rev. Respir. Dis.*, **135**, 639–42.

36. Robbins R.A., Russ, W.D., Rasmussen, J.K. and Clayton, M.M. (1987) Activation of the complement system in the adult respiratory distress syndrome. *Am. Rev. Respir. Dis.*, **135**, 651–8.

37. Idell, S., Kucich, U. and Fein, A. *et al.* (1985) Neutrophil elastase-releasing factors in bronchoalveolar lavage from patients with adult respiratory distress syndrome. *Am. Rev. Respir. Dis.*, **132**, 1098–105.

38. McGuire, W.W., Spragg, R.G., Cohen, A.B. and Cochrane, C.G. (1982) Studies on the pathogenesis of the adult respiratory distress syndrome. *J. Clin. Invest.*, **69**, 543–53.

39. Braude, S., Apperley, J., Krausz, T. *et al.* (1985) Adult respiratory distress syndrome after allogeneic bone-marrow transplantation: evidence for a neutrophil-independent mechanism. *Lancet* **i**, 239–42.

40. Ognibene, F.P., Martin, S.E., Parker, M.M., *et al.* (1986) Adult respiratory distress syndrome in patients with severe neutropenia. *N. Engl. J. Med.*, **315**, 547–51.

41. Cochrane, C.G., Spragg, R.G. and Revak, S.D. *et al.* (1983) The presence of neutrophil elastase and evidence of oxidation activity in bronchoalveolar lavage fluid of patients with adult respiratory distress syndrome. *Am. Rev. Respir. Dis.*, **127**, 525–7.

42. Haagsman, H.P. and van Golde, L.M. (1985) Lung surfactant and pulmonary toxicology. *Lung*, **163**, 275–303.

43. Lachmann, B. (1989) Animal models and clinical pilot studies of surfactant replacement in adult respiratory distress syndrome. *Eur. Respir. J. [Suppl.]*, **3** 98s–103s.

44. Duane, P.G., Rubins, J.B., Weisel, H.R. and Janoff, E.N. (1993) Identification of hydrogen peroxidase as a *Streptococcus pneumoniae* toxin for rat alveolar epithelial cells. *Infect. Immun.*, **61**, 4392–7.

45. Pacht, E.R., Timerman, A.P., Lykens, M.G. and Merola, A.J. (1991) Deficiency of alveolar fluid glutathione in patients with sepsis and the adult respiratory distress syndrome. *Chest*, **100**, 1397–403.

46. Katsura, K., Kawada, H. and Konno, K. (1993) Rat surfactant apoprotein A (SP-A) exhibits antioxidant effects on alveolar macrophages. *Am. J. Respir. Cell Mol. Biol.*, **9** 520–5.

47. Horowitz, S., Watkins, R.H. and Auten, R.L. Jr *et al.* (1991) Differential accumulation of surfactant protein A, B, and C mRNAs in two epithelial cell types of hyperoxic lung. *Am. J. Respir. Cell Mol. Biol.*, **5**, 511–5.

48. Nash, J., McLaughlin, P., Hoyle, C. and Roberts, D. (1991) Immunolocalization of tumour necrosis factor alpha in lung tissue from patients dying with adult respiratory distress syndrome. *Histopathology*, **19**, 395–402.

49. Lewis-Molock, Y., Suzuki, K., Taniguchi, N. *et al.* (1994) Lung manganese superoxide dismutase increases during cytokine-mediated protection against pulmonary oxygen toxicity in rats. *Am. J. Respir. Cell Mol. Biol.*, **10**, 133–41.

50. Braude, S., Nolop, K.B., Hughes, J.M. *et al.* (1986) Comparison of lung vascular and epithelial permeability indices in the adult respiratory distress syndrome. *Am. Rev. Respir. Dis.*, **133**, 1002–5.

51. Coates, G. and O'Brodovich, H. (1986) Measurement of pulmonary epithelial permability with 99mTc-DTPA aerosol. *Semin. Nucl. Med.*, **16**, 275–84.

52. Rinaldo, J.E., Borovetz, H.S., Mancini, M.C. *et al.* (1986) Assessment of lung injury in the adult respiratory distrss syndrome using multiple dilution curves. *Am. Rev. Respir. Dis.*, **133**, 1006–10.

53. Tennenberg, S.D., Jacobs, M.P. and Solomkin, J.S. (1987) Complement-mediated neutrophil activation in sepsis- and trauma-related adult respiratory distress syndrome. Clarification

with radioaerosol lung scans. *Arch. Surg.*, **122**, 26–32.

54. Tennenberg, S.D., Jacobs, M.P. and Solomkin, J.S. *et al.* (1987) Increased pulmonary alveolar-capillary permeability in patients at risk for adult respiratory distress syndrome. *Crit. Care Med.*, **15**, 289–93.

55. Matthay, M.A. and Wiener-Kronish, J.P. (1990) Intact epithelial barrier function is critical for the resolution of alveolar edema in humans. *Am. Rev. Respir. Dis.*, **142**, 1250–7.

56. Eiermann, G.J., Dickey, B.F. and Thrall, R.S. (1983) Polymorphonuclear leukocyte participation in acute oleic-acid-induced lung injury. *Am. Rev. Respir. Dis.*, **128**, 845–50.

57. Hall, S.B., Notter, R.H., Smith, R.J. and Hyde, R.W. (1990) Altered function of pulmonary surfactant in fatty acid lung injury. *J. Appl. Physiol.*, **69**, 1143–9.

58. Holter, J.F., Weiland, J.E. and Pacht, E.R. *et al.* (1986) Protein permeability in the adult respiratory distrss syndrome. Loss of size selectivity of the alveolar epithelium. *J. Clin. Invest.*, **78**, 1513–22.

59. Byrne, K., Carey, P.D., Sielaff, T.D. *et al.* (1991) Ibuprofen prevents deterioration in static transpulmonary compliance and transalveolar protein flux in septic porcine acute lung injury. *J. Trauma*, **31**, 155–64.

60. Matthay, M.A., Eschenbacher, W.L. and Goetzl, E.J. (1984) Elevated concentrations of leukotriene D$_4$ in pulmonary edema fluid of patients with the adult respiratory distress syndrome. *J. Clin. Immunol.*, **4**, 479–83.

61. Taylor, L., Polgar, P., McAteer, J.A. and Douglas, W.H.J. (1979) Prostaglandin production by type II alveolar epithelial cells. *Biochim. Biophys. Acta*, **572**, 502–8.

62. Suarez, M. and Krieger, B.P. (1986) Bronchoalveolar lavage in recurrent aspirin-induced adult respiratory distress syndrome. *Chest*, **90**, 452–3.

63. Hallman, M., Maasilta, P., Sipila, I. and Tahvanainen, J. (1989) Composition and function of surfactant in adult respiratory distress syndrome. *Eur. Respir. J. [Suppl.]*, **3**, 104s–108s.

64. Weaver, T.E. (1988) Pulmonary surfactant-associated proteins. *Gen. Pharmacol.*, **19**, 361–8.

65. Kuan, S.F., Rust, K. and Crouch, E. (1992) Interactions of surfactant protein D with bacterial lipopolysaccharides. Surfactant protein D is an *Escherichia coli*-binding protein in

bronchoalveolar lavage. *J. Clin. Invest.*, **90** 97–106.

66. Wright, J.R. and Dobbs, L.G. (1991) Regulation of pulmonary surfactant secretion and clearance. *Annu. Rev. Physiol.*, **53**, 395–414.

67. Brown, L.S. and Longmore, W.J. (1981) Adrenergic and cholinergic regulation of lung surfactant secretion in the isolated perfused rat lung and in the alveolar type II cell in culture. *J. Biol. Chem.*, **256**, 66–72.

68. Sano, K., Voelker, D.R. and Mason, R.J. (1987) Tetradecanoylphorbol acetate and terbutaline stimulate surfactant secretion in alveolar type II cells without changing the membrane potential. *Biochim. Biophys. Acta*, **902**, 317–26.

69. Brown, L.S. and Wood, L.H. (1989) Stimulation of surfactant secretion by vasopressin in primary cultures of adult rat type II pneumocytes. *Biochim. Biophys. Acta*, **1001**, 76–81.

70. Oyarzun, M.J. and Clements, J.A. (1978) Control of lung surfactant by ventilation, adrenergic mediators, and prostaglandins in the rabbit. *Am. Rev. Respir. Dis.*, **117**, 879–91.

71. Wirtz, H. and Schmidt, M. (1992) Ventilation and secretion of pulmonary surfactant. *Clin. Invest.*, **70**, 3–13.

72. Chander, A. (1989) Regulation of lung surfactant secretion by intracellular pH. *Am. J. Physiol.*, **257**, L354–60.

73. Burkhardt, R., Von Wichert., P., Batenburg, J.J. and Van Golde, L.M. (1988) Fatty acids stimulate phosphatidylcholine synthesis and CTP:choline-phosphate cytidylyltransferase in type II pneumocytes isolated from adult rat lung. *Biochem. J.*, **254**, 495–500.

74. Gilfillan, A.M. and Rooney, S.A. (1985) Arachidonic acid metabolites stimulate phosphatidylcholine secretion in primary cultures of type II pneumocytes. *Biochim. Biophys. Acta*, **833**, 336–41.

75. Wali, A., Beers, M.F. and Dodia, C. *et al.* ATP and adenosine 3', 5'-cyclic monophosphate stimulate the synthesis of surfactant protein A in rat lung. *Am. J. Physiol.*, **264**, L431–7.

76. Rannels, D.E. and Rannels, S.R. (1989) Influence of the extracellular matrix on type 2 cell differentiation. *Chest*, **96**, 165–73.

77. Shannon, J.M., Jennings, S.D. and Nielsen, L.D. (1992) Modulation of alveolar type II cell differentiated function *in vitro*. *Am. J. Physiol.*, **262**, L427–36.

78. Shannon, J.M., Mason, R.J. and Jennings, S.D. (1987) Functional differentiation of alveolar

type II epithelial cells *in vitro*: effects of cell shape, cell – matrix interactions, and cell–cell interactions. *Biochim. Biophys. Acta*, **931**, 143–56.

79. Dobbs, L.G., Wright, J.R. and, Hawgood, S. *et al.* (1987) Pulmonary surfactant and its components inhibit secretion of phosphatidylcholine from cultured rat alveolar type II cells. *Proc. Natl Acad. Sci. USA*, **84**, 1010–4.

80. Chander, A. and Sen, N. Inhibition of phosphatidylcholine secretion by stilbene disulfonates in alveolar type II cells. *Biochem. Pharmacol.*, **45**, 1905–12.

81. Lewis, J.F. and Jobe, A.H. (1993) Surfactant and the adult respiratory distress syndrome. *Am. Rev. Respir. Dis.*, **147**, 18–33.

82. Seeger, W., Gunther, A., Walmrath, H.D. *et al.* (1993) Alveolar surfactant and adult respiratory distress syndrome. Pathogenetic role and therapeutic prospects. *Clin. Invest.*, **71**, 177–90.

83. Wichert, P. and Kohl, F.V. (1977) Decreased dipalmitoyllecithin content found in lung specimens from patients with so-called shocklung. *Intensive Care Med.*, **3**, 27–30.

84. Hallman, M., Spragg, R. and Harrell, J.H. *et al.* (1982) Evidence of lung surfactant abnormality in respiratory failure. *J. Clin. Invest.*, **70**, 673–83.

85. Pison, U., Seeger, W., Buchhorn, R. *et al.* (1989) Surfactant abnormalities in patients with respiratory failure after multiple trauma. *Am. Rev. Respir. Dis.* **140**, 1033–9.

86. Gregory, T.J., Longmore, W.J., Moxley, M.A., *et al.* (1991) Surfactant chemical composition and biophysical activity in acute respiratory distress syndrome. *J. Clin. Invest.*, **88**, 1976–81.

87. von Wichert, P., Weigers, U. and Stephan, W. *et al.* (1978) Altered metabolism of phosphpolpids in the lung of rats with peritonitis. *Res. Exp. Med.*, **172**, 223–9.

88. Wilke, A., Muller, B. and von Wichert, P. (1987) Ambroxol increases the choline but not the fatty acid incorporation into lung phospholipids in experimental lung disorders. *Respiration*, **52**, 129–36.

89. Petty, T.L., Silvers, G.W., Paul, G.W. and Stanford, R.E. (1979) Abnormalities in lung elastic properties and surfactant function in adult respiratory distress syndrome. *Chest*, **75**, 571–4.

90. Idell, S. and Cohen, A.B. (1985) Bronchoalvear lavage in patients with the adult respiratory distress syndrome. *Clin. Chest Med.*, **6**, 459–71.

91. Holm, B.A. and Matalon, S. (1989) Role of pulmonary surfactant in the development and treatment of adult respiratory distress syndrome. *Anesth. Analg.*, **69**, 805–18.

92. Jacobson, W., Park, G., Saich, T. and Holcroft, J. (1993) Surfactant and the adult respiratory distress syndrome. *Br. J. Anaesth.*, **70**, 522–6.

93. Mason, R.J. (1987) Surfactant in adult respiratory distress syndrome. *Eur. J. Respir. Dis.*, **153**, 229–36.

94. Casals, C., Herrera, L., Miguel, E. *et al.* (1989) Comparison between intra- and extracellular surfactant in respiratory distress induced by oleic acid. *Biochim. Biophys. Acta*, **1003**, 201–3.

95. King, R.J., Coalson, J.J., Seidenfeld, J.J. *et al.* (1989) O_2^- and pneumonia-induced lung injury. II. Properties of pulmonary surfactant. *J. Appl. Physiol.*, **67** 357–65.

96. Rauvala, H. and Hallman, M. (1984) Glycolipid accumulation in bronchoalveolar space in adult respiratory distress syndrome. *J. Lipid Res.*, **25**, 1257–62.

97. Kuroki, Y., Gasa, S., Ogasawara, Y. *et al.* (1992) Binding specificity of lung surfactant protein SP-D for glucosylceramide. *Biochem. Biophys. Res. Commun.*, **187** 963–9.

98. Pison, U., Obertacke, U., Seeger, W. and Hawgood, S. (1992) Surfactant protein A (SP-A) is decreased in acute parenchymal lung injury associated with polytrauma. *Eur. J. Clin. Invest.*, **22**, 12–8.

99. Gross, N.J. (1991) Inhibition of surfactant subtype convertase in radiation model of adult respiratory distress syndrome. *Am. J. Physiol.*, **260**, L311–7.

100. Minoo, P., King R.J. and Coalson, J.J. (1992) Surfactant proteins and lipids are regulated independently during hyperoxia. *Am. J. Physiol.*, **263** 291–8.

101. Massaro, D., Thet, L.A., Massaro, G.D. and Frank, L. (1980) hypothesis relating breathing pattern to some forms of the 'adult respiratory distress syndrome'. *Am. J. Med.*, **69**, 113–5.

102. Li, J.J., Bramlet, S.G., Carter, E.A. and Burke J.F. (1991) The rat lung organotypic culture: an *in vitro* model for studying surfactant metabolism abnormalities. *J. Trauma*, **31**, 174–81.

103. O'Brodovich, H.M., Weitz, J.I. and Possmayer, F. (1990) Effect of fibrinogen degradation products and lung ground substance on surfactant function. *Biol. Neonate*, **57**, 325–33.

104. Vadas, P. (1984) Elevated plasma phospholipase A$_2$ levels: correlation with the hemodynamic and pulmonary changes in Gram-negative septic shock. *J. Lab. Clin. Med.*, **104**, 873–81.

105 Stommer, P. and Steinmann, U. (1989) Phospholipase A$_2$ induced diffuse alveolar damage – effect of indomethacin and dexamethasone upon morphology and plasma-histamine level. *Klin. Wochenschr.*, **67**, 171–6.

106. Cockshutt, A.M. and Possmayer F. (1991) Lysophosphatidylcholine sensitized lipid extracts of pulmonary surfactant to inhibition by serum proteins. *Biochim. Biophys. Acta*, **1086**, 63–71.

107. Guy, J., Dhanireddy, R. and Mukherjee, A.B. (1992) Surfactant-producing rabbit pulmonary alveolar cells synthesize and secrete an antiinflammatory protein, uteroglobin. *Biochem. Biophys. Res. Commun.*, **189**, 662–9.

108. Dobbs, L.G. (1989) Pulmonary surfactant. *Ann. Rev. Med.*, **40**, 431–46.

109. Lachmann, B. (1989) Surfactant therapy. *Resuscitation*, **18**, S37–49.

110. Merritt, T.A., Hallman, M., Spragg, R. *et al.* (1989) Exogenous surfactant treatments for neonatal respiratory distrss syndrome and their potential role in the adult respiratory distress syndrome. *Drugs*, **38**, 591–611.

111. Richman, P.S., Spragg, R.G., Robertson, B *et al.* (1989) The adult respiratory distress syndrome: first trials with surfactant replacement. *Eur. Respir. J. [Suppl.]*, **3**, 109s–111s.

112. Spragg, R.G., Richman, P., Gilliard, N. *et al.* (1989) The use of exogenous surfactant to treat patients with acute high-permeability lung edema. *Prog. Clin. Biol. Res.*, **308**, 791–6.

113. van Daal, G.J., So, K.L. and Gommers, D. *et al.* (1991) Intratracheal surfactant administration restores gas exchange in experimental adult respiratory distress syndrome associated with viral pneumonia. *Anesth. Analg.*, **72**, 589–95.

114. Pinkerton, K.E., Lewis, J., Mulder, A.M. *et al.* (1993) Surfactant treatment effects on alveolar type II cell morphology in rabbit lungs. *J. Appl. Physiol.*, **74**, 1240–7.

115. Lewis, J.F., Ikegami, M. and Jobe, A.H. (1990) Metabolism of exogenously administered sur-

factant in the acutely injured lungs of adult rabbits. *Am. Rev. Respir. Dis.*, **145**, 19–23.

116. Merritt, T.A., Strayer, D.S., Hallman, M *et al.* (1988) Immunologic consequences of exogenous surfactant administration. *Semin. Perinatol.*, **12**, 221–30.

117. Suzuki, Y., Robertson, B., Fujita, Y. and Grossman, G. (1988) Respiratory failure in mice caused by a hybridoma making antibodies to the 15 kDa surfactant apoprotein. *Acta Anaesthesiol. Scand.*, **32**, 283–9.

118. Eijking, E.P., Strayer, D.S., van Daal, G.J. and Lachmann, B. (1991) Effects of antisurfactant antibodies on the course of mild respiratory distress syndrome. *Pathobiology*, **59**, 96–101.

119. Kuhn, C. 3rd, (1991) Patterns of lung repair. A morphologist's view. *Chest*, **99**, 11S–14S.

120. Marinelli, W.A., Henke, C.A., Harmon, K.R. *et al.* (1990) Mechanisms of alveolar fibrosis after acute lung injury. *Clin. Chest Med.*, **11**, 657–672.

121. Snyder, L.S., Hertz, M.I., Harmon, K.R. and Bitterman, P.B. (1990) Failure of lung repair following acute lung injury. Regulation of the fibroproliferative response (Part 1). *Chest*, **98**, 733–8.

122. Kuhn, C. 3rd, Boldt, J., King, J.T.E. *et al.* (1989) An immunohistochemical study of architectural remodeling and connective tissue synthesis in pulmonary fibrosis. *Am. Rev. Respir. Dis.*, **140**, 1693–703.

123. Christner, P., Fein, A., Goldberg, S. *et al.* (1985) Collagenase in the lower respiratory tract of patients with adult respiratory distress syndrome. *Am. Rev. Respir. Dis.*, **131**, 690–5.

124. Raghu, G., Striker, L.J., Hudson, L.D. and Striker, G.E. (1985) Extracellular matrix in normal and fibrotic human lungs. *Am. Rev. Respir. Dis.*, **131**, 281–9.

125. Griffin, M., Bhandari, R. and Hamilton, G. *et al.* (1993) Alveolar type II cell-fibroblast interactions, synthesis and secretion of surfactant and type I collagen. *J. Cell Sci.*, **105**, 423–32.

126. Leslie, C.C., McCormick-Shannon, K. and Mason, R.J. (1990) Heparin-binding growth factors stimulate DNA synthesis in rat alveolar type II cells. *Am. J. Respir. Cell Mol. Biol.*, **2** 99–106.

127. Leslie, C.C., McCormick-Shannon, K., Robinson, P.C. and Mason, R.J. (1985) Stimulation of DNA synthesis in cultured rat alveolar type II cells. *Exp. Lung Res.*, **8** 53–66.

128. Mescher, E.J., Dobbs, L.G. and Mason, R.J.

(1983) Cholera toxin stimulates secretion of saturated phosphatidylcholine and increases cellular cyclic AMP in isolated rat alveolar type II cells. *Exp. Lung Res.*, **5**, 173–82.

129. Leslie, C.C., McCormick-Shannon, K. and Mason, R.J. (1989) Bronchoalveolar lavage fluid from normal rats stimulates DNA synthesis in rat alveolar type II cells. *Am. Rev. Respir. Dis.* **139** 360–6.

130. Fraslon, C. and Bourbon, J. (1992) Comparison of effects of epidermal and insulin-like growth factors, gastrin releasing peptide and retinoic acid on fetal lung cell growth and maturation *in vitro*. *Biochim. Biophys. Acta*, **1123**, 65–75.

131. Mason, R., Leslie, C., McCormick-Shannon, K., *et al.* (1994) Hepatocyte growth factor is a growth factor for rat alveolar type II cells. *Am. J. Respir. Cell Mol. Biol.*, **11**, 561–7.

132. Lin, C.Q. and Bissell, M.J. (1993) Multi-faceted regulation of cell differentiation by extracellular matrix. *FASEB J.*, **7**, 737–43.

133. Pilewski, J. and Abelda, S. (1993) Adhesion molecules in the lung. An overview. *Am. Rev. Respir. Dis.*, **148**, S31–7.

134. Sugahara, K., Kiyota, T., Clark, R.A. and Mason, R.J. (1993) The effect of fibronectin on cytoskeletal structure and transepithelial resistance of alveolar type II cells in primary culture. *Virchows Arch. [B]*, **64**, 115–22.

135. Palmgren, M.S., deShazo, R.D., Carter, R.M. *et al.* (1992) Mechanisms of neutrophil damage to human alveolar extracellular matrix: the role of serine and metalloproteases. *J. Allergy Clin. Immunol.*, **89**, 905–15.

136. Kang, B.H., Crapo, J.D., Wegner, C.D. *et al.* (1993) Intercellular adhesion molecule-1 expression on the alveolar epithelium and its modification by hyperoxia. *Am. J. Respir. Cell Mol. Biol.*, **9**, 350–5.

137. Christensen, P.J., Kim, S., Simon, R.H. *et al.* (1993) Differentiation-related expression of ICAM-1 by rat alveolar epithelial cells. *Am. J. Respir. Cell Mol. Biol.*, **8**, 915.

MECHANISMS OF SCARRING

13

Patricia J. Sime and Jack Gauldie

Pulmonary injury in the syndrome of acute respiratory distress in adults (ARDS) results in disruption of the alveolar-capillary membrane by mechanisms acting directly via the airway or indirectly via the bloodstream [1]. Indeed, within hours of injury there is epithelial and endothelial cell damage and denudation, with exposure and disruption of the epithelial and endothelial basement membranes. Microthrombi form in damaged pulmonary capillaries [2], and breakdown of the alveolar-capillary membrane occurs allowing protein-rich interstitial fluid to flood the alveolus and severely impair gas exchange [3]. Hyaline membranes form [1], and inflammatory cells, initially predominantly activated neutrophils, accumulate in the lung, particularly in the alveolar space (Chapter 4). These cells are an important source of proteolytic enzymes, activated oxygen species and cytokines, which further damage the lung and act as chemoattractants and growth factors for other inflammatory and mesenchymal cells [4,5]. Following this phase of acute lung injury two possible outcomes occur: in those patients who survive, there is effective resolution of the inflammation and repair with restoration of structure and function of the gas exchange unit; whereas in some of those who die a respiratory death, an acute fibroproliferative response involving the alveolar space, interstitium and intra-acinar microvasculature supervenes [3]. Such fibrosis can occur within one week of injury

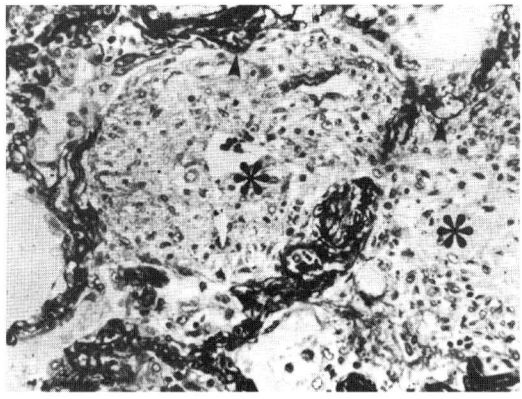

Figure 13.1 Diffuse intra-alveolar fibrosis obliterating the air space after severe acute lung injury. (×150). The epithelial basement membranes (arrows) define the border between the intra-alveolar fibrosis and the alveolar wall. (Reproduced from Fukuda *et al.* [1].)

[2]. During effective repair, type II epithelial cells replicate and differentiate into type I cells, repairing the epithelium; mesenchymal cells proliferate and secrete extracellular matrix in a tightly controlled fashion, repairing the interstitium; and endothelial cells replicate and recanalise to restore vascular patency. By contrast, when a maladaptive fibroproliferate response occurs (Figure 13.1), the alveolar space becomes filled with mesenchymal cells, their connective tissue products and new blood vessels, i.e. the air space becomes granulated [6]. Fibroblasts and myofibroblasts in the interstitium become acti-

ARDS Acute Respiratory Distress in Adults. Edited by Timothy W. Evans and Christopher Haslett. Published in 1996 by Chapman & Hall, London. ISBN 0 412 56910 8

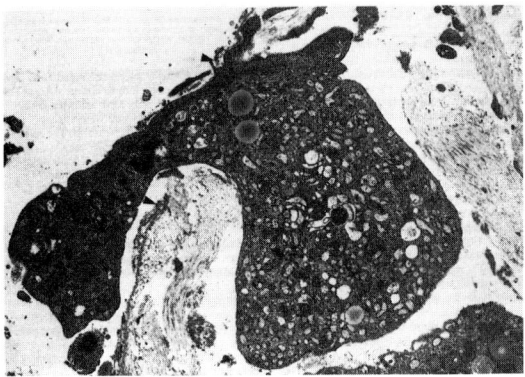

Figure 13.2 A myofibroblast passing through the gap (arrow) in the epithelial basement membrane into the alveolar space. (×100). (Reproduced from Fukuda *et al.* [1].)

vated, migrate through gaps in the damaged basement membrane (Figure 13.2) and attach to the luminal surface of this membrane, where they replicate and secrete matrix elements, including collagens and proteoglycans [1,7]. In patients surviving for more than 10 days there is a 2–3-fold increase in collagen content of the lung [8], particularly the I and III isotypes [9]. Much of this increased collagen is located in the alveolar space [7]. Fibronectin, a potent chemoattractant and growth factor for mesenchymal cells, is also abundant in these areas of intra-alveolar fibrosis [1]. Capillary networks grow into the fibrosing alveolus to form an integral part of the granulation tissue in the air space [10]. This granulation tissue is very similar to that found during dermal injury and repair, but because of its physical situation in the air space there are disastrous physiological consequences due to impaired gas exchange. Fibroproliferative responses also occur in the interstitium and in the vascular intima and media, with resultant luminal narrowing [6], contributing to the production of a lung incapable of efficient gas exchange. The mesenchymal cell response is therefore a vital determinant of the outcome of acute lung injury in ARDS. In this chapter we discuss our current understanding of the mechanisms controlling this mesenchymal response using data from patients with ARDS, from animal models of acute lung injury, and from models of dermal wound healing because of the pathophysiological and morphological similarities of this process to those involved in acute lung injury.

ROLE OF CYTOKINES AND EXTRACELLULAR MATRIX IN THE CONTROL OF INFLAMMATION AND FIBROSIS

The reason(s) why the inflammation in ARDS is followed by resolution and repair in some patients, while others develop persisting inflammation and fibrosis, is unclear. Continuing insult is one possibility, but is not often clinically evident in patients with ARDS. Rather, changes intrinsic to the pulmonary tissue itself in terms of production of cytokines and growth factors and/or changes in the phenotype of inflammatory and structural cells (fibroblasts, endothelial, epithelial and smooth muscle cells) are more likely. Indeed, there is much data from studies *in vitro* and *in vivo* implicating cytokines in the regulation of the inflammatory response which contributes to fibrosis, and in the regulation of the structural cell response. Cytokines are released in a co-ordinated sequence. Early in the course of the acute inflammatory response cytokines such as interleukin (IL)-1α and β, tumor necrosis factor (TNF)α, IL-8 and monocyte chemotactic protein (MCP)-1, are released and participate in the accumulation of monocytes and neutrophils (Chapter 7). Later, when inflammation is full blown, other cytokines, including platelet derived growth factor (PDGF), colony stimulating factors (CSFs) and insulin-like growth factors (IGFs) are produced, followed in some cases by transforming growth factor expression (TGF)β [11]. These act locally within the extracellular microenvironment and elements of this extracellular microenvironment also have effector functions relevant to the control of inflammation and fibrosis.

INTERLEUKIN 1

There are two distinct IL-1 proteins, IL-1α and IL-1β, encoded by separate genes on chromosome 2. They are secreted as 31 kDa precursors that are then processed to 17.5 kDa peptides [12]. IL-1α is usually cell associated [13] and IL-β is the predominant form secreted into the extracellular fluid [13]. They bind to two IL-1 receptors with equal affinity, and have identical biological activities [14]. As mentioned earlier, IL-1 is produced early in the inflammatory process and is vitally important in amplifying the response by recruiting and activating the tissue structural cells. Upon stimulation by IL-1, fibroblasts and other tissue structural cells secrete IL-1, IL-6, IL-8, MCP-1, PDGF, CSFs and TGFβ [15–18], and IL-1 can induce the autocrine production of PDGF by fibroblasts [19]. IL-1 stimulates collagen and glycosaminoglycan formation and also enhances collagenase production by fibroblasts [14]. It increases vascular permeability, induces procoagulant activity by endothelial cells and is important in leukocyte accumulation by induction of the adhesion molecules ICAM-1 and ELAM-1 in the vasculature [20]. IL-1 promotes lymphocyte proliferation, differentiation and immunoglobulin production and activates natural killer (NK) cells, monocytes and macrophages [21]. It can also induce an acute phase response by a direct or indirect (via IL-6) action on hepatocytes [22]. We and others have demonstrated that the cellular sources of IL-1 include monocytes/macrophages, neutrophils and IL-1 and TNFα stimulated structural cells [23,24]. IL-1 is certainly capable of inducing acute pulmonary injury, as seen when it is infused intravenously into rabbits [25]. In our own model of acute lung injury induced by intratracheal lipopolysaccharide (LPS) in rats we found an early rise in

IL-1 mRNA expression in both neutrophils and macrophages, suggesting an association between IL-1 production and lung injury [24]. Using a bleomycin model of pulmonary fibrosis, Phan and Kunkel [26] also indicated a role for IL-1 in the generation of fibrosis. There was increased IL-1 production by alveolar macrophages in (CBA) mice susceptible to bleomycin induced fibrosis, but no increases in IL-1 in macrophages in a strain (BALB/c) not susceptible to such fibrosis. IL-1 levels are elevated in the bronchoalveolar lavage fluid (BAL) of patients with ARDS [27], and macrophages isolated from such patients show increased spontaneous and LPS stimulated release of IL-1 *in vitro* [28]. IL-1 is therefore associated with injury in ARDS, although its role in the pathogenesis of fibrosis is at present unknown. Nevertheless, in other diseases such as idiopathic pulmonary fibrosis (IPF), where fibrosis is the predominant pathological abnormality, there is also evidence of increased IL-1 production [29].

TUMOR NECROSIS FACTOR

Tumor necrosis factor exists in two forms: TNFα and TNFβ. They share the same receptors and have similar biological activities, although TNFα is more potent. TNFα is produced by monocytes, macrophages, neutrophils and activated tissue structural cells [30]. TNFα is not normally constitutively expressed *in vivo* but is induced rapidly following injury. For example, we have detected mRNA and protein for TNFα within one hour in an endotoxin model of acute lung injury in the rat [23]. This early upregulation of TNFα (mRNA changes as early as 30 minutes) occurs in concert with IL-1, and indeed TNFα and IL-1 share many of the same biological activities. TNFα acts synergistically with IL-1 to amplify the local inflammatory response by recruiting tissue structural cells and inducing their production of cytokines, including IL-1, IL-6, IL-8, MCP-1, CSFs, PDGF and TGFβ [11,31,32]. Because of their large number these cells are a huge potential source of cytokine producing effector cells. TNFα also activates monocytes, macrophages and neutrophils *in vitro* and has similar effects to IL-1 on endothelial cells, increasing vascular permeability, procoagulant activity and expression of adhesion molecules. These actions on leukocytes and endothelial cells are likely to be important in the mechanism of production of injury in ARDS. TNFα is angiogenic *in vitro* and *in vivo* [33], and may therefore also be important in the production of the vascular component of the granulation tissue that fills the air space in patients with ARDS. BAL fluids from patients with ARDS certainly show increased levels of TNFα and its inhibitors [27,34]. Evidence for a direct role for TNFα in the sequence of events leading to fibrosis comes from studies using anti-TNFα pretreatment of animals challenged with fibrogenic agents, such as bleomycin or silica dust, where pretreatment abrogates hydroxyproline accumulation, a marker of collagen deposition and hence fibrosis [35,36]. However, transient TNFα administration alone is insufficient for fibrosis in experimental animal systems, and in the LPS model of acute lung injury we found transient TNFα expression which was compatible with rapid repair without fibrosis [24]. By contrast, the prolonged elevations of TNFα which occur in silica induced pulmonary fibrosis may be important [36]. In patients with the fibrotic conditions pneumoconiosis and sarcoidosis there are also reports that stimulated alveolar macrophages produce increased levels of TNFα [37,38]. However, data concerning the role of TNF in the fibrosis of ARDS are not yet available and a role for TNFα remains speculative.

INTERLEUKIN 8

Interleukin 8 is an 8.4 kDa protein that is relatively resistant to proteolysis and denaturation. It functions as a potent and relatively selective chemoattractant for neutrophils [39]. It also activates neutrophils, increasing expression of the integrins CD11b/CD18, initiating a respiratory burst, promoting exocytosis of damaging lysosomal enzymes and increasing production of lipid mediators of inflammation such as leukotriene (LT)B$_4$ [40]. Fibroblasts are an important source of IL-8 as they make large quantities of this cytokine after stimulation by IL-1 or TNF [41]. Alveolar macrophages and stimulated human endothelial and smooth muscle cells can also produce IL-8 [42]. Neutrophil accumulation and activation are the hallmarks of the early changes in ARDS [4,43], and recently Donnelly *et al.* have demonstrated increased levels of IL-8 in the BAL of patients at the earliest stages of the risk period of ARDS [44]. In patients with the chronic fibrotic pulmonary disorder IPF, increased IL-8 mRNA production has also been detected, and Strieter *et al.* [42] have shown a correlation between the level of IL-8 mRNA expression and the percentage of polymorphonuclear neutrophils in the BAL of these patients. However, while a role for IL-8 seems likely in the acute injury of ARDS, its role in inducing fibrosis is uncertain.

MONOCYTE CHEMOATTRACTANT PROTEIN 1 AND MACROPHAGE INFLAMMATORY PROTEINS 1α AND 2

Monocyte chemoattractant protein (MCP)-1 and macrophage inflammatory proteins (MIP)-1α and -2 are members of the C-C chemokine family. They are chemotactic for mononuclear cells, and MCP-1 can produce activation of monocytes *in vitro* [45,46]. MCP-1 is produced by stimulated monocytes and IL-1 or TNF stimulated fibroblasts, endothelial cells and alveolar epithelium [47]. MCP-1, like MIP-1α, is involved in the production of granulomatous inflammation.

Fibroblasts isolated from schistosomal induced hepatic granulomas have recently been shown to produce increased MCP-1 and MIP-α *in vitro* [48], and neutralization of MIP-1α *in vivo* can alter granuloma growth and development [49]. In models of pulmonary fibrosis in rats induced by silica and titanium dioxide, increased MIP-1α and MIP-2 mRNA and protein have been found in lung [50] and a role has been postulated for these mediators in inflammatory cell recruitment. In patients with pulmonary fibrosis MIP-1α expression was identified in the BAL and lung tissue of 22 of 23 patients with sarcoid, and 9 of 9 patients with IPF, but in only one healthy subject [51], and MCP-1 has been found in the BAL and lung tissue of patients with IPF [52]. In the latter study the increase in MCP in BAL was correlated with the absolute increase in mononuclear phagocytes, and the authors suggested that the levels of MCP were sufficient to lead to recruitment and activation of mononuclear cells *in vivo*. It therefore seems likely that these chemokines are important in mononuclear cell accumulation and granuloma formation and it would not be surprising if these cytokines were important in the formation of granulation tissue in patients with ARDS.

PLATELET DERIVED GROWTH FACTOR

Platelet derived growth factor is a highly cationic glycoprotein of 28–35 kDa composed of two polypeptide chains (A and B) linked as a dimer by disulfide bonds. Three forms of the dimer have been described: AA and BB homodimers and an AB heterodimer [53]. They have similar biological effects. The major action of PDGF is as a mitogen for fibroblasts and smooth muscle cells by initiating their transition from quiesent nonreplicating cells into the G_1 phase of the cell cycle [54]. PDGF is also a chemoattractant for fibroblasts and smooth muscle cells, and is important in autocrine loops as a secondary mediator of the mitogenic effects of weakly mitogenic cytokines such as IL-1, TNF and TGFβ [19,55]. PDGF was originally detected in the α granules of platelets, and is also produced by activated fibroblasts, smooth muscle cells, endothelial and epithelial cells,

macrophages and monocytes [56,57]. PDGF and PDGF-like moities have been found in BAL fluid during the course of ARDS. In a study of 26 patients, fibroblast proliferation and migration promoting activity was found in BAL fluids, attributed to three peptides related to PDGF [58]. While it is tempting therefore to suggest a role for PDGF in intra-alveolar fibrosis, it is unlikely that a transient elevation of PDGF alone is sufficient for fibrogenesis, as a substantial number of such patients will go on to repair their lung tissues effectively without fibrosis. Indeed, in a model of hyperoxia induced acute lung injury there was transient elevation of PDGF mRNA but no fibrosis [59], and following acute cutaneous injury in which PDGF mRNA is rapidly induced, it is also rapidly suppressed when normal healing is complete [60]. Little evidence is available on the expression of PDGF in patients with chronic lung disease, but elevated levels of PDGF mRNA (in alveolar macrophages and epithelial cells) have been found in four patients with IPF, but not in normal lung [61]. Therefore, although transient PDGF expression is insufficient for production of fibrosis, prolonged PDGF expression or PDGF expression in the context of an altered structural cell phenotype may be important in the type of fibroproliferative response which occurs in patients with ARDS.

COLONY STIMULATING FACTORS

Colony stimulating factors are acidic glycoproteins defined by the type of granulocyte colonies which they induce from blood or bone marrow precursors. Three different CSFs are recognized: macrophage colony stimulating factor (M-CSF), granulocyte colony stimulating factor (G-CSF), and granulocyte-macrophage colony stimulating factor (GM-CSF). G-CSF is an 18 kDa glycosylated polypeptide that functions to induce granulocytic neutrophil differentiation from marrow stem cells. It also activates mature neutrophils with the release of activated oxygen species and increased antibody dependent cytotoxicity. M-CSF (CSF-1) is a dimer of 80 kDa that selectively stimulates monocyte differentiation from stem cells. It activates macrophages and monocytes, increasing the production of proteinases and cytokines, including IL-1 and TNF. GM-CSF is a 15 – 30 kDa glycoprotein that induces differentiation of neutrophils, eosinophils, monocytes/macrophages, megakaryocytes and early erythroid cells from stem cell progenitors [62]. LPS and cytokine stimulated macrophages and monocytes are major sources of all the CSFs [63] and we have recently shown that, like other tissues, respiratory tract fibroblasts and epithelial cells constitutively produce all three CSFs *in vitro* [64,65]. Vascular smooth muscle and endothelial cells are also capable of releasing CSFs, and production of these by the tissue structural cells is increased through stimulation by IL-1 and TNF [66]. We have shown that conditioned media from respiratory derived epithelial cells and fibroblasts can prolong the survival of peripheral blood neutrophils, eosinophils and monocytes due to the content of the three CSFs [62]. Such prolongation of survival of inflammatory cells, through avoidance of normal apoptotic mechanisms, may also be important *in vivo*, allowing increased activation of these cells by cytokines and increased tissue damage. Most inflammatory cells are derived from bone marrow, but CSFs may also be able to act locally within the tissue to provide the terminal differentiation step for peripheral blood granulocyte precursors which also exist. Evidence for a role of CSFs in the production of fibrosis *in vivo* comes from studies in which GM-CSF was infused by the subcutaneous route in rats for 7 days using a mini-osmotic pump, and a significant accumulation of fibroblasts, a moderate leukocyte infiltration and neovascularization were found [67]. Few studies of the role of CSFs in pulmonary inflammation and fibrosis have been performed, although increased mRNA for GM-CSF in TNF induced pulmonary inflammation [68] and immunoreactive GM-CSF have been identified in the BAL of asthmatic patients [69]. Nevertheless it is likely that GM-CSF plays a role in establishing and maintaining chronic inflammation in patients with ARDS.

TRANSFORMING GROWTH FACTOR β

Transforming growth factor β (TGFβ) is a 25 kDa protein that was first identified as conferring anchorage independent growth or a 'transformed' phenotype to stromal cells. There are five subtypes, but only TGFβ1, TGFβ2 and TGFβ3 are found in mammalian tissue. TGFβ is produced in a latent form that requires cleavage by proteases or acids for activation. It has important effects on stromal cells *in vitro* and these effects may be important in promoting fibrosis in the lungs of patients with ARDS. TGFβ is chemotactic for fibroblasts and can cause fibroblasts from both normal and remodeling lung to proliferate [70]. This mitogenic effect is mediated through the induction of PDGF [71] in the responding cells in an autocrine fashion. TGFβ can also induce its own synthesis in target cells, resulting in the production of a cell with a potentially aggressive autostimulatory phenotype. However, not all cells respond to TGFβ by proliferating. The effect depends on the tissue of origin of the responding cell, the presence of other cytokines and culture conditions. Production of many extracellular matrix components, including collagens [72], fibronectin [73] and fibronectin receptor, chondroitin- and dermatan-sulfate proteoglycans [74], hyaluronan [75] and integrins are all stimulated by TGFβ. Conversely, TGFβ decreases synthesis of matrix degrading enzymes, such as collagenases, and increases the synthesis of protease inhibitors, and therefore has great potential for stimulating the deposition of extracellular matrix components important in producing a rigid, fibrotic lung. TGFβ also has an immunomodulatory role *in vitro*, enhancing monocyte functions and suppressing lymphocyte functions, and has anti-inflammatory activities including downregulation of macrophages [76], direct TNFα antagonism, and inhibition of neutrophil and T lymphocyte adhesion to endothelium. The importance of the anti-inflammatory role of TGFβ is emphasized by studies of TGFβ deficient mice who die of a wasting syndrome and widespread inflammation about 20 days after birth [77]. The neonatal protection seen in these animals derives from placental transfer of TGFβ from the mother [78]. TGFβ is produced *in vitro* by activated macrophages, neutrophils and fibroblasts [70]. TGFβ expression in pulmonary tissues has been most extensively studied in the rodent bleomycin model. Many authors have found increased TGFβ production in animals developing fibrosis [79,80], and maximal TGFβ expression has been shown at one week, preceding the increase in gene expression for procollagens, fibronectin and laminin [81]. This temporal relationship would be in keeping with a role for TGFβ in inducing expression of these extracellular matrix genes *in vivo*. Our own studies, using a cadmium chloride model of pulmonary fibrosis, showed an increase in TGFβ gene expression four days after instillation. By contrast, in the LPS model of acute lung injury, where healing and repair occur without fibrosis, we found no such TGFβ gene induction. TGFβ can also produce granulation tissue formation when infused subcutaneously in rats [82]. This tissue is rich in α smooth muscle actin-expressing myofibroblasts, which may be important in the generation of fibrotic tissue (discussed later). In humans, lung biopsies of four patients with IPF were found to have TGFβ mRNA localized to areas of macrophage aggregation, and TGFβ protein in alveolar buds populated by fibroblasts [83]. In other human studies, TGFβ production was shown in bronchiolar epithelium of patients with IPF, but not in normal subjects [84], and TGFβ mRNA and TGFβ protein have been found in tissue sites where active extracellular matrix deposition is occurring in patients with IPF but not in biopsies of patients who had ongoing inflammation but little or no associated fibrosis [85]. Based on this *in vivo* and *in vitro* data it would seem very likely that TGFβ has an important role in controlling fibrosis and inflammation in ARDS.

FIBROBLAST DERIVED GROWTH FACTOR AND INSULIN-LIKE GROWTH FACTORS

A number of other cytokines and growth factors may also be important in the production of fibrosis in ARDS. Fibroblast growth factors (FGFs) have been identified in lung. They are produced *in vitro* by fibroblasts and vascular smooth muscle cells and can regulate the proliferation and differentiation of a variety of mesenchymal cells [86]. FGFs can also stimulate angiogenesis both *in vitro* and *in vivo* [87] and basic FGF has been detected in the BAL of patients with ARDS [88]. The IGFs are another family of small peptides which may have a role in control of mesenchymal cell proliferation as they are cellular mitogens [89]. They, too, are produced by fibroblasts and can stimulate these cells in an autocrine and paracrine fashion [90]. Exaggerated amounts of IGF-1 have been demonstrated in alveolar macrophages in patients with chronic fibrotic lung disorders [91] but further studies are required to establish a role, if any, for these factors in lung cell biology and in pathological conditions such as ARDS.

EXTRACELLULAR MATRIX AS AN EFFECTOR

There is increasing evidence that components of the extracellular matrix have effector functions during the processes of inflammation and fibrosis through direct binding of cytokines, and by direct effects on structural cells. Both glycosaminoglycans and proteoglycans can bind cytokines, possibly protecting them from proteolytic degradation, and controlling their local concentration. The glycosaminoglycan heparan sulfate, for example, binds FGF [92], GM-CSF and IL-3 [93], and this binding is important in the interaction of FGF with its receptor [94]. TGFβ binds at the cell surface to the proteoglycan betaglycan (which acts as a nonsignal transducing receptor), and in the extracellular matrix to another proteoglycan decorin [95]. Decorin neutralizes the activity of TGFβ, and as the synthesis of decorin by various cell types is stimulated by TGFβ itself, decorin is an effector molecule in a negative feedback loop regulating TGFβ activity [96]. Such a role for decorin as a feedback regulator for TGFβ would be a possible area for investigation, particularly in situations where prolonged expression of active TGFβ occurs in the tissue, as seen in IPF [84,85] or liver fibrosis [97,98]. Fibronectin, another component of the extracellular environment, also has a potential effector role as it is both chemotactic and mitogenic for fibroblasts *in vitro*. Its deposition is certainly prominent in the hyaline membranes of patients with ARDS [1].

CELLULAR INTERACTIONS IN INFLAMMATION AND FIBROSIS

Subsequent to the trauma and/or infective processes seen in ARDS, a number of cells become involved in propagation of the host response and have profound impact on the outcome of the process. Infectious agents can directly activate alveolar macrophages, interstitial macrophages and dendritic cells, such that they release not only the small molecular weight elements of the arachidonic acid cascade along with other vasoactive mediators, but also the early acting cytokines, including IL-1 and TNF, resulting in the initiation of a very potent cytokine and cellular cascade. Trauma can result in similar activation, but may also include mediators such as PDGF and TGFβ released from platelets, as they too

can enter into the progression of the host response.

The response to this tissue injury is inflammation followed by repair, and in the context of a scarring response the most significant mediators are those of the cytokine families described previously. Thus, while the monocyte macrophage can release a very broad spectrum of fibrogenic cytokines, it is the immediate and early release of IL-1 and TNF that likely have the most profound effect, through activation of adjacent cells to release a further spectrum of factors influencing recruitment, growth and repair, and resulting in marked augmentation of the signals from the inflammatory foci in the tissue. IL-1 and TNF are capable of eliciting cytokine responses from adjacent endothelial cells, smooth muscle cells and fibroblasts as well as epithelial cells. The second wave cytokines include a spectrum of growth factors, including PDGF, FGF, IGFs and TGFβ, chemokines such as IL-8 for neutrophils, MCP-1 for monocytes and other mononuclear cells and immune regulatory molecules, such as the many interleukins, suggesting that the entire tissue becomes the source of the mediators, resulting in the accumulation of further inflammatory cells and further tissue damage [3,6].

As a result of this propagation of inflammation, mediators released by the full spectrum of cells involved in the trauma act not only in an endocrine fashion on distal organs and tissues, but importantly can also affect the behavior of local mesenchymal cells in a paracrine and even autocrine fashion. It thus appears logical that factors resulting in local scarring subsequent to ARDS are generated locally and may function solely within the environment of the parenchymal tissue and have little or no apparent impact on events and organs throughout the organism.

While the outcome of the scarring response implies that cells such as the fibroblast may be the target for many of the factors released within the tissue, it must also be assumed that

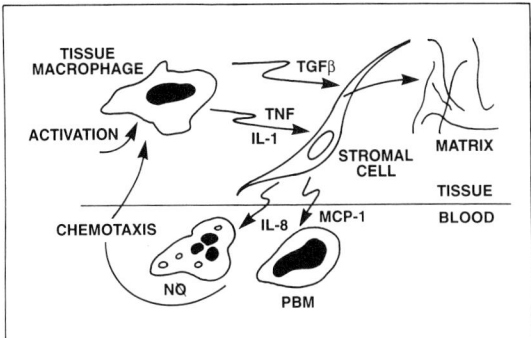

Figure 13.3 Cell and cytokine cascades with resultant modulation of matrix deposition. Activation of tissue macrophages releases IL-1 and TNF, which in turn activate stromal cells to release chemokines that bring further inflammatory cells to the tissue and release matrix stimulating cytokines (TGFβ) to act further on the stromal cell. NØ, peripheral blood neutrophil; PBM, peripheral blood monocyte.

these same target cells contribute to the propagation of the response through feedback cascades on inflammatory and other tissue cells, thereby amplifying the overall effect on their own behavior. Figure 13.3 demonstrates conceptually how factors released from inflammatory cells can regulate the behavior of mesenchymal cells and in turn how second wave factors from the mesenchyme can control the behaviour of inflammatory cells, thus establishing a positive cascade, which, if allowed to continue unchecked, would result in profound tissue remodeling.

RESPONSE OF THE STROMA

In examining the morphology of the scarring events in ARDS, it is evident that there is both a proliferative response of fibroblasts as well as a change in the phenotype of these cells, resulting in marked tissue alteration and disordered collagen deposition typical of fibroblastic scarring. We shall attempt to separate these two events but it is recognized that factors which mediate proliferation may also

mediate phenotype alteration and thus involve similar kinetics in the development of the scarring response.

Proliferation

A number of the cytokines described above have profound effects on the proliferation of fibroblasts. PDGF, IGFs and FGFs can all influence the proliferative capacity of mesenchymal cells. Fibroblasts that repopulate an area after pulmonary tissue destruction appear to involve both chemotaxis of adjacent cells and local proliferation [6]. In models of dermal wound healing, which can arguably represent similar events throughout mesenchymal tissues [99], there is a profound temporal association between the appearance of fibroblast modulating cytokines and the appearance of increased numbers of fibroblasts, as well as the demonstration of products made by these same cells, such as collagen and other extracellular matrix proteins [60]. Since the skin has much easier access for experimental examination, one must assume that a similar temporal association exists within the injured lung, as there are limited studies outlining such findings in ARDS. Most situations in which tissue has been obtained have progressed significantly beyond the early stage of healing and therefore do not represent what could best be described as a true physiologic response. However, examination of the dermal wound system reveals that molecules expected to be present, such as IGF and FGF, are indeed demonstrated (Figure 13.4) and from other data it can be inferred that interrupting this sequence of cytokine and cell interactions results in aberrant wound healing and possible scarring [35,36]. Keloid scars may be visible examples of this disordered process and may be akin to fibrotic changes seen in extensive scarring within the lung.

After acute injury the repair process invariably involves proliferation of mesenchymal cells. One expects PDGF to be a prominent

bFGF

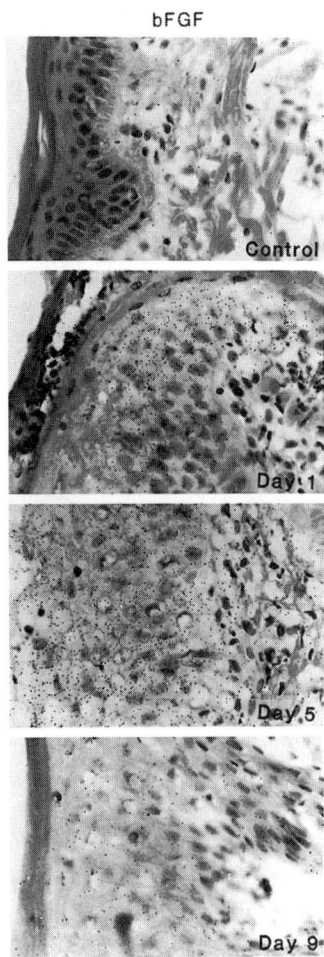

Figure 13.4 Expression of bFGF mRNA in skin epithelial cells before and after cutaneous injury. There is no significant expression of bFGF mRNAs in the epithelial cells of control, uninjured tissue. Expression can be seen within 1 day of injury, remaining strong for about 5 days, declining by day 9, and was completely suppressed by day 17 after injury. (×630). (Reproduced from Antoniades *et al.* [60].)

component of this response [100] and PDGF may, in and of itself, be an obligatory component of repair but need not be a component of fibrosis or scarring. Taking data from a variety of sources it could be argued that further cytokines such as TGFβ, or CSFs like GM-CSF, may be more likely involved in the

scarring response. Examination of damage to fetal skin shows that these wounds heal without scarring. It is only in the neonatal stage or adult stage that dermal tissue injury leads to scar formation [101–103]. Fetal skin does not demonstrate TGFβ production or presence during or after wound responses, whereas in the neonatal and/or adult tissue the presence of TGFβ is always associated with the scarring outcome. Moreover, data [85] showing a temporal and spatial association of the presence of TGFβ with activation of collagen gene expression in IPF tissue imply a special role for this cytokine in fibrogenic responses [102,104,105]. Indeed, in examining the temporal expression of cytokines associated with cadmium chloride administration to rat lung, we found that, early on, molecules such as TNF are significantly expressed and this 'early wave' of gene expression is followed by a 'secondary wave' of expression of PDGF. Subsequent to the decrease in expression of PDGF, a rise in the expression of TGFβ is then seen associated with fibrotic changes in this particular model [106]. Furthermore, the demonstration that prolonged expression of TGFβ leads to a fibrogenesis associated with fibroblast accumulation and phenotype alteration [82,87], and similar outcomes seen in chronic administration of GM-CSF [67,107], make a case that proliferation subsequent to injury is a normal and expected response mediated through the expression of cytokine genes such as PDGF and FGF. However, the switching on of enhanced expression of genes such as TGFβ and/or GM-CSF is associated with the more chronic stage of scarring and fibrotic response as seen in the sequelae of acute lung injury [79]. Proliferation, therefore, is the necessary response to repair the tissue. Chronic proliferation, mesenchymal cell phenotype alteration and matrix gene enhanced expression may be regulated by growth factors such as TGFβ that are inappropriately expressed or not suppressed in a normal fashion [102,108].

Mesenchymal cell phenotype

Morphologic examination of repairing tissue demonstrates that fibroblasts, smooth muscle cells and endothelial cells (and where appropriate epithelial cells) all appear to be involved in proliferation and restructuring of the tissue. However, it has become clear recently, through more detailed examination of the cells that make up granulation tissue, that the mesenchymal cells exhibit considerable heterogeneity and phenotypic differences. In recovering from acute injury, lung tissue contains fibroblasts that exhibit enhanced proliferative capacity *in vitro* [109], and examination of chronically inflamed lung tissue, such as seen in human IPF and animal models, demonstrates that cells that have repopulated the damaged area are morphologically fibroblasts with an enhanced proliferative capacity and altered gene expression, and may be more akin to myofibroblasts [110–113]. If the lung is injured, such as in the experimental bleomycin model, the areas of tissue damage are areas in which fibroblasts begin to express genes of a smooth muscle nature, that is the presence of α smooth muscle actin in cells that morphologically are fibroblasts [111]. Other evidence implies that the conversion from fibroblast-type cells to myofibroblasts can occur in cells, even though they do not express smooth muscle actin [114]. In other words, injury leads to repair but repair may involve prominent myofibroblast presence in the granulation tissue, which may derive from pre-existing fibroblasts or other cells such as the pericyte [115], or even smooth muscle cells themselves. Evidence for this interaction is scanty but the presence of myofibroblasts in repairing tissue is striking and, as their appearance is transient, the derivation of the cell likely is from local tissue. However, little is known of the true nature of the stem cell for the fibroblast and thus the direct differentiation pathway *in vivo* must remain an open question.

If normal lung fibroblasts are placed in culture and exposed to varying concentrations of TGFβ we can demonstrate that they acquire the ability to express α smooth muscle actin and can therefore be classified as myofibroblasts [116]. The fact that this cytokine is one prominent in scarring tissue and that myofibroblasts are associated with granulation and scarring tissue might imply that the overexpression of, or presence of, TGFβ gives rise to the phenotypic differentiation of some mesenchymal cells. These cells in turn play a prominent role in the response of the tissue, resulting in the enhanced presence of mesenchymal cells and disordered extracellular matrix production. Indeed, administration of TGFβ or GM-CSF to tissue results in myofibroblast appearance (α smooth muscle actin-positive cells) and this temporal appearance of phenotypically altered cells may again indicate that any situation resulting in the overexpression of molecules such as TGFβ or GM-CSF could lead to prolonged fibrogenic cellular responses and scarring [67,83,117]. How these particular cytokines are initiated in their expression and why they are not controlled adequately to result in repair without scarring is an unknown and interesting area for investigation.

SUMMARY

Since the mid-1980s the cloning and identification of a large number of biologically important molecules or cytokines released from many cells during inflammatory responses at times appear to complicate our understanding of physiologic processes. Injury, repair and scarring are outcomes of a spectrum of responses mediated by these various factors. Injury leads to activation of the alarm systems in the lung and release of molecules such as IL-1 and TNF. Normally this would activate adjacent mesenchymal cells, repair the damaged tissue and return the lung to normal function. This would involve expression of other 'second wave' cytokines, resulting in homeostatic responses, and include expression of PDGF and FGF and proliferative activation of mesenchymal cells such as fibroblasts and smooth muscle cells. However, if the process proceeds to the next stage, in which there is overexpression of other cytokines such as TGFβ and/or CSFs, this leads to the stage of chronic proliferation, mesenchymal cell phenotypic alteration and finally matrix gene expression resulting in scar formation, and this fibrotic outcome is associated with altered lung function.

Obviously there are processes we poorly understand which would also contribute to these outcomes. Aspects of scar resolution are not well understood. How and why scar tissue is removed or why these normal processes are not switched on in the chronic stage all require intense investigation. Recently, data were presented indicating a role for apoptosis in the resolution of repairing tissue in the lung [118]. This is likely to be a further area for investigation because destruction of this normal resolving process would lead to constant tissue accumulation and fibrotic sequelae. Whether molecules such as TGFβ can interfere with this normal resolving process is unknown; however, we do know that molecules such as GM-CSF can interfere with normal apoptotic mechanisms in hemopoietic cells [62]. It is possible therefore that overexpression of these molecules in the chronic stage of tissue injury could interfere with the normal resolving processes mediated by mechanisms such as apoptosis, and lead to the constant accumulation of phenotypically altered mesenchymal cells, resulting in the presence of disordered matrix deposition and altered organ function. Obviously there is considerable room for the investigation of these possibilities but it would suggest that treatment regimens aimed at restoring normal apoptotic processes or interfering with the expression of genes such as TGFβ or GM-CSF might have a beneficial effect in the treatment of scarring associated with ARDS.

REFERENCES

1. Fukuda, Y., Ishizaki, M., Masuda, Y. *et al.* (1987) The role of intraalveolar fibrosis in the process of pulmonary structural remodeling in patients with diffuse alveolar damage. *American Journal of Pathology,* **126**, 171–82.

2. Jones, R., Langleben, D. and Reid, L.M. (1985) Patterns of remodeling of the pulmonary circulation in acute and subacute lung injury, in *The Pulmonary Circulation and Acute Lung Injury* (ed. S.I. Said), Futura, Mount Kisco, NY, pp. 137–88.

3. Snyder, L.S., Hertz, M.I., Harmon, K.R. *et al.* (1990) Failure of lung repair following acute lung injury. Regulation of the fibroproliferative response (part 1). *Chest,* **98**, 733–8, 989–93.

4. Donnelly, S.C., and Haslett, C. (1992) Cellular mechanisms of acute lung injury; implications for future treatment in the adult respiratory distress syndrome. *Thorax,* **47**, 260–3.

5. Lloyd, A.R. and Oppenheim, J.J. (1992) Poly's lament: the neglected role of the polymorphonuclear neutrophil in the afferent limb of the immune response. *Immunology Today,* **13**, 169–72.

6. Bitterman, P.B. (1992) Pathogenesis of fibrosis in acute lung injury. *American Journal of Medicine,* **92** (suppl. 6A), 39S–43S.

7. Kuhn, C. (1991) Patterns of lung repair. A morphologists view. *Chest,* **99** (suppl.), 11S–14S.

8. Zapol, W.M., Trelstad, R.L., Coffey, J.W. *et al.* (1979) Pulmonary fibrosis in severe acute respiratory failure. *American Review of Respiratory Disease,* **119**, 547–54.

9. Ragu, G., Striker, L.J., Hudson, L.D. *et al.* (1985) Extracellular matrix in normal and fibrotic human lungs. *American Review of Respiratory Disease,* **131**, 281–9.

10. Hasleton, P.S. (1983) Adult respiratory distress syndrome – a review. *Histopathology,* **7**, 307–32.

11. Jordana, M., Ohno, I., Zing, Z. *et al.* (1993) Cytokines in lung and airway fibrosis. *Regional Immunology,* **5**(3–4), 201–6.

12. Schmidt, J.A. (1984) Purification and partial characterisation of normal human IL1. *Journal of Experimental Medicine,* **160**, 772–87.

13. Hazuda, D.J., Lee, J.C. and Young, P.R. (1980) The kinetics of IL1 secretion from activated monocytes. Differences between interleukin 1

alpha and interleukin 1 beta. *Journal of Biological Chemistry*, **263**, 8473–9.

14. Elias, J.A., Zitnik, R.J. and Ray, P. (1992) Fibroblast immune-effector function, in *Pulmonary Fibroblast Heterogeneity* (ed. R.P. Phipps), CRC Press, Boca Raton, pp. 295–322.

15. Cox, G., Gauldie, J. and Jordana, M. (1992) Bronchial epithelial cell derived cytokines (G-CSF and GM-CSF) promote the survival of peripheral blood monocytes *in vitro*. *American Journal of Respiratory Cell and Molecular Biology*, **7**, 507–13.

16. Elias, J.A., Trinchieri, G., Beck, J. *et al*. (1989) A synergistic interaction between IL6 and IL1 mediates the thymocyte-stimulating activity produced by recombinant IL1 stimulated fibroblasts. *Journal of Immunology*, **142**, 509–14.

17. Strieter, R.M., Wiggins, R., Phan, S.H. *et al*. (1989) Monocyte chemotactic protein gene expression by cytokine treated human fibroblasts and endothelial cells. *Biochemical and Biophysical Research Communications*, **162**, 694–700.

18. Gauldie, J., Torry, D, Cox, G. *et al*. (1993) Effector function of tissue structural cells in inflammation, in *Asthma: Physiology, Immunopharmacology and Treatment. Fourth International Symposium* (eds S.T. Holgate, K.F. Austen, L.M. Lichtenstein, and A.B. Kay), Academic Press, London, pp. 211–25.

19. Raines, E.W., Dower, S.K. and Ross, R. (1989) 1L-1 mitogenic activity for fibroblasts and smooth muscle cells is due to PDGF-AA. *Science*, **243**, 393–6.

20. Dejana, E., Brevarto, F., Erroi, A. *et al*. (1987) Modulation of endothelial cell functions by different molecular species of interleukin-1. *Blood*, **69**, 695–9.

21. Aksamit, T.R. and Hunninghake G.W. (1993) Interleukin-1 in *Cytokines of the Lung* (ed. J. Kelley), Marcel Dekker, New York, pp. 185–228.

22. Richards, C., Gauldie, J. and Baumann, H. (1991) Cytokine control of acute phase protein expression. *European Cytokine Network*, **2**, 89–98.

23. Xing, Z., Jordana, M., Kirpalani, H. *et al*. (1994) Cytokine expression by neutrophils and macrophages *in vivo*: endotoxin induces tumor necrosis-α, macrophage inflammatory protein-2, interleukin-1β and interleukin-6 but not RANTES or transforming growth factor-β1 mRNA in acute lung inflammation. *American Journal of Respiratory Cell and Molecular Biology*, **10**, 148–53.

24. Xing, Z., Kirpalani, H., Torry, D. *et al*. (1993) Polymorphonuclear leucocytes as a significant source of tumor necrosis factor-α in endotoxin challenged lung tissue. *American Journal of Pathology*, **143**, 1009–15.

25. Goldblum, S.E., Jay, M., Yoneda, K. *et al*. (1987) Monokine induced acute lung injury in rabbits. *Journal of Applied Physiology*, **63**, 2093–100.

26. Phan, S.H. and Kunkel, S.L. (1992) Lung cytokine production in bleomycin-induced pulmonary fibrosis. *Experimental Lung Research*, **18**, 29–43.

27. Suter, P.M., Suter, S., Girardin, E. *et al*. (1992) High bronchoalveolar levels of tumor necrosis factor and its inhibitors, interleukin-1, interferon, and elastase, in patients with the adult respiratory distress syndrome after trauma, shock or sepsis. *American Review of Respiratory Disease*, **145**, 1016–22.

28. Jacobs, R.F., Tabor, D.R., Burks, W. *et al*. (1989) Elevated interleukin-1 release by human alveolar macrophages during the adult respiratory distress syndrome. *American Review of Respiratory Disease*, **140**, 1686–92.

29. Yamaguchi, E., Okazaki, N., Tsuneta, Y. *et al*. (1988) Interleukins in pulmonary sarcoidosis. Dissociative correlations of lung interleukins 1 and 2 with the intensity of alveolitis. *American Review of Respiratory Disease*, **138**, 645–51.

30. Ulich, T.R. (1992) Tumor necrosis factor, in *Cytokines of the Lung* (ed. J. Kelley), Marcel Dekker, New York, pp. 307–32.

31. Le, J., Weinstein, D., Gubler, V. *et al*. (1987) Induction of membrane associated interleukin-1 by tumor necrosis factor in human fibroblasts. *Journal of Immunology*, **138**, 2137–42.

32. Zucali, J.R., Broxmeyer, H.E., Gross, M.A. *et al*. (1988) Recombinant human tumor necrosis factors α and β stimulate fibroblasts to produce hemopoietic growth factors *in vitro*. *Journal of Immunology*, **140**, 840–4.

33. Leibovich, S.J., Polverini, P.J., Shepard, M.H. *et al*. (1987) Macrophage-induced angiogenesis is mediated by TNF α. *Nature*, **329**, 630–2.

34. Roberts, D.J., Davies, J.M. and Evans, C.C.

(1989) TNF and adult respiratory distress syndrome. *Lancet*, **ii**, [8670] 1043–4.

35. Piguet, P.F., Collart, M.A., Grau, G.E. *et al.* (1990) Tumor necrosis factor plays a key role in bleomycin induced pneumopathy and fibrosis. *Journal of Experimental Medicine*, **170**, 755–63.

36. Piguet, P.F., Collart, M.A., Grau, G.E. et al. (1990) Requirement of TNF for development of silica induced pulmonary fibrosis. *Nature*, **344**, 245–7.

37. Borm, P.J.A., Palmen, N., Engelen, J.J.M. et al. (1988) Spontaneous and stimulated release of TNF from monocytes of miners with coal workers' pneumoconiosis. *American Review of Respiratory Disease*, **138**, 1589–94.

38. Bachwich, P.R., Lynch, J.P., Larrick, J. *et al.* (1981) TNF production by human sarcoid alveolar macrophages. *American Journal of Pathology*, **125**, 421–5.

39. Matsushima, K., Morishita K., Yoshimura, T. *et al.* (1988) Molecular cloning of a human monocyte-derived neutrophil chemotactic factor (MDNCF) and the induction of MDNCF mRNA by interleukin-1 and tumor necrosis factor. *Journal of Experimental Medicine*, **167**, 1883–93.

40. Baggiolini, M., Walz, A. and Kunkel, S.L. (1989) Neutrophil-activating peptide-1/interleukin 8, a novel cytokine that activates neutrophils. *Journal of Clinical Investigation*, **84**, 1045–9.

41. Strieter, R.M., Phan, S.H., Showell, H.J. *et al.* (1989) Monokine-induced neutrophil chemotactic factor gene expression in human fibroblasts. *Journal of Biological Chemistry*, **264**, 10621–6.

42. Strieter, R.M., Standiford, T.J., Rolfe, M.W. *et al.* (1993) Interleukin 8, in *Cytokines of the Lung*, 1st edn (ed. J. Kelley), Marcel Dekker, New York, pp. 281–305.

43. Weiland, J.E., Davis, W.B., Holter, J.F. *et al.* (1986) Lung neutrophils in the adult respiratory distress syndrome. Clinical and pathological significance. *American Review of Respiratory Disease*, **133**, 218–25.

44. Donnelly, S.C., Strieter, R.M., Kunkel, S.L. *et al.* (1993) Interleukin-8 and development of adult respiratory distress syndrome in at-risk patient groups. *Lancet*, **341**, 643–7.

45. Schall, T.J. (1991) Biology of RANTES/sis cytokine family. *Cytokine*, **3**, 165–83.

46. Jiang, Y., Beller, D.I., Frendl, G. *et al.* (1992) Monocyte chemoattractant protein-1 regulates adhesion molecule expression and cytokine production in human monocytes. *Journal of Immunology*, **145**, 2423–8.

47. Rolfe, M.W., Kunkel, S.L., Standiford, T.J. *et al.* (1992) Expression and regulation of human pulmonary fibroblast-derived monocyte chemotactic peptide 1. *American Journal of Physiology*, **263**, L536–45.

48. Lukacs, N.W., Chensue, S.W., Smith, R.E. *et al.* (1994) Production of monocyte chemoattractant protein-1 and macrophage inflammatory protein-1α by inflammatory granuloma fibroblasts. *American Journal of Pathology*, **144**, 711–8.

49. Lukacs, N.W., Kunkel, S.L., Strieter, R.M. *et al.* (1993) The role of macrophage inflammatory protein 1 alpha in *Schistosoma mansoni* egg-induced granulomatous inflammation. *Journal of Experimental Medicine*, **177**, 1551–9.

50. Driscoll, K.E., Hassenbein, D.G., Carter, J. *et al.* (1993) Macrophage inflammatory proteins 1 and 2: expression by rat alveolar macrophages, fibroblasts, and epithelial cells in rat lung after mineral dust exposure. *American Journal of Respiratory Cell and Molecular Biology*, **8**, 311–8.

51. Standiford, T.J., Rolfe, M.R., Kunkel, S.L. *et al.* (1993) Altered production and regulation of monocyte chemoattractant protein-1 from pulmonary fibroblasts isolated from patients with idiopathic pulmonary fibrosis. *Chest*, **103** (suppl. 2), 121S.

52. Strieter, R.M., Koch, A.E., Antony, V.B. *et al.* (1994) The immunopathology of chemotactic cytokines: the role of interleukin-8 and monocyte chemoattractant protein-1. *Journal of Laboratory and Clinical Medicine*, **123**, 183–97.

53. Johnsson, A., Heldin, C.H., Westermark, G. *et al.* (1982) Platelet derived growth factor: identification of constituent polypeptide chains. *Biochemical and Biophysical Research Communications*, **104**, 66–74.

54. Larsson, O., Latham, C., Zicket, P. *et al.* (1989) Cell cycle regulation of human diploid fibroblasts: possible mechanisms of platelet-derived growth factor. *Journal of Cell Physiology*, **139**, 477–83.

55. Paulsson, Y., Austgulen, R., Hofsli, E. *et al.* (1989) Tumor necrosis factor-induced expression of platelet derived growth factor A-chain messenger RNA in fibroblasts. *Experimental Cell Research*, **180**, 490–6.

56. Fabisiak, J.P. and Kelley, J. (1992) Platelet derived growth factor, in *Cytokines of the Lung* (ed. J. Kelley), Marcel Dekker, New York, pp. 3–39.

57. Albelda, S.M., Elias, J.A., Levine, E.M. *et al.* (1989) Endotoxin stimulates platelet-derived growth factor production from cultured human pulmonary endothelial cells. *American Journal of Physiology*, **257**, L65–70.

58. Snyder, L.S., Hertz, M.I., Peterson, M.S. *et al.* (1991) Acute lung injury. Pathogenesis of intraalveolar fibrosis. *Journal of Clinical Investigation*, **88**, 663–73.

59. Fabisiak, J.P., Evans, J.N. and Kelley, J. (1989) Increased expression of PDGF-B(c-sis) mRNA in rat lung preceeds DNA synthesis and tissue repair during chronic hyperoxia. *American Journal of Respiratory Cell and Molecular Biology*, **1**, 181–9.

60. Antionades, H.N., Galanopoulos, T., Neville-Golden, J. *et al.* (1993) Expression of growth factor and receptor mRNAs in skin epithelial cells following acute cutaneous injury. *American Journal of Pathology*, **142**, 1099–110.

61. Antionades, H.N., Bravo, M.A., Avila, R.E. *et al.* (1990) Platelet-derived growth factor in idiopathic pulmonary fibrosis. *Journal of Clinical Investigation*, **86**, 1055–64.

62. Gauldie, J., Jordana, M. and Cox, G. (1992) Myeloid growth factors in the lung, in *Cytokines of the Lung* (ed. J. Kelley), Marcel Dekker, New York, pp. 383–402.

63. Lee, M.-T., Kaushansky, K., Ralph, P. *et al.* (1990) Differential expression of M-CSF, G-CSF and GM-CSF by human monocytes. *Journal of Leukocyte Biology*, **47**, 275–82.

64. Ohtoshi, T., Vancheri, C., Cox, G. *et al.* (1991) Monocyte-macrophage differentition induced by human upper airway epithelial cells. *American Journal of Respiratory Cell and Molecular Biology*, **4**, 255–63.

65. Vancheri, C., Ohtoshi, T., Cox, G. *et al.* (1991) Neutrophilic differentiation induced by human upper airway fibroblast-derived granulocyte/macrophage colony stimulating factor (GM-CSF). *American Journal of Respiratory Cell and Molecular Biology*, **4**, 11–17.

66. Seelentag, W., Mermot, J. and Vassali, P. (1989) Interleukin 1 and tumor necrosis factor α additively increase the levels of granulocyte-macrophage and granulocyte colony-stimulating factor (CSF) mRNA in human fibroblasts. *European Journal of Immunology*, **9**, 209–12.

67. Rubbia-Brandt, L., Sappino, A.-P. and Gabbiani, G. (1991) Locally applied GM-CSF induces the accumulation of α-smooth muscle actin containing myofibroblasts. *Virchows Archiv. B. Cell Pathology*, **60**, 73–82.

68. Kaushansky, K., Lin, N. and Adamson, J.W. (1988) Interleukin 1 stimulates fibroblasts to synthesize granulocyte-macrophage and granulocyte colony-stimulating factors. *Journal of Clinical Investigation*, **81**, 92–7.

69. Mattoli, S., Mattoso, V.L., Solaperto, M. *et al.* (1991) Cellular and biochemical characteristics of bronchoalveolar lavage fluid in symptomatic non-allergic asthma. *Journal of Allergy and Clinical Immunology*, **87**, 794–802.

70. Kelley, J. (1992) Transforming growth factor-β, in *Cytokines of the Lung* (ed. J. Kelley), Marcel Dekker, New York, pp.101–32.

71. Leof, E.B., Proper, J.A., Goustin, A.S. *et al.* (1986) Induction of c-sis mRNA and activity similar to platelet-derived growth factor by transforming growth factor β: a proposed model for indirect mitogenesis involving autocrine activity. *Proceedings of the National Academy of Sciences of the USA*, **83**, 2453–7.

72. Fine, A., and Goldstein, R.H. (1987) The effect of transforming growth factor-β on cell proliferation and collagen formation by lung fibroblasts. *Journal of Biological Chemistry*, **262**, 3897–902.

73. Dean, D.C., Newby, R.F. and Bourgeois, S. (1988) Regulation of fibronectin biosynthesis by dexamethasone, transforming growth factor-β, and cAMP in human cell lines. *Journal of Cell Biology*, **106**, 2159–70.

74. Bassols, A. and Massague, J. (1988) Transforming growth factor beta regulates the expression and structure of extracellular matrix chondroitin/dermatan sulfate proteoglycans. *Journal of Biological Chemistry*, **263**, 3039–45.

75. Westergren-Thorsson, G., Sarnstrand, B., Fransson, L.A. *et al.* (1990) TGF-beta enhances the production of hyaluronan in human lung but not in skin fibroblasts. *Experimental Cell Research*, **186**, 192–5.

76. Tsunawaki, S., Sporn, M., Ding, A. *et al.* (1988) Deactivation of macrophages by transforming growth factor-β. *Nature*, **334**, 260–2.

77. Shull, M.M., Ormsby, I., Kier, A.B. *et al.* (1992) Targeted disruption of the mouse transform-

ing growth factor-β1 gene results in multi-focal inflammatory disease. *Nature*, **359**, 693–9.

78. Letterio, J.J., Geiser A.G., Kulkarni A.B. *et al.* (1994) Maternal rescue of transforming growth factor-β1 null mice. *Science*, **264**, 1936–7.

79. Raghow, R., Irish, P. and Kang, A.H. (1989) Coordinate regulation of transforming growth factor gene expression and cell proliferation in hamster lungs undergoing bleomycin-induced pulmonary fibrosis. *Journal of Clinical Investigation*, **84**, 1836–42.

80. Khalil, N., Bereznay, O., Sporn, M. *et al.* (1989) Macrophage production of transforming growth factor β and fibroblast collagen synthesis. *Journal of Experimental Medicine*, **170**, 727–37.

81. Hoyt, D.G. and Lazo, J.S. (1988) Alterations in pulmonary mRNA encoding procollagens, fibronectin and transforming growth factor β precede bleomycin-induced pulmonary fibrosis in mice. *Journal of Pharmacology and Experimental Therapeutics*, **246**, 765–71.

82. Desmoulière, A., Geinoz, A. and Gabbiani, F. (1993) Transforming growth factor-β1 induces α-smooth muscle actin expression in granulation tissue myofibroblasts and in quiescent and growing cultured fibroblasts. *Journal of Cell Biology*, **122**, 103–11.

83. Limper, A.H., Broekelmann, T.J., Colby, T.V. *et al.* (1991) Analysis of local mRNA expression for extracellular matix proteins and growth factors using in situ hybridisation in fibroproliferative lung disorders. *Chest*, **99**, 55S–6S.

84. Khalil, N., O'Connor, R.N., Unruh, H.W. *et al.* (1991) Increased production and immunohistochemical localisation of transforming growth factor-β in idiopathic pulmonary fibrosis. *American Journal of Respiratory Cell and Molecular Biology*, **5**, 155–62.

85. Broekelmann, T.J., Limper, A.H., Colby, T.V. *et al.* (1991) Transforming growth factor-β1 is present at sites of extracellular matrix gene expression in human pulmonary fibrosis. *Proceedings of the National Academy of Sciences of the USA*, **88**, 6642–6.

86. Gospodarowicz, D., Neufeld, G. and Schweigerer, L. (1987) Fibroblast growth factor: structural and biological properties. *Journal of Cellular Physiology*, **5S**, 15.

87. Pierce, G.F., Tarpley, T.E., Yanagihara, D. *et al.* (1992) Platelet-derived growth factor (BB homodimer), transforming growth factor-β1, and basic fibroblast growth factor in dermal wound healing. *American Journal of Pathology*, **140**, 1375–88.

88. Henke, C., Fiegel, V., Peterson, M. *et al.* (1991) Identification and partial characterisation of angiogenesis bioactivity in the lower respiratory tract after acute lung injury. *Journal of Clinical Investigation*, **88**, 1386–95.

89. Leof, E.B., Wharton, W., Van Wyk, J.J. *et al.* (1982) Epidermal growth factor and somatomedin C regulate G1 progression in competent BALB-C 3T3 cells. *Experimental Cell Research*, **141**, 107–15.

90. Stiles, A.D., Smith, B.T. and Post, M. (1986) Reciprocal autocrine and paracrine regulation of growth of mesenchymal and alveolar epithelial cells from fetal lung. *Experimental Lung Research*, **11**, 165–177.

91. Rom, W.N., Basset, P., Fells, G.A. *et al.* (1988) Alveolar macrophages release an insulin like growth factor 1-type molecule. *Journal of Clinical Investigation*, **82**, 1685–93.

92. Burgess, W.H. and Maciag, T. (1989) The heparin-binding (fibroblast) growth factor family of proteins. *Annual Review of Biochemistry*, **58**, 575–606.

93. Roberts, R., Gallagher, J., Spooncer, E. et al. (1988) Heparan sulphate bound growth factors: a mechanism for stromal cell mediated haemopoiesis. *Nature*, **332**, 376–8.

94. Yayon, A., Klagsbrun, M., Esko, J.D. *et al.* (1991) Cell surface heparin-like molecules are required for binding of basic fibroblast growth factor to its high affinity receptor. *Cell*, **64**, 841–8.

95. Ruoslahti, E. and Yamaguchi, Y. (1991) Proteoglycans as modulators of growth factor activities. *Cell*, **64**, 867–9.

96. Yamaguchi, Y., Mann, D.M. and Ruoslahti E. (1990) Negative regulation of transforming growth factor-β by the proteoglycan decorin. *Nature*, **346**, 281–4.

97. Seyer, J.M. and Raghow, R. (1992) Hepatic fibrosis, in *Wound Healing: Biochemical and Clinical Aspects* (eds I.K. Cohen, R.F. Diegelmann and W.J. Lindblad), W.B. Saunders, Philadelphia, pp. 416–32.

98. Raghow, R. (1994) The role of extracellular matrix in postinflammatory wound healing and fibrosis. *FASEB Journal*, **8**, 823–31.

99. Martin, P., Hopkinson-Woolley, J. and McCluskey, J. (1992) Growth factors and cuta-

neous wound repair. *Progress in Growth Factor Research*, **4**, 25–44.

100. Walsh, J., Absher, M. and Kelley, J. (1993) Variable expression of platelet-derived growth factor family proteins in acute lung injury. *American Journal of Respiratory Cell and Molecular Biology*, **9**, 637–44.

101. Whitby, D.J. and Ferguson, M.W.J. (1991) Immunohistochemical localisation of growth factors in fetal wound healing. *Developmental Biology*, **147**, 207–15.

102. Border, W.A. and Ruoslahti, E. (1992) Transforming growth factor-β in disease: the dark side of tissue repair. *Journal of Clinical Investigation*, **90**, 1–7.

103. Mast, B.A. Diegelmann, R., Krummel, T.M. *et al.* (1992) Scarless wound healing in the mammalian fetus. *Surgery, Gynecology and Obstetrics*, **174**, 441–51.

104. Postlethwaite, A.E., Keski-Oja, J., Moses, H.L. *et al.* Stimulation of chemotactic migration of human fibroblasts by transforming growth β. *Journal of Experimental Medicine*, **165**, 251–6.

105. Ignotz R.A. and Massagué, J. (1986) Transforming growth factor-β stimulates the expression of fibronectin and collagen and their incorporation into the extracellular matrix. *Journal of Biological Chemistry*, **261**, 4337–45.

106. Ohno, I., Driscoll, K.E., Hassenbein, D. *et al.* (1993) Sequential expression of cytokines in lung tissues from rats exposed to cadmium chloride ($CdCl_2$). *American Review of Respiratory Disease*, **147**, A734.

107. Vyalov, S.L., Gabbiani, G. and Kapanci, Y. (1993) Rat alveolar myofibroblasts acquire α-smooth muscle actin expression during bleomycin-induced pulmonary fibrosis. *American Journal of Pathology*, **143**, 1754–65.

108. McCartney, N.L. and Wahl, S.M. (1994) Transforming growth factor β a matter of life and death. *Journal of Leukocyte Biology*, **55**, 401–9.

109. Chen, B., Polunovsky, V., White, J. *et al.* (1992) Mesenchymal cells isolated after acute lung injury manifest an enhanced proliferative phenotype. *Journal of Clinical Investigation*, **90**, 1778–85.

110. Sappino, A.P., Schurch, W. and Gabbiani, G. (1990) Biology of disease. Differentiation repertoire of fibroblastic cells: expression of cytoskeletal proteins as marker of phenotypic modulations. *Laboratory Investigation*, **63**, 144–61.

111. Darby, I., Skalli, O. and Gabbiani, G. (1990) α-Smooth muscle actin is transiently expressed by myofibroblasts during experimental wound healing. *Laboratory Investigation*, **63**, 21–9.

112. Jordana, M., Kirpalani, H. and Gauldie, J. (1992) Fibroblast immune-effector function, in *Pulmonary Fibroblast Heterogeneity* (ed. R.P. Phipps), CRC Press, Boca Raton, pp. 229–49.

113. Torry, D.T., Richards, C.D., Podor, T.J. *et al.* (1994) Anchorage-independent colony growth of pulmonary fibroblasts derived from fibrotic human lung tissue. *Journal of Clinical Investigation*, **93**, 1525–32.

114. Brewster, C.E.P., Howarth, P.H., Djukanovic, R. *et al.* (1990) Myofibroblasts and subepithelial fibrosis in bronchial asthma. *American Journal of Respiratory Cell and Molecular Biology*, **3**, 507–11.

115. Sundberg, C., Ljungström, M. and Lindmark, G. (1993) Microvascular pericytes express platelet-derived growth factor-β receptors in human healing wounds and colorectal adenocarcinoma. *American Journal of Pathology*, **143**, 1377–88.

116. Tremblay, G.M., Nonaka, M., Särnstrand, B. *et al.* (1994) Myofibroblast differentiation in nasal polyposis: down-regulation by topical steroids. *American Journal of Respiratory and Critical Care Medicine*, **149**, A632.

117. Vyalov, S., Desmoulière, A. and Gabbiani, G. (1993) GM-CSF-induced granulation tissue formation: relationships between macrophage and myofibroblast accumulation. *Virchows Archiv. B. Cell Pathology*, **63**, 231–9.

118. Polunovsky, V.A., Chen, B., Henke, C. *et al.* (1993) Role of mesenchymal cell death in lung remodeling after injury. *Journal of Clinical Investigation*, **92**, 388–97.

SECONDARY INFECTIONS IN ACUTE LUNG INJURY

14

Galen B. Toews

Infection and sepsis syndrome were recognized as common and severe complications of the syndrome of acute respiratory distress in adults (ARDS) shortly after the term ARDS was coined [1]. Infections, particularly pulmonary infections, are the leading cause of death in patients who survive for more than 3 days after the onset of their ARDS [2]. This association between secondary infections and lung injury probably results because: (1) the presence of a critical illness is a predisposing factor for the entry of microbes into the lung; and/or (2) the lung injury of ARDS impairs pulmonary host defenses. The interaction between microbes and the pulmonary defenses is dynamic. During this interaction the host utilizes many defensive strategies to prevent microbes from getting a foothold within the respiratory tract. To achieve optimal defense against microbes all components of the response must be functional and coordinated.

HOST DEFENSE

The host defenses are spaced along the airways from the naso-oropharyngeal surface to the lower respiratory tract [3–5]. In the upper respiratory tract, aerodynamic filtration and impaction, mucociliary clearance and cough remove large particulates; neurological reflexes are important in the prevention of aspiration. The naso-oropharyngeal surface has a complex microbial flora of aerobic and anaerobic bacteria that symbiotically exist in normals. This flora is present without untoward effects and for, as yet, an unknown purpose. While this flora is quite varied, the prevalence of aerobic Gram-negative bacilli such as *Enterobacteriaceae* and *Pseudomonas sp.* is low [6].

The host employs several strategies to keep the oropharynx clear of Gram-negative bacilli. Cellular desquamation removes organisms that attach to the outer mucosal surface. Nasopharyngeal secretions which bathe the respiratory mucosa contain proteins such as lysosyme, lactoferrin and lactoperoxidase, all of which have bactericidal effects. Salivary IgA is also important in the prevention of bacterial binding to epithelial cell surfaces [7]. Finally, healthy oral mucosal cells bind Gram-negative bacilli poorly [8,9]. The oropharyngeal defenses of healthy individuals are remarkably efficient. Only 1% of the originally inoculated bacteria, delivered by gargling with a suspension of Gram-negative bacteria, are recoverable by culturing the pharynx 3 hours after inoculation [7].

The conducting airways are endowed with both humoral and cellular defense mechanisms (Figure 14.1). The pseudostratified ciliated epithelium, which lines the conducting

ARDS Acute Respiratory Distress in Adults. Edited by Timothy W. Evans and Christopher Haslett. Published in 1996 by Chapman & Hall, London. ISBN 0 412 56910 8

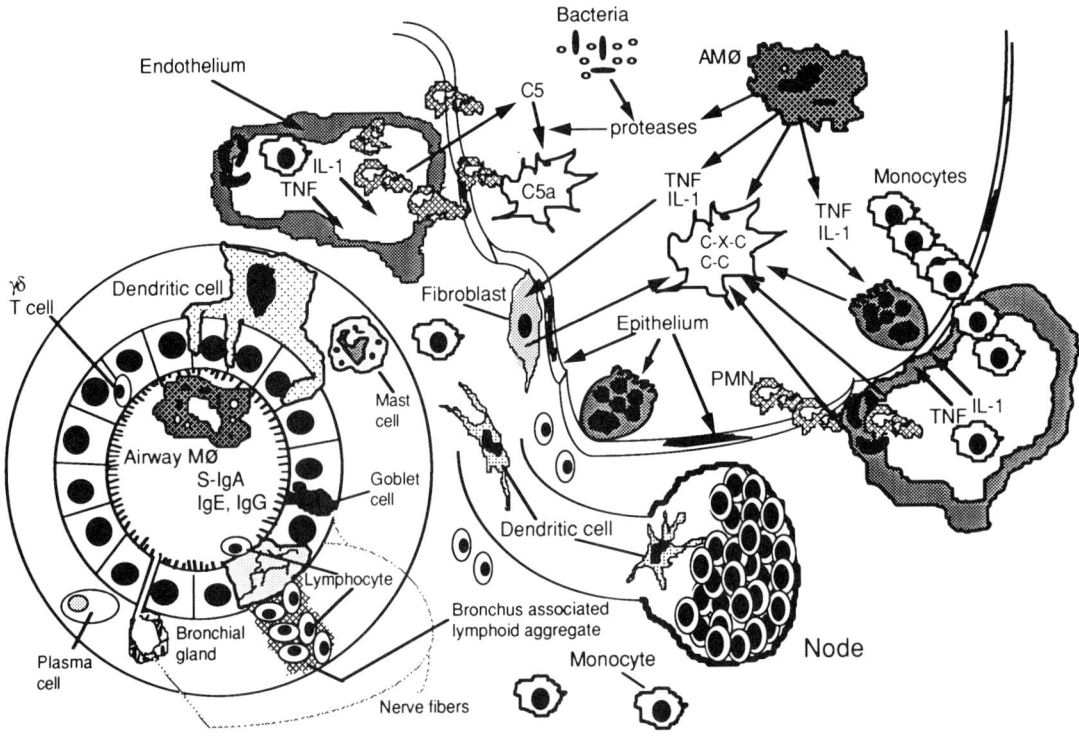

Figure 14.1 Pulmonary host defenses against microbes. AMØ = alveolar macrophage.

airways, is covered by a layer of mucus (produced by goblet cells and bronchial glands) and fluid that contains immunoglobulin (IgA) and various iron binding proteins (transferrin, lactoferrin) which inhibit bacterial growth [10–13]. Macrophages are present on the epithelial surface and are probably involved in the removal of foreign debris and destruction of microbes that are deposited on the epithelial surface [14]. Among the epithelial cells of the conducting airway are dendritic cells, which are important in the initiation of cellular immune responses to microbial antigens [15]. Plasma cells which secrete local immunoglobulins such as IgA, and mast cells which secrete mediators such as histamine, are located in the submucosa below the basement membrane. Airway nerves might be important in linking these glandular and cellular networks together [16]. Nervous control might be achieved through neuropeptide and/or by adrenergic and cholinergic nerve fibers [16,17].

In critically ill patients, bacteria often reach the lower respiratory tract (Figure 14.1). Alveolar macrophages are important in the clearance of micro-organisms, particulates and macromolecular debris from the epithelial surface of the lower respiratory tract. Recognition of microbes is greatly enhanced by specific antibody, complement fragments, fibronectin and surfactant components. Following recognition, the macrophage engulfs the organism and kills it within the phagolysosome, utilizing oxidative and nonoxidative processes [14,18,19]. Oxidative killing can also take place outside the cell since oxygen radicals are released outside alveolar macrophages. Extracellular substances such as surfactant, lysozymes, iron binding proteins and defensins are also important in the extracellular killing of microbes [19,20].

The effective clearance of most microbes from the lower respiratory tract requires the generation of an inflammatory response. Chemotaxins are present in bronchoalveolar lavage after bacterial inoculation and the number of granulocytes present correlates positively with the amount of chemotactic activity [21]. Complement fragments are important early chemotaxins [22,23]. Complement activation might occur via the alternative pathway in the absence of specific IgG or via the classic pathway if specific IgG is present. The interaction of microbial products with alveolar macrophages is probably important in the initiation of this response. Lipopolysaccharide (LPS) stimulates alveolar macrophage production of chemokines such as interleukin (IL)-8, and monocyte chemotactic peptide (MCP) [24,25]. Lipopolysaccharide also stimulates macrophages to produce tumor necrosis factor (TNF) and IL-1β, agents which recruit cells from the alveolar capillary wall (fibroblasts, epithelial cells, endothelial cells) to the process of chemokine production [26–29]. Chemotaxins are probably generated sequentially, with some factors contributing importantly during the early phases, whereas others are involved at later time points and/or in chronic responses. The generation of both acute (polymorphonuclear leukocytes, PMNs) and chronic (monocytes, macrophages, lymphocytes) inflammatory responses is the end result of a complex cytokine mediated cell–cell communication network involving mononuclear phagocytes, endothelial cells, fibroblasts and alveolar epithelial cells.

Specific pulmonary immune responses are essential for the elimination of certain infectious organisms, particularly virulent encapsulated bacteria, viruses and intracellular organisms that survive in normal resident macrophages (Figure 14.1). The activation of T cells is an early event in most immune responses. Activation of T cells results when appropriate antigen is recognized by the T cell receptor/CD3 complex. Activation of T cells requires the participation of antigen presenting cells which recognize and process the antigen, present the antigen on their surface in association with major histocompatability complex molecules, interact with T cell receptor, and deliver necessary cytokine mediated activation signals to responding lymphocytes [30]. Pulmonary dendritic cells, found in the interstitium of the lung and dispersed throughout the columnar epithelium of bronchi, are important antigen presenting cells in the lung [15,31–33]. Dendritic cells are involved in the initiation of primary immune responses involving CD4 and CD8 lymphocytes, both of which have key roles in pulmonary defenses against microbes [34,35]. CD4 T cells in some species (e.g. mouse) can be functionally divided into two mutually exclusive subsets, Th1 cells and Th2 cells; but the exclusiveness of these subsets in humans is less clear at present. Th1 cells produce interferon-γ and IL-2. Th1 cells mediate delayed-type hypersensitivity reactions and activate macrophages for microbicidal activity. Th2 cells produce IL-4, IL-5 and IL-10. Th2 cells provide help for antibody responses [36]. CD8 lymphocytes function as suppressor cells, cytotoxic cells and cytokine secreting cells. Cytotoxic CD8 lymphocytes can lyse cells which contain microbes. CD4 and CD8 cells cooperate in the eradication of many pathogens, including *Cryptococcus neoformans* and *Mycobacterium tuberculosis* [37–40].

Humoral immune responses significantly enhance antimicrobial defenses in the lower respiratory tract. Microbes become coated with specific IgG antibody if appropriate humoral immunity exists. The interaction between the antibody and the microbe might activate a complement sequence which results in bacterial lysis. More commonly, immunoglobulin and complement fragments serve as opsonins which facilitate the ingestion of microbes by phagocytic cells. Humoral immune responses enhance the clearance of most Gram-positive and Gram-negative microbes from the lower respiratory tract.

PNEUMONIA

The incidence of pneumonia in patients with ARDS is difficult to assess for two reasons. First, few series have actually evaluated the incidence of pneumonia in ARDS; most series have evaluated pneumonia in mechanically ventilated patients. Secondly, the difficulty in diagnosing nosocomial pneumonia in ARDS has made studies to determine the exact incidence of secondary pulmonary infection difficult. Early studies observed that 70% of patients with ARDS had pneumonia, but this study did not make a distinction between pneumonia as a cause of ARDS and pneumonia which complicated ARDS [1]. Several studies have evaluated the incidence of pneumonia in nonsurvivors of ARDS. In an initial study, 24 of 47 nonsurvivors had pneumonia on postmortem examination [41]. In a larger series of 129 patients with ARDS, pneumonia emerged as a secondary infection in 53% of patients who did not survive [42]. If all nosocomial infections that were identified during the course of ARDS were considered, the lung was the most common site, being affected three times more often than the next most common site, the abdomen.

The incidence of pneumonia has also been evaluated in patients with endotracheal tubes undergoing mechanical ventilation. The risk of pneumonia in these patients is 7- to 21-fold greater than in other hospitalized individuals [43–45] and is related to the duration of mechanical ventilation. The risk of nosocomial pneumonia was 6.5% after 10 days, 19% at 20 days and 28% at 30 days, suggesting a 1% chance of developing pneumonia per day on mechanical ventilation [46].

Pneumonia is the secondary infection most likely to lead to the death of the patient [42,47,48]. In those treated with mechanical ventilation, the mortality rate of pneumonia has been reported as being between 55% and 75% [49,50]. If pneumonia occurs in the context of ARDS, the fatality rates are probably even higher; the presence of infection of any type has been associated with poor outcome and with the development of multiple system organ failure (chapter 18). In patients with ARDS, the survival rate was 67% in the absence of infection versus 21% when infection of any type was present. When pneumonia was the infection which complicated ARDS, the mortality rate was 88%. Bacteremia complicated pneumonia in 27% of cases; *Pseudomonas* sp. were the responsible pathogens in 58% of these [42]. These findings have been confirmed in a study designed to identify the causes of death in patients with ARDS [2]. Patients who eventually develop ARDS were compared with a controlled population of patients with similar underlying illnesses or injuries, but who did not develop acute respiratory failure. Mortality in the critically ill control group was high (34%) but doubled (68%) if ARDS developed. One third of patients with ARDS died of causes associated with their underlying illness or injury and only 16% from irreversible respiratory failure. The remainder of the patients died of complications related to the development of ARDS. Of 20 patients who developed sepsis syndrome as a complication of ARDS, 17 had a probable pulmonary source of infection prior to meeting the criteria of sepsis syndrome. Thus, patients with lung injury frequently develop pulmonary infection and have a high incidence of sepsis syndrome. These data suggest that patients with lung injury not only are predisposed to pulmonary infection, but are unable to limit this infection to the lungs by usual host defense mechanisms. This probably accounts for the high incidence of multiple system organ failure and mortality observed in these patients.

PATHOGENESIS OF SECONDARY INFECTION

Since aerobic Gram-negative bacteria cause most secondary pulmonary infections in ARDS, attention will be directed to the pathogenesis of these infections. The pathogenic

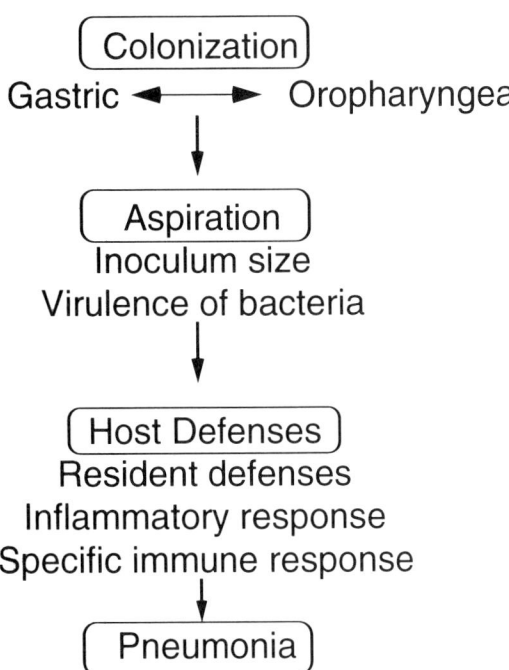

Figure 14.2 Pathogenesis of pneumonia in acute lung injury.

steps involved include: (1) colonization of the host with microbes; (2) aspiration of microbes; and (3) bacterial interaction with the host defenses (Figure 14.2). Pneumonia results if the inoculum is large, if the organisms are virulent and/or the pulmonary defenses are impaired.

COLONIZATION

The normal oropharyngeal surface supports a complex microbial flora of anaerobic and aerobic bacteria. The common isolates in cultures of the upper respiratory tract include *Branhamella catarrhalis, Staphylococcus sp., Streptococcus sp.* and *Neisseria sp.* Large numbers of anaerobic bacteria are present around teeth in gingival crevices (10^8 micro-organisms/ml of oral secretions). These are present for an unknown purpose and have no deleterious effects on the host or the oropharyngeal mucosa [6].

The prevalence of aerobic Gram-negative bacilli, such as *Enterobacteriaceae* and *Pseudomonas sp.* in the upper respiratory tract is low, around 2% in normal persons [51]. However, colonization by these microbes occurs in chronically debilitated or seriously ill patients. The prevalence of such colonization correlates with the severity of the patient's illness; approximately 50% of the patients requiring care in intensive care units are eventually colonized [52]. Risk factors for upper and lower respiratory tract colonization have been identified and include chronic renal failure, diabetes, hypertension, coma, advanced age, smoking and pre-existing lung disease. A variety of factors associated with therapeutic interventions also promote colonization of the oropharynx and tracheobronchial tree, including antibiotic therapy, endotracheal intubation, therapy to neutralize gastric acid, general surgery and malnutrition. Nosocomial pneumonia is preceded by oropharyngeal colonization and occurs almost exclusively in individuals who are colonized. Additionally, the organisms causing the pneumonia are identical to those with which the patient is colonized. The close association of upper respiratory tract colonization with subsequent lower respiratory tract infection implies that colonization of the upper respiratory tract is an important pathogenetic feature of these infections [52,53].

Host defenses can be altered in several fashions to allow microbes to gain a foothold on the mucosa. Endotracheal intubation might promote colonization by: (1) injuring the mucosa, thus making it more susceptible to bacterial growth and/or invasion; (2) interfering with the function of the mucociliary escalator; or (3) providing organisms with direct access to the tracheobronchial tree. Whether endotracheal intubation itself can alter mucosal cells to allow adherence in critically ill patients is unclear. While increases in tracheal cell adherence have been noted when intubated patients are compared with healthy individuals, this increased adherence could not be related to the duration of intubation. The endotracheal tube and its connecting ventilator tubing can serve as the source of organisms. The internal surface of most endotracheal tubes (84%) removed from critically ill patients after an average of 9 days was completely covered with a biofilm containing bacteria [54]. During endotracheal suctioning, and perhaps mechanical ventilation, this biofilm could be inoculated into the airway. Ventilator tubing also frequently harbors large numbers of the patient's own bacteria within its condensate. Inoculation of this condensate via the endotracheal tube could deposit a large endotracheal bolus of microbes.

Antibiotics may promote Gram-negative colonization by interfering with the growth of normal flora in the airway. The mechanisms whereby normal flora prevent Gram-negative colonization are uncertain, but normal flora might inhibit their growth. An inverse relationship between the presence of α *streptococcus* and enteric Gram-negative bacilli has been noted in cultures of oral secretions [55]. While the mechanisms of this interaction are poorly understood, normal flora may release toxic exoproducts that inhibit the proliferation of pathogens or may alternatively occupy all of the existing binding sites on the mucosal surface. The removal of the normal oral flora would thus permit vacant binding sites on the oral mucosa to become occupied by Gram-negative bacteria. The importance of these mechanisms remains uncertain, since some studies have found no role for a lack of inhibitory bacteria in the colonization seen in alcoholics and diabetics [56].

Gastric alkalinization may promote oropharyngeal and tracheobronchial colonization by a complex mechanism. At a pH of 1, the stomach is normally sterile because hydrochloric acid has potent bactericidal activity. Increases in gastric colonization occur with achlorhydria, advanced age and malnutrition [57]. Reduced amounts of gastric acid are present in critically ill patients as a result of

impaired acid production, decreased secretion due to H_2-blockers or regimens of antacids given to neutralize secreted acid [58]. Enteric bacterial growth is noted particularly when gastric pH rises above 4. Gastric cultures are seldom positive at a pH $\leq$ 4 but are frequently positive (59%) for Gram-negative bacilli with a pH $\geq$ 4. Numbers of Gram-negative bacilli may reach 10^8/ml at a gastric pH of 6 [59]. Since gastric organisms have been demonstrated to move retrograde to the oral pharynx, the stomach may serve as a reservoir for Gram-negative organisms that eventually colonize the airway [60]. Increased rates of pneumonia in patients who have received agents that alter gastric pH are probably related to the increased burden of organisms that colonize the stomach and to their spread to the upper respiratory tract.

Bacterial adherence to epithelial cells is critical for colonization, since only adherent bacilli escape removal by clearance mechanisms and therefore proliferate. Adherence to epithelial cells allows bacteria to obtain nutrients from underlying cells and establish microcolonies. Synthesis of proteins necessary for continued adherence and tissue invasion are induced by interaction with epithelial surfaces. Thus, colonization results in the introduction of large amounts of virulent microbes in the upper respiratory tract of the host.

Adherence of *Pseudomonas aeruginosa* to epithelial cells requires a change in the mucosal cells (Figure 14.3). Such changes occur in the mucosal cells of critically ill patients; more Gram-negative bacilli adhere to epithelial cells from critically ill patients than to those of healthy subjects. The increased adherence measured *in vitro* occurs early and precedes colonization *in vivo*. Mechanisms of bacterial attachment to epithelial cells appear to involve the binding of specific adhesins on bacterial pili to binding sites on the epithelial cell. The binding site appears to be present on the pili because non-piliated strains of bacteria fail to adhere. Microbes probably adhere to buccal cells via sugar-

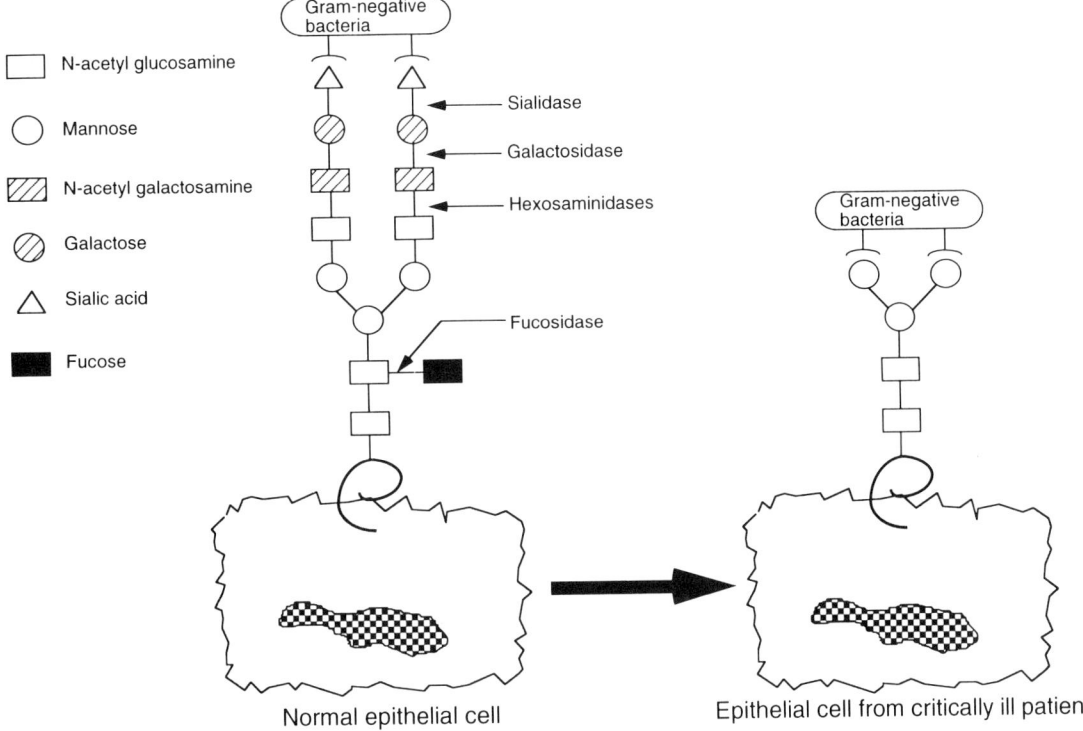

Figure 14.3 Mechanisms of alterations of epithelial cell glycocalyx associated with Gram-negative bacterial adherence.

containing binding sites on the epithelial cell surface [61].

The outer surface of respiratory epithelial cells, from the oropharynx to the alveoli, are covered by a carbohydrate-rich glycocalyx layer [62,63]. Glycosylation of cells is believed to be required for appropriate receptor function, cellular adherence and protection against proteolytic degradation [64]. Six monosaccharides, including mannose, fucose, galactose, sialic acid and the amino sugars, *N*-acetylgalactosamine and *N*-acetylglucosamine, are present on respiratory epithelial cells. These form oligosaccharide chains attached to both membrane proteins and membrane lipids. *N*-linked oligosaccharide structures may contain over 15 monosaccharides arranged in an elaborate branching structures projecting out from the cell surface. Oligosaccharides are the major component of

the outermost cell surface. In most oligosaccharides, sialic acid is present as the terminal sugar at the peripheral, nonreducing end of the oligosaccharide [62,64].

The loss of terminal sugars from the epithelial cell glycocalyx may account for the increased adherence noted in epithelial cells obtained from acute ill patients. The removal of peripheral monosaccharides from the oligosaccharide chain increases bacterial adherence to cell monolayers *in vitro* and to normal rat tracheal epithelium [65,66]. Buccal cells obtained from patients in the medical intensive care unit contain significantly less sialic acid than normal cells [67]; stressed rat buccal epithelial cells and tracheal epithelial cells contain decreased amounts of sialic acid and fucose [66]. Loss of sialic acid may uncover normally internal carbohydrates, such as *N*-acetylglucosamine and mannose

[64]. *N*-acetylglucosamine is a ligand for *Pseudomonas aeruginosa* and D-mannose is the ligand for type I piliated Gram-negative bacteria, which are the most common respiratory tract isolates from patients in the intensive care unit. Thus, sialic acid normally present as the peripheral sugar in oligosaccharides may function to prevent pathogenic bacteria from adhering to respiratory epithelial surfaces by masking internal carbohydrate ligands for pathogenic microbes.

The mechanisms by which respiratory cell surface oligosaccharides become altered are unknown, but several possibilities exist. Oligosaccharide synthesis might be altered by hormones and/or cytokines present in critically ill patients. Formation of oligosaccharides is dependent upon the coordinated action of a number of cytoplasmic enzymes; altered intracellular processing might lead to the formation of glycocompounds with abnormal carbohydrate composition. Alternatively, oligosaccharides might be altered after their transport to the cell surface by enzymes present in respiratory tract secretions. Proteases or glycosidases may be important in this alteration.

ROUTES OF ORGANISM ENTRY INTO THE LUNG

The most important route of entry of bacteria into the lower respiratory tract is the aspiration of a liquid bolus of oropharyngeal secretions. Aspiration of oropharyngeal contents is probably common. Seventy percent of patients with impaired consciousness have aspiration of oropharyngeal secretions during sleep, as do 50% of normal persons [68]. Only small volumes of oropharyngeal secretions are required to deliver a significant bacterial inoculum. Only 0.0001 ml would be required to inoculate the tracheal bronchial tree with 10^4 organisms, as 10^8 Gram-negative bacilli per milliliter of upper respiratory tract secretions have been noted. Inoculation of the lower airway of experimental animals with a liquid bolus containing 10^4 Gram-negative organisms is highly likely to produce pneumonia. Microbes may also enter the respiratory tract by: (1) inhalation of organisms; (2) direct extension from contiguous sites; and (3) hematogenous spread from distant sites. Nebulizer devices contaminated with aerobic Gram-negative bacteria were a common cause of airborne inoculation of bacteria in the 1960s. Contamination of respiratory therapy equipment is now uncommon, largely because most is disposable. *Legionella*, *M. tuberculosis*, *Aspergillus* and viral infections can all be acquired by aerosol inhalation.

PULMONARY DEFENSE IMPAIRMENTS

Whether or not pneumonia develops in a given patient ultimately depends upon the interaction between invading bacteria and host defenses. Pneumonia may develop in acute lung injury because some element of host defense is impaired in most patients. Abnormalities may result from the pulmonary injury itself, from the presence of coexistent disease or because of the therapeutic interventions employed.

ACUTE LUNG INJURY

ARDS itself probably predisposes the host to infection because the inflammatory mediators of this disease adversely alter pulmonary defenses against microbes. The role of the inflammatory response in causing endothelial and epithelial injury in ARDS has been studied extensively, but the effect of this inflammatory response on the host's abilities to defend itself against microbes have not been explored in depth.

Acute lung injury can impair the host's response to intrapulmonary bacteria. Clearance of *Staph. aureus* was impaired in animals treated with α-naphtholthiourea [69]. Similar findings were noted in a rat model of pulmonary edema [70]. Clearance of both *Staph.*

aureus and *Step pneumoniae* was impaired in animals with pulmonary edema. The mortality rate was also increased in an animal model if both pulmonary infection and lung injury were present [71].

The mechanisms whereby acute lung injury/pulmonary edema impair bacterial clearance are not fully understood. Decreased numbers of alveolar macrophages are recoverable by lavage from animals with lung injury. The recovered alveolar macrophages have reduced *in vitro* bactericidal capacities. In addition to altering resident macrophage function, acute lung injury may also adversely alter alveolar lining material [69]. Alveolar lining material from normal animals can enhance the *in vitro* function of alveolar macrophages by promoting phagocytosis and augmenting the intracellular killing of *Staph. aureus* [72,73]. In addition, surfactant has an important role in the extracellular killing of many microbes through its detergent effect [74]. Alteration of normal alveolar lining material during lung injury may lead to depression of phagocytosis, and both intracellular and extracellular killing.

Abnormalities in alveolar neutrophil function have also been noted [75]. Alveolar neutrophils from patients with ARDS were significantly impaired with respect to their production of reactive oxygen species (Chapter 11), microbicidal activity and chemotaxis when compared with neutrophils obtained simultaneously from the pulmonary artery. While the mechanism(s) responsible for the altered alveolar neutrophil function are incompletely understood, it is probable that the alveolar milieu plays an important role. Concentrated lavage fluid from patients with ARDS did not induce changes in neutrophil function, but exposure of normal neutrophils to the oxidants generated in a glucose:glucose oxidant system caused a concentration dependent reduction in superoxide anion production and chemotaxis similar to that noted in ARDS neutrophils. Both H_2O_2 and myeloperoxidase are present in the air spaces of patients with ARDS [76,77] but would not have been concentrated in lavage fluids with the methods used.

These studies suggest a hypothesis to explain neutrophil dysfunction in ARDS (Chapter 8). While newly recruited alveolar neutrophils are known to generate normal amounts of $O_2^{\bullet-}$ and to migrate normally to chemotaxins [78], these newly recruited cells might lose their functional activity because of exposure to oxidants produced in the ongoing inflammatory response. The rate at which neutrophils move along a continuum from 'functional' to 'dysfunctional' cells might be related to the severity of the local inflammatory response. If this were true, patients with the most severe injury would have the most impaired alveolar neutrophils and be the most compromised in their ability to respond to microbes that are present in the airway.

Elastase has been shown to be the predominant protease in the airway lining fluid of patients with ARDS [79] (Chapter 10). While elastase cleavage products derived from Hageman factor, plasminogen, prekallikrein and complement components may have a role in amplifying lung inflammation, elastase may also play a role in impairing microbial defenses. Elastase-rich sputum reduces the beat frequency of ciliated epithelial cells [80], an effect abolished when α_1-antiprotease is preincubated with sputum. Interference with ciliary function might decrease the rate of mucociliary removal of bacteria from airways or may also allow prolonged mucosal contact, thereby predisposing the epithelium to colonization. Elastase can also cleave functional immunoglobulin molecules into nonfunctional low molecular weight fragments. Neutrophil elastase can cleave secretory IgA, which may lead to adverse effects on IgA mediated defenses. IgA is known to inhibit bacterial binding to airway epithelium. An inverse relationship has been observed between sputum elastase and IgA levels and between IgA levels and tracheal cell bacterial adherence [81]. Elastase is also known to cleave IgG [82,83]. IgG cleavage could have devastating effects on lung defenses against Gram-negative microbes, since IgG is required as an opsonin for phagocytosis of these microbes by both alveolar macrophages and granulocytes.

COEXISTENT DISEASE

The presence of an infection at a site distant from the lung or the presence of sepsis can impair pulmonary host defenses. Systemic endotoxin pretreatment adversely altered bacterial clearance of aerosol or intratracheally inoculated *Staph. aureus* from rat lungs [84]. Fewer neutrophils were recruited to the air spaces following intrapulmonary infection with *Staph. aureus* in animals which received LPS than were recruited in those which received systemic placebo treatment. In endotoxin treated animals, neutrophils sequestered in the pulmonary vasculature but did not enter the alveolar spaces. Similar results have been reported in an animal model of experimental bacterial peritonitis [85]. Animals with bacterial peritonitis cleared *Staph. aureus* and *P. aeruginosa* from their lungs less effectively than control animals without peritonitis. While controls could clear *P. aeruginosa*, this bacterium proliferated in the lungs of animals with peritonitis such that 100-fold more bacteria were noted at 24 hours than had been originally inoculated. While all animals challenged with either *Staph. aureus* or *P. aeruginosa* survived in the absence of peritonitis, increased mortality was noted in those which received *P. aeruginosa* in the presence of peritonitis. In animals with peritonitis alone, 35% died, compared with 88% of those with peritonitis who were challenged with *pseudomonas*. The proliferation of *P. aeruginosa* in mice with peritonitis was associated with impaired recruitment of PMNs into the lung. The reduction in numbers of recruited pulmonary PMNs was not due to a depletion of intravascular PMNs by

recruitment to the peritoneal cavity, since a noninfectious peritonitis induced a large PMN response in the peritoneum but did not impair pulmonary recruitment of PMNs.

The impaired recruitment of PMNs is probably related to the systemic effects of sepsis, which may be related to the compartmentalized production of cytokines [86]. Intravenous administration of LPS significantly increases serum but not alveolar TNF content. Alternatively, intratracheal LPS administration increases levels of TNF in bronchoalveolar lavage fluid and in lavaged alveolar macrophages without changing levels of TNF in the vascular space. Thus, in some circumstances, increases in TNF levels can be confined to the LPS challenged compartment. Intravenously challenged animals sequester neutrophils within the pulmonary vasculature while intratracheally LPS challenged animals elicit an intra-alveolar inflammatory response. It is possible that massive activation of inflammatory mediators within the vascular compartment, which accompanies sepsis, causes a diminution of neutrophil migration to the lung by the abnormal sequestration of these cells within the microvasculature.

The functions of resident alveolar macrophages are also impaired in animals with sepsis [87], having a markedly reduced capacity for phagocytosis. Macrophages removed from the septic microenvironment and placed in conditions of optimal oxygen and opsonin content have their phagocytic function restored. Opsonin depletion would be one possibility for these findings. Sepsis is known to deplete complement and has also been shown to deplete fibronectin [88,89]. Both complement and fibronectin are crucial opsonins for optimal alveolar macrophage interaction with microbes. Animals with intra-abdominal sepsis have also been reported to have a decreased ability to kill organisms once they are ingested [85]. Thus, sepsis may alter the ability of alveolar macrophages to recognize and engulf pathogens as well as decrease their ability to kill ingested microbes.

The presence of hemorrhagic shock has also been shown to alter microbial clearance in experimental models [90]. Sublethal inocula of bacteria caused 100% mortality in rats which were fluid resuscitated following exposure to hemorrhagic shock. While the mechanisms of the enhanced bacterial virulence after resuscitation from hemorrhagic shock have not been clearly defined, impaired phagocytic function has been reported following hemorrhagic shock [87,91]. Depletion of opsonic components may also play an important role in this circumstance.

Hypoxia has also been shown to impair alveolar macrophage phagocytosis and killing [92]. Impaired clearance of *Staph. aureus*, *Escherichia coli* and *Klebsiella pneumoniae* has been observed in the hypoxic microenvironment which exists within air spaces that are fluid filled and/or collapsed as a result of lung injury.

Many other coexisting diseases could alter host defenses in critically ill patients who are at risk for the development of ARDS. Abnormalities of chemotaxis have been reported in patients with diabetes mellitus, after burns, after ethanol exposure and in hypophosphatemic patients.

IMPAIRMENTS RELATED TO THERAPEUTIC INTERVENTIONS

Patients with ARDS are universally treated with oxygen therapy. Hyperoxia can clearly contribute to the risk of infection (Chapter 11). Animals exposed to 100% oxygen for as short a period as 24 hours had impaired *in vivo* pulmonary bactericidal activity when exposed to aerosolized *Staph. aureus* [93]. Macrophages from these animals showed no functional deficits after removal from the hyperoxic environment [94]. Furthermore, hyperoxia-exposed alveolar macrophages had decreased bacterial uptake, reduced superoxide and peroxide generation and impaired

intracellular killing *in vitro* [95]. Hyperoxia also impairs mucociliary clearance and leads to surfactant loss [94,96]. The minimal inspired oxygen concentration at which these effects occur is presently unknown.

The effect of pharmacological agents on antimicrobial defenses is difficult to evaluate. Their effect in animal models of bacterial clearance is usually small, but most studies have evaluated single agents, while patients with ARDS are exposed to polypharmacy at any one time. Accordingly, any interactive effects of medications may have been underestimated in these animal studies. Several agents influence host defenses, which might be important in the pathogenesis of secondary infections. Mucociliary function can be impaired by pentobarbital, atropine and morphine [96,97]. Sedation clearly increases the likelihood of aspiration and suppressed cough. Corticosteroids and salicylates impair macrophage and neutrophil phagocytosis as well as the killing function of these cells [98]. Similarly, corticosteroids and anti-inflammatory agents can interfere with granulocyte and macrophage accumulation and oxidant generation.

ACKNOWLEDGEMENTS

This chapter was supported in part by National Institutes of Health Grants, Specialized Center of Research in Occupational and Immunologic Lung Disease Grant #1 P50 HL46487, RO1 HL51082 and a Veterans Affairs Medical Service Merit Review Grant.

REFERENCES

1. Ashbaugh, D.G. and Petty, T.L. (1972) Sepsis complicating the acute respiratory distress syndrome. *Surgery, Gynecology and Obstetrics*, **135**, 865–9.
2. Wimberley, N.M., Bass, J.B., Boyd, B.W. *et al.* (1982) Use of a bronchoscopic protected catheter brush for the diagnosis of pulmonary infections. *Chest*, **81**, 556–62.
3. Green, G.B., Jakab, G.J., Low, R.B. *et al.* (1977) Defense mechanisms of the respiratory mem-

brane. *American Review of Respiratory Disease*, **115**, 479–514.

4. Reynolds, H.Y. (1989) Pulmonary host defense – state of the art. *Chest*, **95**, 223S–30S.

5. Toews, G.B. (1989) Pulmonary clearance of infectious agents, in *Respiratory Infections: Diagnosis and Management* (ed. J.E. Pennington), Raven Press, New York, pp. 41–51.

6. Mackowiak, P.A. (1982) The normal microbial flora. *New England Journal of Medicine*, **307**, 83–93.

7. LaForce, F.M., Hopkins, J., Trow, R. *et al.* (1976) Human oral defenses against Gram-negative rods. *American Review of Respiratory Disease*, **114**, 929–35.

8. Johanson, W.G. Jr, Higuchi, J.H., Chaudhuri, T.R. *et al.* (1980) Bacterial adherence to epithelial cells in bacilliary colonization of the respiratory tract. *American Review of Respiratory Disease*, **121**, 55–63.

9. Johanson, W.G. Jr, Woods, D.E. and Chaudhuri, T. (1979) Association of respiratory tract colonization with adherence of Gram-negative bacilli to epithelial cells. *Journal of Infectious Disease*, **139**, 667–73.

10. Reynolds, H.Y. and Newball, H.H. (1974) Analysis of proteins and respiratory cells obtained from human lungs by bronchial lavage. *Journal of Laboratory and Clinical Medicine*, **84**, 559–73.

11. Mestecky, J. and McGhee, J.R. (1987) Immunoglobulin A: molecular and cellular interactions involved in IgA biosynthesis and immune response. *Advances in Immunology*, **40**, 153–245.

12. Bell, D.Y., Haseman, J.A., Spock, A. *et al.* (1981) Plasma proteins of the bronchoalveolar surface of the lungs of smokers and non-smokers. *American Review of Respiratory Disease*, **124**, 72–9.

13. Thompson, A.B., Bohling, T., Payvandi, F. *et al.* (1990) Lower respiratory tract lactoferrin and lysozyme arise primarily in the airways and are elevated in association with chronic bronchitis. *Journal of Laboratory and Clinical Medicine*, **115**, 148–50.

14. Sibille, Y. and Reynolds, H.Y. (1990) Macrophages and polymorphonuclear neutrophils in lung defense and injury. *American Review of Respiratory Disease*, **141**, 471–500.

15. Sertl, K., Takemura, T., Tschachler, E. *et al.* (1986) Dendritic cells with antigen-presenting capability reside in airway epithelium, lung parenchyma, and visceral pleura. *Journal of Experimental Medicine*, **163**, 436–51.

16. Barnes, P.J. (1986) Neural control of human airways in health and disease. *American Review of Respiratory Disease*, **134**, 1289–314.

17. Barnes, P.J. (1989) Airway neuropeptides: roles in fine tuning and in disease. *News of Physiological Science*, **4**, 116–20.

18. Klebanoff, S.J. (1988) Phagocytic cells: products of oxygen metabolism, in *Inflammation: Basic Principles and Clinical Correlates* (eds J.I. Gallin, I.M. Goldstein and R. Synderman), Raven Press, New York, pp. 291–344.

19. Henson, P.M., Henson, J.E., Fittschen, C. *et al* (1988). Phagocytic cells: degranulation and secretion, in *Inflammation: Basic Principles and Clinical Correlates* (eds J.I. Gallin, I.M. Goldstein and R. Synderman), Raven Press, New York, pp. 363–90.

20. Leher, R.I., Lichtenstein, A.K. and Ganz, T. (1993) Defensins: antimicrobial and cytotoxic peptides of mammalian cells. *Annual Review of Immunology*, **11**, 105–28.

21. Vial, W.C., Toews, G.B. and Pierce, A.K. (1984) Early pulmonary granulocyte recruitment in response to *Streptococcus pneumonia. American Review of Respiratory Disease*, **129**, 87–91.

22. Larsen, G.L., Mitchel, B.C., Harper, T.B. *et al.* (1982) The pulmonary response of C5 sufficient and deficient mice to *Pseudomonas aeruginosa. American Review of Respiratory Disease*, **126**, 306–11.

23. Toews, G.B. and Vial, W.C. (1984) The role of C5 in polymorphonuclear leukocyte recruitment in response to *Streptococcus pneumoniae. American Review of Respiratory Disease*, **129**, 82–86.

24. Strieter, R.M., Chensue, S.W., Basha, M.A. *et al.* (1990) Human alveolar macrophage gene expression of interleukin-8 by TNF-α, LPS, and IL-1β. *American Journal of Respiratory Cell and Molecular Biology*, **2**, 321–6.

25. Leonard, E.J. and Yoshimura, T. (1990) Human monocyte chemoattractant protein-1 (MCP-1). *Immunology Today*, **11**, 97–101.

26. Colotta, F., Borre, A., Wang, J.M. *et al.* (1992) Expression of a monocyte chemotactic cytokine by human mononuclear phagocytes. *Journal of Immunology*, **148**, 760–5.

27. Rolfe, M.W., Kunkel, S.L., Standiford, T.J. *et al.* (1992) Expression and regulation of human pulmonary fibroblast-derived monocyte chemotactic peptide (MCP-1). *American Journal of Physiology*, **263**, L536–45.

28. Standiford, T.J., Kunkel, S.L., Phan, S.H. *et al.*

(1991) Alveolar macrophage-derived cytokines induce monocyte chemoattractant protein-1 expression from human pulmonary type II like epithelial cells. *Journal of Biological Chemistry*, **266**, 9912–8.

29. Standiford, T.J., Kunkel, S.L. and Basha, M.A. *et al.* (1990) Interleukin-8 gene expression by a pulmonary epithelial cell line: a model for cytokine networks in the lung. *Journal of Clinical Investigation*, **86**, 1945–53.

30. Hance, A.J. (1991) Accessory cell–lymphocyte interactions, in *Lung: Scientific Foundations* (eds R.G. Crystal and J.B. West), Raven Press, New York, pp. 483–98.

31. Holt, P.G., Schon-Hegrad, M.A. and Oliver, J. (1988) MHC class II antigen-bearing dendritic cells in pulmonary tissues of the rat. *Journal of Experimental Medicine*, **167**, 262–74.

32. Nicod, L.P., Lipscomb, M.F., Toews, G.B. *et al.* (1989) Separation of potent and poorly functional human lung accessory cells based on autofluorescence. *Journal of Leukocyte Biology*, **45**, 458–65.

33. Pollard, A.A. and Lipscomb, M.F. (1990) Characterization of murine lung dendritic cells: similarities to Langerhans cells and thymic dendritic cells. *Journal of Experimental Medicine*, **172**, 159–67.

34. Inaba, K., Young, J.W.E. and Steinman, R.M. (1987) Direct activation of CD8$^+$ cytotoxic T lymphocytes by dendritic cells. *Journal of Experimental Medicine*, **166**, 182–94.

35. Peeler, J.S. and Niederkorn, J.Y. (1986) Antigen presentation by Langerhans cells *in vivo*: donor-derived Ia + Langerhans cells are required for induction of delayed-type hypersensitivity but not by cytotoxic T lymphocyte responses to alloantigens. *Journal of Immunology*, **136**, 4362–71.

36. Mosmann, T.R. and Coffman, R.L. (1989) Th1 and Th2 cells: different patterns of lymphokine secretion lead to different functional properties. *Annual Review of Immunology*, **7**, 145–73.

37. De Libero, G., Flesch, I. and Kaufmann, S.H. (1988) Mycobacteria-reactive LyT-2 + T cell lines. *European Journal of Immunology*, **18**, 59–66.

38. Mody, C.H., Lipscomb, M.F., Street, N.E. *et al.* (1990) Depletion of CD4 + (L3T4 +) lymphocytes *in vivo* impairs murine host defense to *Cryptococcus neoformans*. *Journal of Immunology*, **144**, 1472–7.

39. Mody, C.H., Chen, C.G., Jackson, C. *et al.* (1993)

Depletion of murine CD8 + T cells *in vivo* decreased pulmonary clearance of a moderately virulent strain of *Cryptococcus neoformans*. *Journal of Laboratory and Clinical Medicine*, **121**, 765–72.

40. Huffnagle, G.B., Yales, J.L. and Lipscomb, M.F. (1991) Immunity to a pulmonary *Cryptococcus neoformans* infection requires both CD4 + and CD8 + T cells. *Journal of Experimental Medicine*, **173**, 793–800.

41. Bell, R.C., Coalson, J.J., Smith, J.D. *et al* (1983) Multi-organ system failure and infection in adult respiratory distress syndrome. *Annals of Internal Medicine*, **99**, 293–8.

42. Seidenfeld, J.J., Pohl, D.F., Bell, R.D. *et al.* (1986) Incidence site, and outcome of infections in patients with the adult respiratory distress syndrome. *American Review of Respiratory Disease*, **134**, 12–16.

43. Celis, R., Torres, A., Gatell, J.M. *et al.* (1988) Nosocomial pneumonia: a multi-variate analysis of risk and prognosis. *Chest*, **93**, 318–24.

44. Cross, A.S. and Roup, B. (1981) Role of respiratory assistance devices in endemic nosocomial pneumonia. *American Journal of Medicine*, **70**, 681–5.

45. Haley, R.W., Hooton, T.M., Culver, D.H. *et al.* (1981) Nosocomial infections in US hospitals, 1975–1976: estimated frequency by selected characteristics of patients. *American Journal of Medicine*, **70**, 947–59.

46. Fagon, J.Y., Chastre, J., Domart, Y. *et al* (1989) Nosocomial pneumonia in patients receiving continuous mechanical ventilation: prospective analysis of 52 episodes with use of a protected specimen brush and quantitative culture techniques. *American Review of Respiratory Disease*, **139**, 877–84.

47. Gross, P.A. and Van Antwerpen, C. (1983) Nosocomial infections and hospital deaths: a case–control study. *American Journal of Medicine*, **75**, 658–62.

48. Gross, P.A., Neu, H.C. Aswapokee, P. *et al.* (1980) Deaths from nosocomial infection: experience in a university hospital and a community hospital. *American Journal of Medicine*, **68**, 219–23.

49. Craven, D.E., Kunches, L.M., Kilinsky, V. *et al.* (1986) Risk factors for pneumonia and fatality in patients receiving continuous mechanical ventilation. *American Review of Respiratory Disease*, **133**, 792–6.

50. Fagon, J.Y., Chastre, Y., Hance, A.J. *et al.* (1988)

Detection of nosocomial lung infection in ventilated patients: use of a protected specimen brush and quantitative culture technique in 147 patients. *American Review of Respiratory Disease*, **138**, 110–6.

51. Johanson, W.G., Pierce, A.K. and Sanford, J.P. (1969) Changing pharyngeal flora of hospitalized patients: emergence of Gram-negative bacilli. *New England Journal of Medicine*, **281**, 1137–40.

52. Johanson, W.G. Jr, Pierce, A.K., Sanford, J.P. *et al.* (1972) Nosocomial respiratory infection with gram-negative bacilli: the significance of colonization in the respiratory tract. *Annals of Internal Medicine*, **77**, 701–6.

53. Reynolds, H.Y. (1987) Bacterial adherence to respiratory tract mucosa: a dynamic interaction leading to colonization. *Seminars in Respiratory Infections*, **2**, 8–19.

54. Sottile, F.D., Marrie, T.J., Prough, D.S. *et al.* (1986) Nosocomial pulmonary infection: possible etiologic significance of bacterial adhesion to endotracheal tubes. *Critical Care Medicine*, **14**, 265–70.

55. Sprunt, K. and Redman, W. (1968) Evidence suggesting importance of role of interbacterial inhibition in maintaining balance of normal flora. *Annals of Internal Medicine*, **68**, 579–90.

56. Mackowiak, P.A., Martin, R.M. and Smith, J.W. (1979) The role of bacterial interference in the increased prevalence of oropharyngeal gram-negative bacilli among alcoholics and diabetics. *American Review of Respiratory Disease*, **120**, 589–93.

57. Craven, D.E., Barber, T.W., Steja, K.A. *et al.* (1990) Nosocomial pneumonia in the 1990s: update of epidemiology and risk factors. *Seminars in Respiratory Infection*, **5**, 157–72.

58. Higuchi, J.H. and Johanson, W.G. Jr (1982) Colonization and bronchopulmonary infection. *Clinics in Chest Medicine*, **3**, 133–42.

59. Higuchi, J.H. and Johanson, W.G. (1980) The relationship between adherence of *Pseudomonas aeruginosa* to upper respiratory cells *in vitro* and susceptibility to colonization *in vivo*. *Journal of Laboratory Clinical Medicine*, **95**, 698–705.

60. Higuchi, J.H., Coalson, J.J. and Johanson, W.G. (1982) Bacteriologic diagnosis of nosocomial pneumonia in primates: usefulness of the protected specimen brush. *American Review of Respiratory Disease*, **125**, 53–7.

61. Finlay, B.B. and Falkow, S. (1989) Common theme in microbial pathogenecity. *Microbiology Review*, **53**, 210–30.

62. Spicer, S.S., Schulte, B.A. and Thomopoulos, G.N. (1983) Histochemical properties of the respiratory tract epithelium in different species. *American Review of Respiratory Disease*, **128**, S20–6.

63. Loveless, R.W., and Feizi, T. (1989) Sialo-oligosaccharide receptors for *Mycoplasma pneumoniae* and related oligosaccharides of poly-*N*-acetyllactosamine series are polarized at the cilia and apical-microvillar domains of the ciliated cells in human bronchial epithelium. *Infection and Immunity*, **57**, 1285–9.

64. Varki, A. (1993) Biological roles of oligosaccharides: all of the theories are correct. *Glycobiology*, **3**, 97–130.

65. Dal Nogare, A.R. and Azizi, S.Q. (1992) Chinese hamster ovarian cell glycoproteins that mediate type 1 piliated Gram-negative bacterial adherence. *American Journal of Respiratory Cell and Molecular Biology*, **7**, 399–405.

66. Mason, C.M., Azizi, S.Q. and Dal Nogare, A.R. (1992) Respiratory epithelial carbohydrate levels of rats with Gram-negative bacillary colonization. *Journal of Laboratory and Clinical Medicine*, **120**, 740–5.

67. Woods, D.E., Straus, D.C., Johnson, W.G. Jr *et al.* (1981) Role of fibronectin in the prevention of adherence of *Pseudomonas aeruginosa* to buccal cells. *Journal of Infectious Disease*, **143** 784–90.

68. Huxley, E.J., Viroslaw, J., Gray, W.R. *et al.* (1978) Pharyngeal aspiration in normal adults and patients with depressed consciousness. *American Journal of Medicine*, **64**, 564–8.

69. LaForce, F.M., Mullane, J.F., Boehme, R.F. *et al.* (1973) The effect of pulmonary edema on antibacterial defenses of the lung. *Journal of Clinical and Laboratory Medicine*, **82**, 634–48.

70. Harris, G.D., Woods, D.E., Fine, R. *et al.* (1980) The effect of intra-alveolar fluid on lung bacterial clearance. *Lung*, **158**, 91–100.

71. Seidenfeld, J.J., Mullins, R.C., Fowler, S.R. *et al.* (1986) Bacterial infection and acute lung injury in hamsters. *American Review of Respiratory Disease*, **134**, 22–6.

72. LaForce, F.M. (1976) Effects of alveolar lining material on phagocytic and bacterial activity of lung macrophages against *Staphylococcus aureus*. *Journal of Laboratory and Clinical Medicine*, **88**, 691–9.

73. Juer, J.A., Roger, R.M., McCurdy, J.B. *et al.*

(1976) Enhancement of bactericidal capacity of alveolar macrophages by human alveolar lung material. *Journal of Clinical Investigation*, **58**, 271–5.

74. Coonrod, J.D., Lester, R.L. and Hsu, L.C. (1984) Characterization of the extracellular bactericidal factors of rat alveolar lung material. *Journal of Clinical Investigation*, **74**, 1269–79.

75. Martin, T.R., Pistorese, B.P., Hudson, L.D. *et al.* (1991) The function of lung and blood neutrophils in patients with adult respiratory distress syndrome: implications for the pathogenesis of lung infections. *American Review of Respiratory Disease*, **144**, 254–62.

76. Baldwin, S.R., Simon, R.H., Grum. C.A. *et al.* (1986) Oxidant activity in expired breath from patients with adult respiratory syndrome. *Lancet*, **i**, 11–14.

77. Weiland, J.E., Davis, W.B., Holler, J.F. *et al.* (1986) Lung neutrophils in the adult respiratory distress syndrome. Clinical and pathophysiologic syndrome. *American Review of Respiratory Disease*, **133**, 218–25.

78. Martin, T.R., Pistorese, B.P., Chi, E.Y. *et al.* (1989) Effect of leukotriene B$_4$ in the human lung: recruitment of neutrophils into the alveolar spaces without a change in protein permeability. *Journal of Clinical Investigation*, **84**, 1609–19.

79. Lee, C.T., Fein, A.M., Lippmann, M. *et al.* (1981) Elastolytic activity in pulmonary lavage fluid from patients with adult respiratory distress syndrome. *New England Journal of Medicine*, **304**, 192–6.

80. Smallman, L.A., Hill, S.L. and Stockley, R.A. (1984) Reduction of ciliary beat frequency *in vitro* by sputum from patients with bronchiectasis: a serine proteinase effect. *Thorax*, **39**, 663–7.

81. Niederman, M.S., Merrill, W.W., Polomski, L. *et al.* (1986) Influence of sputum IgA and elastase on tracheal cell bacterial adherence. *American Review of Respiratory Disease*, **133**, 255–60.

82. Fick, R.B. Jr, Baltimore, R.S., Squier, S.U. *et al.* (1985) IgG proteolytic activity of *Pseudomonas aeruginosa* in cystic fibrosis. *Journal of Infectious Disease*, **151**, 589–98.

83. Fick, R.B. Jr, Naegel, G.P., Squier, S.U. *et al.* (1984) Proteins of the cystic fibrosis respiratory tract: fragmented immunoglobulin G opsonic antibody causing defective opsonophagocytosis. *Journal of Clinical Investigation*, **74**, 236–48.

84. Harris, S.E., Nelson, S., Astry, C.L. *et al.* (1988) Endotoxin-induced suppression of pulmonary antibacterial defenses against *Staphylococcus aureus*. *American Review of Respiratory Disease*, **138**, 1439–43.

85. White, J.C., Nelson, S., Winkelstein, J.A. *et al.* (1986) Impairment of antibacterial defense mechanisms of the lung by extrapulmonary infection. *Journal of Infectious Disease*, **153**, 202–8.

86. Nelson, S., Bagby, G.J., Bainton, B.G. *et al.* (1989) Compartmentalization of intraalveolar and systemic lipopolysaccharide-induced tumor necrosis factor and the pulmonary inflammatory response. *Journal of Infectious Disease*, **159**, 189–94.

87. Shennib, H., Chiu, R.C.J., Mulder, D.S. *et al.* (1984) Pulmonary bacterial clearance and alveolar macrophage function in septic shock lung. *American Review of Respiratory Disease*, **130**, 444–9.

88. Hammerschmidt, D.E., Weaver, L.J., Hudson, L.D. *et al.* (1980) Association of complement activation and elevated plasma-C5a with adult respiratory distress syndrome. *Lancet*, **i**, 947–9.

89. Todd, T.R., Glynn, M.F.X., Silver, E. *et al.* (1984) A randomized trial of cryoprecipitate replacement of fibronectin deficiencies in the critically ill. *American Review of Respiratory Disease*, **129**, A102.

90. Esrig, B.C., Frazee, L., Stephenson, S.F. *et al.* (1977) The predisposition to infection following hemorrhagic shock. *Surgery, Gynecology and Obstetrics*. **144**, 915–7.

91. Saba, T.M. (1978) Prevention of liver reticuloendothelial systemic host defense failure after surgery by intravenous opsonic glycoprotein therapy. *Annals of Surgery*, **188**, 142–52.

92. Harris, G.D., Johanson, W.G. Jr, and Pierce, A.K. (1977) Determinants of lung bacterial clearance in mice after acute hypoxia. *American Review of Respiratory Disease*, **116**, 671–7.

93. Huber, G.L., LaForce, F.M. and Mason, R. (1970) Impairment and recovery of pulmonary antibacterial defense mechanisms after oxygen administration. *Journal of Clinical Investigation*, **49**, 47a.

94. Murphy, S.A., Hyams, J.S., Fisher, A.B. *et al.* (1975) Effects of oxygen exposure on *in vitro* function of pulmonary alveolar macrophages. *Journal of Clinical Investigation*, **56**, 503–11.

95. Suttorp, N. and Simon, L.M. (1983) Decreased

bacteridicidal function and impaired respiratory burst in lung macrophages after sustained *in vitro* hyperoxia. *American Review of Respiratory Disease*, **128**, 486–90.

96. Newhouse, M., Sanchis, J. and Bienenstock, J. (1976) Lung defense mechanisms. *New England Journal of Medicine*, **295**, 990–8, 1045–52.

97. Tubaro, E., Borelli, G., Croce, C. *et al.* (1983) Effect of morphine on resistance to infection. *Journal of Infectious Disease*, **148**, 656–66.

98. Esposito, A.L. (1984) Aspirin impairs antibacterial mechanisms in experimental pneumococcal pneumonia. *American Review of Respiratory Disease*, **130**, 857–62.

PART THREE
PHYSIOLOGY

Peter D. Macnaughton

Regardless of the precipitating cause, the pathophysiology of acute lung injury is relatively uniform and characterized by an abnormal increase in pulmonary endothelial and epithelial permeability [1] (Chapter 4). This results in the accumulation of fluid in the pulmonary interstitial and alveolar spaces, reducing ventilated lung volume and resulting in impaired gas exchange, a large increase in intrapulmonary shunt and reduced lung compliance [2]. Other processes including damage to the surfactant system [3] (Chapter 17) and progressive pulmonary fibrosis [4] may further influence gas exchange and lung compliance adversely.

THE ALVEOLAR-CAPILLARY BARRIER

PHYSIOLOGY

The barrier separating the pulmonary capillary lumen and the alveolar space comprises the capillary endothelium and the alveolar epithelium. The interstitial space which lies between is asymmetrically arranged around the capillaries. Thus, on one side of the capillary the interstitial space is obliterated and the width of the barrier is less than 0.5 μm, which facilitates efficient gas exchange. On the other, the space is larger (1–2 μm) and is thought to be the site of fluid flux between the capillary and interstitium [5] (Chapter 21). The Starling relationship describes the factors that affect the net filtration of fluid (F) across the pulmonary endothelial barrier into the interstitial space:

$$F = K[P_c - P_i] - \sigma [\pi_c - \pi_i], \qquad (1)$$

where K = permeability of endothelium to water and small solutes, P_c = capillary pressure, P_i = interstitial space pressure, π_c = plasma protein oncotic pressure, π_i = interstitial oncotic pressure. The reflection coefficient (σ) is a measure of the permeability of the endothelial barrier to plasma proteins. The endothelium is usually relatively impermeable and σ approaches 1, which maintains the oncotic pressure gradient between the interstitial and intravascular compartments and minimizes net fluid flux. However, the endothelial damage associated with acute lung injury results in a large increase in permeability to plasma proteins and the loss of the normal oncotic pressure gradient. Accumulation of fluid in the interstitial space occurs when the maximal lymphatic drainage rate of the pulmonary interstitium has been exceeded; which is approximately eight times basal flow rates [6].

It is thought that the epithelium represents the chief barrier to the leakage of fluid into the alveolar space [7]. The junction between adjacent endothelial cells is 5 nm, compared with the 1 nm tight junction observed between epithelial cells [8]. This suggests that

ARDS Acute Respiratory Distress in Adults. Edited by Timothy W. Evans and Christopher Haslett. Published in 1996 by Chapman & Hall, London. ISBN 0 412 56910 8

the epithelial barrier is highly impermeable to proteins, which maintains a dry alveolar space due to the oncotic pressure gradient across the epithelium [9]. However, when alveolar flooding occurs during hydrostatic pulmonary edema the composition of fluid entering the airways is almost identical to that of the interstitial space, implying that the epithelium can become freely permeable [10]. It has been postulated that the alveolar space is normally kept dry by the water repellant properties of alveolar surfactant [11]. Mild lung injury can result in interstitial edema formation which may not affect gas exchange significantly [12]. With more severe injury, increased fluid filtration into the interstitial compartment combined with epithelial damage causes alveolar flooding and marked impairment of oxygenation. Associated abnormalities of surfactant function [3] may impair its water repellant properties and potentiate flooding of the alveolar space.

ASSESSMENT OF ALVEOLAR-CAPILLARY PERMEABILITY

A number of techniques have been described to assess the permeability of the alveolar-capillary barrier [13]. The net fluid flux into the interstitium can be measured if the pulmonary lymphatics are cannulated, a procedure limited to animal models of lung injury [14]. Increased permeability of the alveolar capillary unit can be demonstrated if intravenously injected human serum albumin labeled with iodine-131 is recovered from the bronchoalveolar space [15]. The albumin clearance can be calculated if the radioactivity in samples of blood and tracheal aspirate is subsequently quantified. Using this technique a highly significant increase in albumin clearance rates has been demonstrated in patients with pulmonary insufficiency associated with sepsis compared with a group with left ventricular failure [15]. Albumin clearance measured by this method probably reflects epithelial barrier function as this is the rate

limiting component of the overall permeability of the alveolar-capillary unit.

More recently, a double isotope technique to quantify pulmonary endothelial permeability has been described [16]. Transferrin, which has a similar molecular weight to albumin, is labelled with indium-113m and red blood cells with technetium-99m. A protein accumulation index (PAI) can be derived from the relative accumulation in the lungs of transferrin compared with red blood cells and can be measured at the bedside using either a gamma camera or miniscintillation counters [17]. By using an intravascular marker the technique corrects for changes in pulmonary vascular surface area. The technique appears both highly sensitive and specific in quantifying the permeability defect that characterizes acute lung injury [18] and is uninfluenced by cardiogenic pulmonary edema. However, although an abnormal increase in permeability may precede the clinical recognition of pulmonary edema [19], there is considerable overlap in permeability measurements obtained from adult patients with the syndrome of acute respiratory distress (ARDS) and other critically ill patients [20]. Thus, the absolute value of PAI does not appear to predict outcome. Moreover, it has been demonstrated that the improvement in lung function during the recovery phase of ARDS appears to occur while measurable abnormalities of endothelial permeability persist [21]. These observations support the concept that the epithelial barrier is crucial in maintaining a dry alveolar space and that improvement in lung function from pulmonary edema occurs due to recovery of epithelial active transport mechanisms [22].

The permeability of the epithelial barrier can be assessed from the rate of disappearance from the lungs of inhaled ^{99m}Tc-labeled diethylenetriaminepenta-acetate (DTPA) [23]. DTPA clearance is expressed as a half life in minutes with normal nonsmoking subjects having a value of approximately 60 minutes. ARDS is associated with an increased clearance of DTPA with a mean half life of 20 minutes, although there is considerable overlap with values obtained in smokers without lung injury [24]. However, in ARDS the disappearance of DTPA from the lungs often follows a biexponential pattern which is thought to be always abnormal.

DTPA clearance is influenced by a range of both pathological and physiological states [25]. Thus the increase in lung volume that follows the application of positive end expiratory pressure (PEEP) accelerates DTPA clearance [25]. This lack of specificity has limited the clinical utility of the technique, although serial measurements in individual patients, combined with a correction for changes in lung volume, could be used to demonstrate recovery of epithelial integrity.

LUNG WATER

TECHNIQUES OF MEASUREMENT

The pulmonary edema that characterizes acute lung injury results in a large increase in extravascular lung water (EVLW) which can be estimated by a number of methods [26] (Chapter 21).

The thermal dye or dual indicator technique involves the injection of ice cold indocyanine green into a central vein with subsequent sampling from the femoral artery [27]. Heat is the diffusible indicator that distributes to the extravascular volume and indocyanine green is the nondiffusible indicator that remains within the intravascular space. The difference in the volumes of distribution of the two reflects lung tissue volume and appears to correlate with gravimetric estimation of EVLW [28]. However, the technique assumes that lung perfusion is homogenous, which is clearly not the case in ARDS. This may explain the observation that PEEP appears to increase EVLW measured by this technique [29] and that the results obtained are sensitive to hemodynamic change [30].

The soluble inert gas technique is attractive, being noninvasive and relatively simple to perform. The subject breathes a mixture of moderately soluble (acetylene or freon) and insoluble (helium or argon) gases and either breath holds, or more conveniently rebreathes [31]. The initial fall in concentration of the soluble gas represents its dilution by the alveolar volume (V_A) and rapid uptake into the pulmonary tissue. Any subsequent fall is attributable to lung perfusion. From differences in the initial alveolar concentrations of soluble and insoluble gases (the insoluble gas is only distributed to V_A), an estimate of lung tissue volume is obtained, of which more than 80% is water. Animal studies suggest that the technique underestimates EVLW in severe lung injury when ventilation is unevenly distributed [32]. The technique has not been extensively evaluated in the intensive care unit (ICU). Changes in lung water have been inferred from alterations in thoracic impedance [33], although any process that affects thoracic gas (e.g. atelectasis) or fluid volumes (e.g. pleural effusion) influences the result [34]. The recent development of digital radiography for use in the ICU may result in more accurate quantification of lung water from portable chest radiographs [35], but to date the thermal dye method has been used in the majority of clinical studies.

CLINICAL STUDIES

Thermal dye estimates of EVLW have been compared in patients with radiographic pulmonary edema of either cardiac or noncardiac (permeability) origin [36]. Mean EVLW was 15.8 ml/kg in those with permeability pulmonary edema, which was significantly greater than the mean value of 10.2 ml/kg in those with cardiac failure. Patients without radiographic evidence of pulmonary edema had a mean EVLW of 5.6 ml/kg. In addition to defining the 'normal' range of EVLW measurements, this study demonstrated a correlation between EVLW and chest radiograph score. A second study from the same group examined the influence of pulmonary artery occlusion pressure (PAOP) measurements on EVLW [37]. Increases in PAOP resulted in a larger increase in EVLW in patients with permeability pulmonary edema compared with those with left ventricular failure. These observations are supported by the Starling relationship, which predicts that when permeability is increased the most important factor in controlling net fluid flux is the capillary hydrostatic pressure. The clinical role and utility of EVLW measurements is unclear. A measurement of less than 7 ml/kg, used as a goal in a controlled trial of fluid therapy (diuresis and fluid restriction compared with standard fluid therapy) in 101 patients at risk of acute lung injury, resulted in a significant reduction in EVLW, fewer days on the ventilator and a shorter ICU stay [38], although it is unclear whether the same results could have been obtained without such monitoring.

LUNG VOLUMES

ARDS causes a severe restrictive respiratory defect. Vital capacity (VC) can be measured at the bedside with a spirometer, although many critically ill patients are unable to perform a meaningful measurement, such that VC is more a measure of patient cooperation and respiratory muscle strength. The inspiratory capacity and expiratory reserve volume can be measured by alternatively occluding the expiratory and inspiratory limbs respectively on the breathing circuit of a spontaneously breathing patient [39], thereby allowing a more accurate estimate of VC to be obtained in an uncooperative patient.

Functional residual capacity (FRC), which represents the volume of gas remaining in the lungs at the end of a normal expiration, is markedly reduced in ARDS [40] and a number of methods have been described to estimate FRC in patients with acute respiratory failure. The nitrogen washout technique derives FRC from the volume of nitrogen released when the inspired oxygen tension (F_{IO_2}) is increased by more than 20% from its baseline value [41]. The technique is inaccurate when performed in those requiring high F_{IO_2} and its use on the ICU is therefore limited. An adaptation of the nitrogen washout principle has been described using sulfur hexaflouride (SF_6) [42]. The technique has been successfully undertaken in the ICU and can be performed at high F_{IO_2}. Inert gas dilution methods have been performed but have usually required rather complex and unwieldy equipment [43]. More recently, a simple inert gas rebreathing technique has been described in which an accurate and reproducible value of FRC can be derived from the change in helium concentration that occurs after rebreathing six breaths from a 1 liter anesthetic bag [44].

The normal value of FRC of between 2.5 and 3 liters is reduced to less than 1 liter in patients with ARDS [45], due to alveolar flooding by edema fluid and inflammatory exudate and secondary to collapse consequent upon alterations in the mechanical properties of the lungs [4]. The lungs become very heavy due to the widespread infiltration with fluid and inflammatory debris, and computed tomographic (CT) studies have demonstrated the preponderance of areas of high density (representing fluid and collapse) in the dependent regions, with relatively normal lung in the nondependent regions [46] (Figure 15.1). Following the application of PEEP, the areas of high density diminish in number suggesting re-expansion of collapsed lung (recruitable). Other high density regions remain, regardless of the level of applied PEEP (nonrecruitable) [47]. An optimal level of PEEP that caused maximal recruitment of collapsed lung on CT without overdistension of normal lung could be defined for each patient.

Improvement in lung function in ARDS is associated with an increase in FRC [45]. Re-expansion of recruitable lung results in ven-

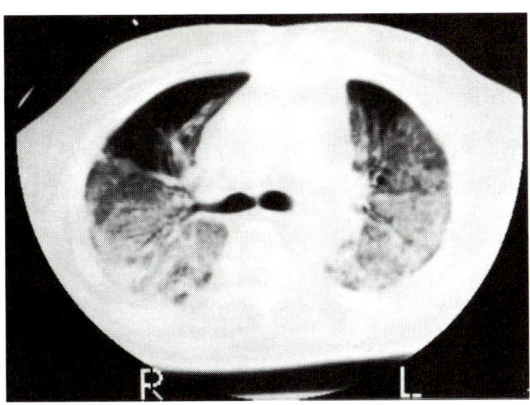

Figure 15.1 Thoracic CT scan of patient with ARDS. Note the presence of areas of normal lung, particularly in the nondependent regions.

tilation of previously collapsed areas and reversal of shunt. However, there have been few studies to assess the clinical utility measurements of FRC in ventilated subjects, largely due to the lack of readily applicable techniques.

GAS EXCHANGE

CAUSES OF GAS EXCHANGE IMPAIRMENT

The impaired gas exchange that occurs in acute lung injury is characterized by refractory hypoxemia and inefficient clearance of CO_2. A number of mechanisms can cause hypoxemia, including diffusion impairment, ventilation perfusion ($\dot{V}/\dot{Q}$) mismatch and shunt. An increase in alveolar dead space reduces the effective minute volume and impairs CO_2 clearance [48]. In addition, the increase in basal metabolic rate which often accompanies ARDS results in an increase in O_2 utilization and CO_2 production, adding to the demands on the respiratory system.

Studies using the multiple inert gas technique have confirmed that the abnormalities of gas exchange which occur in ARDS are attributable mainly to a marked increase in intrapulmonary shunt and dead space [48].

The loss of lung volume due to alveolar flooding and atelectasis results in areas of the lung which are unventilated, the persistence of perfusion to which results in significant intrapulmonary shunt. This also implies that the reflex of hypoxic pulmonary vasoconstriction (HPV) is abolished. Animal studies suggest that a number of mechanisms may be important in inhibiting HPV, including the release of vasodilator prostanoids [49] and the release of endogenous nitric oxide [50]. Both these substances are endothelially derived and their release is influenced by endothelial damage.

The presence of interstitial fluid should increase the distance of the diffusion path for gas exchange between the alveolus and capillary lumen, but although gas transfer, as measured by the carbon monoxide transfer factor (TLCO), is markedly impaired in ARDS [45], it is unclear whether this reflects diffusion impairment or a reduction in pulmonary blood volume.

The increased dead space could result from a number of causes. Areas of inadequate pulmonary perfusion may result from obliteration of the pulmonary vasculature secondary to capillary thrombosis and embolic phenomena, combined with the release of vaso active mediators, producing pulmonary vasoconstriction [51]. The mode of ventilation employed and the level of PEEP applied may also adversely affect perfusion and therefore increase alveolar dead space [52].

ASSESSMENT OF GAS EXCHANGE

The assessment of gas exchange in patients with acute lung injury is often limited to the measurement of arterial blood gas tensions. However, the interpretation of a particular value of Pa_{O_2} is influenced by both pulmonary (Pa_{CO_2}, FI_{O_2}, V/Q match, shunt) and non pulmonary (cardiac output, peripheral oxygen utilization) factors [53]. The alveolar-arterial oxygen tension gradient (A-a gradient) can be calculated using the simplified alveolar gas equation:

$$P_{AO_2} - P_{ao_2} = F_{IO_2} - (\frac{P_{aco_2}}{RQ}) - P_{ao_2} \quad (2)$$

which attempts to correct P_{ao_2} for changes in P_{aco_2} and F_{IO_2}. However, the A-a gradient is influenced by F_{IO_2}, such that the normal value (< 1 kPa breathing air) rises considerably whilst breathing 100% O_2. The ratio of P_{ao_2} to the alveolar P_{O_2} (aA ratio) is not as dependent upon F_{IO_2} [54], but is still influenced by changes in mixed venous P_{O_2} (P_{vo_2}), which in turn is affected by cardiac output and peripheral oxygen utilization (V_{O_2}). These non pulmonary factors can be controlled for by estimating the venous admixture or overall shunt-like effect [55]. A simultaneous measurement of the mixed venous gas tensions in blood obtained via a pulmonary artery catheter enables venous admixture to be estimated as follows:

$$\frac{\dot{Q}s}{\dot{Q}t} = \frac{(Cc_{O_2} - Ca_{O_2})}{(Cc_{O_2} - Cv_{O_2})}, \quad (3)$$

where Cc_{O_2} is the oxygen content of capillary blood, Ca_{O_2} the oxygen content of arterial blood and Cv_{O_2} the oxygen content of mixed venous blood. Cc_{O_2} cannot be measured directly, but is derived from the calculated alveolar P_{O_2}. If a normal value for Cv_{O_2} is assumed, shunt can be estimated from the P_{ao_2} and F_{IO_2} alone using isoshunt plots [56]. However, this approach is invalid in the critically ill, where the values for cardiac output and peripheral oxygen utilization may vary considerably from normal values such that Cv_{O_2} cannot be estimated, and a mixed venous blood sample should be obtained. The calculation of venous admixture has been used to quantify the severity of lung injury [57] and guide therapy, but requires the insertion of a pulmonary artery catheter.

PULMONARY MECHANICS

PRESSURE–VOLUME RELATIONSHIPS

Compliance and acute lung injury

A marked reduction in pulmonary compliance was observed in the first description of ARDS [58]. In most series published since, a reduction in total pulmonary compliance (usually to less than 30 ml/cmH$_2$O, normal > 100 ml/cmH$_2$O) has been a diagnostic requirement. Total compliance (C_T) can be considered as the sum of the reciprocal of chest wall (C_W) and lung (C_L) compliances (elastance):

$$\frac{1}{C_T} = \frac{1}{C_W} + \frac{1}{C_L}. \quad (4)$$

Chest wall compliance is probably unaffected in ARDS, such that a marked reduction in lung compliance principally determines C_T. Contributory factors include the presence of interstitial fluid and fibrosis, abnormalities of surfactant structure and function, and the loss of lung volume [59]. Surfactant changes are probably most relevant at low lung volumes when alveolar dimensions are least and the law of Laplace predicts that surface tension forces are at their greatest. At high lung volumes changes in the lung intersititium are more influential in reducing C_L.

In addition, particularly in the early stages of ARDS, the reduction in compliance may be explained by the reduction in ventilated lung volume. Although C_T may be significantly reduced, the specific compliance (compliance corrected for the absolute volume of aerated lung) may therefore be within normal limits [60]. This is illustrated by considering a patient with normal lungs undergoing pneumonectomy. If the total compliance before operation was 100 ml/cmH$_2$O, after pneumonectomy, when approximately 50% of the aerated lung volume is removed, compliance will fall to 50 ml/cmH$_2$O. However, specific compliance will be unchanged. Thus, in early

ARDS, applying PEEP to recruit collapsed areas of lung may increase C_T towards normal values [60]. These observations support the 'baby lung' concept proposed by Gattinoni and others [46], whereby ARDS does not affect the lung in a uniform manner but rather is heterogenous, allowing the presence of normal areas of lung. The application of large tidal volumes to these small volume lungs may result in excessive peak alveolar pressure and the attendant risks of barotrauma and exacerbation of lung injury.

Measurement

In order to measure C_L an estimate of the alveolar-pleural pressure gradient is required. In clinical practice this is undertaken by inserting an esophageal balloon and using the pressure measured as an estimate of pleural pressure [61]. However, the technique is relatively invasive and may be inaccurate in the supine posture when cardiac artifact is greatest. As C_W is unaffected by ARDS, it is acceptable to measure C_T using airway pressure as an estimate of alveolar pressure.

The airway pressure generated during inspiration depends on a number of factors, considered as follows [62]:

$$P = \dot{V}R + \frac{V}{C} + P_{\text{exp}}, \qquad (5)$$

where P = airway pressure, $\dot{V}$ = rate of gas flow, R = resistive forces including airway resistance and inertia of the system, V = tidal volume, C = total compliance and Pexp = total PEEP (applied + intrinsic). If peak airway pressure after delivering a measured tidal volume is recorded, dynamic compliance can be calculated simply (Figure 15.2). This value will include a significant resistive component, and parameters such as the inspiratory flow rate, endotracheal tube diameter and airway resistance will influence the result [63]. If the pause or plateau pressure is recorded, resistive forces should be mini-

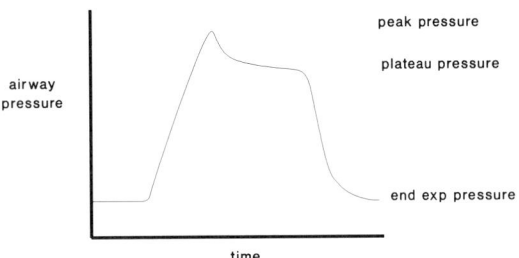

Figure 15.2 Airway pressure–time curve and derivation of dynamic (tidal volume/peak pressure – PEEP) and static (tidal volume/plateau pressure – PEEP) compliances.

mized such that a reasonable estimate of static compliance can be obtained (Figure 15.2). However, if there are marked regional variations in airways resistance and compliance, such as occur in chronic airways disease, a prolonged pause is required to allow equalization of alveolar pressures. The presence of intrinsic or auto PEEP leads to underestimations of compliance if not accounted for [64]. Intrinsic PEEP is greatest in patients with obstructive airways disease where values in excess of 20 cmH_2O have been reported [65], although significant levels may also occur in ARDS [66]. Total PEEP (external + intrinsic) can be measured simply by noting the maximum airways pressure following an end expiratory pause [65].

Accurate and reproducible measurements of compliance require that the subject is paralyzed with neuromuscular blocking agents in order to prevent respiratory muscle activity. However, the resultant loss of chest wall muscle tone increases C_T and should be considered when comparing measurements made under different conditions. A number of workers have described techniques for constructing a complete static inspiratory and expiratory pressure volume curve [67]. Following neuromuscular blockade, the static airway pressure changes that occur after 100 ml volume increments from a large syringe (supersyringe) are recorded during inspiration and expiration.

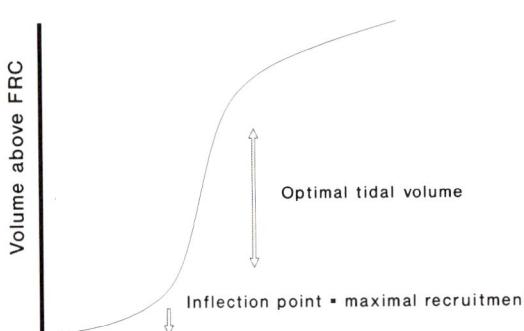

Figure 15.3 Static lung pressure–volume curve of patient with ARDS. Note the inflection point representing maximal recruitment of collapsed lung and the optimal tidal volume avoiding pulmonary overdistension.

Clinical application

Although measurements of compliance are invariably included in the diagnostic criteria for ARDS, it is not always clear if static or dynamic values have been obtained or whether neuromuscular blocking agents have been employed. The lung injury score described by Murray and colleagues includes estimates of dynamic compliance, and is therefore influenced by changes in tracheal tube diameter and inspiratory flow rate [68]. In assessing the severity of lung injury and the requirement for extracorporeal support, Gattinoni utilized measurements of static compliance undertaken with the patient paralyzed [69]. More recently the pressure-volume (*P-V*) curve has been used to titrate ventilator therapy [70].

In ARDS the *P-V* curve may show an inflection point where the slope is shifted upwards, representing an increase in lung compliance due to the recruitment of collapsed alveoli [67,71,72] (Figure 15.3). With increasing airway pressures, the curve flattens, reflecting a reduction in compliance as maximal alveolar recruitment occurs and pulmonary over distension develops. Applying PEEP equal to the pressure at the inflection point produces max-

imal recruitment and therefore the largest reduction in intra pulmonary shunt [70,71]. Tidal volume should then be reduced, such that plateau pressures do not impinge upon the flat portion of the curve, thereby preventing overdistension, barotrauma and a possible paradoxical increase in shunt. The reduction in tidal volume may be associated with an increase in Pa_{CO_2}, a technique termed 'permissive hypercapnia'. Pa_{CO_2} at tensions greater than 12 kPa have been tolerated without adverse affect; an improved outcome has been claimed in patients with ARDS ventilated to minimize maximal airway pressure without regard for the Pa_{CO_2} compared with historical controls [73].

AIRWAY RESISTANCE

Inspiratory airway resistance is most commonly measured from changes in airway pressures that occur following end inspiratory occlusion [74]. Using this technique, a sixfold increase in inspiratory airway resistance in subjects with ARDS compared with normal controls has been described [75]. Airway hyperactivity may occur due to the actions of the various pro-inflammatory mediators that cause acute lung injury [76], and increased airway resistance may result from edema of the airway wall and the presence of fluid and/or secretions within the airway lumen. A further factor that may contribute to an increase in total airway resistance is the decrease in the number of airways available for gas exchange secondary to a loss of functional lung volume. Such a mechanism will reduce resistance without necessarily affecting individual airway diameter. However, as no study has documented specific resistance (resistance per unit lung volume) it is unclear whether the increase in airway resistance observed in ARDS reflects a true reduction in effective airway diameter.

Although the very low lung compliance that occurs in ARDS results in high expiratory driving pressures and flow rates, the measured expiratory resistance may actually be increased [77]. In contrast to patients with obstructive airways disease, where PEEP may prevent dynamic airways collapse and therefore reduces expiratory resistance, the application of PEEP does not reduce expiratory resistance in patients with ARDS.

SUMMARY

Although significant progress has been made in understanding the processes that underlie acute lung injury, therapy remains essentially supportive. By understanding the physiological processes that underlie the abnormalities of pulmonary function such treatment can be applied to maximal effect. Moreover, there is an increasing body of evidence that conventional methods of respiratory support may actually exacerbate lung injury [78].

By guiding ventilatory therapy, both by assessment of arterial blood gas tensions and by analysis of the static pressure – volume curve of the lungs, adverse affects should be minimized. Although CT studies may reveal unexpected abnormalities (e.g. pneumothorax, abscess), they are not a practical method of assessing ventilatory therapy in the majority of centers. Recent studies have confirmed the benefits of maintaining a negative fluid balance, and accurate methods of measuring lung water may improve outcome. Further research is required to identify methods of predicting those patients with lung injury who will develop full blown ARDS. Unfortunately, the measurements of alveolar-capillary permeability that have been developed so far do not appear to fulfill this role.

REFERENCES

1. Brigham, K.L., Woolverton, W., Blake, L. and Staub, N.C. (1974) Increased sheep lung vascular permeability caused by psuedomonas bacteraemia. *Journal of Clinical Investigation* **54**, 792–804.
2. Lamy, M., Fallat, R.J., Koeniger, E. *et al.* (1976) Pathologic features and mechanisms of hypoxemia in adult respiratory distress syndrome. *American Review of Respiratory Disease*, **114**, 267–84.
3. Hallman, M., Spragg, R., Harrell, J.H. *et al.* (1982) Evidence of lung surfactant abnormality in respiratory failure. Study of broncho-alveolar lavage phospholipids, surface activity, phospholipase activity and plasma myoinositol. *Journal of Clinical Investigation*, **70**, 673–83.
4. Tomashefski, J.F. (1990) Pulmonary pathology of the adult respiratory distress syndrome. *Clinics in Chest Medicine*, **11**, 593–619.
5. Weibel, E.R. (1973) Morphological basis of alveolar-capillary gas exchange. *Physiology Review*, **53**, 419–95.
6. Erdmann, J.A., Vaughan, T.R., Brigham, K.L. *et al.* (1975) Effect of increased vascular pressure on fluid balance in unanesthetized sheep. *Circulation Research*, **37**, 271–84.
7. Schneeberger, E.E. (1979) Barrier function of intracellular junctions in adult and fetal lungs, in *Pulmonary Edema* (eds A.P. Fishman and E.M. Renkin), American Physiological Society, Washington, pp. 21–37.
8. DeFouw, D.O. (1983) Ultrastructural features of alveolar epithelial transport. *American Review of Respiratory Disease*, **127**, S9–13.
9. Egan, E.A. (1983) Fluid balance in the air-filled space. *American Review of Respiratory Disease*, **127**, 537–9.
10. Vreim, C.E., Snashall, P.D. and Staub, N.C. (1976) Protein composition of lung fluids in anaesthetised dogs. *American Journal of Physiology*, **230**, 376–9.
11. Hills, B.A. (1988) *The Biology of Surfactant*, Cambridge University Press, Cambridge.
12. Staub, N.C., Nagano, H. and Pearce, M.L. (1967) Pulmonary edema in dogs, especially the sequence of fluid accumulation in lungs. *Journal of Applied Physiology*, **22**, 227–40.
13. Hunter, D.N., Morgan, C.J. and Evans, T.W. (1990) The use of radionuclide techniques in the assessment of alveolar – capillary permeability on the intensive care unit. *Intensive Care Medicine*, **16**, 363–71.
14. Woolverton, W.C., Brigham, K.L. and Staub, N.C. (1978) Effect of positive pressure breathing on lung lymph flow and water content in sheep. *Circulation Research*, **42**, 550–7.
15. Anderson, R.R., Holliday, R.L., Driedger, A.A. *et al.* (1979) Documentation of pulmonary capillary permeability in the adult respiratory dis-

tress syndrome accompanying human sepsis. *American Review of Respiratory Disease*, **119**, 869–77.

16. Gorin, A.B., Kohler, J. and DeNardo, G. (1980) Noninvasive measurement of pulmonary transvascular protein flux in normal man. *Journal of Clinical Investigation*, **66**, 869–77.

17. Hunter, D.N., Lawrence, R., Morgan, C.J. and Evans, T.W. (1990) The use of caesium iodide mini scintillation counters for dual isotope pulmonary capillary permeability studies. *Nuclear Medicine Communications*, **11**, 879–88.

18. Dauber, I.M., Pluss, W.T., VanGrondelle, A. *et al.* (1985) Specificity and sensitivity of non-invasive measurement of pulmonary vascular protein leak. *Journal of Applied Physiology*, **59**, 564–74.

19. Braude, S., Baudouin, S. and Evans, TW. (1992) Serial assessment of pulmonary microvascular permeability in a patient developing the adult respiratory distress syndrome. *European Respiratory Journal*, **5**, 500–2.

20. Rocker, G.M., Wiseman, M.S., Pearson, D. and Shale, D.J. (1989) Diagnostic criteria for ARDS: time for reappraisal. *Lancet*, **i**, 120–3.

21. Calandrino, F.S., Anderson, D.J., Mintun, M.A. and Schuster, D.P. (1988) Pulmonary vascular permeability during the adult respiratory distress syndrome. A positron emission tomographic study. *American Review of Respiratory Disease*, **138**, 421–8.

22. Matthay, M.A. and Wiener-Kronish, J.P. (1990) Intact epithelial barrier function is critical for resolution of alveolar edema in humans. *American Review of Respiratory Disease*, **142**, 1250–7.

23. O'Brodovich, H. and Coates, G. (1987) Pulmonary clearance of ^{99m}Tc-DTPA: a non-invasive assessment of epithelial integrity. *Lung*, **165**, 1–16.

24. Braude, S., Nolop, K.B., Hughes, J.M.B. *et al.* (1986) Comparison of lung vascular and epithelial permeability indices in the adult respiratory distress syndrome. *American Review of Respiratory Disease*, **133**, 1002–5.

25. Nolop, K.B., Maxwell, D.L., Royston, D. and Hughes, J.M.B. (1986) Effect of raised thoracic pressure and volume on ^{99m}Tc-DTPA clearance in humans. *Journal of Applied Physiology*, **60**, 1493–7.

26. Cutillo, A.G. (1987) The clinical assessment of lung water. *Chest*, **92**, 319–25.

27. Lewis, F.R., Elings, V.B. and Storm, J.A. (1979) Bedside measurement of lung water. *Journal of Surgical Research*, **27**, 250–61.

28. Mihm, F.G., Feeley, T.W. and Jamieson, S.W. (1981) Comparison of thermal dye indicator dilution with gravimetric lung water measurement in humans. *Critical Care Medicine*, **9**, 256 (abstract).

29. Carlile, P.V., Lowery, D.D. and Gray, B.A. (1986) Effect of PEEP and type of injury on thermal-dye estimation of pulmonary edema. *Journal of Applied Physiology*, **60**, 22–31.

30. Fallon, K.D., Drake, R.E., Laine, G.A. and Gabel, J.C. (1985) Effect of cardiac output on extravascular lung water estimates made with the Edwards® lung water computer. *Anesthesiology*, **62**, 505–8.

31. Overland, E.S., Gupta, R.N., Huchon, G.J. and Murray, J.F. (1981) Measurement of pulmonary tissue volume and blood flow in persons with normal and edematous lungs. *Journal of Applied Physiology*, **51**, 1375–83.

32. Peterson, B.T., Petrini, M.F., Hyde, R.W. and Schreiner, B.F. (1978) Pulmonary tissue volume in dogs during pulmonary edema. *Journal of Applied Physiology*, **44**, 782–95.

33. Zellner, J.L., Spinale, F.G. and Crawford, F.A. (1990) Bioimpedance: a novel method for the assessment of extravascular lung water. *Journal of Surgical Research*, **48**, 454–59.

34. Van de Water, J.M., Mount, B.E., Bareca, J.R. *et al.* (1973) Monitoring the chest with impedance. *Chest*, **64**, 597–603.

35. Aberle, D.R., Hansell, D. and Huang, H.K. (1990) Current status of digital projectional radiography of the chest. *Journal of Thoracic Imaging*, **5**, 10–20.

36. Sibbald, W.J., Warshawski, F.J., Short, A.K. *et al.* (1983) Clinical studies of measuring extravascular lung water by the thermal dye technique in critically ill patients. *Chest*, **83**, 725–31.

37. Sibbald, W.J., Short, A.K., Warshawski, F.J. *et al.* (1985) Thermal dye measurement of extravascular lung water in critically ill patients. *Chest*, **5**, 585–92.

38. Mitchell, J.P., Schuller, D., Calandrino, F.S. and Schuster, D.P. (1992) Improved outcome based on fluid management in critically ill patients requiring pulmonary artery catheterisation. *American Review of Respiratory Disease*, **145**, 990–8.

39. Marini, J.J., Rodriguez, R.M. and Lamb, V.J. (1986) Involuntary breathstacking. An alter-

native method for vital capacity estimation in poorly cooperative subjects. *American Review of Respiratory Disease*, **134**, 694–8.

40. Mancebo, J. (1991) Functional residual capacity measurement in acute respiratory failure. Methods of measurement in ventilated patients and their clinical utility, in *Update in Intensive Care and Emergency Medicine, 13. Pulmonary Function in Mechanically Ventilated Patients* (eds S. Benito and A. Net), Springer, Berlin, pp. 155–66.

41. Benis, A.M. and Commerton, T.C. (1980) Validation of an oxygen washing method for the measurement of functional residual capacity in the intensive care unit, In *Proceedings of 2nd International Congress on Computers in Critical Care and Pulmonary Medicine* (eds O. Prakash, A.A. Spence and J.P. Payne), Plenum Press, New York.

42. East, T.D., Wortelboer, P.J.M., Van Ark, E. *et al.* (1990) Automated sulfur hexafluoride washout functional residual capacity measurement system for any mode of mechanical ventilation as well as spontaneous respiration. *Critical Care Medicine*, **18**, 84–91.

43. Weaver, L.J., Pierson, D.J., Kellier, R. *et al.* (1981) A practical procedure for measuring functional residual capacity during mechanical ventilation with or without PEEP. *Critical Care Medicine*, **9**, 873–7.

44. Macnaughton, P.D., Morgan, C.J., Denison, D.M. and Evans, T.W. (1993) Simple technique of measurement of lung volume and carbon monoxide transfer in ventilated subjects. *European Respiratory Journal*, **6**, 231–6.

45. Macnaughton, P.D. and Evans, T.W. (1995) Lung function in ARDS. *American Journal of Respiratory and Critical Care Medicine*, **150**, 770–5.

46. Gattinoni, L., Pesenti, A. and Torresin, A. (1986) Adult respiratory distress syndrome profiles by computed tomography. *Journal of Thoracic Imaging*, **1**, 25–30.

47. Gattinoni, L., Pesenti, A. and Bombino, M. (1988) Relationships between lung computed tomographic density, gas exchange and PEEP in acute respiratory failure. *Anesthesiology*, **60**, 824–32.

48. Dantzker, D.R., Brook, C.J., Dehart, P. *et al.* (1979) Ventilation perfusion distributions in the adult respiratory distress syndrome. *American Review of Respiratory Disease*, **120**, 1039–52.

49. Yamaguchi, K., Mori, M., Kawai, A. *et al.* (1992) Attenuation of hypoxic pulmonary vasoconstriction in acute oleic acid lung injury: significance of vasodilator prostanoids. *Advances in Experimental Medical Biology*, **316**, 299–309.

50. Liu, S., Crawley, D.E., Barnes, P.J. and Evans, T.W. (1991) Endothelial-derived relaxing factor inhibits hypoxic pulmonary vasoconstriction in rats. *American Review of Respiratory Disease*, **143**, 32–7.

51. Zapol, W.M. and Jones, R. (1987) Vascular components of ARDS: clinical pulmonary haemodynamics and morphology. *American Review of Respiratory Disease*, **136**, 471–4.

52. Dueck, R., Wagner, P.D. and West, J.B. (1977) Effects of PEEP on gas exchange in dogs with normal and edematous lungs. *Anesthesiology*, **47**, 359–66.

53. Rodriguez-Rosin, R., Roca, J. and Barbera, J.A. (1991) Extrapulmonary and intrapulmonary determinants of pulmonary gas exchange, in *Update in Intensive Care and Emergency Medicine 15: Ventilatory Failure* (eds J.J. Marini and G. Roussos), Springer, Berlin, pp. 18–35.

54. Gilbert, R. and Keighley, J.F. (1974) The arterial/alveolar oxygen tension ratio. An index of gas exchange applicable to varying inspired oxygen concentrations. *American Review of Respiratory Disease*, **109**, 142–5.

55. Nunn, J.F. (1987) Distribution of pulmonary ventilation and perfusion, in *Applied Respiratory Physiology*, 3rd edn (ed. J.F. Nunn), Butterworth, London, pp. 140–183.

56. Benator, S.R., Hewlett, A.M. and Nunn, J.F. (1973) The use of iso-shunt lines for the control of oxygen therapy. *British Journal of Anaesthesia*, **45**, 711–8.

57. Laghi, F., Siegel, J.H., Rivkind, A.I. *et al.* (1989) Respiratory index/pulmonary shunt relationship. *Critical Care Medicine*, **17**, 1121–8.

58. Ashbaugh, D.G., Bigelow, D.B., Petty, T.L. and Levine, B.E. (1967) Acute respiratory distress in adults. *Lancet*, **ii**, 319–23.

59. Marini, J. (1990) Lung mechanics in ARDS. *Clinics in Chest Medicine*, **11**, 673–90.

60. Benito, S. and Lemaire, F. (1990) Pulmonary pressure–volume relationship in acute respiratory distress syndrome in adults. *Journal of Critical Care*, **5**, 27–34.

61. Anthonisen, N.R. (1986) Tests of mechanical function, in *Handbook of Physiology, sect. 3 The Respiratory System, vol. 3 The Mechanics of Breathing* (eds P.T. Macklem and J. Mead),

American Physiological Society, Bethesda, pp. 753–84.

62. Ottis, A.B., Fenn, W.O. and Rahn, H. (1950) Mechanics of breathing in man. *Journal of Applied Physiology,* **2**, 592–607.

63. Bone, R.C. (1976) Diagnosis of causes for acute respiratory distress by pressure volume curves. *Chest,* **70**, 740–6.

64. Rossi, A., Gottfried, S.B., Zocchi, L. *et al.* (1985) Measurement of static compliance of the total respiratory system in patients with acute respiratory failure during mechanical ventilation. The effect of intrinsic positive end expiratory pressure. *American Review of Respiratory Disease,* **131**, 672–7.

65. Pepe, P.E. and Marini, J.J. (1982) Occult PEEP in mechanically ventilated patients with airflow obstruction. *American Review of Respiratory Disease,* **126**, 166–70.

66. Bernasconi, M., Ploysongsang, Y., Gottfried, S.B. *et al.* (1988) Respiratory compliance and resistance in mechanically ventilated patients with acute respiratory failure. *Intensive Care Medicine,* **14**, 547–53.

67. Matamis, D., Lemaire, F., Hart, A. *et al.* (1984) Total respiratory pressure volume curves in the adult respiratory distress syndrome. *Chest,* **86**, 58–66.

68. Murray, J.F., Mathay, M.A., Luce, J.M. and Flick, M.R. (1988) Pulmonary perspectives. An expanded definition of the adult respiratory distress syndrome. *American Review of Respiratory Disease,* **138**, 720–3.

69. Gattinoni, L., Pesenti, A. and Caspani, M.L. (1984) Role of static lung compliance in the management of severe ARDS unresponsive to conventional treatment. *Intensive Care Medicine,* **10**, 121–6.

70. Roupie, E., Dambrosio, M., Mentec, H. *et al.* (1993) Titration of tidal volume reduction and permissive hypercapnia in adult respiratory distress syndrome. *American Review of Respiratory Disease,* **147**, A351 (abstract).

71. Ranieri, V.M., Eissa, N.T., Corbeil, C. *et al.* (1991) Effects of positive end-expiratory pressure on alveolar recruitment and gas exchange in patients with the adult respiratory distress syndrome. *American Review of Respiratory Disease,* **144**, 544–51.

72. Gattinoni, L., Pesenti, A., Avalli, L. *et al.* (1987) Pressure volume curve of total respiratory system in acute respiratory failure. *American Review of Respiratory Disease,* **136**, 730–6.

73. Hickling, K.G., Henderson, S.L. and Jackson, R. (1990) Low mortality associated with low volume pressure limited ventilation with permissive hypercapnia in severe ARDS. *Intensive Care Medicine,* **16**, 372–7.

74. Bates, J.H.T., Rossi, A. and Milic-Emili, J. (1985) Analysis of the behaviour of the respiratory system with constant inspiratory flow. *Journal of Applied Physiology,* **58**, 1840–8.

75. Wright, P.E. and Bernard, G.R. (1989) The role of airflow resistance in patients with the adult respiratory distress syndrome. *American Review of Respiratory Disease,* **139**, 1169–74.

76. Hutchinson, A.A., Hinson, J.M., Brigham, K.L. *et al.* (1983) Effect of endotoxin on airway hyper-responsiveness to aerosol histamine in sheep. *Journal of Applied Physiology,* **54**, 1463–8.

77. Pesenti, A., Pelosi, P., Rossi. N. *et al.* (1991) The effects of positive end expiratory pressure on respiratory resistance in patients with the adult respiratory distress syndrome and in normal anesthetised subjects. *American Review of Respiratory Disease,* **144**, 101–7.

78. Hickling, K.G. (1990) Ventilatory management of ARDS: can it affect outcome? *Intensive Care Medicine,* **16**, 219–26.

Patricia L. Haslam

The search for therapeutic agents to improve the clinical outcome in adult patients with the acute respiratory distress syndrome (ARDS) has focused on early intervention. A variety of approaches have been attempted using methods that modulate the components of the systemic inflammatory response, but none has led to a major breakthrough. However, early intervention is difficult to achieve for the majority of patients with ARDS who present with the syndrome fully established. Consequently, therapeutic approaches for rescue therapy also need to be developed. This requires a knowledge of events associated with progression and prognosis. The development of ARDS is characterized by damage to the pulmonary vascular endothelium. This is followed by leakage of proteins from the damaged vessels and extravasation of activated neutrophils causing interstitial inflammation and edema. Damage to the alveolar epithelium then occurs, resulting in accumulation of proteins and neutrophils within the alveolar spaces. These changes within the alveoli have important pathophysiological consequences. In particular, they cause dysfunction of the pulmonary surfactant system which amplifies the injury (Figure 16.1).

Pulmonary surfactant dysfunction can lead to alveolar instability, flooding and collapse, and in these respects the catastrophic acute lung injury that occurs in ARDS shows many similarities to the infantile syndrome (IRDS). This can develop in premature neonates because of surfactant deficiency due to immaturity of the lungs at the time of birth [1]. The lungs fail to inflate adequately, resulting in alveolar flooding and collapse. Various types of exogenous surfactant have been developed for treatment of IRDS and are of established benefit [2,3]. This has provoked interest in the potential for surfactant replacement therapy in ARDS [4]. However, while surfactant deficiency is the primary etiologic factor in IRDS, alterations in the surfactant system in ARDS develop as a secondary consequence of lung injury. The mechanisms involved and the precise approaches to therapy in the two disorders therefore differ in a number of respects. The aim of this chapter is to describe the composition and functions of normal human pulmonary surfactant, and to review the alterations which develop in ARDS. The current status of exogenous surfactant therapy in ARDS is also reviewed.

NORMAL PULMONARY SURFACTANT

ROLE IN REGULATION OF ALVEOLAR SURFACE TENSION

Pulmonary surfactant is a complex, highly surface active material that spreads to cover the alveolar epithelial surfaces of the lungs [5]. Phospholipids account for about 85% of the composition, the main component being dipalmitoylphosphatidylcholine (DPPC), which is also the main surface active com-

ARDS Acute Respiratory Distress in Adults. Edited by Timothy W. Evans and Christopher Haslett. Published in 1996 by Chapman & Hall, London. ISBN 0 412 56910 8

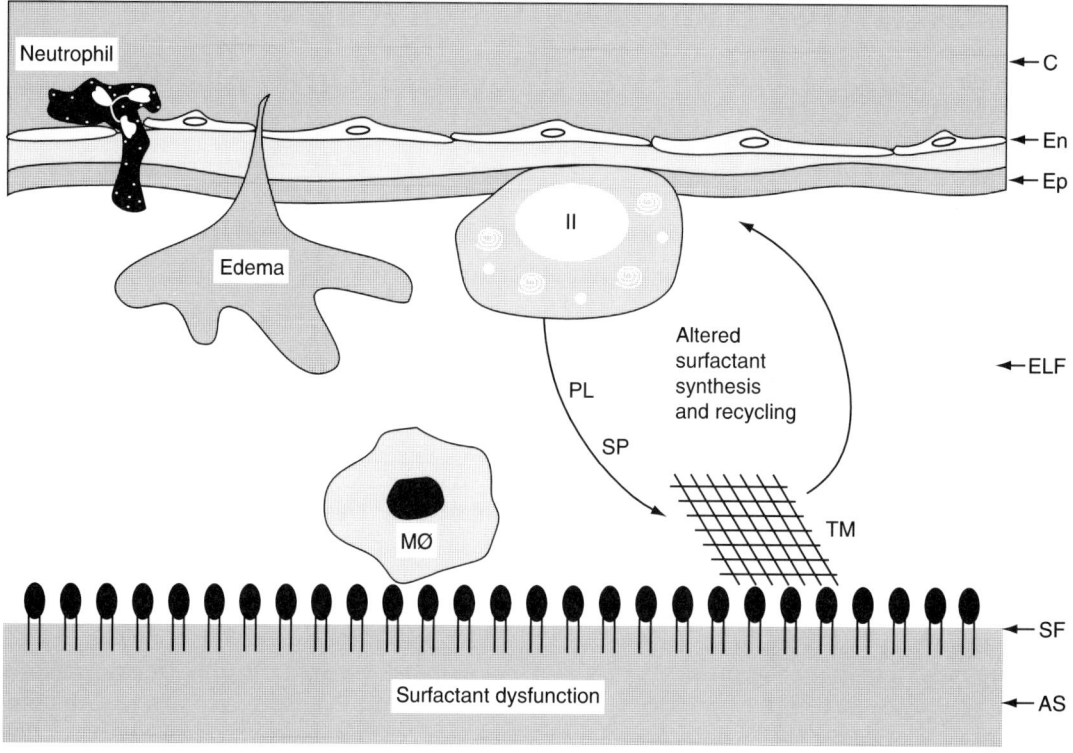

Figure 16.1 Events that lead to dysfunction of the pulmonary surfactant system in patients with ARDS. C = capillary; En = endothelium; Ep = epithelium; ELF = epithelial lining fluid; SF = surface film indicating phospholipid monolayer; AS = alveolar space; II = Type II cell; PL = phospholipid; SP = surfactant-specific apoprotein; MØ = macrophage; TM = tubular myelin.

ponent. In addition, the surfactant system contains about 8% proteins, 5% neutral lipids and 2% carbohydrates [1,4–6]. These components interact together in a highly organized manner to form a monolayer film of phospholipid over the surface of the alveolar epithelium. This film plays an important role in lung function by generating a 'film-pressure' which opposes and reduces the surface tension of the alveolar epithelial lining fluid to maintain it at near zero throughout the whole cycle of breathing. This counteracts the differences in pressure between alveolar spaces and tissues which would otherwise cause the alveoli to flood and the lungs to collapse, especially at low lung volumes when the intra-alveolar pressures are very

low. There is still controversy as to the exact mechanism by which surfactant stabilizes the alveoli and prevents flooding and collapse, and the various hypotheses proposed have been reviewed in detail elsewhere [7]. The conventional and most widely accepted hypothesis is the 'bubble' model. This assumes that the alveoli are lined with a continuous layer of liquid, and that they behave like bubbles in terms of their inherent stability. Mathematically, the collapsing pressure (Δp) of a bubble is related to the surface tension (γ) and the radius of curvature (r) by the law of Young and Laplace $\Delta p = 2\gamma/r$. Bubble stability is established when the air inside has been compressed until its pressure is raised above the pressure outside by an amount (Δp) which opposes further collapse. Equilibrium is established when Δp equals the recoil pressure of the bubble ($2\gamma/r$). Because alveoli are networks of interacting 'bubbles' of differing sizes that change during breathing, Clements *et al.* [8] proposed that the alveoli might remain stable despite the variation in their radii if surfactant is able to progressively vary surface tension to decrease bubble recoil ($2\gamma/r$), then further reduce surface tension as the bubble starts to collapse until $2\gamma/r$ of each bubble is the same for all. In this way a whole range of bubbles of widely differing diameters can be brought to equilibrium with the same external air source and, hence, with each other.

The 'bubble' hypothesis is based on the view that a 'continuous' layer of fluid lines the alveolar surfaces. However, alternative theories suggest that the fluid lining is 'discontinuous' with dry and wet patches [7]. The 'water repellent model' postulates that the fluid is confined to 'pools' and 'pits' from which it can tension dry patches of the alveoli by pulling in excess epithelial membrane as 'pleats' [9]. The gas transfer surface is kept essentially dry by water repellency induced by a monolayer of surfactant directly adsorbed on to the epithelial surface. The 'pools' assume a convex profile and act as 'corner pumps' to return fluid to the interstitium. If flooding continues, the 'pools' will link to form the 'bubble' model, but only in a pathological and not the physiological state [9].

The monolayer film of surfactant phospholipid is able to modulate surface tension because of the highly polar nature of the molecules (Figure 16.2). This causes them to align at the air–liquid interface, with their hydrophilic phosphatidyl head groups in the liquid and their hydrophobic fatty acid tails in the air space. The compression of these molecules during expiration generates the increasing film pressure which opposes, and reduces, the force of surface tension at the air–liquid interface. As the radii of the alveoli

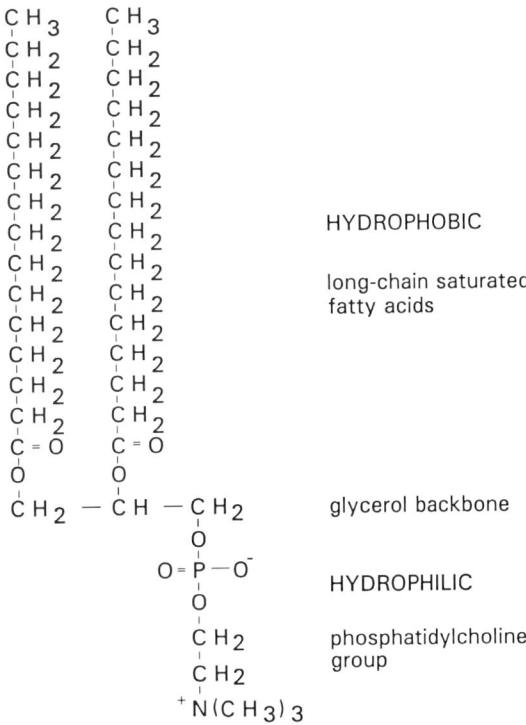

Figure 16.2 Chemical structure of dipalmitoyl-phosphatidylcholine (DPPC) showing the highly polar nature of the molecule.

increase on inspiration the pressure between the molecules decreases, allowing the surface tension to increase. The ability of pulmonary surfactant to lower surface tension under dynamic compression *in vitro* can be assessed in a variety of ways, but problems of reproduciblity can arise because the measurements are very sensitive to variability in concentration and contamination [10]. The two methods most commonly used are the Langmuir–Wilhelmy balance [11] and more recently the oscillating bubble apparatus of Enhörning [12]. Thus, Clements used a modified Wilhelmy balance to confirm the hypothesis that pulmonary surfactant was capable of lowering surface tension when the film it formed was compressed into a smaller area [11]. Both methods can generate similar information, but the oscillating bubble

Table 16.1 Surfactant-specific apoproteins

Apoprotein	Biochemical properties	Molecular weight (kDa)	Selected references
SP-A	Hydrophilic glycoprotein	26–36	23–25
SP-B	Hydrophobic protein	7.5–9	28–33
SP-C	Hydrophobic protein	3.5	28–33
SP-D	Hydrophilic glycoprotein	43	26,27

method has the advantage that surface tension measurements can be continuously determined between maximum and minimum bubble size for very small volumes of surfactant material (25 μL). This makes it a convenient method for clinical studies of pathological events which disturb the biophysical function of the surfactant system.

BIOCHEMICAL COMPOSITION

Clinical studies of the composition, as well as the function, of human pulmonary surfactant in health and disease have been facilitated by the technique of bronchoalveolar lavage (BAL) which enables components to be sampled from the air spaces of the lungs of humans with safety [13,14]. BAL is conducted using a standardized procedure, by instilling and aspirating aliquots of physiological saline (typically, 4 × 60 ml in adults) via a fiberoptic bronchoscope placed into a defined segment of the lung, usually the right middle or lateral segment of the right lower lobe [15]. The recovered BAL samples are examined to determine the number of cells present, then spun immediately at low speed ($\leq$ 300 g) for 10 minutes at 4°C to separate the cells from the cell-free supernatant fluid. For lipid studies it is essential to remove rapidly cells which might otherwise contaminate the surfactant components in the supernatants with cell derived lipids and proteins. High centrifugation forces must not be used because, apart from inducing cell damage, these can sediment and cause loss of aggregates of surfactant phospholipids and proteins. To evaluate surfactant phospholipid composition,

lipids are extracted from the cell-free BAL fluids using conventional methods, for example chloroform–methanol extraction. The main phospholipid classes are separated and quantified by thin layer or high pressure liquid chromatography [5,16,17].

On average, phosphatidylcholine (PC) accounts for 73% of the phospholipid in lavage samples from normal, healthy, non smoking human volunteers, and it is mostly in the form of saturated DPPC which is highly surface active. Phosphatidylglycerol (PG) is the second major phospholipid component, accounting for on average 12% of the phospholipid, while the remainder include the minor components phosphatidylinositol (PI), phosphatidylethanolamine (PE), phosphatidylserine (PS), sphingomyelin (SM), cardiolipin, and lysophosphatidylcholine, none of which usually account for more than 3% of the total phospholipid. By contrast, phospholipids in lung tissue and blood plasma contain lower proportions of PC (mean < 50%) with a higher content of unsaturated fatty acids, and much lower proportions of PG (< 2%). Lung tissue also contains higher proportions of PE (mean 17%), and both lung tissue and blood plasma contain higher proportions of SM (mean 11% and 24% respectively). In pathological situations, components from damaged tissue and exudation of plasma into the alveolar spaces can contaminate the surfactant system [18]. This can result in abnormal elevations in PE and SM (as well as in proteins and other tissue or plasma-derived components) in BAL samples. Cigarette smoking must be taken into account in clinical studies of surfactant,

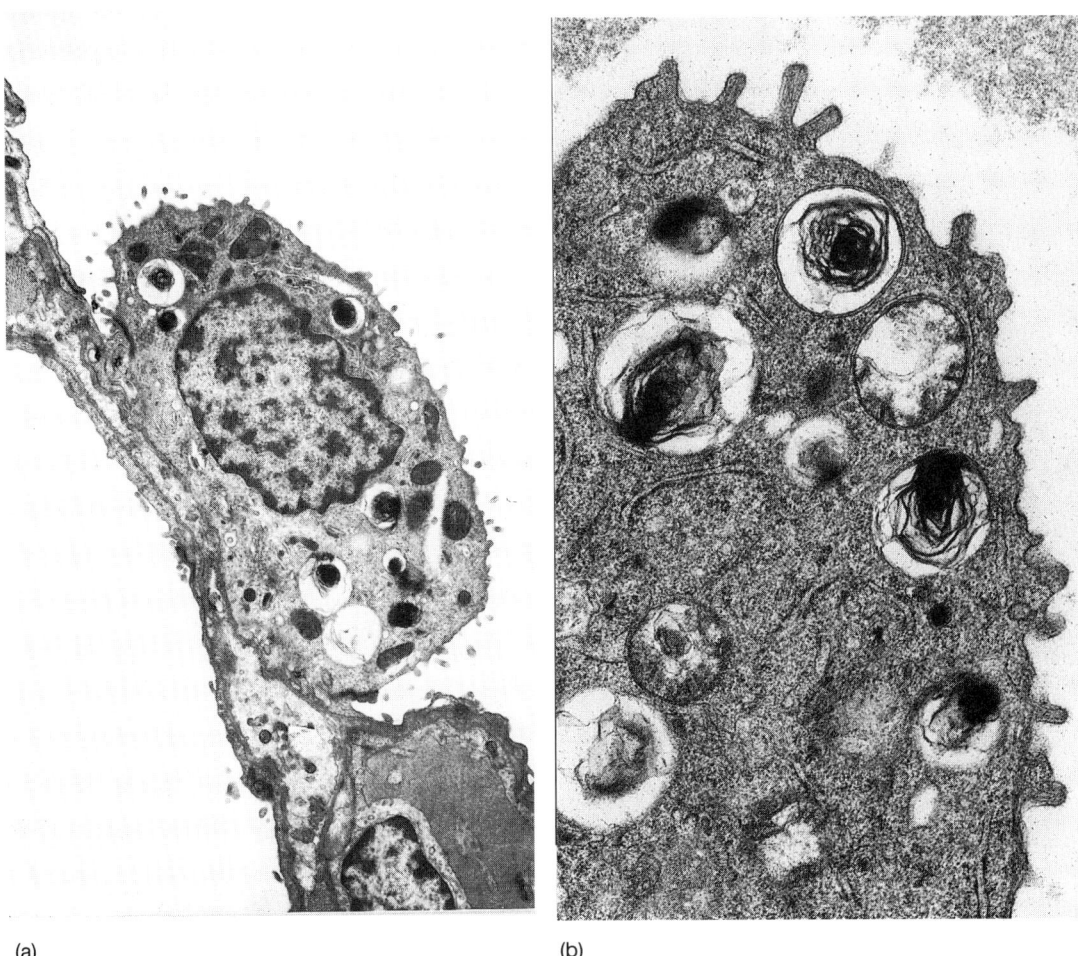

(a)   (b)

Figure 16.3 (a) Electron micrograph showing the ultrastructural appearance of a human type II alveolar epithelial cell (×6500). (b) Higher power view of the cytoplasm of the cell showing the characteristic lamellar bodies containing phospholipids (×19 500). (By courtesy of Ann Dewar, National Heart & Lung Institute, London, UK.)

because BAL samples from apparently healthy cigarette smokers contain significantly higher proportions of PE and SM compared with healthy nonsmoking volunteers [19]. This indicates that smoking related tissue damage is sufficient to have a measurable effect on surfactant composition. The functional consequences have not been investigated. However, pulmonary vascular permeability is increased in cigarette smokers compared with nonsmokers [20]. Dysregula-

tion of surface tension due to surfactant alterations could be relevant to this observation.

Apart from phospholipids, about 2% of the proteins in normal alveolar lining fluid are specific to the surfactant system. These are termed the surfactant apoproteins. They have been studied less than the phospholipids because they have been discovered more recently [6,21,22]. Four surfactant-specific proteins have been identified including the

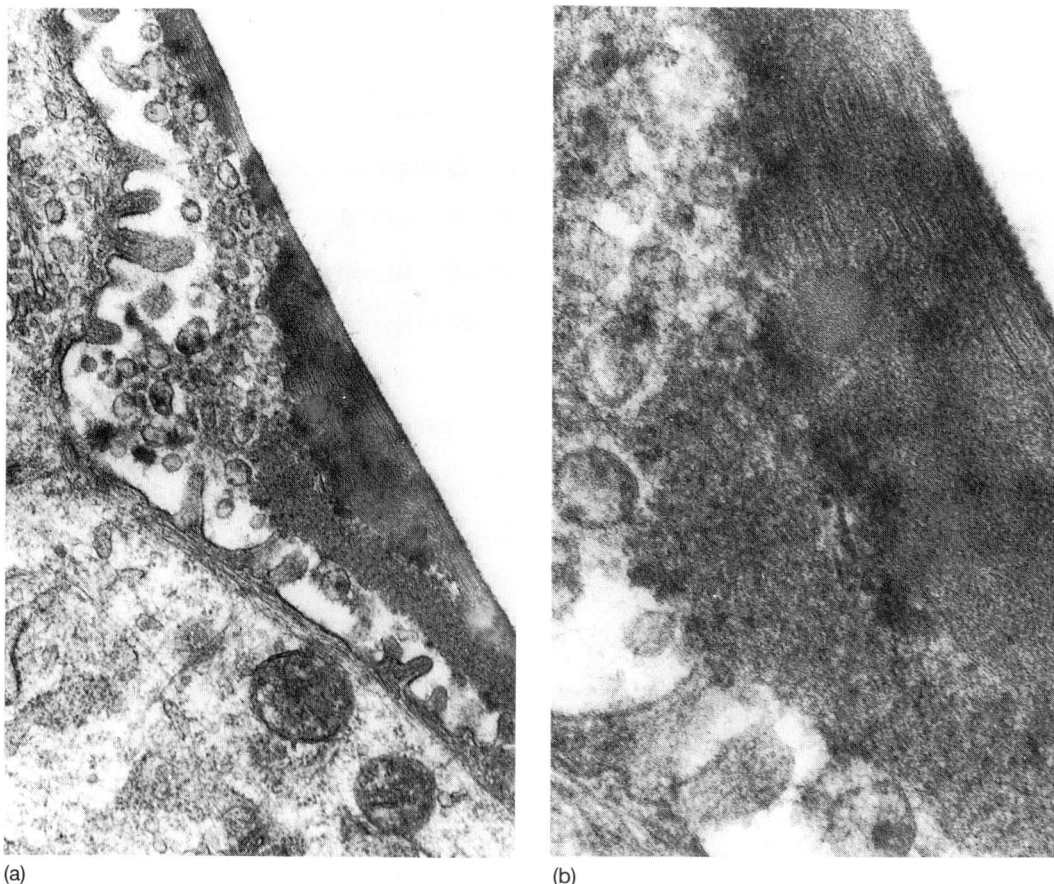

(a)

(b)

Figure 16.4 (a) Electron micrograph showing the membranes and part of the cytoplasm of two human alveolar epithelial cells covered by a layer of alveolar lining fluid containing surfactant. The lung was fixed *in situ* to preserve the surfactant layer. A large tubular myelin aggregate composed of phospholipids and apoproteins is demonstrated (×32 000). (b) Higher power view of the surfactant layer showing the tubular myelin aggregate together with smaller aggregates in the liquid hypophase (×85 500). (By courtesy of Ann Dewar, National Heart & Lung Institute, London, UK.)

higher molecular weight hydrophilic glycoproteins Sp-A [23–25] and Sp-D [26,27], and the low molecular weight hydrophobic proteins Sp-B and Sp-C [28–33] (Table 16.1). These proteins, as well as the phospholipids, are essential for the efficient functioning and turnover of the surfactant system. The main phospholipid and specific protein components are synthesized and secreted by the type II alveolar epithelial lining cells. After synthesis, the phospholipids are stored within the cytoplasm of the cells in specialized organ-

elles termed lamellar bodies (Figure 16.3), from which they are released on to the alveolar epithelial surfaces. The surfactant-specific proteins are transported separately to the cell surface in multivesicular bodies, although some Sp-A may be present in lamellar bodies. The phospholipids and proteins aggregate extracellularly to form lattice structures known as tubular myelin [34–38] (Figure 16.4). These aggregates are the most highly surface active fraction of surfactant and they aid the spreading of phospholipid to form a monolayer film over the surface of the epithelial lining. Sp-A is the major surfactant apoprotein and plays a very important role in tubular myelin formation by interacting with phospholipids, Sp-B, Sp-C and calcium ions [35,36,39,40]. Sp-B and Sp-C play a further essential role in enhancing the adsorption and spreading of the monolayer of phospholipid at the air–liquid interface of the lung lining fluid [29,30,41]. Sp-B also promotes the squeezing out of impurities and 'exhausted' phospholipids from the lipid monolayer [30]. Sp-A then regulates phospholipid recycling to type II cells for resynthesis [42] and it plays a role in regulating secretion [43]. There is also evidence that Sp-A plays a role in host defense by enhancing the phagocytosis and killing of micro-organisms by alveolar macrophages [44]; and recent evidence suggests that Sp-D may play a similar role in host defense [45]. Compared to phospholipids, the importance of the apoproteins in the surfactant system has been recognized relatively recently and this is an active field of current research. In particular, it is hoped that synthetic surfactants containing recombinant surfactant apoproteins or their functional analogs plus synthetic phospholipids, now being developed for therapeutic use [46,47], will provide an advance over current artificial surfactants containing phospholipid because they should more closely mimic the natural product.

SYNTHESIS AND TURNOVER

The synthesis and turnover of surfactant components is a highly dynamic process [48,49]. This is necessary because the cycles of contraction and expansion which occur during breathing have an adverse effect on the surface phospholipid which is continuously expelled from the monolayer and replaced with newly synthesized material [50]. Ultrastructural examination of lungs fixed to preserve surfactant show the presence of small aggregates distinct from the larger aggregates of tubular myelin [51] (Figure 16.4). These small aggregates have poor surface activity and are thought to represent spent phospholipid. Some of the material expelled from the monolayer is recycled back to type II alveolar epithelial cells for resynthesis, while some is phagocytosed by alveolar macrophages and removed [48,52,53]. Phospholipid recycling to type II cells is aided by the main surfactant specific protein Sp-A, which can interact with phospholipid and attach to Sp-A receptors on the surface of the type II cells [42,54]. Sp-A also appears to play a role in modulating the release of phospholipid by type II cells [43,55]. The highly dynamic nature of synthesis and turnover of surfactant components means that the system is susceptible to disturbance not only due to contaminants, degradative processes or loss by increased diffusion across the damaged epithelial and endothelial barriers, but also by any interference with synthesis or turnover.

MECHANISMS OF SURFACTANT DYSFUNCTION

Surfactant deficiency caused by immaturity of type II alveolar epithelial cells is the primary etiological factor in IRDS [56]. The levels and relative proportions of the two major phospholipids PC and PG are markedly reduced, while the levels and proportions of the phospholipids PI and SM are increased [1] (Figure 16.5). In fetal lung, PI is produced preferentially to PG from the common precursor CDP diacylglycerol, but in full term infants there is a switch to preferential production of PG prior to birth. The risk of surfactant deficiency is higher with increasing prematurity and, while IRDS occurs in about 20% of infants born at 30–32 weeks gestational age, the incidence is 60–80% in those of 26–28 weeks gestational age [57,58]. Fetal lung immaturity also results in a deficiency in apoprotein components of surfactant [59]. The lungs fail to inflate adequately because of the primary lack of phospholipid and apoprotein components, and there is alveolar flooding

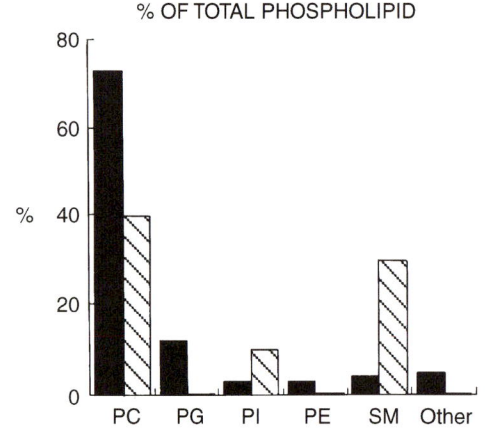

Figure 16.5 Phospholipid compositional alterations in IRDS. ⊠ = IRDS; ■ = normal.

due to leakage of proteins from the plasma into the alveolar spaces. Pulmonary edema then provides a secondary mechanism which further promotes surfactant dysfunction. This occurs because protein contamination can interfere with the surface tension lowering properties of surfactant in a dose dependent manner.

A variety of plasma proteins and proteins such as fibrin degradation products generated by the coagulation processes involved in edema formation have been shown to inhibit surfactant function *in vitro*. Different proteins vary in their inhibitory effects, and in general fibrinogen and fibrin monomers are more inhibitory than serum proteins such as hemoglobin and albumin at comparable doses [60–63]. The levels of inhibition induced by protein are highly dependent on the concentration of surfactant as well as the amount of inhibitory protein. At low surfactant concentrations, plasma proteins significantly inhibit adsorption of the surface film of phospholipid, resulting in an increase in the equilibrium surface tension. However, at higher surfactant concentrations, adsorption is not impaired by the presence of plasma proteins even when their levels are increased proportionately [61,62,64]. Indeed, in experiments

using the pulsating bubble surfactometer to study the effects of plasma derived proteins on the dynamic surface tension lowering ability of lung surfactant, a fourfold increase in surfactant phospholipid concentration to 2 mg/ml reduced the inhibitory effect of even a 20-fold increase in the concentration of inhibitory proteins compared with the marked inhibition observed using a surfactant concentration of 0.5 mg/ml and protein concentrations of 10 mg/ml [64]. *In vitro* experiments have also shown that different formulations of therapeutic surfactant differ markedly in their sensitivity to the effects of inhibitory plasma proteins [65–67]. This is also indicated by *in vivo* studies in experimental models [68,69]. It is clear that such differences may be of considerable importance in selecting a therapeutic formulation appropriate for use in different pathological situations. It is of interest that addition of surfactant apoproteins to various surfactant lipid preparations has recently been shown to increase the resistance of these preparations to plasma protein inhibition [67,70–72]. The possible mechanisms proposed to explain how contaminating proteins might inhibit surfactant function have been reviewed recently [73]. These include physicochemical interactions with surfactant phospholipids or apoproteins, interference by insertion into the intact surface film, or by competition with surfactant molecules for space at the air–liquid interface during adsorption.

Protein contamination due to increased endothelial and epithelial permeability resulting in intra-alveolar edema is probably the main mechanism by which surfactant dysfunction initially occurs in ARDS [4,74]. As the syndrome progresses, surfactant dysfunction will be amplified if damage to type II alveolar epithelial cells results in a quantitative deficiency of surfactant components due to impaired synthesis, secretion and turnover [75]. It has been proposed that additional mechanisms may also contribute to surfactant damage in ARDS. Phospholipases with the capacity to disrupt surfactant function have been found in BAL samples from patients with ARDS [76]; and increased phospholipase A_2 activity correlating with decreased PC levels has been reported in patients with respiratory failure associated with acute pancreatitis [77–79]. In patients with sepsis, it has been suggested that secretion of phospholipases by bacteria should also be considered [80]. Oxidants released by activated neutrophils, monocytes and macrophages are thought to play a role in the pathogenesis of ARDS [81–83], and lipid peroxidation products have been shown to be capable of interfering with the normal surface activity of surfactant *in vitro* [84]. The saturated phospholipids which form the major part of the phospholipid in the surfactant system are resistant to oxidation, but tissue damage may release lipids containing unsaturated fatty acids which can provide a substrate. Activated neutrophils also produce proteases which are capable of damaging the major surfactant apoprotein Sp-A *in vitro*, implying that they might induce such damage *in vivo* in ARDS [85]. This situation might be promoted if the major inhibitor of neutrophil elastase in the air spaces of the lung, α_1-antiprotease, is rendered inactive due to oxidation of methionine in the active site of the inhibitor [81].

Thus, it is clear that surfactant dysfunction is subject to wide variation dependent upon many contributory factors. However, when pathological situations arise where there is an abnormally low available pool of functional surfactant together with increased alveolar protein contamination, there is a high risk of failure of surfactant to regulate alveolar surface tension.

SURFACTANT ALTERATIONS AS A CONSEQUENCE OF LUNG INJURY

ARDS

The risk factors which can precipitate ARDS in previously healthy individuals, and the initial mechanisms involved are described in detail elsewhere (Chapter 2). Risk factors which affect the lungs directly include infectious and aspiration pneumonias and smoke inhalation, while indirect risks include sepsis, sepsis syndrome, multiple blood transfusions, drug overdose, disseminated intravascular coagulation, trauma or multiple fractures, major surgery (including that needing cardiopulmonary bypass) and many other risks [86–89]. These initial insults, by mechanisms not fully understood, may result in increased pulmonary vascular capillary permeability to plasma proteins leading to massive pulmonary edema [90,91]. The prevalence of ARDS in relation to different risk factors and time scale of development of the injury is variable, presumably reflecting differences in the exact mechanisms involved [86]. It is conceivable that risks which directly affect the lungs may lead to epithelial damage and amplified surfactant dysfunction more rapidly than systemic risk factors.

Evidence of surfactant dysfunction

Pulmonary surfactant dysfunction probably first arises during the course of ARDS as a consequence of protein contamination due to edema. It is likely to be enhanced when damage to type II epithelial cells becomes sufficient to result in a deficiency of surfactant components (Figure 16.1). The surfactant dysfunction contributes to the development of the life threatening acute respiratory failure, which in many cases progresses to multi-organ failure and death. The syndrome was described by Ashbaugh *et al.* in 1967, who also first reported that fluid recovered from minced postmortem lung tissue had a reduced ability to lower surface tension *in vitro* (minimum surface tension > 20 dyne/cm) compared with normal values (< 10 dyne/cm) suggesting surfactant dysfunction [92]. This was confirmed by Von Wichert and Kohl, who also showed that lung extracts from patients who died of ARDS had a decreased DPPC content [93]. BAL studies of the composition and surface activity of surfactant from patients with ARDS provided further evidence that the lung injury causes disturbances to the surfactant system [76]. Thus, lavages from postmortem lungs of patients with ARDS have an abnormally increased surface compressibility compared with those from control lungs [94]. Static pressure–volume curves obtained from the intact specimens also showed that the ARDS lungs exhibited lower volumes and decreased compliance compared with normals. The BAL samples from the ARDS lungs had a high protein content, and the authors concluded that this may have been responsible for the decreased compliance recorded for the whole lungs. Studies were subsequently performed on the phospholipid composition and surface activity of surfactant recovered from BAL samples from living patients with a variety of pulmonary diseases including ARDS, pneumonia, malignancy and chronic obstructive lung disease [75]. The surfactant was purified from the BAL samples by sucrose density gradient centrifugation and the pellets solubilized in organic solvents to remove contaminating protein prior to measuring the surface tension lowering ability using a Wilhelmy balance. Despite these steps, the samples from patients with ARDS had little or no surface tension lowering activity compared with normal controls. There was no significant difference in total phospholipid, but the fractional content of PC and PG was reduced and SM increased compared to normal. In ARDS associated with trauma the alterations in surfactant composition and function in BAL were then shown to correlate with the severity of ARDS as assessed by respiratory failure scores [95]. No quantitative abnormality in total phospholipid in BAL was identified, but the fractions of PC and PG were reduced compared with normal controls, and PC was lower in patients with high compared with low respiratory failure scores. Surfactant function assessed by the Wilhelmy balance

also showed a correlation between increasing minimum surface tensions, declining hysteresis areas and the degree of respiratory failure in these patients. In a subsequent study of trauma complicated by sepsis this complication was shown to be associated with further depletion of alveolar phospholipids [96]. These workers also investigated the time course of development of surfactant abnormalities in ARDS associated with trauma, the relationship with levels of protein contamination, and the severity of respiratory failure [97]. A rapid increase in alveolar protein load (demonstrated within the first 48 hours) was followed by progressive decreases in PC and PG and increases in PI, PE and SM. Declining surfactant function correlated with levels of protein leakage, decline in PC, and the severity of respiratory failure assessed by the ARDS score. These observations were confirmed in a prospective study employing serial BAL samples [98]. Plasma protein leakage was more evident than alterations in PC over the first week of the injury. A progressive decrease in PC (percent of total phospholipid) then became increasingly apparent with increasing duration of the injury in patients with a high ARDS score. More recently, the surface tension-lowering ability of the surfactant fraction of BAL samples has been shown to be decreased in patients at risk of developing ARDS, although not to the same extent as in patients with the established syndrome [99].

Although studies of surfactant composition and function in patients with ARDS are relatively few compared with work in experimental models of acute lung injury (see below), they support the view that surfactant abnormalities contribute to the pathophysiology of ARDS. They indicate that protein contamination initially plays the major role, and that alterations in phospholipid composition also develop at a later stage in the course of severe lung injury. Our own observations in a series of patients with severe ARDS associated with a range of risk factors are con-

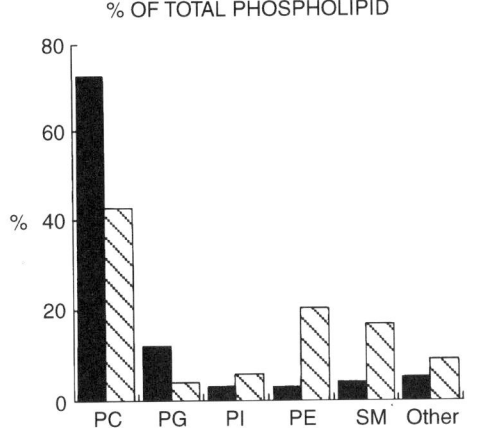

Figure 16.6 Phospholipid compositional alterations in ARDS. ⬚ = ARDS; ■ = normal.

sistent with these conclusions (Figure 16.6). We have also observed notable increases in the nonsurfactant phospholipid SM in the BAL samples from our patients, indicating the presence of contaminants from necrotic tissue or dead inflammatory cells, as has been suggested by Hallman *et al.* [75].

Mechanisms implicated

Many mechanisms are likely to contribute to protein contamination and compositional alterations in surfactant in ARDS. The total protein content of the alveolar lining fluid may be the combined result of plasma leakage, tissue damage, products generated by activation of the humoral clotting, fibrinolytic and complement systems, plus products from inflammatory cells. The alterations in phospholipid composition may be due to the combined effects of damage to type II alveolar epithelial cells, altered synthesis as a result of type II regeneration and hyperplasia, contamination with phospholipids from plasma or necrotic cells, interference with phospholipid recycling from the air spaces due to type II cell dysfunction, or disturbance in the normal mechanisms of clearance of surfactant by alveolar macrophages or via the mucociliary escalator. Damage or dysfunction of type II

alveolar epithelial cells may also explain the reductions in the levels of the surfactant-specific proteins Sp-A and Sp-B reported in patients with ARDS, and the reduced levels of Sp-A in patients at risk of ARDS [99]. Type II cells are the main source of surfactant-specific proteins, and monitoring their levels should provide a sensitive indicator of damage to type II cells because of their specificity to the system. Although *in vivo* studies (supported by evidence from transgenic models) have shown that Sp-B and Sp-C, but not Sp-A, are essential for maximal surface tension lowering efficiency of surfactant [31–33, 70], reductions in Sp-A may have an adverse effect *in vivo*. Sp-A contributes in tubular myelin formation and it also regulates phospholipid recycling to type II cells, which may be important to 'kickstart' the normal dynamic process of phospholipid turnover after injury. Phospholipid recycling and regeneration is essential to maintain normal lung function throughout cycles of compression and expansion. Sp-A also plays an important role in host defense, as described below, and may help to protect patients with ARDS from nosocomial infections.

Protein contaminants

There have been many investigations of total protein in BAL samples from patients with ARDS, but few attempts to identify the range of proteins present. In one of the most detailed [100], the authors explored whether the normal size-selective process that restricts the passage of large molecules from the plasma to the alveolar lining fluid is destroyed by the alveolar-capillary injury of ARDS. They determined the relative concentrations in plasma and BAL of total protein and of seven individual proteins: α_1-antitrypsin (54 000 mol.wt), albumin (68 000 mol.wt), transferrin (90 000 mol.wt), haptoglobin (100 000 mol.wt), ceruloplasmin (150 000 mol.wt), α_2-macroglobulin (820 000 mol.wt) and IgM (900 000 mol.wt). The mean total protein in BAL in eight patients with ARDS was greater than 12 times the level detectable in 11 normal volunteers and three patients with cardiogenic pulmonary edema; and the high molecular weight proteins immunoglobulin M and α_2-macroglobulin were present at greater than 90 times the normal or cardiac edema concentrations. For the seven proteins studied, the distribution coefficients of BAL concentrations versus log molecular weights increased hyperbolically in normals but were flat in ARDS patients. Sodium dodecyl sulfate (SDS) polyacrylamide gel electrophoresis indicated the presence of the full spectrum of plasma proteins in BAL from ARDS, but not normals. This evidence supports the proposal that lung injury in ARDS is associated with a loss of size restriction of the alveolar-capillary barriers so that plasma proteins are distributed more equally between plasma and alveolar lining fluid than in the normal lung. Fowler *et al.* have also demonstrated increases in high molecular weight plasma derived proteins in ARDS lavage fluids [101], including fibrinogen (340 000 mol.wt), which is one of the most potent protein inhibitors of surfactant function [60]. Evidence that proteins from activated inflammatory cells (notably neutrophils and possibly macrophages) also contribute to the increases in total protein in BAL in ARDS patients comes from observations that both collagenase and neutrophil elastase are present in increased amounts in lavage samples from patients with ARDS [102,103]. Apart from interfering in adsorption and function of the surface film of surfactant, proteases have the capacity to degrade surfactant apoproteins *in vitro* [85]. It is possible that such mechanisms may operate *in vivo* if there is deficiency of antiproteases. The acute phase C-reactive protein, which is generated in increased amounts during inflammatory processes, including ARDS, also has the capability to impair the surface tension lowering ability of surfactant *in vitro* [104].

Protein inhibition of surfactant function is reversible in the sense that functional surfactant can be recovered by centrifugation to separate it from the soluble proteins [105]. This approach obviously cannot be exploited for therapeutic purposes *in vivo*, but attempts to increase the relative surfactant concentration to reduce the inhibitory effect of proteins represent one of the major aims of surfactant therapy in ARDS. The therapeutic formulations and doses to achieve this effect may, however, be variable according to the *in vivo* situation. Approaches to therapy are discussed in greater detail in the separate section below.

Phospholipid alterations

The exact mechanisms resulting in the alterations in phospholipid composition seen in patients with ARDS are unclear (Figure 16.6). The reasons for the more pronounced decreases in the second major surfactant phospholipid component, PG, compared with the major phospholipid, PC, are also unknown. A decrease in PG with a relative increase in PI, as observed in some patients, may reflect the pattern of phospholipid production by regenerating type II alveolar epithelial cells, which *in vitro* show a pattern of phospholipid synthesis similar to that of fetal lung [106,107]. Direct damage to type II cells may also contribute to the reductions in levels and proportions of PG and PC. However, proportionate reductions relative to the total phospholipid present may arise due to increased phospholipid contamination of alveolar lining fluid from necrotic cells and edema fluid. Increases in SM and PE in the lavage samples of ARDS patients provide evidence that this mechanism is also involved [75,97]. The functional consequences of decreases in the second major phospholipid component of surfactant PG in adult lungs are unknown, because PG is not essential for the normal biophysical function of surfactant *in vitro* if it is replaced by PI [108,109]. Decreases in the proportions and levels of the major surfactant phospholipid PC, however, parallel the severity of ARDS *in vivo* [97,98]. Contamination of the surfactant system with phospholipids from necrotic cells and edema may explain partly why there have been contradictory reports on surfactant phospholipid pool size in patients with ARDS. Some workers have reported no changes in total phospholipid levels in BAL from ARDS patients compared with controls [75,95], while others have reported decreases [96,98] or increases [110]. This variability may be partly because of a lack of recognition of the contribution of contaminants to the total phospholipid pool, compounded by the lack of accurate markers to assess dilution due to the BAL procedure, and poor standardization of methods for recovery and measurement of phospholipids which are subject to technical variation. These considerations make it difficult to interpret studies of surfactant pool sizes in humans and explain why surfactant dysfunction, including deficient production of surfactant, can occur without an apparent reduction in the total phospholipid pool size.

Experimental models have been used to obtain more standardized information on surfactant pool size, composition and function during the course of acute lung injury, but these models have the limitation that they cannot provide an exact representation of the complexity of the clinical situation. However, they have generated much useful information about the early events involved in the pathogenesis of acute lung injury, and have enabled a number of new therapeutic approaches, including the use of therapeutic surfactants, to be explored.

EXPERIMENTAL MODELS OF ACUTE LUNG INJURY

Many experimental models of acute lung injury have been developed which exhibit the histological and pathophysiological features of ARDS [111]. A detailed description is beyond the scope of this chapter, but they have been of great importance in elucidating the wide range of mechanisms involved in pathogenesis [4,74,90]. Different insults are used to induce the injury and, as in the clinical syndrome, the damaging mechanisms are variable. A number of the models closely mimic certain of the clinical risk factors. They have confirmed that functional deficiency of surfactant develops as a common consequence of severe acute lung injury, and that the reasons for the dysfunction vary dependent upon the nature of the injury. Surfactant replacement therapy has improved gas exchange and reduced the severity of the injury in several of these models, as described in the following section.

SURFACTANT REPLACEMENT THERAPY

THERAPEUTIC SURFACTANTS

The recognition that pulmonary surfactant deficiency is the primary etiological factor in the pathogenesis of IRDS [1] led to the development of a variety of exogenous surfactant preparations, which are of established benefit both for prophylaxis and for rescue therapy in premature infants [2,3]. Initial attempts at therapy employed pure DPPC, which had by then been identified as the major surface active phospholipid in pulmonary surfactant [112]. The results were very disappointing [113,114] and almost discouraged further trials. It was then discovered that DPPC alone is not suitable for use in therapy because additional components are required to enable it to adsorb rapidly and spread to form a surface film, and to stabilize the film during repeated cycles of expansion and compression [115]. The breakthrough in therapy came when Enhörning and Robertson used natural surfactant extracts from the lungs of adult rabbits to treat premature rabbit pups and showed a marked improvement in lung function [116,117]. This was confirmed in models using other species [118]. In 1980, Fujiwara *et al.* reported the first successful treatment of newborn infants with respiratory distress syndrome [119]. They achieved striking improvements in arterial oxygenation using a saline extract of minced bovine lung enriched with synthetic lipids. Therapeutic surfactants obtained from mammalian sources are termed 'natural' surfactants, but the methods of preparation usually result in some 'modification' compared with normal pulmonary surfactant. A range of 'natural' and 'modified natural' surfactants from mammalian sources have been developed for therapeutic use in IRDS and shown to be efficacious [2]. These include extracts from minced bovine lung [119–124], from porcine lung [125–129], calf lung lavages [130–138] and surfactant recovered from human amniotic fluid [139–141]. Surfactant recovered from alveolar lavage or amniotic fluid is similar to the natural material, consisting mainly of surface active phospholipid, together with both hydrophobic and hydrophilic proteins. The 'modified natural' surfactants are lung minces or lavages that have been extracted with organic solvents to remove hydrophilic proteins. They contain mainly phospholipids and hydrophobic surfactant apoproteins, and are usually reconstituted in physiological saline before use. The lung tissue extracts contain nonsurfactant lipid contaminants from cell membranes, and they are often supplemented with additional components, for example synthetic DPPC, to optimize the surface activity [119,120].

Because of concerns about the risk of infection, potential immunogenicity of proteins and the limited supply of material from natural sources, artificial surfactants were also developed for therapeutic use in IRDS [3]. Two are in current use, and both contain synthetic phospholipid and are protein free. The artificial surfactant Exosurf consists of synthetic DPPC, to which is added the alcohol hexadecanol, and the mucolytic agent tyloxapol to aid liquefaction and adsorption of the surface film of phospholipid. These components are mixed in weight proportions 30.5:1.5:1 and suspended in 0.1M sodium chloride at a DPPC concentration of 13.5 mg/ml [142–146]. The other artificial surfactant used for treatment of IRDS is ALEC (Artificial Lung Expanding Compound; Britannia Pharmaceuticals, Redhill, Surrey, UK), which is a 3:1 mixture of synthetic DPPC and PG prepared from egg [115]. It was initially used as a dry powder [147] but is now prepared for clinical use as a 100 mg/ml suspension in saline [148–150].

The consensus of many clinical trials of surfactant therapy in IRDS is that prophylactic treatment using 'natural', 'modified natural' or artificial surfactants can reduce mortality by up to 50% [1–3]. Moreover, 'natural' or 'modified natural' surfactants can also reduce mortality by up to 40% when used as rescue therapy in infants with established IRDS [1,2]. New therapeutic surfactants are still being developed because of the recognition of the importance of the apoproteins in surfactant function. Attempts are being made to produce synthetic surfactants which more closely resemble the natural material [46,47]. The genes for the surfactant-specific apoproteins have been cloned [151–155] and recombinant apoproteins have been produced [156]. Synthetic analogs of apoproteins have also been developed [157–159]. It is hoped that mixtures of synthetic phospholipids and recombinant apoproteins or their analogs will be more efficacious than current protein-free artificial surfactants. The advantage of synthetic materials is that they can be produced in large quantities, without risk of infection, and at lower cost than the natural products. A summary of some of the main types of exogenous therapeutic surfactants currently used in IRDS, and synthetic products in development, is given in Table 16.2.

EXPERIENCE IN EXPERIMENTAL MODELS OF ACUTE LUNG INJURY

The benefit of surfactant replacement therapy in IRDS has raised much interest in its poten-

Table 16.2 Therapeutic surfactants used in IRDS and synthetic products in development

Main groups	Main components	Examples of preparations	Selected references
Natural or modified natural surfactants	Phospholipids/neutral lipids/ proteins	Human amniotic fluid	139–141
		Lung tissue extracts:	
		Surfactant-TA (bovine)	119,120
		Survanta (bovine)	121–124
		Curosurf (porcine)	125–129
		Lung lavage extracts:	
		Infasurf (bovine)	130–133
		CLSE (bovine)	134–136
		Alveofact (bovine)	137,138
Artificial surfactants	DPPC/hexadecanol/tyloxapol	Exosurf	142–146
	DPPC/PG	ALEC	147–150
Synthetic 'natural' surfactants	Phospholipids/Recombinant apoproteins or analogs	Phospholipids/rSpC	46
		Phospholipid/KL$_4$	47

rSpC, recombinant SpC.

tial for treatment of other disorders where surfactant dysfunction is a contributory factor, particularly ARDS. However, because the causes of surfactant dysfunction in ARDS differ from those in IRDS and vary during the course of the syndrome, the optimal approaches to therapy are likely to differ and need to be defined. Important questions yet to be resolved are the following.

1. What is the optimal time to commence therapy after the patient has encountered the risk factor triggering ARDS?
2. What is the optimal formulation of therapeutic surfactant and will this be influenced by the risk factor?
3. Is the optimal formulation likely to differ at different stages in the development of ARDS?
4. What is the optimal method of delivery?
5. What is the optimal dose?
6. Are multiple doses likely to be required and for what duration?
7. Is anti-inflammatory therapy also needed to reduce the risk of damage to the instilled material by products of inflammation such as oxidants and proteolytic enzymes?
8. Can replacement therapy also promote endogenous surfactant synthesis?

These questions have not yet been answered definitively, but the results of surfactant therapy in experimental models indicate that it can reduce the severity of injury and improve oxygenation.

The models of ARDS in which a beneficial effect of exogenous surfactant administration has been demonstrated (Table 16.3) include acute lung injury induced by saline whole lung lavage in guinea pigs and other species [160–166], influenza A pneumonia and other infections in mice and rats [167–169, 111], injection of antilung serum in guinea pigs [170], vagotomy in rabbits [105], *N*-nitroso-*N*-methylurethane injection in rats and rabbits [171–172], prolonged hyperoxia in rabbits and baboons [173–177] and hydrochloric acid instillation in rabbits [178–179].

Saline lung lavage

Repeated *in vivo* whole lung lavage causes acute lung injury by removing most of the alveolar lining fluid, including the surfactant. This results in reduced lung compliance and severe hypoxemia ($Pa_{O_2} < 60$ mmHg (5 kPa)) despite ventilation with 100% oxygen. Lachmann *et al.* conducted one of the first studies

Table 16.3 Experimental models of ARDS in which a beneficial effect of exogenous surfactant administration has been demonstrated

Model	Species	Surfactant	Delivery	Reference
Saline lung lavage	Guinea pigs	Porcine modified natural	Instilled	160–163
	Rabbits	Sheep (164) or porcine (165) modified natural	Instilled	164,165
	Sheep	Bovine modified natural (Survanta)	Instilled and aerosolized	166
Infections				
Influenza-A pneumonia	Mice	Bovine modified natural	Instilled	167
Sendai virus pneumonia	Rats	Bovine modified natural	Instilled	168
Pneumocystis carinii pneumonia	Rats	Bovine modified natural	Instilled	109
Streptococcus pneumonia	Mice	Bovine modified natural	Instilled	111
Antilung serum	Guinea pigs	Bovine modified natural	Instilled	170
Bilateral vagotomy	Rabbits	Sheep natural	Instilled	105
N-Nitroso-N-methylurethane	Rats	Bovine modified natural (Survanta)	Instilled	171
	Rabbits	Bovine modified natural (Survanta)	Instilled and aerosolized	172
Prolonged hyperoxia	Rabbits	Calf lung surfactant extract (CLSE)	Instilled	173–175
	Baboons	Artificial surfactant (Exosurf)	Aerosolized	176,177
Hydrochloric acid	Rabbits	Bovine (Survanta, 178) or porcine (179) modified natural	Instilled	178,179

to explore the benefit of surfactant replacement in ARDS using a saline lavage model in guinea pigs [161]. Intratracheal administration of 50 mg of natural surfactant immediately and 30 minutes after lavage resulted in a rapid and dramatic improvement in gas exchange and lung function, maintained over the 5 hour period of the experiment. In subsequent studies they showed that improvement was obtained even if the treatment was given up to 2 hours after the lavage [162,163].

Histologically, saline lavage results in extensive atelectasis, marked necrosis and desquamation of type I alveolar epithelial cells but lesser damage to type II cells, and hyaline membrane formation [160]. The histological changes in surfactant treated animals are minimal by comparison [162]. The benefit of tracheal instillation of exogenous natural surfactant has also been demonstrated in lavage models using adult rabbits [164,165], and more recently in a lavage model using adult sheep in which the efficacy of tracheal

instilled was compared with aerosolized exogenous surfactant given by nebulizer [166]. Both preparations improved oxygenation and lung compliance but the levels of improvement were greater for instilled delivery [166]. However, in a study using a different model nebulized delivery was superior [172]. The authors concluded that different delivery approaches may be required dependent upon the nature of the underlying injury.

Saline lung lavage models of ARDS have been criticized because the injury is homogeneous rather than inhomogeneous, as in the clinical syndrome; and because the marked deficiency of surfactant produced is more similar to the primary surfactant deficiency of IRDS than the mechanisms causing surfactant functional deficiency in ARDS. Despite these criticisms such studies have been important in providing a standard model for the testing and comparison of different preparations of therapeutic surfactants, which is essential for pharmacological development.

Other models

There are a number of other experimental models of ARDS which induce surfactant deficiency as a secondary consequence of lung injury, thereby resembling the mechanisms in ARDS, although the insults used are not necessarily comparable to the clinical risk factors. Surfactant replacement therapy has been shown to be of benefit in several of these models.

Infections

Various models mimicking the development of ARDS in patients with pneumonias or systemic infections are available. In 1987, acute lung injury in mice with influenza A pneumonia was shown to be improved by instillation of 200 mg/kg natural bovine surfactant [180]. The infection is normally lethal within 6 days, but both thoracic lung compliance and survival were improved by therapy. Therapy with natural surfactant (200 mg/kg) has also been reported to improve arterial oxygenation in rats with pneumonia induced by nebulized live Sendai virus [168]. In this model, abnormalities in surfactant function are associated with increased total protein in BAL. Instillation of natural bovine surfactant (200 mg/kg) has also improved gas exchange in experimental models of respiratory failure induced by *Pneumocystis carinii* pneumonia in rats [169] and *Streptococcus pneumoniae* infection in mice (111). Experimental models mimicking ARDS associated with Gram-negative septicemia are also available. These models have been induced, for example, by intravenous or intraperitoneal injection of live *Escherichia coli* or *E. coli* endotoxin in a variety of species [181–183]. The features are similar to those of the clinical syndrome and include alterations in surfactant function associated with high permeability edema and reduced synthesis of DPPC. Although sepsis is one of the most common and severe risks associated with the clinical development of ARDS, the

benefit of surfactant replacement therapy in these models has yet to be investigated.

Antilung serum

A different model of acute lung injury can be induced by injection of antilung serum containing antibodies to surfactant associated proteins and to antigens of alveolar-capillary basement membrane [170]. Inactivation of surfactant function occurs due to edema and decreased lung phospholipid content. Evidence was obtained using this model suggesting that some alveolar phospholipid is lost by leakage into the blood across the damaged capillaries [111,170]. This identifies another mechanism which may contribute to alterations in surfactant composition after acute lung injury. Tracheal instillation of natural surfactant (350 mg/kg) soon after exposure to antilung serum was able to induce a significant improvement in gas exchange [170].

Bilateral vagotomy

Bilateral vagotomy in rabbits induces severe hypoxemia and reduced lung compliance within 4 hours [105]. The histological features show interstitial and intra-alveolar edema and hyaline membrane formation; and impaired surfactant function develops due mainly to protein inhibition. Tracheal instillation of natural surfactant (50 mg/kg) has also been reported to improve gas exchange and lung compliance in this experimental model of acute lung injury [105].

N-nitroso-N-methylurethane:

Changes very similar to those in ARDS can be induced in animals by subcutaneous injection of *N*-nitroso-*N*-methylurethane (NNNMU). The changes develop within a few days, and include alterations in BAL phospholipid composition resembling those in ARDS, and increased BAL protein [184]. A beneficial effect of instilled natural surfactant (100 mg/

kg) has been reported using this model in rats [171] and in rabbits using either instilled or aerosolized surfactant [172]. More recently the metabolism of exogenously administered surfactant has been investigated in NNNMU injured rabbits [185]. The clearance of ^{3}H-labeled surfactant from the alveolar wash and lung tissue was the same in both the normal and NNNMU injured groups, suggesting similar catabolic pathways [184,185]. However, the levels of DPPC were lower in the alveoli and lung tissue of the injured compared with the control animals 24 hours after treatment suggesting decreased endogenous surfactant synthesis and/or secretion [185]. This and other [173] studies indicate that a single dose of instilled surfactant is unlikely to result in prolonged supplementation of the intra-alveolar pool of DPPC because of its rapid clearance and catabolism. It is important to bear this in mind when devising optimal approaches to surfactant therapy in ARDS. Even in IRDS, rescue therapy after the development of lung injury often requires several instilled doses given over the first 24 hours (1).

Hyperoxia

Reactive oxidants (e.g. superoxide anion (O_2^-), hydrogen peroxide (H_2O_2), hydroxyl radicals (OH^-), singlet oxygen and other free radicals) released from activated inflammatory cells are thought to play a role in the pathogenesis of ARDS [81–83]. They may contribute to tissue damage by oxidation of thiol groups on proteins, peroxidation of cell membrane associated fatty acids, and by generating reactive products that can cause further damage. Prolonged exposure to hyperoxia (100% O_2) can be used to produce experimental models of oxidant induced ARDS [186–188]. Injury develops after 24–48 hours of exposure, when the Pa_{O_2} drops acutely shortly before death [189–191]. There is a progressive increase in alveolar permeability, a fall in BAL phospholipid content, an increase in BAL proteins and impaired surfactant function [186]. Matalon *et al.* [173] reported that intratracheal instillation of a saline suspension of 125 mg of calf lung surfactant extract (CLSE) (an organic extract of alveolar lavage containing 99% lipid and 1% hydrophobic proteins) after 64 hours of O_2 exposure could improve hyperoxia induced lung injury in rabbits. A second dose was given 12 hours after the first to maintain supplementation. Prolonged survival in rabbits with oxygen induced lung injury has also been achieved by prophylactic instillation of 125 mg of CLSE after 24 hours of 100% O_2 exposure before evidence of injury, followed by repeated doses at 24 hourly intervals [174]. Others have also reported a beneficial effect of early treatment with instilled surfactant in the rabbit model [175]. More recently, it has been demonstrated that administering exogenous surfactant by aerosol at the start of exposure to hyperoxia can improve oxygenation and reduce alveolar epithelial cell damage in adult baboons [176,177]. However, late stage treatment of oxygen induced lung injury does not necessarily achieve response [192], and the timing of surfactant therapy after injury is likely to be of considerable importance in relation to the benefit achieved. Moreover, the optimal timing may differ for different risk factors where the mechanisms and rate of development of lung injury are variable.

Oleic acid induced lung injury

ARDS can develop in patients who suffer fat embolism due to the release of fatty acids from fractured long bones after trauma. An experimental model of this type of injury has been developed using intravenously injected oleic acid [193,194]. Surfactant dysfunction appears to be mainly due to increased contamination of the alveolar lining fluid with protein and unsaturated fatty acid [195–197]. An attempt has been made to treat oleic acid induced lung injury in sheep with an aerosolized preparation of the artificial surfactant Exosurf (mainly DPPC), but no response was achieved [198]. There is much controversy over the comparative advantages and disadvantages of aerosolized versus instilled delivery of therapeutic surfactants. It is also possible that protein-free artificial surfactants may not be able to counteract the complex disturbances of the surfactant system which occur in ARDS. These difficulties are discussed below in relation to the few clinical trials of surfactant replacement therapy in ARDS.

Installation of hydrochloric acid

ARDS can be induced by aspiration of gastric contents; and an experimental model mimicking this situation has been produced by intrabronchial instillation of hydrochloric acid [178,179]. Interestingly, the efficacy of surfactant therapy (modified natural porcine surfactant 75 mg/kg) was improved in this model by prelavaging the damaged lung with saline

to remove inhibitory proteins before instillation of the therapeutic surfactant [179]. This suggests that whole lung lavage immediately before therapy could be considered in clinical situations where there is protein inhibition, if no response is achieved using the conventional approaches.

These experimental models mimicking different risk factors associated with clinical ARDS help to define better the rationale for surfactant replacement therapy in a variety of circumstances leading to surfactant deficiency. The findings justify the continuation of efforts to develop further this approach for the treatment of patients with ARDS.

CLINICAL EXPERIENCE OF SURFACTANT REPLACEMENT IN ARDS

Despite encouraging results in experimental models of ARDS, there have been only a few clinical trials of surfactant replacement therapy in patients with ARDS to date (Table 16.4). The major difficulty in designing clin-

Table 16.4 Clinical trials of surfactant replacement therapy in ARDS

Number of patients	Risk factor	Surfactant	Delivery	Reference
Case reports				
1 child	Viral and bacterial pneumonia	Bovine modified natural, 300 mg/kg	Instilled	199
3 adults	Sepsis Pancreatitis Aspiration pneumonia	Porcine modified natural (Curosurf) approx. 60 mg/kg within 72 h of onset	Instilled	200
2 adults	Burn injury Cardiopulmonary bypass	Bovine modified natural (Surfactant-TA) 240 mg/day	Instilled repeated doses	201
7 children	?	Bovine modified natural, 100 mg lipid/kg of a lipid extract from alveolar lavage at 6–8 h intervals to max. 4 doses	Instilled repeated doses	202
Controlled trials				
49 adults	Sepsis	Artifical (Exosurf), 40.5 or 81 mg/ml for up to 5 days after onset	Nebulized	203
498 adults	Sepsis	Artificial (Exosurf), 13.5 mg DPPC/ml for up to 5 days after onset	Nebulized	204
59 adults	Trauma Multiple blood transfusions Sepsis Aspiration pneumonia	Bovine modified natural (Survanta) 50 mg PL/kg at minimum 6 h intervals to max. 8 doses; or 100 mg PL/kg to max. 4 doses; or 100 mg PL/kg to max. 8 doses	Instilled repeated doses	205,206

PL = total phospholipid

ical trials is due to the lack of knowledge of the precise nature of surfactant alterations at different stages during the course of ARDS, and the influence of the different risk factors. The first clinical trials reported in the literature were mainly uncontrolled case reports of empirical treatment early after the onset of ARDS [199–201]. At this early stage, protein contamination often makes the major contribution to surfactant dysfunction [97,98]. The first report was of a terminally ill child with viral and bacterial pneumonia treated with instilled natural bovine surfactant, 300 mg/kg [199]. There was a dramatic improvement in arterial oxygen tension (Pa_{O_2}) which rose from 19 to 240 mmHg (2.5 to 32 kPa) within 4 hours of treatment. The chest radiograph also showed a marked improvement. The second report was of three patients with severe ARDS related to sepsis, pancreatitis or aspiration pneumonia, treated by tracheal instillation with 4 g (approximately 60 mg/kg) of the modified natural porcine surfactant Curosurf in 50 ml volume within 72 hours of onset [200]. Treatment was well tolerated and produced a transient improvement in gas exchange. Nosaka *et al.* then reported that repeated instilled doses (240 mg/day) of the modified bovine natural surfactant Surfactant-TA approximately 15 times over 38 days in a 66 year old woman who developed ARDS after severe burn injury, and three times in a 51 year old man who developed ARDS after cardiopulmonary bypass, achieved more persistent improvement in gas exchange [201].

In 1992, the preliminary results of the first multicenter, randomized, placebo controlled trial of exogeneous surfactant therapy in ARDS were presented [203]. A nebulized preparation of the artificial surfactant Exosurf was used in this trial, aiming to achieve more prolonged delivery and even distribution. Nebulized doses (40.5 or 81 mg/ml) were given over the first 5 days after onset to patients with sepsis induced ARDS. The initial results on an intake of 49 cases indicated a trend towards reduced mortality and improved physiology at 14 days. However, results recently reported for a larger intake of 498 patients revealed no significant improvement in any parameter compared with the matched controls [204]. Patients were stratified by risk of mortality (APACHE-III score) and randomized to receive either Exosurf (13.5 mg DPPC/ml) or placebo (0.45% saline) aerosolized for up to 5 days; 249 of the patients received surfactant (138 males and 111 females, mean age 49 years ± 17) and 249 received placebo (141 males and 108 females, mean age 53 years ± 18). At entry to the study, both groups had similar histories and APACHE-III score distribution. Twenty-eight percent of patients did not complete the full 5 days of therapy due to early discontinuation of ventilation or death, but the surfactant was well tolerated and safety assessments showed no consistent differences between the groups. Improvement was judged by the assessment of mortality at 30 days for the group overall, for the patients stratified according to APACHE-III distribution, and for the subset of patients with pneumonia. Treatment had no significant effect on 30 day mortality, or on physiological measurements over the 5 days of treatment in any of these groups.

By contrast with the Exosurf trial, more encouraging results have been obtained in another multicenter, randomized controlled trial in progress using the modified natural bovine surfactant Survanta, employing multiple instilled doses, and comparing several dosing strategies [205,206]. Patients with ARDS associated with trauma, multiple blood transfusions, sepsis sydrome and/or witnessed aspiration of gastric contents are being studied and the preliminary results have recently been presented [205,206]. Patients were included in the trial within 48 hours of onset if the $Pa_{O_2}/F_{I_{O_2}}$ ratio was < 200 and positive end expiratory pressure PEEP > 10 cmH$_2$O, and four groups were compared. One ($n = 8$) received doses of 50 mg phospholipid/kg, repeating this dose at a minimum dosing interval of 6 hours to a maximum of eight doses according to prospectively determined criteria (Pa_{O_2}/F_{IO_2} falling to below 250). A second group ($n = 16$) were given 100 mg phospholipid/kg, employing a maximum of four doses, while a third group ($n = 19$) were given 100 mg phospholipid/kg to a maximum of eight doses. The fourth ($n = 16$) was treated in the standard way without surfactant supplementation. Response was determined from arterial blood gas tensions and ventilator settings recorded at baseline and 120 hours after the initial dose of surfactant. Patient outcome at 28 days was also recorded. Evaluation of the changes from baseline to 120 hours indicated that a significant improvement in ventilatory requirements was achieved using 100 mg phospholipid/kg to a maximum of four doses ($P < 0.05$ compared with standard therapy). Twenty-eight day mortality was significantly decreased, and this trend was also observed using 100 mg phospholipid/kg to a maximum of eight doses. BAL samples were obtained at baseline and 120 hours after the initial dose of surfactant to evaluate the surface active function and chemical composition of surfactant before and after Survanta supplementation. The highest supplementation was obtained using 100 mg phospholipid/kg to a maximum of eight doses [206]. In another recent study, preliminary results showing improvement have also been obtained using repeated instilled doses of bovine natural surfactant (100 mg lipid/kg of a lipid extract from alveolar lavage) in an uncontrolled trial in seven pediatric patients with ARDS [202]. Up to four doses were given at 6–8-hourly intervals depending on oxygen criteria. Four of the seven patients had significant improvements in oxygenation ($Pa_{O_2}/F_{IO_2} > 200$ in three, and > 150 in one) peaking within 2 hours after the first dose. These patients also had improvements in ventilation efficiency and peak inspiratory pressure values. On the basis of these results, it was proposed that a randomized double blind clinical trial of exogenous surfactant therapy should be performed in pediatric patients with ARDS.

There are many possible explanations for the contradictory results obtained in the first two multicenter, randomized controlled trials of surfactant therapy in ARDS. The formulations of the two surfactants used differed in major respects, as did the modes of delivery and doses. The patient selection criteria also differed; the Exosurf trial included only patients with sepsis associated ARDS, while the Survanta trial included patients with ARDS associated with a range of risk factors. Regarding the influence of different formulations, many clinical trials in IRDS have indicated that 'natural' or 'modified natural' surfactants are more efficacious for rescue therapy than the protein-free artifical surfactants [1]. The results of the first two controlled trials suggest that this may also be the case in ARDS. Regarding methods of delivery, the proposal that nebulized delivery might have significant advantages was not validated by the Exosurf trial [166,204], but the efficacy of natural surfactant preparations using this method of delivery is unknown. Nebulization has the advantage that surfactant can be delivered continuously during ventilation (linked with cycles of inspiration) to maintain supplementation over prolonged periods but it has the disadvantage that $< 30\%$ of the administered dose is deposited within the lungs [207]. There is also evidence that the process of nebulization may cause foaming, which reduces the surface tension lowering ability of surfactant preparations *in vitro* [208]. Preferential delivery to more normal areas of the lungs is also a potential problem [209]. If instilled multiple doses prove inadequate to maintain supplementation at optimal levels, it is possible that a combined approach to delivery, commencing with high dose instilled surfactant to achieve maximal initial supplementation followed by nebulization to maintain supplementation, may be an appropriate way to achieve optimal delivery of therapeutic surfactants to adult lungs.

The timing of treatment after encountering the initiating risk factor is likely to be of great importance in relation to the response achieved. Prophylactic therapy is more efficacious than rescue therapy in IRDS [1], and this raises the question of whether prophylactic use of surfactant replacement therapy can reduce the development of acute lung injury in patients at risk of ARDS. To address this question, a clinical trial has been conducted recently to determine the effect of exogenous surfactant therapy (3.2 g of ALEC instilled 60 minutes after bypass) on lung function after cardiopulmonary bypass [210]. No improvement was detected in eight treated compared with eight untreated control patients monitored at regular intervals up to 180 minutes after bypass. Moreover, the carbon monoxide transfer factor (TLCO) was significantly lower in the treated group at 120 minutes after therapy, raising the question whether treatment may be disadvantageous in individuals who may not require it. This emphasizes the need for early prognostic indicators to identify and select those patients especially at risk.

There is very little information on surfactant replacement therapy in patients at a late stage of severe ARDS, when there is deficient surfactant production as well as excessive protein contamination of the system [97,98]. We investigated the effect of single dose intrabronchial instillation of the artificial surfactant ALEC (75 mg/kg) in four such patients [211]. There was no sustained clinical improvement, but BAL samples before and at 24 hours after treatment showed that measurable supplementation of *in vivo* PC and PG levels and proportions had been achieved. ALEC is composed of 70% DPPC and 30% PG, but BAL levels of PC at 24 hours were increased up to 4.4-fold and PG levels up to 34.7-fold. PC proportions (percent of total phospholipid) remained below the normal range, but PG increased to above the normal

range in three patients. These findings are consistent with experimental evidence that PC is cleared from the air spaces of the lungs more rapidly than PG [1,212–214]. This suggests that doses and formulations of therapeutic surfactant to produce greater and more sustained supplementation of PC are required in patients with late stage ARDS. These findings demonstrate the value of BAL in monitoring the levels of supplementation and other *in vivo* effects of surfactant therapy, to guide therapeutic modifications that may be required to optimize response.

Our study in patients with late stage ARDS [211] also indicated that surfactant therapy does not reduce neutrophil counts in BAL. This suggests that combined treatment with anti-inflammatory drugs may be advisable to prevent further damage to intrinsic or instilled surfactant by oxidants and proteases from such cells. Many clinical trials of corticosteroids have been conducted in ARDS with the aim of suppressing neutrophils [215]. Most were trials of prophylactic treatment of patients with sepsis at risk of ARDS, or early stage treatment after onset of the syndrome. They concluded that early treatment with corticosteroids is of no therapeutic benefit. The only exception to this was a trial in patients with ARDS associated with fat embolism [216]. However, recent evidence suggests that corticosteroids can be of value in patients at a later stage of ARDS who develop the complication of pulmonary fibrosis [217]. We have had the opportunity to study one such case and observed that BAL neutrophil counts, phospholipid levels and proportions of PC and PG normalized after commencement of treatment in association with a striking clinical response [218]. This suggests that the benefit of corticosteroids may be due not only to their anti-inflammatory effects but also to their ability to stimulate surfactant phospholipid production by type II alveolar epithelial cells, either directly or by stimulating fibroblasts to produce a 'fibroblast pneumocyte factor' which can enhance surfactant synthesis [219].

Suppression of neutrophils in ARDS may also reduce damage to surfactant-specific proteins which have been shown to be susceptible to degradation by neutrophil derived proteases *in vitro* [85]. There is little information on *in vivo* levels of surfactant-specific proteins in ARDS, but a recent report indicates that BAL levels of Sp-A and Sp-B are significantly decreased, and Sp-A levels are also decreased in patients at risk [99]. These reductions are likely to contribute to surfactant dysfunction because of the importance of these molecules in surfactant biophysical function and turnover. Sp-A and Sp-D also have antimicrobial functions (see below) which could be of relevance to the increased susceptibility of patients with ARDS to nosocomial infections. In the light of these observations, it is probable that more complete formulations of natural or synthetic therapeutic surfactants containing surfactant associated proteins and phospholipids will prove to be of greatest benefit for the treatment of ARDS.

ROLE IN HOST DEFENSE

The pulmonary surfactant system plays an important role in pulmonary immune defense mechanisms, although less is known about these functions than its biophysical properties. Normal surfactant enhances the innate 'nonspecific' immune defense mechanisms which clear inhaled particles and microbes from the lungs, and suppresses the development of specific T lymphocyte mediated immune responses to inhaled antigens, preventing a constant state of immune hyperreactivity detrimental to life. Lymphocytes from the alveolar spaces of normal lungs are less responsive to mitogenic and antigenic stimulation than their counterparts in blood [220]. In 1979, Ansfield *et al.* first reported that normal surfactant from canine lungs suppresses the proliferation of canine blood lymphocytes [221]. Work from our group has shown subsequently that normal pulmonary surfactant from humans, pigs and rabbits also suppresses human blood lymphocyte proliferation to mitogens and alloantigens [222]. The major phospholipid components, PC and PG, are highly immunosuppressive, but the minor components, SM and PE (which increase during tissue damage), are highly immunostimulatory [223]. This suggests that the alterations in surfactant composition which develop during acute lung injury could have an influence on the regulation of pulmonary inflammatory responses.

By contrast with its immunosuppressive effects on T lymphocytes, normal pulmonary surfactant enhances 'nonspecific' pulmonary immune defense mechanisms. It aids mechanical clearance of cells and particles from the air spaces by its biophysical properties which promote movement towards the mucociliary escalator at end expiration, due to the increasing film pressure exerted by the surface monolayer of phospholipids. It is also thought to play a role in recruiting alveolar macrophages to the air spaces of the lungs, as both natural surfactant and Sp-A are chemotactic for alveolar macrophages *in vitro* [224–226]. Alveolar macrophages are the main phagocytes responsible for the immune defense of normal lungs, and it has been demonstrated that Sp-A and Sp-D can enhance the phagocytosis and killing of micro-organisms by these cells [44,45, 227–230]. Neutrophils recruited during inflammatory responses also phagocytose and kill bacteria, and assist wound healing through their scavenger functions by degrading and removing products of tissue damage. However, an excessive neutrophil response, as occurs in ARDS, can have adverse effects which outweigh the advantages [231]. It is not known whether pulmonary surfactant plays a role in regulating neutrophil responses, but a study using the porcine modified natural surfactant Curosurf indicates that this has no effect on neutrophil adherence or migration and may slightly reduce bacterial phagocytosis and killing by these cells [232]. Surfactant has also been reported to enhance CD11b/CD18 adhesion molecule expression on neutrophils *in vitro* [233] and we have observed that there is no reduction in BAL neutrophil counts after ALEC therapy in patients with ARDS [211], suggesting that surfactant may not inhibit neutrophil activation nor recruitment to the lungs. Elucidation of the effect of surfactant on neutrophils is an important area for future research, especially in relation to ARDS. On the other hand, the synthetic surfactant Exosurf has been reported to inhibit secretion of the cytokines tumor necrosis factor (TNF)α, interleukin (IL)-1 and IL-6 by activated human alveolar macrophages *in vitro* in a dose dependent manner [234]. Decreased secretion of TNFα after preincubation of human blood monocytes with the natural porcine surfactant Curosurf has also been reported [235]. These and other cytokines are thought to play an important role in the inflammatory mechanisms involved in the pathogenesis of ARDS [90,91,231,236–238]. The mechanisms are described in detail elsewhere.

Apart from providing information on surfactant composition and function, BAL investigations have the potential to clarify the relationship between changes in levels of inflammatory cells and their products, and the development of surfactant dysfunction in ARDS. New therapeutic agents are being developed to modulate the effects of inflammatory mediators, including antibodies to endotoxin or cytokines [239–241], low molecular weight antagonists of cytokines or cytokine receptors [242] and agents to modulate expression or block interaction with adhesion molecules [243–245]. These developments, together with the research in progress to produce more efficient synthetic therapeutic surfactants, appear to offer better prospects for the future.

SUMMARY

Alterations in pulmonary surfactant are an important contributory factor in the pathogenesis of ARDS. Their consequences on rate of progression of the syndrome, prognosis and increased susceptibility to nosocomial infection need to be better elucidated. Continuing work on surfactant therapy, including efforts to develop synthetic surfactants which more closely emulate natural surfactant, is important, as this has the potential to improve survival and/or speed recovery by reducing ventilatory requirements.

ACKNOWLEDGEMENTS

The author thanks the British Lung Foundation and The Clinical Research Committee of the Royal Brompton Hospital for their support of our studies of pulmonary surfactant in ARDS, the colleagues who are collaborating, in particular Dr Tim Evans, Cathy Baker, Dr David Hughes and Ann Dewar, and Mrs Joanna Harwood for typing the manuscript.

REFERENCES

1. Jobe, A. and Ikegami, M. (1987) State of the art: surfactant for the treatment of respiratory distress syndrome. *Am. Rev. Respir. Dis.*, **136**, 1256–75.
2. Smith, B.T. (1992) Clinical experience with modified natural surfactant, in *Pulmonary Surfactant: From Molecular Biology to Clinical Practice* (eds B. Robertson, L.M.G. Van Golde and J.J. Batenburg), Elsevier, Amsterdam, pp. 593–604.
3. Morley, C.J. (1992) Clinical experience with artificial surfactants, in *Pulmonary Surfactant: From Molecular Biology to Clinical Practice* (eds B. Robertson, L.M.G. Van Golde and J.J. Batenburg), Elsevier, Amsterdam, pp. 605–33.
4. Lewis, J.F. and Jobe, A.H. (1993) Surfactant and the adult respiratory distress syndrome. *Am. Rev. Respir. Dis.*, **147**, 218–33.
5. King, R.J. and Clements, J.A. (1972) Surface active materials from dog lung: composition and physiological correlations. *Am. J. Physiol.*, **223**, 715–26.

6. Possmayer, F. (1988) Pulmonary perspective: a proposed nomenclature for pulmonary surfactant associated proteins. *Am. Rev. Respir. Dis.*, **138**, 990–8.

7. Hills, B.A. (1988) *The Biology of Surfactant*, Cambridge: Cambridge University Press.

8. Clements, J.A., Hustead, R.I., Johnson, R.P. and Gribetz, I. (1961) Pulmonary surface tension and alveolar stability. *J. Appl. Physiol.*, **16**, 444–50.

9. Hills, B.A. (1982) Water repellency induced by pulmonary surfactants. *J. Physiol.*, **325**, 175–86.

10. Notter, R.H. and Finkelstein, J.N. (1984) Pulmonary surfactant: an interdisciplinary approach. *J. Appl. Physiol.*, **57**, 1613–24.

11. Clements, J.A. (1957) Surface tension of lung extracts. *Proc. Soc. Exp. Biol. Med.*, **95**, 170–2.

12. Enhorning, G. (1977) Pulsating bubble technique for evaluating pulmonary surfactant. *J. Appl. Physiol.*, **43**, 198–203.

13. Klech, H. and Pohl, W. (eds) (1989) Technical recommendations and guidelines for bronchoalveolar lavage (BAL): report of the European Society of Pneumology Task Group on BAL. *Eur. Respir. J.*, **2**, 561–85.

14. The BAL Co-operative Group Steering Committee (1990) Bronchoalveolar lavage constituents in healthy individuals, idiopathic pulmonary fibrosis, and selected comparison groups. *Am. Rev. Respir. Dis.*, **141 (suppl.)**, S169–202.

15. Hughes, D.A. and Haslam, P.L. (1989) Changes in phosphatidylglycerol in bronchoalveolar lavage fluids from patients with cryptogenic fibrosing alveolitis. *Chest*, **95**, 82–9.

16. King, R.J. and Clements, J.A. (1972) Surface active materials from dog lung. Method of isolation. *Am. J. Physiol.*, **223**, 704–14.

17. Pison, U., Gono, E., Joka, K. and Obladen, M. (1986) High performance liquid chromatography of adult human bronchoalveolar lavage: assay for phospholipid lung profile. *J. Chromatogr.*, **377**, 79–89.

18. King, R.J. (1984) Isolation and chemical composition of pulmonary surfactant, in *Pulmonary Surfactant* (eds B. Robertson, L.M.G. Van Golde and J.J. Batenburg), Elsevier, Amsterdam, pp. 1–15.

19. Hughes, D.A. and Haslam, P.L. (1990) Effect of smoking on the lipid composition of lung lining fluid and relationship between immunostimulatory lipids, inflammatory cells and foamy macrophages in extrinsic allergic alveolitis. *Eur. Respir. J.*, **3**, 1128–39.

20. Minty, B.D., Jordan, C. and Jones, J.G. (1981) Rapid improvement in abnormal epithelial permeability after stopping cigarettes. *BMJ*, **282**, 1183–7.

21. Weaver, T.E. (1988) Pulmonary surfactant-associated proteins. *Gen. Pharmacol.*, **19**, 361–8.

22. Hawgood, S. (1989) Pulmonary surfactant apoproteins: a review of protein and genomic structure. *Am. J. Physiol.*, **257** L13–22.

23. Whitsett, J.A., Hull, W., Ross, G. and Weaver, T. (1985) Characteristics of human surfactant-associated glycoproteins A. *Pediatr. Res.*, **19**, 501–8.

24. Hawgood, S., Efrati, H., Schilling, J. and Benson, B.J. (1985) Chemical characterization of lung surfactant apoproteins: amino acid composition, N-terminal sequence and enzymic digestion. *Trans. Biochem. Soc.*, **13**, 1092–6.

25. Floros, J., Phelps, D.S., Kourembanas, S. and Taeusch, H.W. (1986) Primary translation products, biosynthesis, and tissue specificity of the major surfactant protein in rat. *J. Biol. Chem.*, **261**, 828–31.

26. Persson, A., Chang, D., Rust, K. *et al.* (1989) Purification and biochemical characterization of CP4 (SP-D): a collagenous surfactant-associated protein. *Biochemistry*, **27**, 6361–7.

27. Rust, K., Grosso, L., Zhang, V. *et al.* (1991) Human surfactant protein D: SP-D contains a C-type lectin carbohydrate recognition domain. *Arch. Biochem. Biophys.*, **290**, 116–26.

28. Curstedt, T., Johansson, J., Persson, P. *et al.* (1990) Hydrophobic surfactant-associated polypeptides. SP-C is a lipopeptide with two palmitoylated cysteine residues, whereas SP-B lacks covalently linked fatty acyl groups. *Proc. Natl. Acad. Sci. USA*, **87**, 2985–9.

29. Whitsett, J.A. Ohning, B.L., Ross, G. *et al.* (1986) Hydrophobic surfactant-associated protein in whole lung surfactant and its importance for biophysical activity in lung surfactant extracts used for replacement therapy. *Pediatr. Res.*, **20**, 460–7.

30. Takahashi, A. and Fujiwara, T. (1986) Proteolipid in bovine lung surfactant: its role in surfactant function. *Biochem. Biophys. Res. Commun.*, **135**, 527–32.

31. Yu, S.H. and Possmayer, F. (1988) Comparative studies on the biophysical activities of the low-molecular-weight hydrophobic proteins purified from bovine pulmonary surfactant. *Biochim. Biophys. Acta*, **961**, 337–50.

32. Yu, S. and Possmayer, F. (1990) Role of bovine pulmonary surfactant-associated proteins in the surface-active property of phospholipid mixtures. *Biochim. Biophys. Acta*, **1046**, 233–241.

33. Takahashi, A., Waring, A.J., Arnirkhaman, J. *et al.* (1990) Structure function relationships of bovine pulmonary surfactant proteins: SP-B and SP-C. *Biochim. Biophys. Acta*, **1044**, 43–9.

34. Williams, M.C. (1977) Conversion of lamellar body membranes into tubular myelin in alveoli of fetal rat lung. *J. Cell Biol.*, **72**, 260–77.

35. Suzuki, Y. Fujita, Y. and Kogishi, K. (1989) Reconstitution of tubular myelin from synthetic lipids and proteins associated with pig pulmonary surfactant. *Am. Rev. Respir. Dis.* **140**, 75–81.

36. Williams, M.C., Hawgood, S. and Hamilton, R.I. (1991) Changes in lipid structure produced by surfactant proteins SP-A, SP-B, and SP-C. *Am. J. Respir. Cell Mol. Biol.*, **5**, 41–50.

37. Hallman, M., Katsumi, M. and Wagner, R.M. (1976) Isolated lamellar bodies from rat lung: correlated ultrastructural and biochemical studies. *Lab. Invest.*, **35**, 79–86.

38. Sanders, R.I., Hassett, R.J. and Vatter, A.E. (1980) Isolation of lung lamellar bodies and their conversion to tubular myelin figures *in vitro*. *Anat. Rec.*, **198**, 485–501.

39. Hawgood, S., Benson, B.J. and Hamilton, R.L. (1985) Effects of a surfactant-associated protein and calcium ions on the structure and surface activity of lung surfactant lipids. *Biochemistry*, **24**, 184–90.

40. King, R.J., Carmichael, M.C. and Horowitz, P.M. (1983) Reassembly of lipid–protein complexes of pulmonary surfactant. Proposed mechanism of interaction. *J. Biol. Chem.*, **258**, 10672–80.

41. Tanaka, Y., Takei, T., Aiba, T. *et al.* (1986) Development of synthetic lung surfactants. *J. Lipid Res.*, **27**; 475–85.

42. Wright, J.R., Wager, R.E., Hawgood, S. *et al.* (1987) Surfactant apoprotein Mr = 26 000–36 000 enhances uptake of liposomes by type II cells. *J. Biol. Chem.* **262**, 2888–94.

43. Dobbs, L.G., Wright, J.R., Hawgood, S. *et al.* (1987) Pulmonary surfactant and its components inhibit secretion of phosphatidylcholine from cultured rat alveolar type II cells. *Proc. Natl. Acad. Sci. USA*, **84**, 1010–4.

44. van Iwaarden, F., Welmers, B., Verhoef, J. *et al.* (1990) Pulmonary surfactant protein A enhances the host-defense mechanism of rat alveolar macrophages. *Am. J. Respir. Cell Mol. Biol.*, **2**, 91–8.

45. Kuan, S.-F., Rust, K. and Crouch, E. (1992) Interactions of surfactant protein D with bacterial lipopolysaccharides. *J. Clin. Invest.*, **90**, 97–106.

46. Hafner, D., Germann, P. and Hauschke, D. (1994) Lung surfactant (LSF) improves gas exchange and histopathology in a model of adult respiratory distress syndrome (ARDS). *Am. J. Respir. Crit Care Med.*, **149**, A126.

47. Sweeney, T.D., Reinisch, U.S., Kirk, J.E. *et al.* (1994) A synthetic phospholipid-KL surfactant improves lung function in a rat model of ARDS. *Am. J. Respir. Crit. Care Med.*, **149**, A126.

48. Wright, J.R. and Clements, J.A. (1987) Metabolism and turnover of lung surfactant. *Am. Rev. Respir. Dis.*, **135**, 426–44.

49. Gross, N.J., Barnes, E. and Narine, K.R. (1988) Recycling of surfactant in black and beige mice: pool sizes and kinetics. *J. Appl. Physiol.*, **64**, 2017–25.

50. Magoon, M.W., Wright, J.R., Bantussio, A. *et al.* (1983) Subfractionation of lung surfactant. Implications for metabolism and surface activity. *Biochim. Biophys. Acta*, **750**, 18–31.

51. Manabe, T. (1979) Freeze-fracture study of alveolar lining layer in adult rat lungs. *J. Ultrastruct. Res.*, **69**, 86–97.

52. Baritussio, A., Carraro, R., Bellina, J. *et al.* (1985) Turnover of phospholipids isolated from fractions of lung lavage fluid. *J. Appl. Physiol.*, **59**, 1055–60.

53. Wright, J.R., Wager, R.E., Hamilton, R.L. *et al.* (1986) Uptake of lung surfactant subfractions into lamellar bodies of adult rabbit lungs. *J. Appl. Physiol.*, **60**, 817–25.

54. Kuroki, Y., Mason, R.J. and Voelker, D.R. (1988) Alveolar type II cells express a high-affinity receptor for pulmonary surfactant protein A. *Proc. Natl. Acad. Sci. USA*, **85**, 5566–70.

55. Rice, W.R., Ross, G.F., Singleton, F.M. *et al.* (1987) Surfactant-associated protein inhibits phospholipid secretion from type II cells. *J. Appl. Physiol.*, **63**, 692–8.

56. Avery, M.E. and Mead, J. (1959) Surface properties in relation to atelectasis and hyaline membrane disease. *Am. J. Dis. Child.*, **97**, 517–23.

57. Verloove-Vanhorick, S.P., Verwey, R.A., Brand, R. *et al.* (1986) Neonatal mortality risk in relation to gestational age and birth weight. *Lancet*, **i**, 55–7.

58. Kitchen, W.H., Doyle, L.W., Ford, G.W. *et al.* (1991) Changing two-year outcome of infants weighing 500 to 999 grams at birth: a hospital study. *J. Pediatr.*, **118**, 938–43.

59. Chida, S., Phelps, D.S., Cordle, C. *et al.* (1988) Surfactant-associated proteins in tracheal aspirates of infants with respiratory distress syndrome after surfactant therapy. *Am. Rev. Respir. Dis.*, **137**, 943–7.

60. Seeger, W., Stöhr, G., Wolf, H.R.D. and Neuhof, H. (1985) Alteration of surfactant function due to protein leakage: special interaction with fibrin monomer. *J. Appl. Physiol.*, **58**, 326–38.

61. Holm, B.A., Notter, R.H. and Finkelstein, JN. (1985) Surface property changes from interactions of albumin with natural lung surfactant extracted lung lipids. *Chem. Phys. Lipids*, **38**, 287–98.

62. Holm, B.A. and Notter, R.H. (1987) Effects of hemoglobin and red blood cell membrane lipids on the biophysical and physiological activity of pulmonary surfactant. *J. Appl. Physiol.*, **63**, 1434–42.

63. Fuchimukai, T., Fujiwara, T., Takahashi, A. and Enhorning, G. (1987) Artificial pulmonary surfactant inhibited by proteins. *J. Appl. Physiol.*, **57**, 1134–42.

64. Holm, B.A., Enhorning, G. and Notter, R.H. (1988) A biophysical mechanism by which plasma proteins inhibit lung surfactant activity. *Chem. Phys. Lipids*, **49** 49–55.

65. Seeger, W. Grube, C., Günther, A. and Schmidt, R. (1993) Surfactant inhibition by plasma proteins: differential sensitivity of various surfactant preparations. *Eur. Respir. J.*, **6**, 971–7.

66. Holm, B.A., Venkitaraman, A.R., Enhorning, G. and Notter, R.H. (1990) Biophysical inhibition of synthetic lung surfactants. *Chem. Phys. Lipids*, **52**, 243–50.

67. Seeger, W. Thede, C. Gunther, A. and Grube, C. (1991) Surface properties and sensitivity to protein-inhibition of a recombinant apoprotein C-based phospholipid mixture *in vitro* – comparison to natural surfactant. *Biochim. Biophys. Acta*, **1081** 45–52.

68. Ikegami, M., Jobe, A., Jacobs, H. and Jones, S. (1981) Sequential treatments of premature lambs with an artificial surfactant and natural surfactant. *J. Clin. Invest.*, **68**, 491–6.

69. Ikegami, M., Agata, Y., Elkady, T. *et al.* (1987) A comparison of four surfactants: *in vitro* surface properties and responses of preterm lambs to treatment at birth. *Pediatrics*, **79**, 38–46.

70. Venkitaraman, A.R., Hall, S.B., Whitsett, J.A. and Notter, R.H. (1990) Enhancement of biophysical activity of lung surfactant extracts and phospholipid-apoprotein mixtures by surfactant proteins. *Chem. Phys. Lipids*, **56**, 1–10.

71. Venkitaraman, A.R., Baatz, J.E., Whitsett, J.A. *et al.* (1990) Biophysical inhibition of synthetic phospholipid-lung surfactant apoprotein admixtures by plasma proteins. *Chem. Phys. Lipids*, **57**, 49–57.

72. Cockshutt, A., Weitz, J. and Possmayer, F. (1990) Pulmonary surfactant-associated protein A enhances the surface activity of lipid extract surfactant and reverses inhibition by blood proteins *in vitro*. *Biochemistry*, **29**, 8424–9.

73. Holm, B.A. (1992) Surfactant inactivation in adult respiratory distress syndrome, in *Pulmonary Surfactant: From Molecular Biology to Clinical Practice* (eds B. Robertson, L.M.G. Van Golde and J.J. Batenburg) Elsevier, Amsterdam, pp. 665–84.

74. Holm, B.A. and Matalon, S. (1989) Role of pulmonary surfactant in the development and treatment of adult respiratory distress syndrome. *Anesth. Analg.*, **69**, 805–18.

75. Hallman, M., Spragg, R., Harrell, J.H. *et al.* (1982) Evidence of lung surfactant abnormality in respiratory failure: study of bronchoalveolar lavage phospholipids, surface activity, phospholipase activity, and plasma myoinositol. *J. Clin. Invest.*, **70**, 673–83.

76. Holm, B.A., Keicher, L., Liu, M. *et al.* (1991) Inhibition of pulmonary surfactant function by phospholipases. *J. Appl. Physiol.*, **71**, 1–5.

77. Passi, R.B. and Possmayer, F. (1981) Surfactant metabolism in acute pancreatitis. *Prog. Respir. Res.*, **15**, 136–40.

78. Vadas, P. (1984) Elevated plasma phospholipase A_2 levels: correlation with the hemodynamic and pulmonary changes in Gram negative septic shock. *J. Lab. Clin. Med.*, **104**, 873–81.

79. Vadas, P. and Pruzanski, W. (1986) Biology of disease: role of secretory phospholipases A_2 in the pathobiology of disease. *Lab. Invest.*, **55**, 391–9.

80. Bejar, R., Curbelo, V., Davis, C. and Gluck, L. (1981) Premature labor. II. Bacterial source of phospholipase. *Obstet. Gynecol.*, **57**, 479–82.

81. Weiss, S.J. (1989) Tissue destruction by neutrophils. *N. Engl. J. Med.*, **320**, 365–76.

82. Henson, P.M. and Johnston, R.B. (1987) Tissue injury in inflammation: oxidants, proteinases and cationic proteins. *J. Clin. Invest.*, **79**, 669–74.

83. Fantone, J.C. and Ward, P.A. (1985) Polymorphonuclear leukocyte-mediated cell and tissue injury: oxygen metabolites and their relation to human disease. *Hum. Pathol.*, **16**, 973–8.

84. Esterbauer, H. (1985) Lipid peroxidation products: formation, chemical properties and biological activities, in *Free Radicals in Liver Injury* (eds G. Poli, K.H. Cheeseman, M.U. Dianzani, *et al.*), IRL Press, Oxford, pp. 29–47.

85. Ryan, S.F., Ghassibi, Y. and Liau, D.F. (1991) Effects of activated polymorphonuclear leukocytes upon pulmonary surfactant *in vitro*. *Am. J. Respir. Cell Mol. Biol.*, **4**, 33–41.

86. Fowler, A.A., Hamman, R.F., Good, J.T. *et al.* (1983) Adult respiratory distress syndrome: risks with common predispositions. *Ann. Intern. Med.*, **98**, 593–7.

87. Montgomery, A.B., Stager, M.A., Carrico, C.J. and Hudson, L.D. (1985) Causes of mortality in patients with the adult respiratory distress syndrome. *Am. Rev. Respir. Dis.*, **132**, 148.

88. Murray, J.F., Matthay, M.A., Luce, J.M. and Flick, M.R. (1988) An expanded definition of the adult respiratory distress syndrome. *Am. Rev. Respir. Dis.*, **138**, 720–3.

89. Bernard, G.R., Artigas, A., Brigham, K.L. *et al.* (1994) Conference report: The American–European Consenus Conference on ARDS. Definitions, mechanisms, relevant outcomes, and clinical trial coordination. *Am. J. Respir. Crit. Care Med.*, **149**, 818–24.

90. Rinaldo, J.E. and Christman, J.W. (1990) Mechanisms and mediators of the adult respiratory distress syndrome. *Clin. Chest Med.*, **11**, 621–32.

91. Donnelly, S.C. and Haslett, C. (1992) Cellular mechanisms of acute lung injury: implications for future treatment in the adult respiratory distress syndrome. *Thorax*, **47**, 260–3.

92. Ashbaugh, D.G., Bigelow, D.B., Petty, T.L. and Levine, B.E. (1967) Acute respiratory distress in adults. *Lancet*, **ii**, 319–23.

93. Von Wichert, P. and Kohl, F.V. (1977) Decreased dipalmitoyllecithin content found in lung specimens from patients with so-called shock-lung. *Eur. Intensive Care Med.*, **3**, 27–30.

94. Petty, T.L., Reiss, O.K., Paul, G.W. *et al.* (1977) Characteristics of pulmonary surfactant in adult respiratory distress syndrome associated with trauma and shock. *Am. Rev. Respir. Dis.*, **115**, 531–6.

95. Pison, U., Seeger, W., Buchhorn, R. *et al.* (1989) Surfactant abnormalities in patients with respiratory failure after multiple trauma. *Am. Rev. Respir. Dis.*, **140**, 1033–9.

96. Pison, U., Obertacke, U., Brand, M. *et al.* (1990) Altered pulmonary surfactant in uncomplicated and septicemia-complicated courses of acute respiratory failure. *J. Trauma*, **30**, 19–26.

97. Seeger, W., Pison, U., Buchhorn, T. *et al.* (1990) Alterations in alveolar surfactant following severe multiple trauma, in *Progress in Respiration Research*, vol. 25 Basic Research on Lung Surfactant (eds P. von Wichert and B. Muller), Karger, Basel, pp. 215–23.

98. Seeger, W., Pison, U., Buchhorn, R. *et al.* (1990) Surfactant abnormalities and adult respiratory failure. *Lung*, **168(suppl.)**, 891–902.

99. Gregory, T. Longmore, W., Moxley, M. *et al.* (1991) Surfactant chemical composition and biophysical activity in acute respiratory distress syndrome. *J. Clin. Invest.*, **88**, 1976–81.

100. Holter, J.F., Weiland, J.E., Pacht, E.R. *et al.* (1986) Protein permeability in the adult respiratory distress syndrome. Loss of size selectivity of the alveolar epithelium. *J. Clin. Invest.*, **78**, 1513–22.

101. Fowler, A.A., Walchak, S., Giclas, P.C. *et al.* (1982) Characterization of antiproteinase activity in the adult respiratory distress syndrome. *Chest*, **81 (suppl.)**, 50S-51S.

102. Lee, C.T. Fein, A.M., Lippman, M. *et al.* (1981) Elastolytic activity in pulmonary lavage fluid from patients with adult respiratory distress syndrome. *N. Engl. J. Med.*, **304**, 192–6.

103. Wewers, M.D., Herzyk, D.J. and Gadek J.E. (1988) Alveolar fluid neutrophil elastase activity in the adult respiratory distress syndrome is complexed to alpha-2-macroglobulin. *J. Clin. Invest.*, **82**, 1260–7.

104. Li, J.J., Sanders, R.L., McAdam, K.P. *et al.* (1989) Impact of C-reactive protein (CRP) on surfactant function. *J. Trauma*, **29**, 1690–7.

105. Berry, D., Ikegami, M. and Jobe, A. (1986) Respiratory distress and surfactant inhibition following vagotomy in rabbits. *J. Appl. Physiol.*, **61**, 1741–8.

106. Liau, D.F., Barrett, C.R., Bell, A.L.L. and Ryan, S.F. (1985) Normal surface properties of phosphatidylglycerol-deficient surfactant from dog after acute lung injury. *J. Lipid Res.*, **26**, 1338–44.

107. Batenburg, J.J., Klazinga, W. and Van Golde, L.M.G. (1985) Regulation and location of phosphatidylglycerol and phosphatidylinositol synthesis in type II cells isolated from fetal rat lung. *Biochim. Biophys. Acta.*, **833**, 17–24.

108. Hallman, M., Enhorning, G. and Possmayer, F. (1985) Composition and surface activity of normal and phosphatidylglycerol-deficient lung surfactant. *Pediatr. Res.*, **19** 286–92.

109. Beppu, O.S., Clements, J.A. and Goerke, J. (1983) Phosphatidylglycerol-deficient lung surfactant has normal properties. *J. Appl. Physiol.*, **55**, 496–502.

110. Gross, N. (1991) Altered surfactant subtypes in an experimental form of ARDS: radiation pneumonitis. *Am. J. Physiol.*, **260**, L302–10.

111. Lachmann, B. and van Daal G-J. (1992) Adult respiratory distress syndrome: animal models, in *Pulmonary Surfactant: from Molecular Biology to Clinical Practice*, (eds B. Robertson, L.M.G. Van Golde and J.J. Batenburg), Elsevier, Amsterdam, pp. 635–63.

112. Klaus, M.H., Clements, J.A. and Havel, H.J. (1961) Composition of surface active material isolated from beef lung. *Proc. Natl. Acad. Sci. USA*, **47**, 1858.

113. Robillard, E., Alarie, Y., Dagenais-Perusse, P. *et al.*, (1964) Microaerosol administration of synthetic β-γ-dipalmotyl-ʟ-α-lecithin in the respiratory distress syndrome. A preliminary report. *Can. Med. Assoc. J.*, **90**, 55–7.

114. Chu, J., Clements, J.A., Cotton, E.K. *et al.* (1967) Neonatal pulmonary ischaemia: clinical and physiologic studies. *Pediatrics*, **40**, 709–82.

115. Bangham, A.D., Morley, C.J. and Phillips, M.C. (1979) The physical properties of an effective lung surfactant. *Biochim. Biophys. Acta*, **573**, 552–6.

116. Enhörning, G. and Robertson, J.B. (1972) Lung expansion in the premature rabbit fetus after tracheal deposition of surfactant. *Pediatrics*, **50**, 55–66.

117. Robertson, B. and Enhörning, G. (1974) The alveolar lining of the premature newborn rabbit after pharyngeal deposition of surfactant. *Lab. Invest.*, **31**, 54–9.

118. Adams, F.H., Towers, B., Osher, A.B. *et al.* (1978) Effects of tracheal instillation of natural surfactant in premature lambs. I. Clinical and autopsy findings. *Pediatr. Res.*, **12**, 841–8.

119. Fujiwara, T., Chida, S., Watabe, Y.J. *et al.* (1980) Artificial surfactant therapy in hyaline membrane disease. Lancet, i, 55–9.

120. Fujiwara, T., Konishi, M., Chida, S. *et al.* (1990) Surfactant replacement therapy with a single postventilatory dose of a reconstituted bovine surfactant in preterm neonates with respiratory distress syndrome: final analysis of a multicenter, double-blind, randomized trial and comparison with similar trials. *Pediatrics*, **86**, 753–64.

121. Soll, R.F., Hoekstra, R.A., Fangmann, J.J. *et al.* (1990) Multicenter trial of single-dose modified bovine surfactant extract (Survanta) for prevention of respiratory distress syndrome. *Pediatrics*, **85**, 1092–102.

122. Horbar, J.D., Soll, R.F., Schachinger, H. *et al.* (1990) A European multicenter randomized trial of single dose surfactant therapy for idiopathic respiratory distress syndrome. *Eur. J. Pediatr.*, **149**, 416–23.

123. Ware, J., Taeusch, H.W., Soll, R.F. and McCormick, M.C. (1990) Health and developmental outcomes of a surfactant controlled trial: follow-up at 2 years. *Pediatrics*, **85**, 1103–7.

124. Hoekstra, R.E., Jackson, J.C., Myers, T.F. *et al.* (1991) Improved neonatal survival following multiple doses of bovine surfactant in very premature neonates at risk for respiratory distress syndrome. *Pediatrics*, **88**, 10–8.

125. Noack, G., Berggren, P., Curstedt, T., *et al.* (1987) Severe neonatal respiratory distress syndrome treated with the isolated phospholipid fraction of natural surfactant. *Acta Paediatr. Scand.*, **76**, 697–705.

126. Collaborative European Multicenter Study Group (1988) Surfactant replacement therapy for severe neonatal respiratory distress syndrome: an international randomized clinical trial. *Pediatrics*, **82**, 683–91.

127. Robertson, B. (1990) European multicenter trials of Curosurf for treatment of neonatal respiratory distress syndrome. *Lung*, **168**, 860–3.

128. Collaborative European Multicenter Study Group (1991) Factors influencing the clinical response to surfactant replacement therapy in babies with severe respiratory distress syndrome. *Eur. J. Pediatr.*, **150**, 433–9.

129. Speer, C.P., Robertson, B., Curstedt, T. *et al.* (1992) Randomized European multicenter trial of surfactant replacement therapy for severe neonatal respiratory distress syndrome: single versus multiple doses of Curosurf. *Pediatrics.*, **89**, 13–20.

130. Yu, S., Harding, P.G.R., Smith, N. and Possmayer, F. (1983) Bovine pulmonary surfactant: chemical and physical properties. *Lipids*, **18**, 522–9.

131. Enhörning, G., Shennan, A., Possmayer, F. *et*

al. (1985) Prevention of neonatal respiratory distress syndrome by tracheal instillation of surfactant: a randomized clinical trial. *Pediatrics*, **76**, 145–53.

132. Dunn, M.S., Shennan, A.T. and Possmayer, F. (1990) Single- versus multiple-dose surfactant replacement therapy in neonates of 30 to 36 weeks' gestation with respiratory distress syndrome. *Pediatrics*, **86**, 564–71.

133. Dunn, M.S., Shennan, A.T. Zayack, D. and Possmayer, F. (1991) Bovine surfactant replacement therapy in neonates of less than 30 week's gestation – a randomized controlled trial of prophylaxis versus treatment. *Pediatrics*, **87**, 377–86.

134. Shapiro, D.L., Notter, R.H., Morin, F.C. *et al.* (1985) Double-blind randomized trial of a calf lung surfactant extract administered at birth to very premature infants for prevention of respiratory distress syndrome. *Pediatrics*, **76**, 593–9.

135. Kwong, M.S., Egan, E.A., Notter, R.H. and Shapiro, D.L. (1985) Double-blind clinical trial of calf lung surfactant extract for the prevention of hyaline membrane disease in extremely premature infants. *Pediatrics*, **76**, 585–92.

136. Kendig, J.W., Notter, R.H., Cox, C. *et al.* (1988) Surfactant replacement therapy at birth: final analysis of a clinical trial and comparisons with similar trials. *Pediatrics*, **82**, 756–62.

137. Disse, B., Gortner, L., Weller, E. *et al.* (1988) Efficacy and standardization of SF-RII: a preparation from bovine lung surfactant, in *Surfactant Replacement Therapy in Neonatal and Adult Respiratory Distress Syndrome* (ed. B. Lachmann), Springer, Berlin, pp. 37–41.

138. Gortner, L., Bernsau, U., Hellwege, H.H. *et al.* (1990). A multicenter randomized controlled clinical trial of bovine surfactant for prevention of respiratory distress syndrome. *Lung*, **168 (suppl.)**, 864–9.

139. Hallman, M., Merritt, T.A., Schneider, H. *et al.* (1983) Isolation of human surfactant from amniotic fluid and a pilot study of its efficacy in respiratory distress syndrome. *Pediatrics*, **71**, 473–82.

140. Hallman, M., Merritt, T.A., Jarvenpaa, A.L. *et al.* (1985) Exogenous human surfactant for treatment of severe respiratory distress syndrome. *J. Pediatr.*, **106**, 963–9.

141. Merritt, T.A., Hallman, M., Berry, C. *et al.* (1991) Randomized, placebo-controlled trials of human surfactant given at birth versus rescue administration in very low birth

weight infants with lung immaturity. *J. Pediatr.*, **118**, 581–94.

142. Durand, D.J., Clyman, R.I., Heymann, M.A. *et al.* (1985) Effects of a protein-free, synthetic surfactant on survival and pulmonary function in preterm lambs. *J. Pediatr.*, **109**, 775–80.

143. Bose, C., Corbet, A. Bose, G. *et al.* (1990) Improved outcome at 28 days of age for very low birth weight infants treated with a single dose of synthetic surfactant. *J. Pediatr.*, **117**, 947–53.

144. Corbet, A., Bucciarelli, R., Goldman, S. *et al.* (1991) Decreased mortality rate among small premature infants treated at birth with a single dose of synthetic surfactant: a multicenter controlled trial. *J. Pediatr.*, **118**, 277–84.

145. Phibbs, R.H., Ballard, R.A., Clements, J.A. *et al.* (1991) Initial trials of Exosurf, a protein-free synthetic surfactant, for the prophylaxis and early treatment of hyaline membrane disease. *Pediatrics*, **88**, 1–9.

146. Long, W., Thompson, T., Sundell, H. *et al.* (1991) Effects of two rescue doses of a synthetic surfactant on mortality rate and survival without bronchopulmonary dysplasia in 700 to 1350-gram infants with respiratory distress syndrome. *J. Pediatr.*, **118**, 595–605.

147. Morley, C.J., Bangham, A.D., Miller, N. and Davis J.A. (1981) Dry artificial surfactant and its effect on very premature babies. *Lancet*, **i**, 64–8.

148. Morley, C.J., Greenough, A., Miller, N.G. *et al.* (1988) Randomised trial of artificial surfactant (ALEC) given at birth to babies from 23 to 34 week's gestation. *Early Hum. Dev.*, **17**, 41–54.

149. Ten-Centre Study Group (1987) Ten-centre trial of artificial surfactant (artificial lung expanding compound) in very premature babies. *BMJ*, **294**, 991–6.

150. Morley, C.J. (1989) The use of artificial surfactant (ALEC) in the prophylaxis of neonatal respiratory distress syndrome. *Eur. Respir. J.*, **3 (suppl.)**, 81s–86s.

151. White, R.T., Damm D., Miller J. *et al.* (1985) Isolation and characterization of the human pulmonary surfactant apoprotein gene. *Nature*, **317**, 361–3.

152. Floros, J., Steinbrink, R. Jacobs, K. *et al.* (1986) Isolation and characterization of cDNA clones for the 35-kDa pulmonary surfactant-associated protein. *J. Biol. Chem.*, **261**, 9029–33.

153. Pilot-Matias, T.J., Kister, S.E., Fox, J.L. *et al.* (1989) Structure and organization of the gene

encoding human pulmonary surfactant pro-teolipid SP-B. *DNA*, **8**, 75–86.

154. Glasser, S.W., Korfhagen, T.R., Weaver, T.E. *et al.* (1988) cDNA deduced polypeptide struc-ture and chromosomal assignment of human pulmonary surfactant proteolipid SPL(pVal). *J. Biol. Chem.*, **263**, 9–12.

155. Glasser, S.W., Korfhagen, T.R., Perme, C.M. *et al.* (1988) Two SP-C genes encoding human pulmonary surfactant proteolipid. *J. Biol. Chem.*, **263**, 10326–31.

156. Voss, T., Melchers, K., Scheirle, G. and Schä-fer, K.P. (1991) Structural composition of recombinant pulmonary surfactant protein SP-A derived from two human coding sequences: implications for the chain compo-sition of natural human SP-A, *Am. J. Respir. Cell Mol. Biol.*, **4** 88–94.

157. Waring, A., Taeusch, W., Bruni, R. *et al.* (1989). Synthetic amphipathic sequences of surfac-tant protein-B mimic several physicochemical and in vivo properties of native pulmonary surfactant proteins. *Peptide Res*; **2** 308–13.

158. Rice, W.R, Sarin, V.K, Fox, JL *et al.* (1989) Surfactant peptides stimulate uptake of phos-phatidylcholine by isolated cells. *Biochim. Bio-phys. Acta*, **1006**, 237–45.

159. Baatz, J.E, Sarin, V. Absolom, D.R. *et al.* (1991) Effects of surfactant-associated protein SP-B synthetic analogs on the structure and surface activity of model membrane bilayers. *Chem. Phys. Lipids*, **60** 163–78.

160. Lachmann, B. Robertson, B. and Vogel, J. (1980). In vivo lung lavage as an experimental model of the respiratory distress syndrome. *Acta Anaesthesiol. Scand.*, **24** 231–6.

161. Lachmann, B., Fujiwara, T., Chida, S., *et al.* (1983) Surfactant replacement therapy in the experimental adult respiratory distress syn-drome (ARDS), in *Pulmonary surfactant system* (eds E.V. Cosmi and E.M. Scarpelli), Elsevier, Amsterdam, pp. 231–5.

162. Berggren, P., Lachmann, B. Curstedt, T. *et al.* (1986) Gas exchange and lung morphology after surfactant replacement in experimental adult respiratory distress induced by repeated lung lavage. *Acta Anaesthesiol. Scand.*, **30** 321–8.

163. Lachmann, B. (1987) Surfactant replacement in acute respiratory failure: animal studies and first clinical trials, in *Surfactant Replace-ment Therapy in Neonatal and Adult RDS* (ed. B. Lachmann), Springer, New York, pp. 207–11.

164. Oetomo Bambang, S., Reijngoud, D-J., Ennema, J. *et al.* (1988). Surfactant replace-ment therapy in surfactant-deficient rabbits: early effects on lung function and biochemical aspects. *Lung*, **166** 65–73.

165. Kobayashi, T., Kataoka, H., Ueda, T. *et al.* (1984). Effects of surfactant supplement and end-expiratory pressure in lung-lavaged rab-bits. *J. Appl. Physiol* **57** 995–1001.

166. Lewis, J.F. Tabor, B., Ikegami, M. *et al.* (1993) Lung function and surfactant distribution in saline lavaged sheep given instilled versus nebulized surfactant. *J. Appl. Physiol* **74** 1256–64.

167. van Daal, G.J. Bos, J.A.H. Eijking, E.P. *et al.* (1992) Surfactant replacement therapy improves pulmonary mechanics in endstage influenza A in mice. *Am. Rev. Respir. Dis.*, **145**, 859–63.

168. van Daal, G.J., So, K.L., Gommers, D. *et al.* (1991) Intratracheal surfactant administration restores gas exchange in experimental adult respiratory distress syndrome associated with viral pneumonia. *Anesth. Analg.*, **72**, 589–95.

169. Eijking, E.P., van Daal, G.J., Tenbrinck, R. *et al.* (1991) Effect of surfactant replacement on *Pneumocystis carinii* pneumonia in rats. *Inten-sive Care Med.*, **17**, 475–8.

170. Lachmann, B., Hallman, M. and Bergmann, K.C. (1987) Respiratory failure following anti-lung serum: study on mechanisms associated with surfactant system damage. *Exp. Lung Res.*, **12** 163–80.

171. Harris, J.D., Jackson, F., Moxley, M.A. and Longmore, W.J. (1989) Effect of exogenous surfactant instillation on experimental acute lung injury. *J. Appl. Physiol.*, **66**, 1846–51.

172. Lewis, J., Ikegami, M., Higucni, R. *et al.* (1991) Nebulized vs instilled exogenous surfactant in an adult lung injury model. *J. Appl. Physiol.*, **71**, 1270–6.

173. Matalon, S., Holm, B.A. and Notter, R.H. (1987) Mitigation of pulmonary hyperoxic injury by administration of exogenous surfac-tant. *J. Appl. Physiol.*, **62** 756–61.

174. Loewen, G.M., Holm, B.A., Milanowski, I. *et al.* (1989) Alveolar hyperoxic injury in rabbit receiving exogenous surfactant. *J. Appl. Phys-iol.*, **66** 1087–92.

175. Engstrom, P.C, Holm, B.A. and Matalon, S. (1989) Surfactant replacement attenuates the increase in alveolar permeability in hyper-oxia. *J. Appl. Physiol.*, **67**, 688–93.

176. Fracica, P.J. Piantadosi, C.A. Young, S.L. and Crapo, J.D. (1992) Artificial surfactant dimin-ishes pathological injury in hyperoxia in pri-mates. *Am. Rev. Respir. Dis.*, **145**, A609.

177. Simonson, S.G., Huang, Y.C., Fracica, P.J. *et al.* (1992) Exogenous surfactant improves oxygenation in hyperoxic lung injury. *Am. Rev. Respir. Dis.*, **145**, A610.

178. Lamm, W.J.E. and Albert, R.K. (1990) Surfactant replacement improves recoil in rabbit lungs after acid aspiration. *Am. Rev. Respir. Dis.*, **142**, 1279–83.

179. Kobayashi, T., Ganzuka, M., Taniguchi, J. *et al.* (1990) Lung lavage and surfactant replacement for hydrochloric acid aspiration in rabbits. *Acta Anaesthesiol. Scand.*, **34**, 216–21.

180. Lachmann, B. and Bergmann, K.C. (1987) Surfactant replacement improves thorax – lung compliance and survival rate in mice with influenza infection. *Am. Rev. Respir. Dis.*, **135**, A6.

181. Rinaldo, J.E., Dauber, J.H., Christman, J. and Rogers, R.M. (1984) Neutrophil alveolitis following endotoxemia. Enhancement by previous exposure to hyperoxia. *Am. Rev. Respir. Dis.*, **130**, 1065–71.

182. Ishizaka, A., Stephens, K.E., Tazelaar, H.D. *et al.* (1988) Pulmonary edema after *Escherichia coli* peritonitis correlates with thiobarbituric-acid-reactive materials in bronchoalveolar lavage fluid. *Am. Rev. Respir. Dis.*, **137**, 783–9.

183. Oldham, K.T., Guice, K.S., Stetson, P.S. and Wolfe, R.R. (1989) Bacteremia-induced suppression of alveolar surfactant production. *J. Surg. Res.*, **47**, 397–402.

184. Lewis, J.F., Ikegami, M. and Jobe, A.H. (1990) Altered surfactant function and metabolism in rabbits with acute lung injury. *J. Appl. Physiol.*, **69**, 2303–10.

185. Lewis, J.F., Ikegami, M. and Jobe, A.H. (1992) Metabolism of exogenously administered surfactant in the acutely injured lungs of adult rabbits. *Am. Rev. Respir. Dis.*, **145**, 19–23.

186. Holm, B.A., Notter, R.H., Seigle, J. and Matalon S. (1985) Pulmonary physiological and surfactant changes during injury and recovery from hyperoxia. *J. Appl. Physiol.*, **59**, 1402–9.

187. Gross, N.J. and Smith, D.M. (1981) Impaired surfactant phospholipid metabolism in hyperoxic mouse lungs. *J. Appl. Physiol.*, **51**, 1198–203.

188. Clark, J.M. and Lambertsen, C.J. (1971) Pulmonary oxygen toxicity: a review. *Pharmacol. Rev.*, **23**, 37–133.

189. Matalon, S. and Egan, E.A. (1981) Effects of 100% oxygen breathing on permeability of

alveolar epithelium to solute. *J. Appl. Physiol.*, **50**, 859–63.

190. Matalon, S. and Egan, E.A. (1984) Interstitial fluid volumes and albumin spaces in pulmonary oxygen toxicity. *J. Appl. Physiol.*, **57**, 1767–72.

191. Matalon, S. and Cesar, M.C. (1985) Effects of 100% oxygen breathing on the capillary filtration coefficient in rabbit lungs. *Microvasc. Res.*, **29**, 70–80.

192. Ennema, J.J., Kobayashi, T., Robertson, B. and Curstedt, T. (1988) Inactivation of exogenous surfactant in experimental respiratory failure induced by hyperoxia. *Acta Anaesthesiol. Scand.*, **32**, 665–71.

193. Ashbaugh, D.G. and Uzawa, T. (1968) Respiratory and hemodynamic changes after injection of free fatty acids. *J. Surg. Res.*, **8**, 417–23.

194. Greenfield, L.J., Barkett, V.M. and Coalson, J.J. (1968) The role of surfactant in the pulmonary response to trauma. *J. Trauma*, **8**, 735–41.

195. Grossman, R.F., Jones, J.G. and Murray, J.F. (1980) Effects of oleic acid-induced pulmonary edema on lung mechanics. *J. Appl. Physiol.*, **48**, 1045–51.

196. Guerrero, M., Donoso, P., Puig, F. and Oyarzun, M.J. (1982) Interference of free fatty acids on pulmonary surfactant in rabbits. *Arch. Biol. Med. Exp.*, **15**, 43–8.

197. Hall, S.B., Notter, R.H., Smith, R.J. and Hyde, R.W. (1990) Altered function of pulmonary surfactant in fatty acid lung injury. *J. Appl. Physiol.*, **69**, 1143–9.

198. Zelter, M., Escudier, J., Hoeffel, J.M. and Murray, J.F. (1991) Effects of aerolized artificial surfactant on repeated oleic acid injury in sheep. *Am. Rev. Respir. Dis.*, **141**, 1014–9.

199. Lachmann, B. (1987) The role of pulmonary surfactant in the pathogenesis and therapy of ARDS, in *Update in intensive care and emergency medicine* (ed. J.L. Vincent), Springer, Berlin, pp. 123–4.

200. Richman, P.S., Spragg, R.G., Robertson, B. *et al.* (1989) The adult respiratory distress syndrome: first trials with surfactant replacement. *Eur. Respir. J.*, **2** (suppl. 3), 109s–111s.

201. Nosaka, S., Sakai, T., Yonekura, M. and Yoshikawa, K. (1990) Surfactant for adults with respiratory failure. *Lancet*, **336**, 947–8, (letter).

202. Lewis, J., Dhillon, J. and Frewen, T. (1994) Exogenous surfactant therapy in pediatric patients with ARDS. *Am. J. Respir. Crit. Care Med.*, **149**, A125.

203. Wiedemann, H., Baughman, R., de Boisblanc,

B. *et al.* (1992) A multi centred trial in human sepsis-induced ARDS of an aerosolized synthetic surfactant (Exosurf). *Am. Rev. Respir. Dis.*, **145 (suppl.)**, A184.

204. Anzueto, A., Baughman, R., Guntupaill, K. *et al.* (1994) An international randomized, placebo-controlled trial evaluating the safety and efficacy of aerosolized surfactant in patients with sepsis-induced ARDS. *Am. J. Respir. Crit. Care Med.*, **149**, A567.

205. Gregory, T.J., Gadek, J.E., Weiland, J.E. *et al.* (1994) Survanta supplementation in patients with acute respiratory distress syndrome (ARDS). *Am. J. Respir. Crit. Care Med.*, **149**, A567.

206. Gregory, T.J., Longmore, W.J., Moxley, M.A. *et al.* (1994) Surfactant repletion following Survanta supplementation in patients with acute respiratory distress syndrome (ARDS). *Am. J. Respir. Crit. Care Med.*, **149**, A124.

207. Clarke, S. (1990) Principles of inhaled therapy, In *Respiratory Medicine* (eds G.J. Gibson, D.M. Geddes and B.A.L. Bretius), Baillière Tindall, London, pp. 386–406.

208. Marks, L.B., Notter, R.H., Oberdorster, G. and McBride, J.T. (1983) Ultrasonic and jet aerosolisation of phospholipids and the effects on surface activity. *Pediatr. Res.*, **17**, 742–7.

209. Lewis, J.F., Ikegami, M., Jobe, A. and Absolom D. (1993) Physiologic responses and distribution of aerosolized surfactant (Survanta) in a nonuniform pattern of lung injury. *Am. Rev. Respir. Dis.*, **147**, 1364–70.

210. Macnaughton, P.D. and Evans, T.W. (1994) The effect of exogenous surfactant therapy on lung function following cardiopulmonary bypass. *Chest*, **105**, 421–5.

211. Haslam, P.L., Hughes, D.A., Macnaughton, P.D. *et al.* (1994) Surfactant replacement therapy in late-stage adult respiratory distress syndrome. *Lancet*, **343**, 1009–11.

212. Oguchi, K., Ikegami, M., Jacobs, H. and Jobe, A. (1985) Clearance of large amounts of natural surfactant and DPPC from lungs of 3-day old rabbits following tracheal injection. *Exp. Lung Res.*, **9**, 221–35.

213. Hallman, M., Merritt, T.A., Pohjavuori, M. and Gluck, L. (1986) Effect of surfactant substitution on lung effluent phospholipids in respiratory distress syndrome: evaluation of surfactant phospholipid turnover, pool size, and the relationship to severity of respiratory failure. *Pediatr. Res.*, **20**, 1228–35.

214. Geiger, K., Gallagher, M.L. and Hedley-Whyte, J. (1975) Cellular distribution and clearance of aerosolized dipalmitoyl lecithin. *J. Appl. Physiol.*, **39**, 759–66.

215. Metz, C. and Sibbald, J. (1991) Anti-inflammatory therapy for acute lung injury. A review of animal and clinical studies. *Chest*, **100**, 1110–19.

216. Schonfeld, S.A., Ploysongsang, Y. DiLisior, D. *et al.* (1983) Fat embolism prophylaxis with corticosteroids. A prospective study in high risk patients. *Ann. Intern. Med.*, **99**, 438–43.

217. Meduri, G.U., Belenchia, J.M., Estes, R.J. *et al.* (1991) Fibroproliferative phase of ARDS. Clinical findings and effects of corticosteroids. *Chest*, **100**, 943–52.

218. Braude, S., Haslam, P.L. Hughes, D.A. *et al.* (1992) 'Chronic' adult respiratory distress syndrome. A role for corticosteroids? *Crit. Care Med.*, **20**, 1187–9.

219. Smith, B.T. and Sabry, K. (1983) Glucocorticoid-thyroid synergism in lung maturation: a mechanism involving epithelial-mesenchymal interaction. *Proc. Natl. Acad. Sci. USA*, **80**, 1951–4.

220. Kaltreider, H.B. and Salmon, S.E. (1973) Immunology of the lower respiratory tract: functional properties of bronchoalveolar lymphocytes obtained from the normal canine lung. *J. Clin. Invest.*, **52**, 2211–7.

221. Ansfield, M.J., Kaltreider, H.B., Benson, B.J. and Caldwell, J.L. (1979) Immunosuppressive activity of canine pulmonary surface active material. *J. Immunol.*, **122**, 1062–6.

222. Wilsher, M.L., Hughes, D.A. and Haslam, P.L. (1988) Immunoregulatory properties of pulmonary surfactant: effect of lung lining fluid on proliferation of human blood lymphocytes. *Thorax*, **43**, 354–9.

223. Wilsher, M.L., Hughes, D.A. and Haslam, P.L. (1988) Immunoregulatory properties of pulmonary surfactant: influence of variations in the phospholipid profile. *Clin. Exp. Immunol.*, **73**, 117–22.

224. Schwartz, L.W. and Christman, C.A. (1979) Alveolar macrophage migration: influence of lung lining material and acute lung insult. *Am. Rev. Respir. Dis.*, **120**, 429–39.

225. Hoffman, R.M., Claypool, W.D., Katyal, S.L., *et al.* (1987) Augmentation of rat alveolar macrophage migration by surfactant protein. *Am. J. Respir. Dis.*, **135**, 1358–62.

226. Wright, J.R. and Youmans, D.C. (1991) Surfactant protein SP-A stimulates migration of alveolar macrophages. *Am. Rev. Respir. Dis.*, **143**, A314.

227. Tenner, A.J., Robinson, S.L., Borchelt, J. and

Wright, J.R. (1989) Human pulmonary surfactant protein (SP-A), a protein structurally homologous to Clq, can enhance FcR- and CRl-mediated phagocytosis. *J. Biol. Chem.*, **264**, 13923–8.

228. van Iwaarden, J.F., van Strijp, J.A., Ebskamp, M.J. *et al.* Surfactant protein A is opsonin in phagocytosis of herpes simplex virus type 1 by rat alveolar macrophages. *Am. J. Physiol.*, **261**, L204–9.

229. LaForce, F.M., Kelly, W.J. and Huber G.L. (1973) Inactivation of *Staphylococci* by alveolar macrophages with preliminary observations on the importance of alveolar lining material. *Am. Rev. Respir. Dis.*, **108**, 784–90.

230. Juers, J.A., Rogers, R.M., McCurdy, T.B. and Cook, W.W. (1976) Enhancement of bactericidal capacity of alveolar macrophages by human alveolar lining material. *J. Clin. Invest.*, **58**, 271–5.

231. Weiland, J.E., Davis, W.B. and Holter, J.F. (1986) Lung neutrophils in the adult respiratory distress syndrome. Clinical and pathological significance. *Am. Rev. Respir. Dis.*, **133**, 218–25.

232. Speer, C.P., Götze, B., Robertson, B. and Curstedt, T. (1991) The effect of natural porcine surfactant (Curosurf) on the phagocytosis-associated functions of human neutrophils, in *The Surfactant System of the Lung. Prevention and Treatment of Neonatal and Adult Respiratory Distress Syndrome* (eds E.V. Cosmi, G.C.Di Renzo and M.M. Anceschi), Macmillan, London, pp. 142–50.

233. Zetterberg, G., Curstedt, T., Eklund, A. *et al.* (1992) Increased expression of adhesion proteins (MAC-1) and altered metabolic response in human leukocytes exposed to surfactant *in vitro*. APMIS, **100**, 695–700.

234. Thomassen, M.J., Meeker, D.P., Antal, J.M. *et al.* (1992) Synthetic surfactant (Exosurf) inhibits endotoxin-stimulated cytokine secretion by human alveolar macrophages. *Am. J. Respir. Cell. Mol. Biol.*, **7**, 257–60.

235. Speer, C.P., Götze, B., Curstedt, T. and Robertson, B. (1991) Phagocytic functions and tumor necrosis factor secretion of human monocytes exposed to natural porcine surfactant (Curosurf). *Pediatr. Res.*, **30**, 69–74.

236. Tracey, K.J., Beutler, B., Lowry, S.F. *et al.* (1986) Shock and tissue injury induced by recombinant human cachectin. *Science*, 234, 470–4.

237. Beutler, B. and Cerami, A. (1987) Cachectin: more than a tumor necrosis factor. *N. Engl. Med.*, **316**, 379–80.

238. Strieter, R.M., Chensue, S.W., Basha, M.A. *et al.* (1990) Human alveolar macrophage gene expression of interleukin-8 by tumour necrosis factor-α, lipopolysaccharide, and interleukin-1β. *Am. J. Respir. Cell. Mol. Biol.*, **2**, 321–6.

239. Ziegler, E.J., Fisher, C.J., Sprung, C.L. *et al.* (1991) Treatment of Gram-negative bacteria and septic shock with HA1A human monoclonal antibody against endotoxin. A randomised double blind, placebo controlled trial. *N. Engl. J. Med.*, **324**, 429–36.

240. Beutler, B., Milsark, I.W. and Cerami, A.C. (1985) Passive immunization against cachectin/tumor necrosis factor protects mice from lethal effect of endotoxin. *Science*, **229**, 869–71.

241. Tracey, K.J., Fong, Y., Hesse, D.G. *et al.* (1987) Anti-cachectin/TNF monoclonal antibodies prevent septic shock during lethal bacteraemia. *Nature*, **330**, 662–4.

242. Suffredini, A.F., Reda, D., Agosti, J. and Banks, S. (1994) Antiinflammatory effects of recombinant tumor necrosis factor receptor (TNFR:Fc) in normal humans following intravenous endotoxin. *Am. J. Respir. Crit. Care Med.*, **149**, A240.

243. Wollner, A., Wollner, S. and Raffin, T.A. (1994) Acting via A_2 receptors, adenosine inhibits the adhesive capacity of CD11b/CD18 on endotoxin-stimulated neutrophils. *Am. J. Respir. Crit. Care Med.*, **149**, A231.

244. Ridings, P.C., Windsor, A.C.J., Jutila, M.A. *et al.* (1994) A dual binding monoclonal antibody to E-selectin and L-selectin receptors prevents sepsis induced lung injury without reducing neutrophil integrin expression. *Am. J. Respir. Crit. Care Med.*, **149**, A429.

245. Karzai, W., Natanson, C., Patterson, M. *et al.* (1994) Effects of a murine monoclonal antibody (MAb) against leukocyte CD11b adhesion protein during toxic oxygen exposure in rats. *Am. J. Respir. Crit. Care Med.*, **149**, A430.

PULMONARY VASCULAR CONTROL MECHANISMS

Nigel A.M. Paterson and David G. McCormack

The important contribution of the pulmonary vasculature to the expression of acute lung injury was recognized in early clinical and experimental studies of the syndrome of acute respiratory distress in adults (ARDS). Acute pulmonary hypertension was shown to be an important early feature with adverse prognostic implications, and persistence of the hypertension was found to be associated with structural vascular changes. More recently, it has been recognized that there is also a profound loss of pulmonary and systemic reactivity, with substantial implications for lung defense, gas exchange, etc.

In this chapter, pulmonary vasomotor control in the normal and acutely injured lung is reviewed. Pulmonary vasomotor responses must be considered in the context of the particular anatomical and physiological features of the pulmonary circulation, including the high capacitance and relatively low resistance and intravascular pressures, plus the relatively greater influence of local, versus central, control mechanisms. To illustrate these features, the acute response to hypoxia will be considered in detail. In examining the pulmonary vasomotor response to injury, both the well characterized early hypertensive response and also the more recently described impairment of vascular reactivity will be reviewed.

PULMONARY VASCULAR CONTROL IN THE NORMAL LUNG

NERVOUS CONTROL

Although adrenergic [1] and cholinergic [2] innervation of the pulmonary circulation in humans and other species has been documented, its significance is uncertain. The role of the sympathetic and parasympathetic nervous systems in controlling resting pulmonary vascular tone is at best minor [3–5]. Furthermore, there is no evidence that these pathways regulate pulmonary blood flow in disease states.

The existence of the nonadrenergic noncholinergic (NANC) nervous system in the pulmonary circulation was first postulated in the 1930s, although its functional role has not been studied extensively until recently. Preliminary reports suggest that NANC neurotransmission is present in the pulmonary circulation. Thus, electrical field stimulation of precontracted guinea pig [6,7] and human [8] pulmonary arteries *in vitro* results in a vasodilatation resistant to adrenergic or cholinergic blockade, but which is abolished by treatment with the neurotoxin tetrodotoxin [9]. The postulated role in the pathogenesis of inflammatory diseases such as asthma [10] has led to speculation of the role of the NANC nervous system in the control of vascular tone in lung injury. At the present time

ARDS Acute Respiratory Distress in Adults. Edited by Timothy W. Evans and Christopher Haslett. Published in 1996 by Chapman & Hall, London. ISBN 0 412 56910 8

however, there are no firm data to support this.

LOCAL CONTROL (ENDOTHELIUM, NITRIC OXIDE)

The endothelium is now known to regulate vascular tone through the production and liberation of vasoconstrictor and vasodilator mediators. An endothelium derived relaxant factor has been identified as nitric oxide (NO) [11,12] (Chapters 29 and 30) and is synthesized from L-arginine [13] through the action of NO synthase (Figure 17.1). NO causes relaxation of vascular smooth muscle by stimulating guanylate cyclase and guanosine 3',5'-cyclic monophosphate (cGMP) production. Synthesis of NO can be blocked by arginine analogs such as N^G-monomethyl-

L-arginine (L-NMMA) [14,15]. Administration of NO synthesis inhibitors to animals has provided evidence for a tonic release of NO in the systemic and (to a much lesser extent) the pulmonary circulation [16,17]. In the pulmonary circulation administration of NO synthesis antagonists such as L-NMMA or N^ω-nitro-L-arginine methyl ester (L-NAME) causes constriction of isolated pulmonary artery rings *in vitro* [18] and a rise in pulmonary vascular resistance when administered *in vivo* [19] (Figure 17.2).

Despite this explosion of knowledge regarding NO in both the pulmonary and systemic circulations, there has been a lack of reported information concerning its action in the human pulmonary circulation. Indeed, it was not until 1987 that Greenberg and coworkers [20] published data showing that it

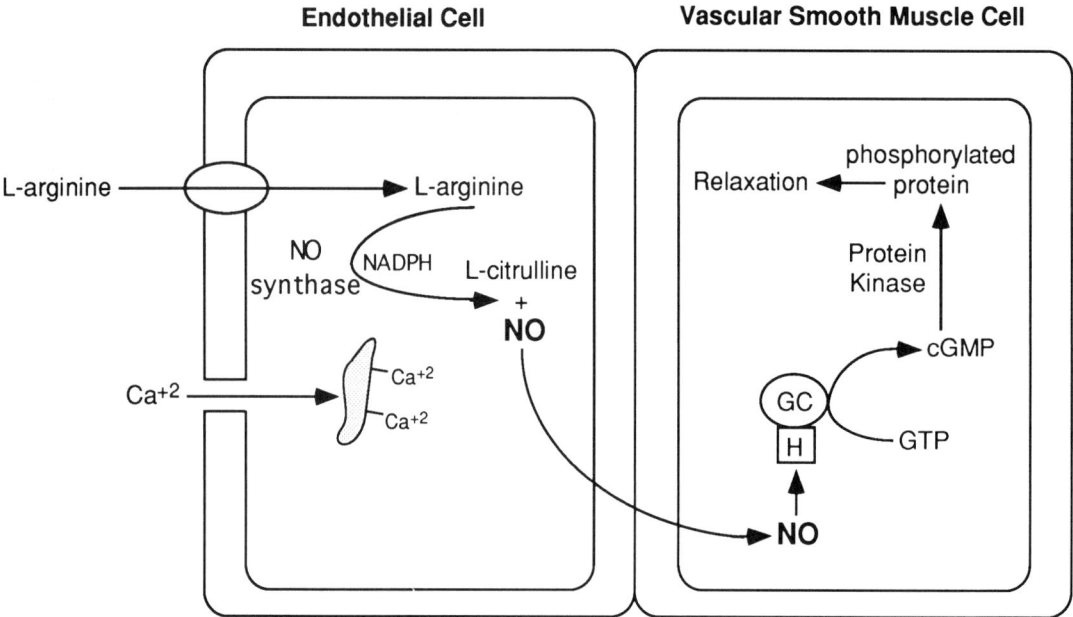

Figure 17.1 Nitric oxide (NO) synthetic pathway. L-arginine is converted into NO and L-citrulline by NADPH dependent NO synthase, which does (constitutive) or does not (inducible) require the presence of calcium. L-arginine enters the cell via amino acid carriers. The NO diffuses readily to the adjacent smooth muscle cell and binds to the heme moiety (H) of soluble guanylate cyclase (GC), causing enzyme activation and cGMP formation. The latter lowers intracellular Ca^{2+} concentration and causes smooth muscle relaxation.

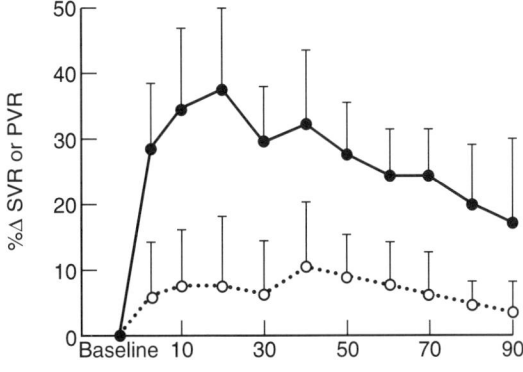

Figure 17.2 Effect of L-NMMA (50 mg/kg) on pulmonary (○) and systemic (●) vascular resistance in rats breathing room air. L-NMMA was administered intravenously to conscious, unanesthetized, hemodynamically monitored rats. The rise in PVR was modest compared to the increase in SVR (unpublished data).

was possible to remove the endothelium from normal human pulmonary arteries mechanically and demonstrated *in vitro* endothelium dependent vasodilatation in response to acetylcholine and ATP. Since then, further studies with human pulmonary arteries *in vitro* have provided evidence that NO mediates the vasodilator response to acetylcholine [21] and attenuates the vasoconstrictor response to phenylephrine *in vitro*. This raises the possibility that endogenous NO may provide a protective mechanism against inappropriate vasoconstriction in lung injury.

HYPOXIC PULMONARY VASOCONSTRICTION

Over 50 years ago, Beyne [22] demonstrated that, in contrast to systemic blood vessels, pulmonary vessels constrict in response to hypoxia. This phenomenon is known as hypoxic pulmonary vasoconstriction (HPV). The predominant stimulus is alveolar hypoxia, although luminal pulmonary arterial (i.e. mixed venous) hypoxemia augments this stimulus [23].

By diverting blood flow from areas of alveolar hypoxia, HPV minimizes the consequences of regional hypoventilation, thereby promoting regional ventilation/perfusion matching and improving gas exchange [24] (Figure 17.3). Furthermore, if alveolar hypoxia is more widespread, such that HPV leads to a rise in pulmonary arterial pressure, vascular surface area is recruited, leading to increased diffusing capacity [25].

Hypotheses of the mechanism of HPV need to incorporate three features. Firstly, neuronal involvement is unlikely. Blockade of the sympathetic and parasympathetic nervous system has no significant effect on HPV [4, 5, 26–28]. Indeed, central neural connections are not a prerequisite since HPV can be reproduced in isolated, perfused lungs from many species [29]. Furthermore, HPV can be demonstrated in the human transplanted (and therefore denervated) lung [30]. Secondly, the time course of HPV is distinctive. The response begins within seconds, reaches a peak within minutes, and is sustained for as long as the hypoxic stimulus persists. With restoration of normoxia, the offset is equally prompt. Thirdly, the major site of HPV, at least in most species, appears to be the small arterial resistance vessels in the 50–200 μm diameter range [23,31–34]. However, hypoxia also causes pulmonary venoconstriction [33–35] and its contribution to HPV may sometimes be substantial [36].

To reconcile these features, two types of mechanism have been proposed. Firstly, hypoxia may be sensed by a cell adjacent to vascular smooth muscle, stimulating the release of a vasoconstrictor which *indirectly* mediates HPV. This would account for both the strikingly different response of systemic and pulmonary vessels to hypoxia and the relationship of HPV to alveolar rather than luminal hypoxia. Alternatively, pulmonary vascular smooth muscle cells may sense the hypoxia *directly* and translate the signal into a constrictor response. These two mechanisms are not mutually exclusive.

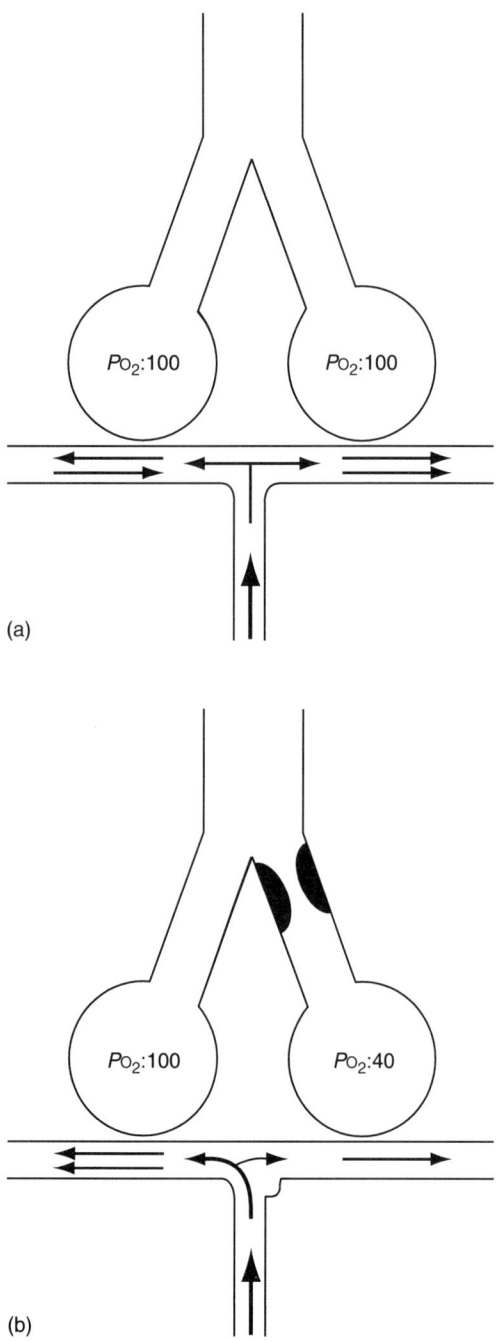

(a)

(b)

Figure 17.3 Hypoxic pulmonary vasoconstriction. (a) Alveoli with normal P_{AO_2} have blood flow equally distributed; (b) underventilation of one alveolus lowers P_{AO_2}. The adjacent pulmonary artery constricts, shunting blood away from the involved portion of lung.

Indirect mediation or amplification of HPV could be due to either increased vasoconstriction or decreased vasodilatation (e.g. by inhibition of tonic vasodilator release). An increased vasoconstrictor effect may in turn reflect either increased levels of vasoconstrictor (stimulated release, or reduced clearance) or increased vasoreactivity to a tonically released vasoconstrictor – for example, hypoxia increases the sensitivity to leukotriene (LT)D_4 [37]. However, most attention has been directed toward vasoconstrictor release or vasodilator suppression by hypoxia.

The search for a vasoconstrictor mediator has been extensive, but inconclusive. There have been tantalizing clues, ranging from the early observation by Lloyd that a cuff of lung parenchyma was necessary to support a vasoconstrictor response *in vitro* [38] to the more recent observation that thoracic lung lymph from hypoxic but not normoxic dogs contracted pulmonary arterial strips *in vitro* [39]. However, over the past 50 years a succession of newly characterized vasoconstrictors have been examined as candidate mediators of HPV, and found wanting. Temporary favourites have included catecholamines, histamine, serotonin, angiotensin II and constrictor cyclo-oxygenase products of arachidonic acid metabolism such as prostaglandin (PG)$F_{2\alpha}$ and thromboxane (Tx) A_2, etc. [40].

More recently the role of the sulfidopeptide leukotrienes (LTC$_4$ and LTD$_4$) has been extensively evaluated. Interest was stimulated by the observation that leukotriene levels were elevated in bronchoalveolar lavage fluid from infants with persistent pulmonary hypertension [41] and in fluid lavaged from isolated rat lung subjected to hypoxia [42]. Furthermore, in several studies HPV was inhibited by leukotriene synthesis inhibitors or receptor antagonists [43–47]. However, hypoxia induced leukotriene release has not been confirmed [48], the effects of 5-lipoxygenase inhibitors have been inconsistent or nonspecific [49–55] and in subsequent studies receptor antagonists failed to inhibit HPV [56,57]. Thus mediation of HPV by leukotrienes now seems unlikely.

Similarly, the possibility that endothelins mediate HPV arose from recognition of their potent pulmonary vasoconstrictor activity, together with the demonstration that hypoxia stimulates endothelin gene expression and release in cultured endothelial cells [58]. However, in contrast to HPV, endothelins cause a characteristically protracted contractile response, with marked tachyphylaxis on repeat challenge. This differs substantially from HPV.

In view of the vasoregulatory role of the endothelium, it might be the source of a constrictor mediator of HPV. Rubyani and Van Houtte reported that an endothelium derived contracting factor (EDCF)-1 was released from systemic vessels in response to hypoxia [59]. However, the mediation of this contractile activity remains uncertain [60]. Further, reports that intact endothelium is required for hypoxic contractions of pulmonary arterial strips *in vitro* [61–63] have not been confirmed [64–67].

Alternatively, HPV may result from suppressed levels of a tonically released vasodilator [68]. NO is an obvious candidate and there is some evidence that hypoxia reduces NO synthesis [69,70]. However, if NO is released tonically, an inhibitor of NO synthesis given during normoxia should reproduce HPV. In fact, as reviewed above, augmentation of resting pulmonary vascular tone by NO synthesis antagonists has been generally modest both *in vivo* [71] and *in vitro* [18,72–75] and the pattern of response to NO inhibitors does not mimic HPV. In addition, if HPV is due to removal of tonically released NO (during normoxia), hypoxia should have little additional pressor effect in the presence of NO synthesis inhibitors. In fact, HPV is generally augmented by NO synthesis inhibitors in isolated arterial segments [65,66], perfused preparations [18,72,75,76] and *in vivo* [19].

Thus, HPV is probably modulated by secondary NO release.

Inhibition of tonic prostacyclin release has also been suggested as a mechanism of HPV. However HPV is not duplicated by cyclooxygenase inhibitors, and although hypoxia inhibits prostacyclin synthesis in pulmonary artery endothelial cells [77], pulmonary prostacyclin levels are increased during hypoxia [78]. Thus like NO, PGI_2 may actually modulate HPV.

The hypothesis that hypoxia *directly* leads to contraction of pulmonary vascular smooth muscle has prompted several studies of isolated pulmonary vessels *in vitro*. In general, the contractile response of isolated vessels to hypoxia has been less impressive, has required more profound hypoxia (or anoxia) and is often delayed and/or transient. Thus, the contractile mechanism may not be identical. One reason for the discrepancy is that the arterial segments or strips studied have often been obtained from larger conduit arteries, i.e. upstream from the presumed major site of HPV. This may be crucial because, in cats, the *in vitro* contractile response to hypoxia of pulmonary arteries over 500 μm in diameter is minimal compared with that of segments of smaller arteries (200–500 μm diameter) [79]. Recently, contractile responses to moderate hypoxia of isolated pulmonary artery smooth muscle cells have been demonstrated [67,80,81]. The contraction is not seen in muscle cells from mesenteric [67] or cerebral [81] arteries, implying that the cellular mechanism is specific for pulmonary artery smooth muscle.

The contraction of arterial strips/segments *in vitro* is associated with membrane depolarization [79,82], is dependent on extracelluar Ca^{2+} [67,82–84], can be inhibited by blockers of voltage gated Ca^{2+} channels [65,82–85], and is augmented by the calcium channel activator BAY K8644 [62,65,86]. These findings have been confirmed using human pulmonary artery rings [65,84]. Studies of cultured pulmonary artery smooth muscle suggest that hypoxia inhibits voltage gated K^+ channels, with opening of voltage gated Ca^{2+} channels as a secondary event [87,88]. The intracellular Ca^{2+} elevation may be due at least partly to Ca^{2+} release from intracellular stores [87]. Elevation of intracellular Ca^{2+} in turn leads to activation of myosin light chain kinase and the contractile response [80].

Thus, the mechanism of HPV remains unclear. A direct mechanism involving membrane depolarization and elevation of intracellular calcium levels, secondary to inhibition of voltage gated K^+ channels, probably contributes to the response. In addition, increased constrictor or decreased dilator release from a nearby oxygen sensing cell, remains attractive as an alternative or additional indirect mechanism. The endothelium appears to down regulate the response, mainly by the secondary release of NO.

ENDOTHELINS

The endothelins are a family of three related 21 amino acid peptides: endothelin (ET)-1, ET-2 and ET-3. ET-1 is derived from a 212 amino acid precursor, preproendothelium 1, which is sequentially cleaved by an endoprotease to the 38 amino acid peptide proendothelin 1, followed by generation of ET-1 via the endothelin converting enzyme [89]. The lung is not only a source of endothelins, but is also a major site of their metabolic clearance [90,91].

Endothelins exhibit potent vasoactivity which can be either constrictor or dilator. ET-1 and ET-2 are potent vasoconstrictors of resistance vessels. The constrictor response is distinctively prolonged and is followed by tachyphylaxis (reduced response) to subsequent exposure. The dilator response to endothelins is generally much more evident with lower doses of ET-1 and ET-2, or with ET-3, which is a weaker constrictor. The dilator response, or at least a substantial component thereof, is mediated by NO release [89].

The vascular actions of endothelin are mediated by at least two receptors: ET-A and ET-B. The ET-A receptor has a high affinity for ET-1 and ET-2, and a much lower affinity for ET-3, whereas the ET-B receptor binds all three endothelins with approximately equal affinity [89]. The ET-A receptor mediates vasoconstriction and is located on vascular smooth muscle cells, whereas the ET-B receptor is found mainly on endothelial cells and mediates ET induced NO release. However, ET-B receptors on vascular smooth muscle can also cause vasoconstriction [89].

ET-1 and ET-2 act mainly as pulmonary vasoconstrictors, via the ET-A receptor. The vasoconstriction may be mediated, at least partially, by TxA_2 generation [92]. The vasoconstrictor response is most prominent at low tone [93] and in these circumstances ET-3 can also cause pulmonary vasoconstriction [94]. At high tone, the dominant effect of ET-1 and ET-2 is dilatorory [95]. The dilator effect is due to release of prostacyclin [96], mediated by the ET-A receptor [97] and/or ET-B receptor mediated NO release [98]. In general, the major site of pulmonary vasoconstriction by endothelins is thought to be the small muscular pulmonary arteries, although in some *in vitro* experiments with isolated vascular segments the pulmonary veins have been more sensitive. The endothelin dependent, NO mediated, pulmonary vasodilator response [99,100] is initiated by binding to endothelial ET-B receptors [101] and is exemplified by ET-3 [94,100], which generally is a weaker constrictor than ET-1 and ET-2 [102]. There is less tachyphylaxis and cross-tachyphylaxis of the dilator response.

CONTROL IN LUNG INJURY

Pulmonary hypertension commonly accompanies ARDS and its magnitude correlates with the overall severity of lung injury [103]. The hypertension is due to a combination of vasoconstriction and mechanical obstruction

Table 17.1 Causes of increased vascular resistance in acute lung injury

Structural
Intraluminal obstruction
  Macrothrombi
  Microthrombi
    Fibrin
    Hyaline (platelet/fibrin)
  Other cell aggregates (white blood cells, red
    blood cells, etc.)
Wall thickening
  Endothelial cell swelling
  Intimal proliferation
  Medial hypertrophy/extension
External compression
  Interstitial/alveolar
  Edema/hemorrhage
  Increased alveolar pressure

Vasomotor
Vasoconstrictor mediators
  Alveolar hypoxia

(Table 17.1), the proportions of which depend on the severity and time course of the insult. As is reviewed below, the use of a profound, acute stimulus of lung injury (such as bolus endotoxin infusion) causes a correspondingly dramatic acute pulmonary vasoconstrictor response. In models employing a more sustained or subtle insult, the vascular response also reflects the structural changes that develop over hours and days. The clinical syndrome of sepsis is characterized by a low systemic vascular resistance (and, if intravascular volume is maintained, high cardiac output) in contrast to the hypotensive, low output, high systemic resistance response to bolus endotoxin. The differences in the hemodynamic profile of clinical sepsis versus endotoxin infusion may be partly due to the additional biological effects of live bacteria. However, most of the variation between various models of sepsis is probably due to differences in time/concentration profiles of the array of mediators contributing to the response.

Since the causes of the structural changes contributing to pulmonary hypertension are dealt with elsewhere (Chapter 4), we focus first on the vasoconstrictor mechanisms involved in the acute phase response and then review the evidence that reduced pulmonary vascular reactivity is an equally important component of the response.

PULMONARY HYPERTENSION IN ACUTE LUNG INJURY

The acute pulmonary hypertensive response to endotoxin [104] or live bacteria [105] has been well characterized [104], consisting of an early peak (within minutes), a decline over a few hours, and then a later sustained response associated with edema and other inflammatory events. The early response is associated with elevated TxA_2 levels and both the pulmonary hypertension and the TxA_2 elevation can be inhibited by pretreatment with thromboxane synthase inhibitors [106,107]. These data suggested that TxA_2 mediates the acute pulmonary hypertensive response to endotoxin.

Subsequently, the role of the sulfidopeptide leukotrienes (LTC_4, LTD_4 and LTE_4) has been evaluated. Circumstantial clinical support for a role of leukotrienes in ARDS was provided by the observation that leukotriene levels are elevated in pulmonary edema fluid [108,109] and urine [110] of patients with ARDS. Similarly, it was found that 5-lipoxygenase metabolites are elevated in lung lymph obtained from sheep challenged with endotoxin [111–113] and in bile after endotoxin challenge of rats [114]. Furthermore, the acute hypertensive response to endotoxin infusion is partially inhibited by 5-lipoxygenase inhibitors [111] or by leukotriene antagonists [115–117]. Since leukotriene antagonists blocked TxA_2 elevation *in vivo*, but not *in vitro*, it has been proposed that pulmonary hypertension may involve the sequential release of leukotrienes, followed by TxA$_2$ [117].

The role of platelet activating factor (PAF) has also attracted attention because it can be released simultaneously with arachidonic acid metabolites whenever phospholipase A$_2$ is activated. PAF infusion causes pulmonary hypertension [118–120] and endotoxin infusion causes elevation of PAF levels [121]. Pretreatment of animals with PAF antagonists inhibits both the rise in TxA$_2$ [122] and the pressor response to endotoxin [122,123]. Finally, PAF can stimulate leukotriene release [124] and vice versa [125].

Taken together, these data suggest that endotoxin infusion stimulates the release of an array of vasoactive lipids, including cyclooxygenase and lipoxygenase arachidonic acid metabolites as well as PAF, which together provoke an acute hypertensive pulmonary vascular response.

Endothelin release may also contribute to the vasoconstrictor response. Release of ET-1 is stimulated by endotoxin [126] and elevated ET-1 levels have been reported in sepsis [127,128]. In a recent clinical study of patients with ARDS [129], increased circulating levels of ET-1 were observed. Comparison of the response to ET-1 infusion in the ARDS group, versus healthy controls, suggested that the increased levels were due to both reduced ET-1 clearance and net ET-1 release by the lungs.

With the passage of time in both clinical ARDS and experimental models, structural events such as endothelial swelling, interstitial edema and the formation of cellular/fibrin thrombi become more important contributions to the hypertensive response (Figure 17.4). Nevertheless, vasomotor influences may persist beyond the first few hours: for example, the pulmonary hypertension observed in dogs 24 hours after intraperitoneal implantation of thrombus containing *Escherichia coli* could be reversed by cyclooxygenase inhibitors [130].

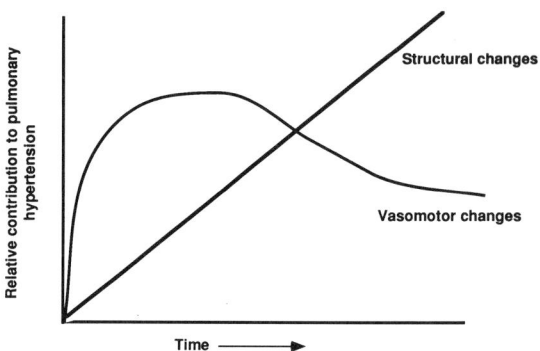

Figure 17.4 Relative importance and temporal progression of vasomotor and structural changes that contribute to the pulmonary hypertension in acute lung injury.

ATTENUATED PULMONARY VASCULAR REACTIVITY IN LUNG INJURY

Despite the pulmonary hypertension associated with acute lung injury, reactivity of the pulmonary circulation is impaired.

Dantzker *et al.* [131] have demonstrated that hypoxemia in ARDS is primarily the result of intrapulmonary shunting. Using the multiple inert gas elimination technique, they showed that this was related to perfusion of lung units characterized by low ventilation ($\dot{V}$)/perfusion ($\dot{Q}$) ratios. The response of the normal lung is to divert blood away from areas of low ventilation by HPV and therefore this normal physiological mechanism must be impaired in lung injury.

Indeed, in animal models of acute lung injury induced by pneumonia [132,133] (Figure 17.5), oxygen toxicity [134], bleomycin [135] (Figure 17.6) or systemic sepsis secondary to peritonitis [136], pulmonary vasoconstrictor responsiveness is substantially attenuated. In particular, the pressor responses to physiological (hypoxia) or pharmacological (phenylephrine, angiotensin II) stimuli are reduced substantially. In a model of acute pneumonia, Light has reported [132] that there is no change in perfusion to consolidated lung and this is likely due to a failure of HPV.

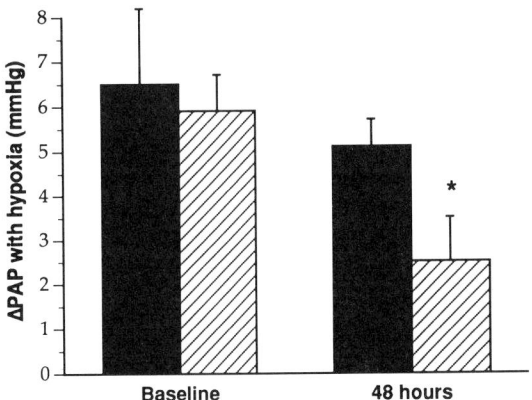

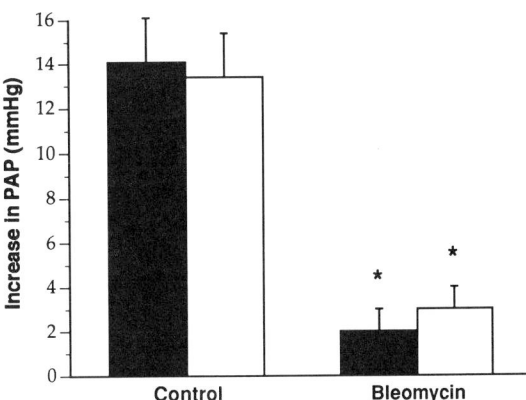

Figure 17.5 Attenuation of the hypoxic pressor response ($\triangle$PAP) in control (solid bars) rats and rats with pneumonia (hatched bars). HPV was induced with the animals breathing 8% oxygen. HPV was recorded in the baseline period and 48 hours after the intratracheal instillation of *Pseudomonas aeruginosa* (pneumonia) or saline (control). There was a significant attenuation in the hypoxic pressor response in animals with penumonia. (* = $P < 0.05$) (unpublished data).

Figure 17.6 Attenuation of two consecutive hypoxic pressor responses in isolated perfused lungs from control rats or rats treated with intratracheal bleomycin 48 hours before study. Lungs were ventilated with 3% oxygen and the maximum rise in PAP ($\triangle$PAP) recorded. Solid bars represent the rise in PAP during the first hypoxic pressor response and open bars represent the rise in PAP during the second hypoxic pressor response. (* = $P < 0.05$). (Redrawn from McCormack *et al.* [135].)

Further, segments of small pulmonary arteries obtained from animals with lung injury exhibit an analogous loss of vasoconstrictor responsiveness *in vitro* (Figure 17.7). A limitation of these *in vitro* experiments is that the vessels studied are conducting vessels (i.e. upstream of the major site of pulmonary vascular resistance *in vivo*). Thus, we cannot conclude that the *in vitro* and *in vivo* observations are due to the same process. Nevertheless, there is a striking correspondence between the two sets of findings and it seems plausible that the same pathological mechanism operates in both conducting vessels (studied *in vitro*) and the microvasculature (responsible for resistance changes *in vivo*). This remains to be established.

With chronic or established ARDS, the associated chronic hypoxia may affect endothelium dependent vasodilatation. Thus, pulmonary vessels from chronically hypoxic rats [138, 139] exhibit reduced vasodilatation in response to acetylcholine, a phenomenon

which may be explained by a selective impairment of soluble guanylate cyclase. Further, isolated pulmonary vessels from patients with chronic hypoxic lung disease also demonstrate reduced endothelium dependent vasodilatation [140]. It has been suggested that this may contribute to the pulmonary hypertension characteristic in chronic lung disease although this hypothesis is not proven.

MECHANISMS OF LOSS OF CONSTRICTOR RESPONSIVENESS

The loss of pulmonary vasoconstrictor responsiveness in systemic sepsis suggests that the defect can be induced by a remote stimulus. This stimulus likely leads to the distant, local release of a 'second messenger' which possesses appropriate biological activity, i.e. the ability to dampen vasoconstrictor

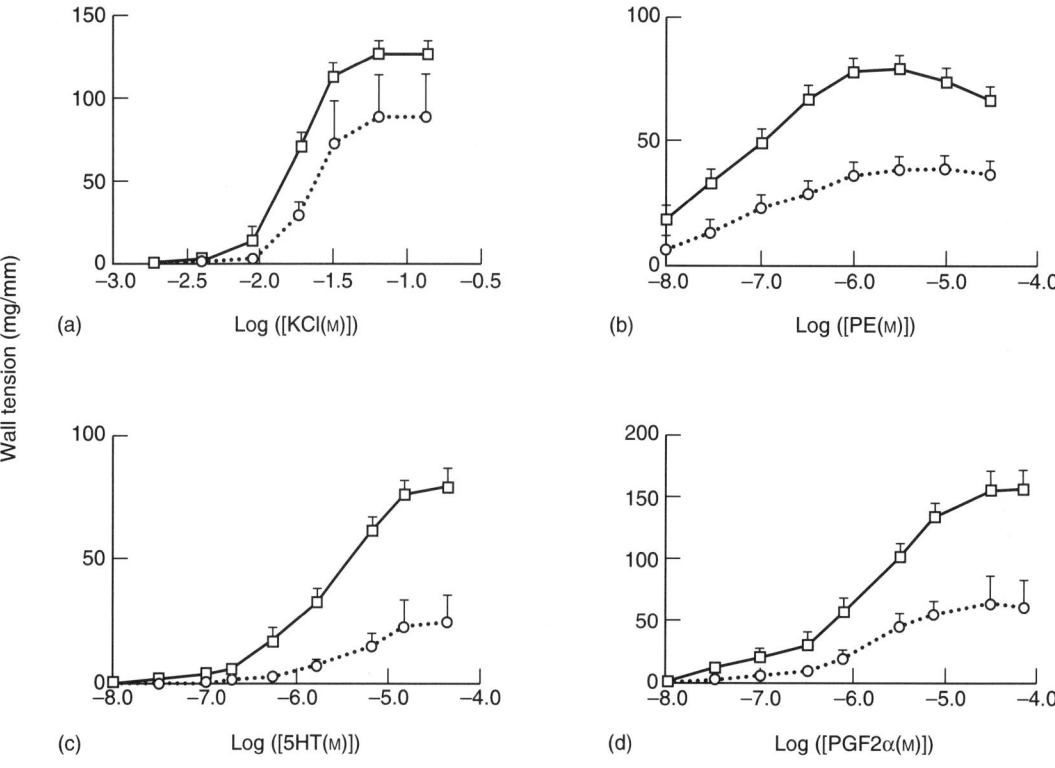

Figure 17.7 Attenuated *in vitro* pulmonary vascular reactivity of pulmonary arteries from rats with pseudomonas pneumonia. Vessels (200–400 μm internal diameter) from the infected segment of lung (□) or from control animals (○) were suspended in an organ bath and contractility to pharmacologic agents recorded: (a) potassium chloride (KCl); (b) phenylephrine (PE); (c) serotonin (5-HT); and (d) prostaglandin $F_{2\alpha}$. The contraction to all agonists was decreased significantly in vessels from pneumonic lungs. (Redrawn from Yaghi *et al.* [137].)

responses to a variety of stimuli. Several known bioactive moieties are logical candidates, and have been proposed as mediators of the vasoconstrictor hyporesponsiveness: prostaglandins [141–143], PAF [144], tumor necrosis factor [145] and interleukin-1 [146]. Participation of these potential mediators is not mutually exclusive since there may either be simultaneous release with additive or synergistic effects, or a sequential cascade of mediator release.

In animal models of acute pneumonia, cyclo-oxygenase blockade results in improved gas exchange, possibly due to inhibition of the synthesis of vasodilator prostaglandins such as prostacyclin [142,143]. The only clinical study to evaluate this examined the effects of indomethacin in patients with acute pneumonia [147]. Treatment with indomethacin improved arterial oxygenation and lowered the Pao_2/Fio_2 ratio, although the response was variable.

There is also considerable evidence that NO contributes to the vascular hypocontractility that follows the administration of endotoxin [148–151], and several of the aforementioned mediators are also capable of stimulating NO synthesis. Further, the expression of the inducible form of NO synthase in vascular smooth muscle and endothelial cells has been reported following exposure to endotoxin [152,153]. Furthermore, increased inducible NO synthase mRNA and protein expression has been found in lung tissue following endotoxin administration [154]. Nevertheless, it remains to be proven whether excess release of NO accounts for the pulmonary vascular hyporeactivity characteristic of acute lung injury. Work done to date has not supported a role for excess production of NO in the abnormal vasoreactivity associated with lung injury [71,137]. It is important to note however that these studies used arginine analogs (which are not selective to the inducible or the constitutive form of NO synthase) to inhibit NO synthase. Further studies using specific inhibitors of the inducible form of this enzyme are needed to clarify the role of NO in disease.

PROSPECTS FOR THERAPY

GENERAL CONSIDERATIONS

The use of vasoactive drugs in pulmonary conditions requires careful consideration of the advantages and disadvantages of the intervention. For example, it is tempting to use a vasodilator to ameliorate the adverse consequences of pulmonary hypertension secondary to acute and chronic hypoxia in chronic obstructive pulmonary disease. How-

ever, the adverse effect on gas exchange of the loss of regional HPV might outweigh the benefit in terms of reduced cardiac afterload. Conversely, the use of a vasoconstrictor to restore (hypoxic) vascular responsiveness in acute lung injury might improve gas exchange by decreasing shunt, but would worsen pulmonary hypertension and might impair host defense by diminishing the inflammatory hyperemia. In addition to local considerations, the systemic effects of the drug may be disadvantageous, and outweigh any local (pulmonary) benefit.

VASODILATORS

Several vasodilators have been studied in ARDS (Table 17.2). PGE_1 has been evaluated in three separate studies [155–157] leading to similar conclusions. Pulmonary vascular resistance falls, but at the cost of increased hypoxemia, due to shunt. Despite the hypoxemia, the increased cardiac index leads to improved oxygen delivery and consumption [157]. However, it is not clear whether there is an overall benefit in terms of recovery or survival [155,157]. The pattern of response to nitroprusside [158] and diltiazem [159] has been similar with reduced pulmonary artery pressure and vascular resistance, but increased hypoxemia due to increased shunt. Thus, a beneficial role for vasodilators in ARDS has not been established.

Table 17.2 Results of vasodilator treatment in acute lung injury in published studies

Vasodilator	CI	$\dot{Q}_{O_2}$	PAP	PVR	Pa_{O_2}	$\dot{Q}s/\dot{Q}t$
Nitroprusside [158]	↑	↓	↓	↓	↓	↑
Diltiazem [159]	↔	NR	↓	↓	↓	↑
Prostaglandin E_1 [155]	NR	NR	NR	NR	↑	NR
Prostaglandin E_1 [157]	↑	↑	NR	↓	NR	NR
Prostaglandin E_1 [156]	↑	NR	↓	NR	↓	↑

CI = cardiac index; $\dot{Q}_{O_2}$ = systemic oxygen delivery; PAP = pulmonary artery pressure; PVR = pulmonary vascular resistance; Pa_{O_2} = partial pressure of oxygen; $\dot{Q}s/\dot{Q}t$ = shunt fraction; NR = not reported; ↑ = increased; ↓ = decreased; ↔ = no change.

NITRIC OXIDE AND PROSTACYCLIN

Given the limitations of current intravenously administered vasodilators a more selective action or delivery mode is highly desirable. The recent recognition that inhaled nitric oxide leads to pulmonary vasodilatation [160] led to the assessment of this therapy in ventilated patients with ARDS [161]. In this group of patients, concentrations of NO as low as 18 p.p.m. have resulted in a fall in pulmonary artery pressure, decreased intrapulmonary shunting and improvement in the efficiency of arterial oxygenation. Inhaled NO has now been reported to be beneficial in a variety of experimental [162,163] and clinical [164–166] scenarios associated with pulmonary hypertension, hypoxemia and acute lung injury (Chapter 29).

Furthermore, aerosolized prostacyclin has been demonstrated to lower pulmonary artery pressure and improve gas exchange in patients with ARDS [167]. Similar to inhaled NO, this beneficial effect has been attributed to the preferential distribution of aerosolized prostacyclin to better ventilated lung units.

The effects of inhaled nitric oxide and aerosolized prostacyclin on patient outcome in ARDS is not yet known and requires careful investigation.

REFERENCES

1. Kai, T. (1969) Distribution of adrenergic nerve fibers in the lungs of rabbit, guinea pig and man as demonstrated by Falck-Hillarp's method. *Bull. Chest Dis. Res.* **2**, 225.
2. Partanen, M., Laitinen, A., Hervonen, A. *et al.* (1982) Catecholamine- and acetylcholinesterase-containing nerves in human lower respiratory tract. *Histochemistry*, **76**, 175–88.
3. Rudolph, A.M., Heyman, M.A. and Lewis, A.B. (1977) Physiology and pharmacology of the pulmonary circulation in the fetus and newborn, in *Lung Biology in Health and Disease. Development of the Lung* (ed. W.A. Hodson), Marcel Dekker, New York, pp. 497–523.
4. Colebatch, H.J.H., Dawes, G.S., Goodwin, J.W. and Nadeau, R.A. (1965) The nervous control of the circulation in the foetal and newly expanded lungs of the lamb. *J. Physiol.*, **178**, 544–62.
5. Malik, A.B. and Kidd, L. (1973) Adrenergic blockade and the pulmonary vascular response to hypoxia. *Respir. Physiol.*, **19**, 96–106.
6. Kubota, E., Hamasaki, Y., Sata, T. *et al.* (1988) Autonomic innervation of pulmonary artery: evidence for a nonadrenergic noncholinergic inhibitory system. *Exp. Lung Res.*, **14**, 349–58.
7. Maggi, C.A., Patacchini, R., Perretti, F. *et al.* (1990) Sensory nerves, vascular endothelium and neurogenic relaxation of the guinea-pig isolated pulmonary artery. *Naunyn Schmiedebergs Arch. Pharmacol.*, **342**, 78–84.
8. Scott, J.A. and McCormack, D.G. (1993) Nitric oxide is a mediator of non-adrenergic, noncholinergic vasodilation of human pulmonary arteries. *Can. Fed. Biol. Soc.*, A243, 89.
9. Liu, S.F., Crawley, D.E., Evans, T.W. and Barnes, P.J. (1992) Endothelium dependent nonadrenergic, noncholinergic neural relaxation in guinea pig pulmonary artery. *J. Pharmacol. Exp. Ther.*, **260**, 541–8.
10. Barnes, P.J. (1986) Asthma as an axon reflex. *Lancet*, **i**: 242–5.
11. Palmer, R.M.J., Ferrige, A.G. and Moncada, S. (1987) Nitric oxide release accounts for the biological activity of endothelium-derived relaxing factor. *Nature*, **327**, 524–6.
12. Ignarro, L.J., Buga, G.M., Wood, K.S. *et al.* (1987) Endothelium-derived relaxing factor produced and released from artery and vein is nitric oxide. *Proc. Natl. Acad. Sci. USA*, **84**, 9265–9.
13. Palmer, R.M.J., Ashton, D.S. and Moncada, S. (1988) Vascular endothelial cells synthesise nitric oxide from L-arginine. *Nature*, **333**, 664–6.
14. Palmer, R.M.J., Rees, D.D., Ashton, D.S. and Moncada, S. (1988) L-arginine is the physiological precursor for the formation of nitric oxide in endothelium-dependent relaxation. *Biochem. Biophys. Res. Commun.*, **153**, 1251–6.
15. Rees, D.D., Palmer, R.M.J., Hodson, H.F. and Moncada, S. (1989) A specific inhibitor of nitric oxide formation from L-arginine attenuates endothelium-dependent relaxation. *Br. J. Pharmacol.*, **96**, 418–24.
16. Persson, M.G., Gustafsson, L.E., Wiklund, N.P. *et al.* (1990) Endogenous nitric oxide as a modulator of rabbit skeletal muscle micro-

circulation *in vivo*. *Br. J. Pharmacol.*, **100**, 463–6.

17. Rees, D.D., Palmer, R.M.J., Schulz, R. *et al.* (1990) Characterization of three inhibitors of endothelial nitric oxide synthase *in vitro* and *in vivo*. *Br. J. Pharmacol.*, **101**, 746–52.

18. Archer, S.L., Tolins, J.P., Raij, L. and Weir, E.K. (1989) Hypoxic pulmonary vasoconstriction is enhanced by inhibition of the synthesis of an endothelium derived relaxing factor. *Biochem. and Biophys. Res. Commun.*, **164**, 1198–205.

19. Persson, M.G., Gustafsson, L.E., Wiklund, N.P. *et al.* (1990) Endogenous nitric oxide as a probable modulator of pulmonary circulation and hypoxic pressor response *in vivo*. *Acta Physiol. Scand.*, **140**, 449–57.

20. Greenberg, B., Rhoden, K. and Barnes, P.J. (1987) Endothelium-dependent relaxation of human pulmonary arteries. *Am. J. Physiol.*, **252**, H434–8.

21. Crawley, D.E., Liu, S.F., Evans, T.W. and Barnes, P.J. (1990) Inhibitory role of endothelium-derived relaxing factor in rat and human pulmonary arteries. *Br. J. Pharmacol.*, **101**, 166–70.

22. Beyne, J. (1942) Influence de l'anoxemie sur la grande circulation et sur la circulation pulmonaire. *C.R. Soc. Biol. (Paris)*, **136**, 399–400.

23. Marshall, C. and Marshall, B.E. (1983) Influence of perfusate P_{O_2} on hypoxic pulmonary vasoconstriction in rats. *Circ. Res.*, **52**, 691–6.

24. von Euler, U.S and Liljestrand, G. (1946) Observations on the pulmonary arterial blood pressure in the cat. *Acta Physiol. Scand.*, **12**, 301–20.

25. Wagner, W.W. Jr, Latham, L.P. and Capen, R.L. (1979) Capillary recruitment during airway hypoxia: role of pulmonary artery pressure. *J. Appl. Physiol.*, **47**, 383–7.

26. Fishman, A.P., Fritts, H.W. and Cournand, A. (1960) Effects of acute hypoxia and exercise on the pulmonary circulation. *Circulation*, **22**, 204–15.

27. Silove, E.D. and Grover, R.F. (1968) Effects of alpha adrenergic blockade and tissue catecholamine depletion on pulmonary vascular response to hypoxia. *J. Clin. Invest.*, **47**, 274–85.

28. Lodato, R.F., Michael, J.R. and Murray, P.A. (1988) Absence of neural modulation of hypoxic pulmonary vasoconstriction in conscious dogs. *J. Appl. Physiol.*, **65**, 1481–7.

29. Peake, M.D., Harabin, A.L., Brennan, N.J. and Sylvester, J.T. (1981) Steady-state vascular responses to graded hypoxia in isolated lungs of five species. *J. Appl. Physiol.*, **51**, 1214–9.

30. Robin, E.D., Theodore, J., Burke, C.M. *et al.* (1987) Hypoxic pulmonary vasoconstriction persists in the human transplanted lung. *Clin. Sci.*, **72**, 283–7.

31. Kato, M. and Staub, N.C. (1966) Response of small pulmonary arteries to unilobar hypoxia and hypercapnia. *Circ. Res.*, **19**, 426–40.

32. Hakim, T.S., Michel, R.P., Minami, H. and Chang, H.K. (1983) Site of pulmonary hypoxic vasoconstriction studied with arterial and venous occlusion. *J. Appl. Physiol.*, **54**, 1298–302.

33. Nagasaka, Y., Bhattacharya, J., Nanjo, S. *et al.* (1984) Micropuncture measurement of lung microvascular pressure profile during hypoxia in cats. *Cir. Res.*, **54**, 90–5.

34. Shirai, M., Sada, K. and Ninomiya, I. (1986) Effects of regional alveolar hypoxia and hypercapnia on small pulmonary vessels in cats. *J. Appl. Physiol.*, **61**, 440–8.

35. Miller, D., Hamilton, J.T. and Paterson, N.A.M. (1989) The role of leukotrienes in hypoxic contractions of isolated porcine pulmonary artery and vein. *Exp. Lung Res.*, **15**, 213–22.

36. Raj, J.V. and Chen, P. (1986) Micropuncture measurement of microvascular pressures in isolated lamb lungs during hypoxia. *Cir. Res.*, **59**, 398–404.

37. Paterson, N.A.M., Hamilton, J.T., Yaghi, A. *et al.* (1988) ERffect of hypoxia on responses of respiratory smooth muscle to histamine and LTD_4. *J. Appl. Physiol.*, **64**, 435–40.

38. Lloyd, T.C. (1968) Hypoxic pulmonary vasoconstriction: role of perivascular tissue. *J. Appl. Physiol.*, **25**, 560–5.

39. Cutaia, M. and Rounds, S. (1990) Hypoxic pulmonary vasoconstriction: physiological significance, mechanism, and clinical relevance. *Chest*, **97**, 706–18.

40. Fishman, A.P. (1985) Pulmonary circulation, in *Handbook of Physiology*, (ed. S.R. Geiger), American Physiological Society, Bethesda, M.D., pp. 93–165.

41. Stenmark, K.R., James, S.J., Voelkel, N. *et al.* (1983) Leukotriene C4 and D4 in neonates with hypoxemia and pulmonary hypertension. *N. Engl. J. Med.*, **309**, 77–80.

42. Morganroth, M.L., Stenmark, K.R., Zirrolli, J.A. *et al.* (1984) Leukotriene C_4 production

during hypoxic pulmonary vasoconstriction in isolated rat lungs. *Prostaglandins*, **28**, 867–5.

43. Morganroth, M.L., Stenmark, K.R., Morris, K.G. *et al.* (1985) Diethylcarbamazine inhibits acute and chronic hypoxic vasoconstriction in awake rats. *Am. Rev. Respir. Dis.*, **131**, 488–92.

44. Goldberg, R.N., Suguihara, C., Ahmed, T. *et al.* (1985) Influence of an antagonist of slow-reacting substance of anaphylaxis on the cardiovascular manifestations of hypoxia in piglets. *Pediatr. Res.*, **19**, 1201–5.

45. Raj, J.U. and Chen, P. (1987) Role of eicosanoids in hypoxic vasoconstriction in isolated lamb lungs. *Am. J. Physiol.*, **253**, H626–33.

46. Schreiber, M.D., Heymann, M.A. and Soifer, S.J. (1985) Leukotriene inhibition prevents and reverses hypoxic pulmonary vasoconstriction in newborn lambs. *Pediatr. Res.*, **19**, 437–41.

47. Voelkel, N.F., Stenmark, K.R., Reeves, J.T. *et al.* (1984) Actions of lipoxygenase metabolites in isolated rat lungs. *J. Appl. Physiol.*, **57**, 860–7.

48. Schnaar, R.L. and Sparks, H.V. (1972) Response of large and small coronary arteries to nitroglycerine, $NaNO_2$, and adenosine. *Am. J. Physiol.*, **223**, 223–8.

49. Gottlieb, J.E., McGeady, M. Adkinson, N.F. Jr and Sylvester, J.T. (1988) Effects of cycloand lipoxygenase inhibitors on hypoxic vasoconstriction in isolated ferret lungs. *J. Appl. Physiol.*, **64**, 936–43.

50. Lonigro, A.J., Sprague, R.S., Stephenson, A.H. and Dahms, T.E. (1988) Relationship of leukotriene C4 and D4 to hypoxic pulmonary vasoconstriction. *J. Appl. Physiol.*, **64**, 2538–43.

51. Leffler, C.W., Mitchell, J.A. and Green, R.S. (1984) Cardiovascular effects of leukotrienes in neonatal piglets. *Cir. Res.*, **55**, 780–7.

52. Garrett, R.C., Foster, S. and Thomas, H.M. III. (1987) Lipoxygenase and cyclooxygenase blockade by BW 755c enhances pulmonary hypoxic vasoconstriction. *J. Appl. Physiol.*, **62**, 129–33.

53. Rubin, L.J., Hughes, J.D. and Lazar, J.D. (1985) The effects of eicosanoid synthesis inhibitors on normoxic and hypoxic pulmonary vascular tone. *Am. Rev. Respir. Dis.*, **132**, 93–8.

54. Schuster, D.P. and Dennis, D.R. (1987) Leukotriene inhibitors do not block hypoxic pulmonary vasoconstriction in dogs. *J. Appl. Physiol.*, **62**, 1808–13.

55. McCormack, D.G. and Paterson, N.A.M. (1989) The contrasting influence of two lipoxygenase inhibitors on hypoxic pulmonary vasoconstriction in anesthetized pigs. *Am. Rev. Respir. Dis.*, **139**, 100–5.

56. Thomas, H.M. III, Sourour, M.S., Lopez, D. and Foster, S.H. (1989) Antagonism of leukotriene receptors and administration of a 5-lipoxygenase inhibitor do not affect hypoxic vasoconstriction. *Lung*, **167**, 187–98.

57. Cassin, S., Gause, G., Davis, T. *et al.* (1989) Do inhibitors of lipoxygenase and cycloxygenase block neonatal pulmonary vasoconstriction? *J. Appl. Physiol.*, **66**, 1779–884.

58. Kourembanas, S., Marsden, P.A., McQuillan, L.P. and Faller, D.V. (1991) Hypoxia induces endothelin gene expression and secretion in cultured human endothelium. *J. Clin. Invest.*, **88**, 1054–7.

59. De Mey, J.G. and Vanhoutte, P.M. (1983) Anoxia and endothelium-dependent reactivity of the canine femoral artery. *J. Physiol. (Lond.)*, **335**, 65–74.

60. Muramatsu, M., Iwama, Y., Shimizu, K. *et al.* (1992) Hypoxia-elicited contraction of aorta and coronary artery via removal of endothelium-derived nitric oxide. *J. Appl. Physiol.*, **263**, H1339–47.

61. Holden, W.E. and McCall, E. (1984) Hypoxia-induced contractions of porcine pulmonary artery strips depend on intact endothelium. *Exp. Lung Res.*, **7**, 101–12.

62. Rodman, D.M., Yamaguchi, T., O'Brien, R.F. and McMurtry, I.F. (1988) Hypoxic contraction of isolated rat pulmonary artery. *J. Pharmacol. Exp. Ther.*, **248**, 952–9.

63. Demiryurek, A.T., Wadsworth, R.M., Kane, K.A. and Peacock, A.J. (1993) The role of endothelium in hypoxic constriction of human pulmonary artery rings. *Am. Rev. Respir. Dis.*, **147**, 283–90.

64. Zhao, Y., Packer, C.S. and Rhoades, R.A. (1992) Pulmonary vein contracts in response to hypoxia. *Am. J. Physiol.*, **265**, L87–92.

65. Ohe, M., Ogata, M., Katayose, D. and Takishima, T. (1992) Hypoxic contraction of prestretched human pulmonary artery. *Respir. Physiol.*, **87**, L05–14.

66. Ogata, M., Ohe, M., Katayose, D. and Takishima, T. (1992) Modulatory role of EDRF in hypoxic contraction of isolated porcine pulmonary arteries. *Am. J. Physiol.*, **262**, H691–7.

67. Yuan, X.-J., Tod, M.L., Rubin, L.J. and Blaus-

tein, M.P. (1990) Contrasting effects of hypoxia on tension in rat pulmonary and mesenteric arteries. *Am. J. Physiol.*, **259**, H281–9.

68. Weir, E.K. (1978) Does normoxic pulmonary vasodilatation rather than hypoxic vasoconstriction account for the pulmonary pressor response to hypoxia? *Lancet*, **i**, 476–7.

69. Rodman, D.M., Yamaguchi, T., Hasunuma, K. *et al.* (1990) Effects of hypoxia on endothelium-dependent relaxation of rat pulmonary artery. *Am. J. Physiol.*, **258**, L207–14.

70. Johns, R.A., Linden, J.M. and Peach, M.J. (1989) Endothelium-dependent relaxation and cyclic GMP accumulation in rabbit pulmonary artery are selectively impaired by moderate hypoxia. *Circ. Res.*, **65**, 1508–15.

71. McCormack, D.G. and Paterson, N.A.M. (1993) Loss of hypoxic pulmonary vasoconstriction in chronic pneumonia is not mediated by nitric oxide. *Am. J. Physiol.*, **265**, H1523–8.

72. Liu, S., Crawley, D.E., Barnes, P.J. and Evans, T.W. (1991) Endothelium-derived relaxing factor inhibits hypoxic pulmonary vasoconstriction in rats. *Am. Rev. Respir. Dis.*, **143**, 32–7.

73. Oka, M., Hasunuma, K., Webb, S.A. *et al.* (1993) EDRF suppresses an unidentified vasoconstriction mechanism in hypertensive rat lungs. *Am. J. Physiol.*, **264**, L587–97.

74. Bansal, V., Toga, H. and Usha Raj, J. (1993) Tone dependent nitric oxide production in ovine vessels *in vitro*. *Respir. Physiol.* **93**, 249–60.

75. Mazmanian, G.-M., Baudet, B., Brink, C. *et al.* (1989) Methylene blue potentiates vascular reactivity in isolated rat lungs. *J. Appl. Physiol.*, **66**, 1040–5.

76. Brashers, V.L., Peach, M.J. and Rose, C.E. Jr (1988) Augmentation of hypoxic pulmonary vasoconstriction in the isolated perfused rat lung by *in vitro* antagonists of endothelium-dependent relaxation. *J. Clin. Invest.* **82**, 1495–502.

77. Madden, M.C., Vender, R.L. and Friedman, M. (1986) Effect of hypoxia on prostacyclin production in cultured pulmonary artery endothelium. *Prostaglandins*, **31**, 1049–62.

78. Voelkel, N.F., Gerber, J.G., McMurtry, I.F. *et al.* (1981) Release of vasodilator prostaglandin, P.G.I.$_2$ from isolated rat lung during vasoconstriction. *Cir. Res.* **48**, 207.

79. Madden, J.A., Dawson, C.A. and Harder, D.R. (1985) Hypoxia-induced activation in small isolated pulmonary arteries from the cat. *J. Appl. Physiol.* **59**, 113–8.

80. Murray, T.R., Chen, L., Marshall, B.E. and Macarak, E.J. (1990) Hypoxic contraction of cultured pulmonary vascular smooth muscle cells. *Am. J. Respir. Cell. Mol. Biol. Mol. Biol.*, **3**, 457–65.

81. Madden, J.A., Vadula, M.S. and Kurup, V.P. (1992) Effects of hypoxia and other vasoactive agents on pulmonary and cerebral artery smooth muscle cells. *Am. Physiol.* **263**, L384–93.

82. Harder, D.R., Madden, J.A. and Dawson, C. (1985) Hypoxic induction of Ca^{2+}-dependent action potentials in small pulmonary arteries of the cat. *J. Appl. Physiol.* **59**, 1389–93.

83. Jin, N., Packer, C.S. and Rhoades, R.A. (1992) Pulmonary arterial hypoxic contraction: signal transduction. *Am. J. Physiol.* **263**, L73–8.

84. Hoshino, Y., Obara, H., Kusunoki, M. *et al.* (1988) Hypoxic contractile response in isolated human pulmonary artery: role of calcium ion. *J. Appl. Physiol.* **65**, 2468–74.

85. Rodman, D.M., Yamaguchi, T., O'Brien, R.F. and McMurtry, I.F. (1989) Hypoxic contraction of isolated rat pulmonary artery. *J. Pharmacol. Exp.* **248**, 952–9.

86. McMurtry, I.F. (1985) Bay K8644 potentiates and A23187 inhibits hypoxic vasoconstriction in rat lungs. *Am. Physiol.* **249**, H741–6.

87. Salvaterra, C.G. and Goldman, W.F. (1993) Acute hypoxia increases cytosolic calcium in cultured pulmonary arterial myocytes. *Am. Physiol.*, **264**; L323–8

88. Yuan, X.-J., Goldman, WF, Tod, ML *et al.* (1993) Hypoxia reduces potassium currents in cultured rat pulmonary but not mesenteric arterial myocytes, *Am. J. Physiol.*, **264**, L116–23.

89. Haynes, W.G. and Webb, D.J. (1993) The endothelin family of peptides: local hormones with diverse roles in health and disease? *Clin. Sci.*, **84**, 485–500.

90. Sirvio, M.L., Matsarinne, K., Saijonmaa, O. and Fyhrquist, F. (1990) Tissue distribution and half life of 125 I-endothelin in the rat: importance of pulmonary clearance. *Biochem. Biophys. Res. Commun.*, **167**; 1191–5.

91. Westcott, J.Y., Henson, J., McMurtry, I.F. and O'Brien, R.F. (1990) Uptake and metabolism of endothelin in the isolated perfused rat lung. *Exp. Lung Res.*, **16** 521–32.

92. Horgan, M.J., Pinheiro, J.M. and Malik, A.B.

(1991) Mechanism of endothelin-1 induced pulmonary vasoconstriction. *Circ. Res.*, **69**; 157–64.

93. Wang, Y. and Coceani, F. (1992) Isolated pulmonary resistance vessels from fetal lambs – contractile behavior and responses to indomethacin and endothelin-1. *Circ. Res.*, **71**; 320–30.

94. Lippton, H.L., Cohen, G.A., McMurtry, I.F. and Hyman, A.L. (1991) Pulmonary vasodilation to endothelin isopeptides is mediated by potassium channel activation. *J. Appl. Physiol.*, **70**; 947–52.

95. Lippton, H.L., Hauth, T.A., Cohen, G.A. and Hyman, A.L. (1993) Functional evidence for different endothelin receptors in the lung. *J. Appl. Physiol.*, **75**; 38–48.

96. De Nucci, G., Thomas, R., D'Orleans-Juste, P. *et al.* Pressor effects of circulating endothelin are limited by its removal from the pulmonary circulation and by the release of prostacyclin and endothelium-derived relaxing factor. *Proc. Natl Acad. Sci. USA* **85**; 9797–800.

97. D'Orleans-Juste, P., Telemaque, S., Claing, A., *et al.* (1992) Human big-endothelin-1 and endothelin-1 release prostacyclin via the activation of ET_1 receptors in the rat perfused lung. *Br. J. Pharmacol.*, **105**; 773–5.

98. Tod, M.L. and Cassin, S. (1992) Endothelin-1-induced pulmonary arterial dilation is reduced by N_w-nitro-L-arginine in fetal lambs. *J. Appl. Physiol.*, **72**; 1730–4.

99. Namiki, A., Hirata, Y., Ishikawa, M. *et al.* Endothelin-1 and endothelin-3-induced vasorelaxation via common generation of endothelium-derived nitric oxide. *Life Sci.*, **50**; 677

100. Crawley, D.E., Liu, S.F., Barnes, P.J. and Evans, T.W. (1992) Endothelin-3 is a potent pulmonary vasodilator in the rat. *J. Appl. Physiol.*, **72**; 1425–31.

101. Hirata, Y., Emori, T., Eguchi, S., *et al.* (1993) Endothelin receptor subtype B mediates synthesis of nitric oxide by cultured bovine endothelial cells. *J. Clin. Invest.*, **91**; 1367–73.

102. Inoue, A., Yanagisawa, M., Simura, S. *et al.* (1989) The human endothelin family: three structurally and pharmacologically distinct isopeptides predicted by three separate genes. *Proc. Natl Acad. Sci. USA*, **86**; 2863–7.

103. Sibbald, W.J., Paterson, N.A.M., Holliday, R.L. *et al.* (1978) Pulmonary hypertension in sepsis: measurement by the pulmonary arterial

diastolic-pulmonary wedge pressure gradient and the influence of passive factors. *Chest*, **73**; 583–91.

104. Snapper, J.R., Bernard, G.R., Hinson, *et al.* (1993). Endotoxemia-induced leukopenia in sheep – correlation with lung vascular permeability and hypoxemia but not with pulmonary hypertension. *Am. Rey. Respir. Dis.* **127**; 306–9.

105. Dehring, D.J., Lowery, B.D., Flynn, J. *et al.* (1983) Indomethacin improvement of septic acute respiratory failure in a porcine model. *J. Trauma*, **23**; 725–9.

106. Winn, R., Harlan, J., Nadir, B. *et al.* (1983) Thromboxane A_2 mediates lung vasoconstriction but not permeability after endotoxin. *J. Clin. Invest.* **72**; 911–8.

107. Watkins, W.D., Huttemeier, P.C., Kong, D. and Peterson, M.B. (1982) Thromboxane and pulmonary hypertension following *E. coli* endotoxin infusion in sheep: effect of an imidazole derivative. *Prostaglandins*, **23**; 273–85.

108. Matthay, M.A., Eschenbacher, W.L. and Goetzel, E.J. (1984) Elevated concentrations of leukotriene D_4 in pulmonary edema fluid of patients with the adult respiratory distress syndrome. *J. Clin. Immunol.*, **4**; 479–83.

109. Ratnoff, W.D., Matthay, M.A., Wong, M.Y.S. *et al.* (1988) Sulfidopeptide-leukotriene peptidases in pulmonary edema fluid from patients with the adult respiratory distress syndrome. *J. Clin. Immunol.*, **8**; 250–8.

110. Bernard, G.R., Korley, V., Chee, P. *et al.* (1991) Persistent generation of peptido leukotrienes in patients with the adult respiratory distress syndrome. *Am. Rev. Respir. Dis.*, **144**, 263–7.

111. Coggeshall, J.W., Christman, B.W., Lefferts, P.L. *et al.* (1988) Effect of inhibition of 5-lipoxygenase metabolism of arachidonic acid on response to endotoxemia in sheep. *J. Appl. Physiol.*, **65**; 1351–9.

112. Olson, N.C., Dobrowsky, R.T. and Fleisher, L.N. (1987) Hydroxyeicosatetraenoic acids are increased in bronchoalveolar lavage fluid of endotoxemic pigs. *Prostaglandins*, **34**; 493–503.

113. Ogletree, M.L., Oates, J.A., Brigham, K.L. and Hubbard, W.C. (1982) Evidence for pulmonary release of 5-hydroxyeicosatetranoic acid (5-HETE) during endotoxemia in unanesthetized sheep. *Prostaglandins*, **23**, 459–8.

114. Hagmann, W., Denzlinger, C. and Keppler, D.

Production of peptide leukotrienes in endo-toxin shock. *FEBS Lett.*, **180**; 309–13.

115. Ahmed, T., Wasserman, M.A., Muccitelli, R., *et al.* (1986) Endotoxin-induced changes in pulmonary hemodynamics and respiratory mechanics – role of lipoxygenase and cyclooxygenase products. *Am. Rev. Respir. Dis.* **134**; 1149–57.

116. Gross, D., Dahan, J.B., Landau, E.H. and Krausz, M.M. (1990) Effect of leukotriene inhibitor LY-171883 on the pulmonary response to *Escherichia coli* endotoxemia. *Crit. Care Med.*, **18**; 190–7.

117. Ahmed, T., Weichman, B., Wasserman, M.A. *et al.* (1988) Prevention and reversal of endotoxin-induced pulmonary hypertension by a leukotriene antagonist. *Eur. Respir. J.*, **1**; 145–52.

118. Hamasaki, Y., Mojarad, M., Saga, T. *et al.* (1984) Platelet-activating factor raises airway and vascular pressures and induces edema in lungs perfused with platelet free solution. *Am. Rev. Respir. Dis.* **129**; 742–6.

119. Christman, B.W., Lefferts, P.L., King, G.A. and Snapper, J.R. (1988) Role of circulating platelets and granulocytes in PAF-induced pulmonary dysfunction in awake sheep. *J. Appl. Physiol.* **64**; 2033–41.

120. Burhop, K.E., van der Zee, H., Bisios, R. *et al.* (1986) Pulmonary vascular responses to platelet-activating factor in awake sheep and the role of cyclooxygenase metabolites. *Am, Rev. Respir. Dis.*, **134**; 548–54.

121. Doebber, T.W., Wu, M.S., Robbins, J.C. *et al.* (1985) Platelet activating factor involvement in endotoxin-induced hypotension in rats: studies with PAF-receptor antagonist kadsurenone. *Biochem. Biophys. Res. Commun.* **127**; 799–808.

122. Christman, BW, Lefferts, P.L., Blair, I.A. and Snapper, J.R. (1990) Effect of platelet-activating factor receptor antagonism on endotoxin-induced lung dysfunction in awake sheep. *Am. Rev. Respir. Dis.*, **142**; 1271–8.

123. Sessler, C.N., Glauser, F.L., Davis, D. and Fowler, A.A.-III. Effects of platelet-activating factor antagonist SRI 63–441 on endotoxemia in sheep. *J. Appl. Physiol.*, **65**; 2624–31.

124. Hsueh, W., Gonzalez-Crussi, F. and Arroyave, J.L. (1986) Release of leukotriene C4 by isolated, perfused rat small intestine in response to platelet-activating factor. *J. Clin. Invest.* **78**; 108–14.

125. McIntyre, T.M., Zimmerman, G.A. and Prescott, S.M. (1986) Leukotrienes C4 and D4 stimulate human endothelial cells to synthesize platelet-activating factor and bind neutrophils. *Proc. Natl Acad. Sci. USA*, **83**; 2304–8.

126. Morel, D.R., Lacroix, J.S., Hemsen, A. *et al.* (1989) Increased plasma and pulmonary lymph levels of endothelin during endotoxin shock. *Eur. J. Pharmacol.*, **167**; 427–8.

127. Pittet, J.F., Morel, D.R., Hemsen, A. *et al.* (1991) Elevated plasma endothelin-1 concentrations are associated with the severity of illness in patients with sepsis. *Ann. Surg.*, **213**; 261–4.

128. Weitzberg, E., Lundberg, J.M. and Rudehill, A. (1991) Elevated plasma level of endothelin in patients with sepsis syndrome. *Circ. Shock*, **33**; 222–7.

129. Druml, W., Steltzer, H., Waldhausl, W. *et al.* (1993) Endothelin-1 in adult respiratory distress syndrome. *Am. Rev. Respir. Dis.*, **148**; 1169–73.

130. Fink, M.P., MacVittie, T.J. and Casey, L.C. (1984) Inhibition of prostaglandin synthesis restores normal hemodynamics in canine hyperdynamic sepsis. *Ann. Surg.*, **200**; 619–26.

131. Dantzker, D.R., Brook, C.J., Dehart, P. *et al.* (1979) Ventilation-perfusion distributions in the adult respiratory distress syndrome. *Am. Rev. Respir. Dis.*, **120**; 1039–52.

132. Light, R.B., Mink, S.N. and Wood, L.D.H. (1981) Pathophysiology of gas exchange and pulmonary perfusion in pneumococcal lobar pneumonia in dogs. *I. Appl. Physiol.*, **50**; 524–30.

133. Graham, L.M., Vasil, A., Vasil, M.L. *et al.* (1990) Decreased pulmonary vasoreactivity in an animal model of chronic pseudomonas pneumonia. *Am. Rev. Respir. Dis.*, **142**; 221–9.

134. Newman, J.H., Loyd, J.E., English, D.K. *et al.* (1983) Effects of 100% oxygen on lung vascular function in awake sheep. *J. Appl. Physiol.* **54**; 1379–86.

135. McCormack, D.G., Crawley, D., Barnes, P.J. and Evans, T.W. (1992) Bleomycin-induced acute lung injury in rats selectively abolishes hypoxic pulmonary vasoconstriction: evidence against a role for platelet-activating factor. *Clin. Sci.*, **82**, 259–64.

136. Martin, C.M., Yaghi, A., Sibbald, W.J. *et al.* (1993) Differential impairment of vascular

reactivity of small pulmonary and systemic arteries in hyperdynamic sepsis. *Am. Rev. Respir. Dis.* **148**; 164–72.

137. Yaghi, A., Paterson, N.A.M. and McCormack, D.G. (1993) Nitric oxide does not mediate the attenuated pulmonary vascular reactivity of chronic pneumonia. *Am. J. Physiol.*, **265**; H943–8.

138. Crawley, D.E., Zhao, L., Giembycz, M.A. *et al.* (1992) Chronic hypoxia impairs soluble guanylyl cyclase-mediated pulmonary arterial relaxation in the rat. *Am. J. Physiol.*, **263**, L325–32.

139. Eddahibi, S., Adnot, S., Carville, C. *et al.* (1992) L-Arginine restores endothelium-dependent relaxation in pulmonary circulation of chronically hypoxic rats. *Am. J. Physiol.*, **263**; L194–200.

140. Dinh-Xuan, A.T., Higenbottam, T.W., Clelland, C.A. *et al.* (1991) Impairment of endothelium-dependent pulmonary-artery relaxation in chronic obstructive lung disease. *N. Engl. J. Med.*, **324**; 1539–47.

141. Parratt, J.R. and Sturgess, R.M. (1975) *E. coli* endotoxin shock in the cat: treatment with indomethacin. *Br. J. Pharmacol.*, **53**; 485–8.

142. Light, R.B. (1986) Indomethacin and acetylsalicylic acid reduce intrapulmonary shunt in experimental pneumococcal pneumonia. *Am. Rev. Respir. Dis.*, **134**; 520–5.

143. Hanly, P., Sienko, A. and Light, R.B. (1987) Effect of cyclooxygenase blockade on gas exchange and hemodynamics in Pseudomonas pneumonia. *J. Appl. Physiol.*, **63**; 1829–36.

144. Heuer, H.O., Darius, H., Lohmann, H.F. *et al.* (1991) Platelet-activating factor type activity in plasma from patients with septicemia and other diseases. *Lipids*, **26**; 1381–5.

145. Tracey, K.J., Stephen, F.L. and Cerami, A. (1988) Cachetin/TNFa in septic shock and septic adult respiratory distress syndrome. *Am. Rev. Respir. Dis.*, **138**; 1377–9.

146. Beasley, D., Cohen, R.A. and Levinsky, N.G. (1989) Interleukin-1 inhibits contraction of vascular smooth muscle. *J. Clin. Invest.* **83**; 331–5.

147. Hanly, P.J., Dobson, K., Roberts, D. and Light, R.B. (1987) Effect of indomethacin on arterial oxygenation in critically ill patients with severe bacterial pneumonia. *Lancet* **i**, 351–4.

148. Julou-Schaeffer, G., Gray, G.A., Fleming, I. *et al.* (1990) Loss of vascular responsiveness induced by endotoxin involves L-arginine pathway. *Am. J. Physiol.*, **259**; H1038–43.

149. Kilbourn, R.G. and Griffith, O.W. (1992) Overproduction of nitric oxide in cytokine-mediated and septic shock. *J. Natl Cancer Inst.*, **84**, 827–31.

150. Wright, C.E., Rees, D.D. and Moncada, S. (1992) Protective and pathological roles of nitric oxide in endotoxin shock. *Cardiovasc. Res.*, **26**; 48–57.

151. Auguet, M., Lonchampt, M.O., Delaflotte, S. *et al.* (1992) Induction of nitric oxide synthase by lipoteichoic acid from staphylococcus aureus in vascular smooth muscle cells. *FEBS Lett.*, **297**; 183–5.

152. Busse, R. and Mulsch, A. (1990) Induction of nitric oxide synthase by cytokines in vascular smooth muscle cells. *FEBS Lett.*, **275**; 87–90.

153. Sato, K., Miyakawa, K., Takeya, M. *et al.* (1995) Immunohistochemical expression of inducible nitric oxide synthase (iNOS) in reversible endotoxic shock studied by a novel monoclonal antibody against rat iNOS. *J. Leukoc. Bioc.*, **57**; 36–44

154. Hom, G., Grant, S., Wolfe, G. *et al.* (1995) Lipopolysaccharide-induced hypotension and vascular hyporeactivity in the rat: tissue analysis of nitric oxide synthase mRNA and protein expression in the presence and absence of dexamethasone, N^G-monomethyl-L-arginine or indomethacin. *J. Pharmacol. Exp. Ther.*, **272**, 452–9.

155. Holcroft, J.W., Vassar, M.J. and Weber, C.J. Prostaglandin E$_1$ and survival in patients with the adult respiratory distress syndrome. *Ann. Surg.*, **85**; 371–8.

156. Melot, C., Lejeune, P., Leeman, M. *et al.* (1989) Prostaglandin E$_1$ in the adult respiratory distress syndrome. *Am. Rev. Respir. Dis.* **139**; 106.

157. Bone, R.C., Slotman, G., Maunder, R. *et al.* (1989) Randomized double-blind, multicenter study of prostaglandin E$_1$ in patients with the adult respiratory distress syndrome. *Chest*, **96**, 114–9.

158. Sibbald, W.J., Driedger, A.A., McCallum, D. *et al.* (1986) Nitroprusside infusion does not improve biventricular performance in patients with acute hypoxemic respiratory failure. *J. Crit. Care*, **1**, 197–203.

159. Melot, C., Naeije, R., Mols, P. *et al.* (1987) Pulmonary vascular tone improves pulmonary gas exchange in the adult respiratory

distress syndrome. *Am. Rev. Respir. Dis.*, **138**, 1232–6.

160. Frostell, C., Fratacci, M.D., Wain, J.C. *et al.* (1991) Inhaled nitric oxide: a selective pulmonary vasodilator reversing hypoxic pulmonary vasoconstriction. *Circulation*, **83**, 2038–47.

161. Rossaint, R., Falke, K.J., Lopez, F. *et al.* (1993) Inhaled nitric oxide for the adult respiratory distress syndrome. *Engl. J. Med.*, **328**, 399–405.

162. Berger, J.I., Gibson, R.L., Redding, G.J. *et al.* (1993) Effect of inhaled nitric oxide during group B streptococcal sepsis in piglets. *Am. Rev. Respir. Dis.*, **147**, 1080–6.

163. Weitzberg, E., Rudehill, A. and Lundberg, J.M. (1993) Nitric oxide inhalation attenuates pulmonary hypertension and improves gas exchange in endotoxin shock. *Eur. J. Pharmacol.*, **233**, 85–94.

164. Abman, S.H., Kinsella, J.P., Schaffer, M.S. and Wilkening, R.B. (1993) Inhaled nitric oxide in the management of a premature newborn with severe respiratory distress and pulmonary hypertension. *Pediatrics*, **92**, 606–9.

165. Haydar, A., Mauriat, P., Pouard, P. *et al.* (1992) Inhaled nitric oxide for postoperative pulmonary hypertension in patients with congenital heart defects. *Lancet*, **340**, 8834–5.

166. Rich, G.F., Murphy, G.D., Roos, C.M. and Johns, R.A. (1993) Inhaled nitric oxide – selective pulmonary vasodilation in cardiac surgical patients. *Anesthesiology*, **78**, 1028–35.

167. Walmrath, D., Schneider, T., Pilch, J. *et al.* (1993) Aerosolised prostacyclin in adult respiratory distress syndrome. *Lancet*, **342**, 961–2.

Ravi S. Gill and William J. Sibbald

The syndrome of acute respiratory distress in adults (ARDS) was first described in 1967 [1]. Classically, ARDS is recognized clinically as acute respiratory failure with bilateral infiltrates on chest radiography, depressed pulmonary compliance and arterial hypoxemia. The terms acute lung injury (ALI) and ARDS have been used interchangeably within the intensive care (ICU) literature; however, their etiologies differ (Table 18.1). In this chapter, we review the concept that ARDS can result from either an alveolar insult (i.e. progression of ALI) or a panendothelial injury secondary to a remote insult (i.e. peritonitis), and discuss how ARDS is related to the multiple organ dysfunction syndrome (MODS) (Figure 18.1).

ARDS is distinct from many other lung disorders in its ability to afflict previously healthy individuals across a diverse range of disease entities. Associated with a mortality of 60% when first described [1], this poor outcome has since remained generally unchanged. However, the cause of death in patients with ARDS is now rarely due to respiratory failure but more frequently attributed to delayed onset, sepsis-related MODS [2–6].

MODS is a syndrome defined by a constellation of clinical signs and symptoms in which multiple organs (kidney, heart, gut, etc.) are in a state of dysfunction or outright failure. Its increasing frequency since the 1970s may be correlated with improvements in resuscitation techniques and the application of newer surgical and medical technologies to a progressively aging society. Nevertheless, after 20 years of research in which improvements in ventilator therapies, cardiovascular management and supportive care have been introduced, why the development of ARDS is still accompanied by such a high mortality remains unclear, [7] (Chapter 2).

The significant and multiple roles played by the lung within the body provide a vast surface area in which essential nutrient exchange takes place. The mechanics of breathing modulate cardiac function, influencing preload, afterload and contractility through changes in intrathoracic pressures and volumes. The lungs are a common site for both metabolic and pathological interactions between cellular and humoral components (e.g. 'sensitization' by external bacteria, production of vasoactive mediators). The injured

Table 18.1 Clinical predispositions to ARDS

Direct (ALI)	Remote (ARDS)
Gastric aspiration	Sepsis
Pneumonia	Trauma
Inhalational injury	Pancreatitis
Pulmonary contusion	Massive blood transfusion
Near drowning	Disseminated intravascular coagulation
Drug overdose	

ARDS Acute Respiratory Distress in Adults. Edited by Timothy W. Evans and Christopher Haslett. Published in 1996 by Chapman & Hall, London. ISBN 0 412 56910 8

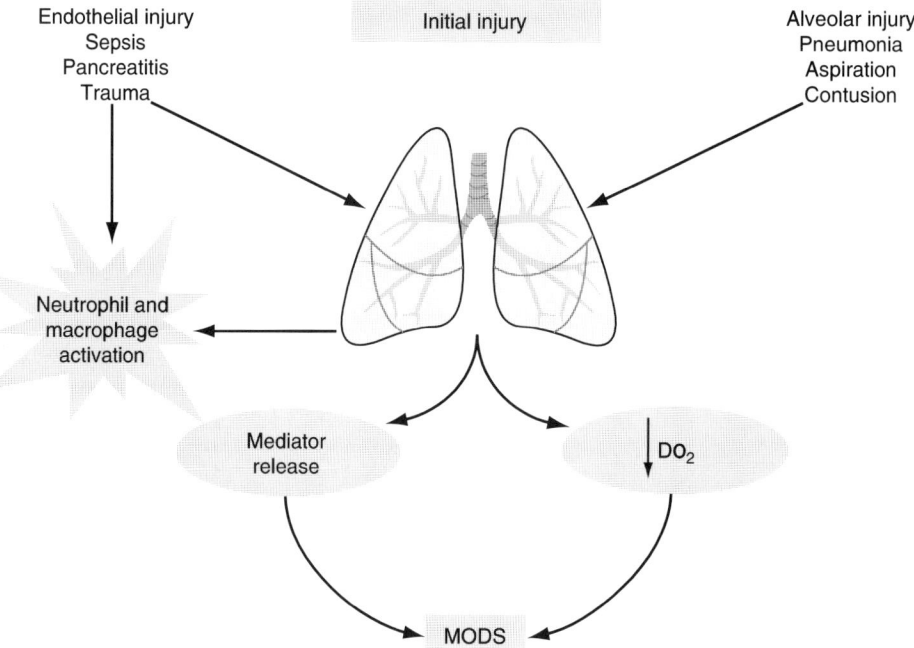

Figure 18.1.

or failing lung may therefore both initiate and amplify the processes that result in MODS.

Most physicians recognize that acute respiratory failure defined as ARDS can complicate tissue destruction accompanied by a generalized inflammatory response (systemic inflammatory response syndrome, SIRS) [8]. MODS is recognized clinically as failure of the lungs (i.e. ALI or ARDS) combined with dysfunction in other organs, including the circulation, the central nervous, hematopoietic, renal and hepatic systems. In this context, the remote effects of severe infection or trauma on the lung is recognized as ARDS, and on other organs as MODS. ARDS may therefore be regarded as but one component of the MOD syndrome.

Additionally, it is now recognized that injury to the alveolar-capillary membrane, through aspiration of gastric contents or smoke inhalation (i.e. ALI), may cause remote organ injury [9]. This may occur in one of two ways. Firstly, aspiration may trigger the release of inflammatory mediators from the lung and thereby injure remote organs, i.e. MODS develops from a lung-initiated inflammatory response. Alternatively, a hospital acquired pneumonia may develop in an injured lung. In this circumstance, sepsis may supervene and lead to ARDS and MODS [10,11] (Figure 18.1).

Following definitions of the terminology used in this chapter, we describe the relationship between ARDS and MODS. Finally, the pathogenesis of ARDS and MODS are discussed with the aim of pointing out similarities and links between these syndromes.

DEFINITIONS

Historically, ARDS has been an ill-defined potpourri of clinical findings indistinguishable from ALI. For the purpose of this chapter, the following definitions are used throughout.

ARDS AND ALI

The recent European – American Consensus Conference on ARDS published the following definitions for acute lung injury (ALI) and ARDS [12]. ALI has three components:

1. **oxygenation:** Pao_2/Fio_2 ratio $\leq$ 300 regardless of the amount of positive end expiratory pressure (PEEP);
2. **chest radiograph:** bilateral infiltrates seen on anteroposterior chest radiograph;
3. **pulmonary artery occlusion pressure:** $\leq$ 18 mmHg when measured or no evidence of left atrial hypertension based on chest radiograph and other clinical data.

ARDS has been given the same definition, except that the Pao_2/Fio_2 ratio is $\leq$ 200 in this syndrome, regardless of the level of PEEP applied.

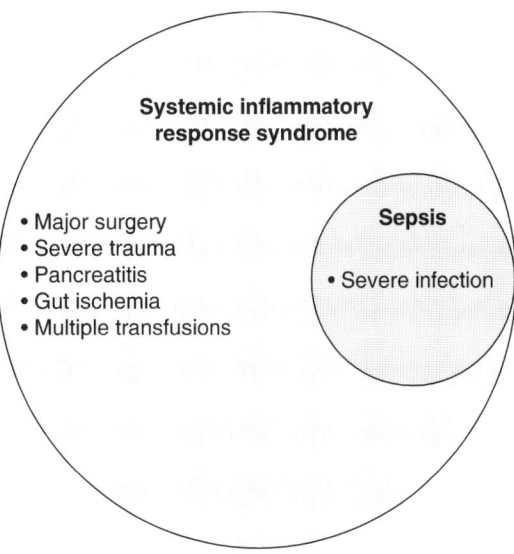

Figure 18.2.

MODS AND SIRS

The clinical pattern of progressive organ dysfunction complicating the post-resuscitative phase of an acute illness is termed MODS [8]. MODS has been previously referred to as multiple organ failure (MOF) or multiple systems organ failure (MSOF).

Sepsis has been defined as the response of the body to infection [8], characterized by certain physiological findings. It is now realized that a hyperdynamic state similar to that seen in sepsis may exist without an infective focus being present. This has been defined as SIRS [8] and represents an abnormal host response (Figure 18.2).

EPIDEMIOLOGY OF ARDS AND MODS

Both ARDS and MODS are characterized by a constellation of clinical and physiological findings resulting from a large number of insults (Chapter 2). Severe trauma, with or without hypotension and/or devitalization of tissue, pancreatitis, severe infection, gut ischemia and massive blood transfusions are clinical predispositions that have been related

to the development of both syndromes [5,13,14]. The ICU literature recognizes SIRS or sepsis-related SIRS from any source as the most common precipitating event leading to ARDS [15], as well as the most frequent clinical association with MODS [16,17]. ARDS has usually been thought of as a distinct disease entity. It has not been recognized as part of the host systemic dysfunction that characterizes MODS.

Existing clinical investigations describing both syndromes have been dogged by a lack of precise definitions. All too often, the abbreviations ALI and ARDS have been used interchangeably, whilst the criteria used to define organ dysfunction or failure differ substantially between published surveys [5,14,18–20]. As uniform criteria for the definition of organ dysfunction have yet to be established, the true incidence and natural history of MODS remains unclear. Despite this inability to describe concisely the epidemiology of MODS, important lessons can be synthesized from the existing literature.

Firstly, the increasing number of cases of MODS seen in conjunction with ARDS has

Table 18.2 Incidence of Organ Dysfunction Associated with ARDS

System	Failure (%)
Hematologic	0–26
Central nervous system	7–30
Gastrointestinal	7–30
Cardiac	10–23
Hepatic	12–95
Renal	40–55

paralleled the therapeutic advances applied to an aging population with life threatening illness and severe coexisting medical disease (e.g. the elderly patient with severe chronic obstructive pulmonary disease who undergoes an emergency laparotomy for peritonitis) [21]. Secondly, individual organ failure rates in association with ARDS have been summarized from various reports (Table 18.2) [20]. This abstracted data has led to the recognition of a 'domino' effect, i.e. organs failing in a sequential pattern following the development of ARDS. However, the mechanism of this organ–organ interaction is still poorly understood. Thirdly, the number of failed organ systems has been shown to be related to mortality. The mortality rate for single organ failure is 15–30% and rises to 45–55% when two organs fail. Once three or more organs have failed, mortality exceeds 80% and reaches 100% if MODS is established beyond 4 days [5]. Finally, with the development of MODS, therapeutic interventions are often necessary for life support and may include diverse pharmacotherapy, novel ventilation and renal dialysis. Paradoxically, all are capable of perpetuating the diffuse inflammatory response which underlies the pathogenesis of MODS.

Traditionally, ARDS has been viewed as a distinct disease entity, perhaps due to its effects on physiological parameters that are easily detected and monitored (i.e. respiratory rate and arterial blood gases) However, both ARDS and MODS are often preceded by similar, precipitating, catastrophic events. This

has led to an increasing belief that ARDS is only a single component of the continuum known as MODS. Although respiratory failure may be the precipitating trigger for an ICU admission, its cause, whether it be direct or secondary to a remote organ injury, may herald an all encompassing inflammatory response that ends in MODS (Figure 18.3).

PATHOPHYSIOLOGY

Infectious and *inflammatory* models have been proposed to describe the evolution of ARDS and MODS in critically ill patients. The progression from a state of relative health and homeostasis, to one of organ dysfunction and ultimately organ failure in critically ill patients admitted to the ICU, was initially thought to be the result of secondary infection following an insult to the host. However, cases of MODS without demonstrable evidence of an infectious focus caused researchers to rethink the concept that infection was invariably present in these circumstances [22]. Thus, SIRS leading to MODS may complicate pancreatitis, severe trauma, or pulmonary aspiration, all of which are injuries without a defined infective focus. Figure 18.4 summarizes some of the components known to be important in the pathogenesis of ARDS and MODS.

INFECTIOUS MODEL

Early research supported an *infectious* model of ARDS/MODS. It was believed that following the development of ARDS, continued pulmonary or nosocomial infection led to MODS [24]. In 18 consecutive patients with ruptured abdominal aneurysms the susequent development of MODS was thought to be the result of a combination of pre-existing disease, hemorrhagic shock and infection [23]. Further evidence supporting an infectious etiology was provided by retrospective review of 399 patients admitted for trauma or intra-abdominal emergencies [24]. In this patient group,

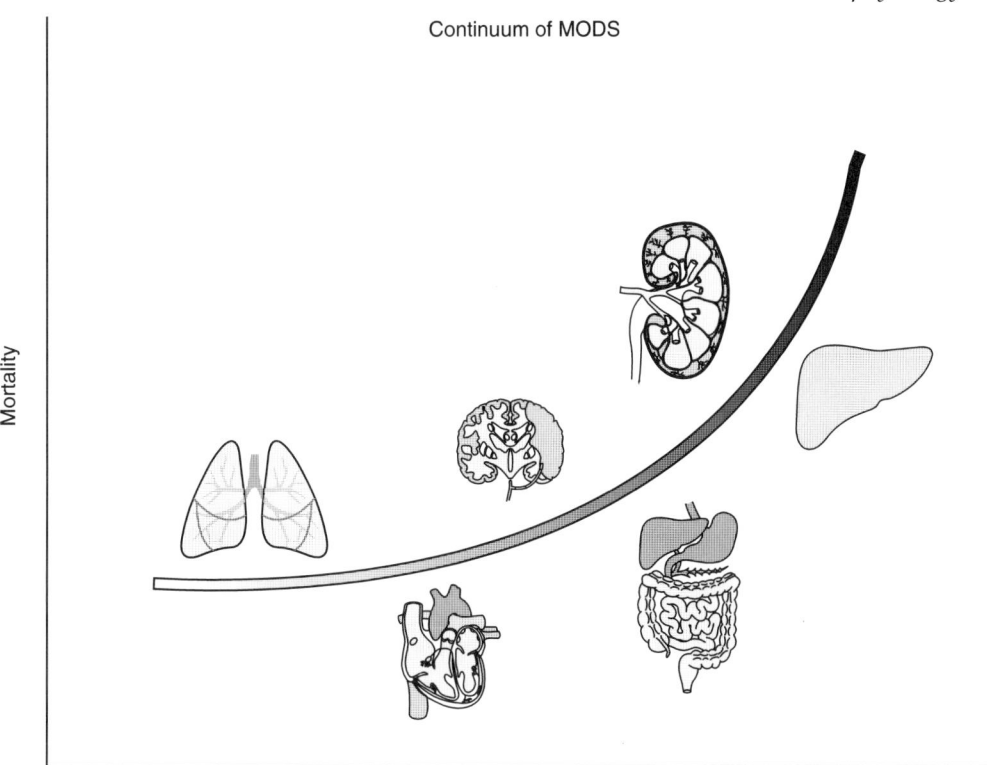

Continuum of MODS

Mortality

Time

Figure 18.3.

11% developed ARDS, of whom 83% were septic either before, or concurrent with, their development of ARDS. In a second study, of 42 patients with MODS, 50% had an intra-abdominal abscess as the precipitating trigger [3]. This *infectious* model was developed further in a retrospective review of 553 patients who required emergency operations. Seven percent developed ARDS/MODS, of whom 90% were thought to be septic at some point [4].

Clinical data until the mid 1980s therefore consistently related the development of ARDS and MODS in critically ill patients to the finding of a well defined infective focus, such as pneumonia, primary or nosocomial, or an intra-abdominal abscess. It was therefore concluded that untreated or inadequately treated infection established a sequence of events which led to progressive widespread organ injury and death (Figure 18.5). Indeed, the diagnosis of MODS at one time was held to be so pathognomonic of 'unrecognized' infection that laparotomy was frequently used as a diagnostic test to rule out the possibility of occult intra-abdominal infection in the presence of progressive MODS.

INFLAMMATORY MODEL

Proponents of this model believe that the host inflammatory response is upregulated following an initial insult such as trauma, severe hypotension or ischemia-reperfusion injury [22,25]; this is appropriate in the area of injured tissue, but clearly inappropriate if normal tissue is involved. In normal circumstances the host limits any potential injury to

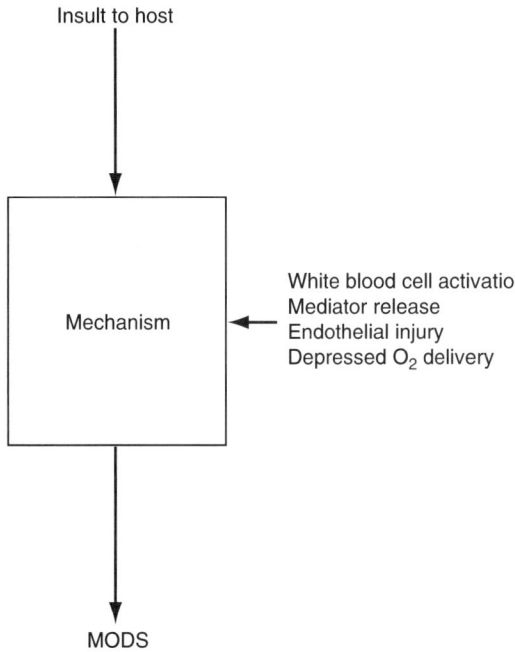

Figure 18.4.

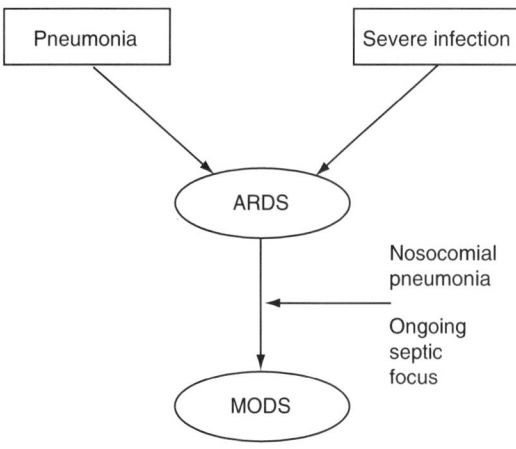

Figure 18.5.

normal tissue by regulating inflammatory responses. However, when these become excessive, or in the face of host defense depression, tissue damage and organ dysfunction may ensue.

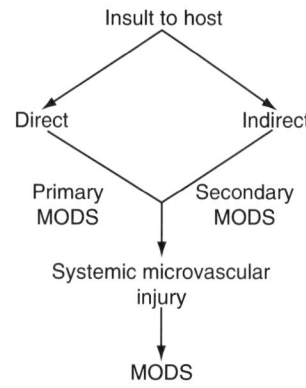

Figure 18.6.

In a survey of 433 trauma patients who required emergency operative procedures, 12% developed ARDS, and 8% MODS [26]. From this data two distinct patterns could be seen in the development of MODS: primary MODS, acute in nature and associated with massive tissue destruction and prolonged hypotension; and secondary MODS, a more insidious process possibly involving priming before further activation of inflammatory cascades (Figure 18.6). The temporal relationship of ARDS/MODS in this model was further explored in 100 multiple trauma patients with infectious complications, 75% of whom developed MODS [25]. However, in patients who developed MODS at or close to the time of the initial insult, virtually all infections were late (primary MODS). By contrast, of those patients who had a prolonged clinical course leading eventually to MODS (secondary MODS), 50% would have fulfilled the criteria for SIRS and ARDS (Figure 18.7). Furthermore, the combination of ARDS and MODS was shown conclusively to occur less frequently in patients without sepsis with trauma compared with patients developing ARDS/MODS from other causes [16].

Finally, cadaveric evidence from patients dying within hours of their injuries suggests that the lungs are not the only organs affected by an uncontrolled inflammatory process typical of MODS [27]. This recent clinical data is

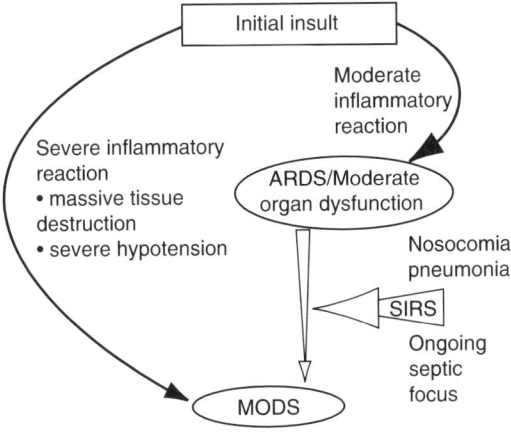

Figure 18.7.

supported by experimental findings describing widespread, early tissue damage in animal models of both sepsis and ARDS [10,11,28]. Therefore, it is probable that MODS follows an insult that activates an unopposed host inflammatory reaction, and that this uncontrolled release of mediators leads to the tissue injury that is seen in MODS.

ARDS, MODS AND THE MICROCIRCULATION

Although respiratory failure secondary to ARDS often predates the failure of other organ systems, it is unclear whether this is a cause and effect relationship. Thus, the lung may act as a focus for inflammatory mediator generation, or might be only a single component of a systemic injury, in which those organs with the least reserve or largest endothelial surface area fail first. Several hypotheses have been put forward to explain how ARDS evolves into MODS. Some are based on macrophage activation, others on ischemia-reperfusion [29] occurring at the time of injury. All discuss the significant role of a diffuse microcirculatory injury [30].

In ARDS, the pathology of the pulmonary microcirculatory injury is evidenced by increased capillary permeability and plug-

ging by activated leukocytes, and is manifested in various animal models by increased wet:dry weight ratios of individual organs [31,32] (Chapter 4). A patchy, widespread injury to both the systemic and pulmonary microcirculations precedes biochemical evidence of organ dysfunction [8, 10, 28]. This type of injury is often seen in conjunction with a loss of cell volume regulation, early mitochondrial disruption in the endothelium and plugging of capillaries by leukocytes. Neutrophil entrapment, initially reported in the pulmonary microcirculation [33], has now been demonstrated in extrapulmonary circulations as MODS evolves [28,32, 34]. The concept that neutrophil-mediated endothelial interaction causes injury to the alveolar-capillary membrane in ARDS [33,35] may therefore be extended to the systemic microcirculation in MODS.

The consequences of a panendothelial injury in MODS are multiple. Tissue edema results from increased microvascular permeability [36–38]. In the lungs, this leads to ventilation–perfusion mismatch and arterial hypoxemia, depressing systemic oxygen delivery (hypoxic hypoxia) and exacerbating tissue hypoxia in remote organs.

The diffuse microcirculatory injury seen in hyperdynamic models of sepsis [39,40] results in a decreased number of perfused capillaries, a phenomenon explained by neutrophil entrapment, endothelial swelling or tissue edema. An already reduced oxygen delivery is further depressed, exacerbating tissue hypoxia, secondary to a reduction in the number of perfused capillaries, increased oxygen carrier-free regions in organs [41] and loss of microvascular control [42]. This results in a broad spectrum of injury within organs ranging from relatively healthy to necrotic tissue.

ARDS AND ORGAN–ORGAN INTERACTIONS

Shock is defined as the failure to provide adequate nutritive flow to tissues. Unrecognized shock in the form of flow-dependent oxygen consumption has been implicated as a possible key factor in patients with ARDS/MODS [43,44]. Flow dependent oxygen consumption was first described in the early 1970s [45–47] and has been observed in patients with high mortality rates, implying that occult tissue hypoxia promotes organ failure [48], (Chapter 20).

Although this phenomenon has been ascribed to technical errors, including measurement techniques and mathematical coupling [49–51], there is still an ongoing debate regarding its significance [52,53] (Chapter 20). Nevertheless, if pathophysiological flow dependency exists in sepsis-related SIRS, organs with marginal nutritive supply may well be rendered hypoxic by the burdens of ARDS and its treatment modalities.

The gastrointestinal tract has been described as the 'motor of MODS', a contention based primarily on epidemiologic data [14]. Further support was added to this hypothesis by the trials of selective decontamination of the digestive tract [54] and research aimed at defining the optimal route for nutrition [55]. These clinical observations were enhanced by research that documented bacterial translocation from the gastrointestinal tract to mesenteric lymph nodes and the portal circulation, a phenomenon shown in a wide variety of rodent models of sepsis [56–58]. However, despite numerous articles describing bacterial translocation, there is as yet no documented link between this event and remote organ failure. It has been suggested that translocation might be a defense mechanism following a stressful insult, leading to initial priming of the immune system [59]. Furthermore, clinical trials have failed to document bacterial translocation in the etiology of MODS [60,61]. Thus, although there is evidence to support the process of bacterial translocation, its true role has yet to be defined. The gastrointestinal tract fails early in MODS and is probably an important

source of ongoing inflammatory mediator generation, which perpetuates the MODS process [62].

Other new evidence also demonstrates that remote organ damage may occur secondary to ALI. Increased wet: dry ratios in the heart, gut and kidneys have been demonstrated in a model of acid aspiration [9]. This study implicated many of the mediators known to be involved in SIRS [63], demonstrated widespread leukosequestration and described a protective role for anti-tumor necrosis factor antiserum in this process. It is therefore quite feasible that, following a direct injury to the lungs, activated neutrophil-endothelial interactions may be responsible for the associated widespread tissue edema [64], remote organ dysfunction and amplification of the systemic inflammatory response that is pathogenic of MODS.

ARDS following a remote systemic insult is therefore the consequence of a panendothelial injury that is within the spectrum of MODS. Acute lung injury that progresses to ARDS from a direct insult may lead to widespread remote organ dysfunction. In this instance the lungs could act as a driving force in a manner similar to Marshall's proposal for the gastrointestinal tract. Although the evidence is equivocal, both probably have a role in the process that ends in MODS. The temporal relationship of remote organ dysfunction to the development of ARDS is also unknown, but may be dependent upon a time differential for different organs to fail.

MANAGEMENT AND FUTURE TRENDS

Prevention, as in so many fields of medicine, should be the aim of therapy. Unfortunately, even in the era of invasive monitoring, rapid surgery, aggressive resuscitation and admission to ICU, the development of MODS appears unrelenting. Despite this, every effort should be made at rapid restoration of oxygen transport where indicated, control and drainage of infective foci and the early aggressive resuscitation of all patients at risk of ARDS, SIRS or MODS.

The lungs play a pivotal role in oxygenation and, when injured, supportive techniques should be aimed at preventing the progression of the disease, not only within the lung but throughout the body. Thus, the management of a patient with ARDS may influence the development of MODS. However, whether the goal of therapy is to prevent MODS in an at risk population or to treat established organ failure, the principle of management are similar.

VENTILATION

The traditional practise of using high inflation pressures to maintain physiological tidal volumes and normalize arterial blood gas tensions has been questioned in recent years. New ventilatory strategies have been developed as the perception of ARDS as a homogeneous injury has been challenged. Computed tomography has demonstrated aerated, compliant areas in nondependant lobes of lungs in patients with ARDS [65] (Chapter 22). These relatively normal units can be damaged by traditional ventilatory techniques, as overt alveolar damage occurs within minutes of exposing normal lungs to high distending pressures [66]. Central to these new therapies has been control of peak airway pressure. Unfortunately, none has proved effective in reducing mortality in well controlled studies. Permissive hypercapnia secondary to pressure controlled, inverse ratio ventilation (PCIRV) has become accepted therapy on the basis of a retrospective study [67] and the value of extracorporeal carbon dioxide removal has fallen into question recently [68]. Although PCIRV is widely used, when it should be instituted is still unclear (Chapters 23 and 24).

HEMODYNAMIC AND FLUID MANAGEMENT

In the management of both hemodynamics and fluid balance in patients with ARDS there are two schools of thought: firstly, whether to pursue normal or supranormal oxygen delivery (DO_2); and, secondly, 'wet versus dry'. Therapy aimed at driving patients to supranormal levels of DO_2 was first described by Shoemaker [69]. No specific trials have addressed this issue in ARDS, although many such patients have been included in trials of the theraputic benefit of supranormal levels of DO_2 [70]. Most of this literature (Chapter 20) has been dogged by experimental errors and inconsistencies of measurement. There is still no definitive evidence that driving patients to supranormal levels of DO_2 improves outcome in the general medical ICU or trauma patient. Clearly, how supranormal levels of DO_2 are attained, using fluids (crystalloid or colloid), blood products or inotropes, must be significant. The majority of trials to date have initially used fluids, attaining a pulmonary artery occlusion pressure of 15–18 mmHg, which would place most of the proponents of supranormal oxygen delivery in to the 'wet' school of therapy.

If the manifestations of ARDS are secondary to permeability pulmonary edema, and fluid flux across the alveolar–capillary membrane follows the Starling equation (Chapters 16, 21 and 28), in theory the intravascular volume should be controlled by fluid restriction. Unfortunately, no definitive clinical trials have resolved this issue. It is conceivable that severe fluid overload influences the onset of MODS in patients with ARDS. A depressed global DO_2 is often seen in conjuction with ARDS, but if the edema that is obvious macroscopically is mirrored within the tissues of vital organs, regional DO_2 would be compromised further; leading to tissue injury. In summary, DO_2 must be maintained and, given an adequate intravascular volume, inotropes should be used to this end.

There is a group of surgical patients to

whom the previously discussed data may not apply. High risk patients undergoing major surgery often develop ARDS and/or MODS. Risk modification in this group of patients emphasizes the early recognition of factors that inappropriately increase postoperative tissue oxygen needs or depress the ability to increase tissue Do_2. Strategies aimed at minimizing intra- and post-operative oxygen deficits may reduce morbidity and mortality. The identification of such patients and the use of the pulmonary artery catheter to guide therapy may reduce tissue oxygen deficit and affect mortality [71].

INFECTION

The inflammatory response to infection (sepsis) is the most frequent precursor of both ARDS and MODS. It is therefore crucial that management strategies exist for preventing and treating infection. These range from policies on hand washing, isolation and room ventilation to intravenous and urinary catheter related sepsis. Whilst selective decontamination of the gut has failed to reduce mortality, it has highlighted the interaction of the gut and bronchial tree in the etiology of nosocomial infections. Early enteral feeding [72] may play a protective role in this area whilst minimizing the loss of gut integrity.

FUTURE THERAPIES

Although the prognosis of ARDS/MODS remains poor, we are entering the decade of immunotherapy. The complex and multiple interactions of inflammatory mediators have ensured that no 'magic bullet' therapy has yet emerged. However, our understanding of these processes is expanding at an unparalleled rate. Monoclonal antibodies have been developed to a number of putative mediators of ARDS/MODS. Despite the failure of the anti-endotoxin antibody HA-1A to fulfill its early promise, clinical trials of an interleukin

receptor antagonist and anti-tumor necrosis factor are underway. Competitive inhibition of platelet activating factor and the use of monoclonal antibodies against neutrophil endothelial interactions are being pursued (Chapter 30).

REFERENCES

1. Asbaugh, D.G., Bigelow, D.B., Petty, T.L. and Levine, B.E. (1967) Acute respiratory distress in adults. *Lancet*, **ii**, 319–23.
2. Dorinsky, P.M. and Gadek J.E. (1990) Multiple organ failure. *Clin. Chest Med.*, **11**, 581–91.
3. Eiseman, B., Beart, R. and Norton L. (1977) Multiple organ failure. *Surg. Gynecol. Obstet.*, **144**, 779–81.
4. Fry, D.E., Pearlstein, L., Fulton, R.L. *et al.* Multiple system organ failure: the role of uncontrolled infection. *Arch. Surg.*, **115**, 136–40.
5. Knaus, W.A., Draper, E.A., Wagner, D.P. and Zimmerman, J.E. (1985) Prognosis in acute organ-system failure. *Ann. Surg.*, **202**, 685–93.
6. Montgomery, A.B., Stager, M.A., Carrico, C.J. *et al.* (1985) Causes of mortality in patients with adult respiratory distress syndrome. *Am. Rev. Respir. Dis.*, **132**, 132–485.
7. Suchyta, M.R., Clemmer, T.P., Elliott, C.G., *et al.* (1992) The adult respiratory distress syndrome: a report of survival and modifying factors. *Chest*, **101**, 74–9.
8. Bone, R. (1992) ACCP/SCCM Consensus Conference. Definitions for sepsis and organ failure and guidelines for the use of innovative therapies in sepsis. *Chest*, **101**, 1644–55.
9. Goldman, G., Shepro, D., Hectman, H.B., *et al.* (1990) Tumor necrosis factor mediates acid aspiration induced systemic organ injury. *Ann. Surg.*, **212**, 513–20.
10. Hersch, M., Berstein, A.D., Neal, A., *et al.* (1989) Quantative evidence of microcirculatory compromise in skeletal muscle of normotensive, hyperdynamic sepsis. *Crit. Care Med.*, **17**, S60.
11. Hersch, M., Gnidec, A.A., Berstein, A.D. *et al.* (1990) Histological and ultrastructural changes in nonpulmonary organs during early hyperdynamic sepsis. *Surgery*, **107**, 397–410.
12. Bernard, G.R. and Artigas, A. (1994) European – American Consensus Conference on ARDS. *Am. J. Respir. Dis. Crit. Care Med.*, **149**, 818–24.
13. Chang, R.W.S., Jacobs, S. and Lee B. (1988)

Predicting outcome among intensive care patients using MSOF scores. *Intensive Care Med.*, **14**, 558–66.

14. Marshall, J.C., Christou, N.V., Horn, R. and Meakins J.L. (1988) The microbiology of multiple organ failure. *Arch. Surg.*, **123**, 309–15.

15. Demling, R.H. (1990) Current concepts on the adult respiratory distress syndrome. *Circ. Shock.* **30**, 297–309.

16. Goris, R.J.A., te Boekhorst, T.P.A., Nuytinch, J.K.S. and Gimbrere, J.S.F. (1985) Multiple-organ failure – generalized autodestructive disease. *Arch. Surg.*, **120**, 1109–15.

17. Marshall, J. and Sweeney, D. (1990) Microbial infection and the septic response in critically ill patients. *Arch. Surg.*, **125**, 17–23.

18. Baue, A.E. (1975) Multiple, progressive or sequential systems failure: a syndrome of the 1970s. *Arch. Surg.*, **110**, 293–8.

19. Crump, J.M., Duncan, D.A. and Wears, R. (1988) Analysis of multiple organ system failure in trauma and non trauma patients. *Am. Surg.*, **54**, 702–8.

20. Seidenfeld, J.J., Pobl, D.F., Bell, R.C. *et al.* (1986) Incidence, site and outcome of infections in patients with adult respiratory distress syndrome. *Am. Rev. Respir. Dis.*, **134**, 12–6.

21. Tran, D.D., Groenveld, A.J., Vandermulen, J. *et al.* (1990) Age, chronic disease, sepsis, organ system failure and mortality in a medical intensive care unit. *Crit. Care Med.*, **18**, 474–9.

22. Pinsky, M. and Matuschak, G. (1990) A unifying hypothesis of multiple systems organ failure: failure of host defense homeostasis. *J. Crit. Care*, **5**, 108–14.

23. Tilney, N., Bailey, G. and Morgan, A. (1973) Sequential systems failure after rupture of abdominal aortic aneurysms: an unsolved problem in postoperative care. *Ann. Surg.*, **178**, 117–2.

24. Fulton, R.L. and Jones, C.E. (1975) The cause of post traumatic pulmonary insufficiency. *Surg. Gynecol. Obstet.*, **140**, 179–86.

25. Waydhas, C., Nast-Kolb, D., Jochum, M. *et al.* (1992) Inflammatory mediators, infection, sepsis, and multiple organ failure. *Arch. Surg.*, **127**, 460–7.

26. Faist, E., Baue, A.E., Dittmer, H. *et al.* (1983) Multiple organ failure in polytrauma patients. *J. Trauma*, **23**, 775–87.

27. Nuytinck, H.K.S., Offermans, C.J.M., Kubat, K. *et al.* (1988) Whole body inflammation in trauma patients: an autopsy study. *Arch. Surg.* **123**, 1517.

28. Mizer, L., Weisbrode, S. and Dorinsky, P.M. (1989) Neutrophil accumulation and structural changes in non-pulmonary organs following phorbol myristate acetate-induced acute lung injury. *Am. Rev. Respir. Dis.*, **139**, 1017–26.

29. Granger, D.N. (1988) Role of xanthine oxidase and granulocytes in ischemia reperfusion injury. *Am. J. Physiol.*, **255**, H1269–75.

30. Dorinsky, P.M. and Gadek J.E. (1989) Mechanisms of multiple nonpulmonary organ failure in ARDS. *Chest*, **96**, 885–92.

31. Eichacker, P.Q., Hoffman, W.D., Farese, A. *et al.* (1991) TNF but not IL-1 in dogs causes lethal lung injury. *J. Appl. Physiol.*, **71**, 1979–89.

32. Natanson, C., Cunnion, R.E., Barrett, D.A. *et al.* (1986) Reversible myocardial dysfunction in a canine model of septic shock is associated with myocardial microcirculatory damage and focal neutrophil infiltration. *Clin. Res.*, **34A**, 639.

33. Warshawski, F., Sibbald, W.J., Driedger, A.A. *et al.* (1986) Abnormal neutrophil-pulmonary interaction in adult respiratory distress syndrome: qualitative and quantitative assessment of pulmonary neutrophil kinetics in humans with *in vivo* 111-indium neutrophil scintigraphy. *Am. Rev. Respir. Dis.*, **133**, 797–804.

34. Welsh, C.H., Lien, D., Worthens, G.S. *et al.* (1988) Pentoxifylline decreases endotoxin induced pulmonary neutrophil sequestration and extravascular protein accumulation in the dog. *Am. Rev. Respir. Dis.*, **138**, 1106.

35. Bersten, A.D., Gnidec, A.A., Rutledge, F.S. *et al.* (1990) Hyperdynamic sepsis modifies a PEEP-mediated redistribution in organ blood flows. *Am. Rev. Respir. Dis.*, **141**, 293–306.

36. Bressack, M.A., Morton, M.S. and Horton, J. (1987) Group streptococcal sepsis in the piglet: effects of fluid therapy on venous return, organ edema and organ blood flow. *Circ. Res.*, **61**: 659–69.

37. Natanson, C., Danner, R.L. and Reilly, J.M. (1990) Antibiotic versus cardiovascular support in a canine model of human septic shock. *Am. J. Physiol.*, **259**, H1140–7.

38. van Lambalgen, A.A., van den Bos, G.C. and Thijs, L. (1989) Blood flow and plasma extravasation in skeletal muscle during endotoxemia. *Int. J. Microcirc. Clin. Exp.*, **8**, 217–32.

39. Farquhar, I., Lam, C., Ellis, C. *et al.* (1992) Intravital microscopy of the mucosal micro-

circulation in sepsis. *Clin. Invest. Med.*, **15**, A25.

40. Lam, C., Tyml, K., Martin, C. and Sibbald W.J. (1994) Microvascular perfusion is impaired in a rat model of normotensive sepsis. *J. Clin. Invest.*, **94**, 2077–83.

41. Gayeski, T.E. (1991) Principal determinants of tissue P_{O_2}, in *Tissue Oxygen Utilization* (eds G. Gutierrez and J.L. Vincent), Springer, Berlin, pp. 56–70.

42. Lewis, D.H. (1987) Disturbances in microcirculatory regulation in septic shock, in *Septic Shock (European View)* (eds J.L. Vincent and L.G. Thijs), Springer, Berlin, pp. 26–34.

43. Moore, F.A., Haenel, J.B., Moore, E.E. *et al.* (1992) Incommensurate oxygen consumption in response to maximal oxygen availability predicts postinjury multiple organ failure. *J. Trauma*, **33**, 58–67.

44. Shoemaker, W.C., Appel, P.L. and Kram, H.B. (1992) Role of oxygen debt in the development of organ failure. *Chest*, **102**, 208–15.

45. Danek, S.J., Lynch, J.P., Weg, J.G., *et al.* (1980) The dependence of oxygen uptake on oxygen delivery in adult respiratory distress syndrome. *Am. Rev. Respir. Dis.*, **122**, 387–95.

46. Powers, S.R., Mannal, R., Neclerio, M. *et al.* (1973) Physiological consequences of positive end expiratory pressure ventilation. *Ann. Surg.*, **178**, 265–72.

47. Rhodes, G.R., Newell, J.C., Shah, D. *et al.* (1978) Increased oxygen consumption accompanying increased oxygen delivery with hypertonic mannitol in adult respiratory distress syndrome. *Surgery*, **84**, 490–7.

48. Bihari, D., Smithies, M., Gimson, A. and Tinker J. (1987) The effects of vasodilation with prostacyclin on oxygen delivery and uptake in critically ill patients. *N. Engl. J. Med.*, **317**, 397–403.

49. Annat, G., Viale, J.P., Percival, C. *et al.* (1986) Oxygen delivery and uptake in adult respiratory distress syndrome. *Am. Rev. Respir. Dis.*, **133**, 999–1001.

50. Ronco, J.J., Phang, P.T., Walley, K.R., *et al.* (1991) Oxygen consumption is independent of increase in oxygen delivery in severe adult respiratory distress syndrome. *Am. Rev. Respir. Dis.*, **143**, 1267–73.

51. Vermeij, C.G., Feenstra, B.W. and Bruining, H.A. (1990) Oxygen delivery and oxygen uptake in post-operative and septic patients. *Chest*, **98**, 415–20.

52. Russell, J.A. and Phang, P.T. (1994) The oxygen delivery/consumption controversy. Approaches to management of the crtically ill. *Am. Rev. Respir. Dis.*, **149**, 533–7.

53. Schumacker, P.T. and Samsel, R.W. (1990) Oxygen supply and consumption in the adult respiratory distress syndrome. *Clin. Chest Med.*, **11**, 715–22.

54. Reidy, J.J. and Ramsay, G. (1990) Clinical trials of selective decontamination of the digestive tract. *Crit. Care Med.*, **18**, 1449–56.

55. Moore, F.A., Feliciano, D.V., Moore, E.E. *et al.* (1992) Early enteral feeding, compared with parenteral reduces postoperative septic complications. *Ann. Surg.*, **216**, 172–83.

56. Deitch, E.A. (1990) The role of intestinal barrier failure and bacterial translocation in the development of systemic infection and multiple organ failure. *Arch. Surg.*, **125**, 403–4.

57. Herndon, D.N. and Zeigler, S.T. (1993) Bacterial translocation after thermal injury. *Crit. Care Med.* **21**, S50–4.

58. Mainous, M.R., Xu, D. and Deitch, E.A. (1993) Role of xanthine oxidase and prostaglandins in inflammatory-induced bacterial translocation. *Circ. Shock*, **40**, 99–104.

59. Wells, C.L. (1990) Relationship between intestinal microecology and the translocation of intestinal bacteria. *Antonie Van Leeuwenhoek*, **58**, 87–93.

60. Cerra, F.B., Maddaus, M.A., Dunn, D.L. *et al.* (1992) Selective gut decontamination reduces nosocomial pneumonia infections and length of stay but not mortality or organ failure in sugical intensive care unit patients. *Arch. Surg.*, **127**, 163–9.

61. Moore, F.A., Moore, E.E., Poggetti, R. *et al.* (1991) Gut bacterial translocation via the portal vein: a clinical perspective with major torso trauma. *J. Trauma*, **31**, 629–36.

62. Marshall, J.C., Christou, N.V. and Meakins J.L. (1993) The gastrointestinal tract: the 'undrained abcess' of multiple organ failure. *Ann. Surg.*, **218**, 111–9.

63. Welbourn, R., Shepro, D., Hectman, H.B. *et al.* (1990) Involvement of thromboxane and neutrophils in multiple systems organ edema with interleukin-2. *Ann. Surg.*, **212**, 728–33.

64. Goldman, G., Shepro, D., Hectman, H.B., *et al.* (1992) Adherent neutrophils mediate permeability after atelectasis. *Ann. Surg.*, **216**, 372–80.

65. Gattinoni, L., Pelosi, P., Pesenti, A. *et al.* (1991)

CT scan in ARDS: clinical and physiopathological insights. *Acta Anaesthesiol. Scand. Suppl.*, **95**, 87–94.

66. Dreyfuss, D., Soler, P., Basser, G. and Saumon, G. (1985) High inflation pressure pulmonary edema. *Am. Rev. Respir. Dis.*, **132**, 880–4.

67. Hickling, K.G., Henderson, S.J. and Jackson, R. (1990) Low mortality associated with low volume pressure limited ventilation with permissive hypercapnia in severe adult respiratory distress syndrome. *Intensive Care Med.*, **16**, 372–7.

68. Morris, A.H., Wallace, J.C., Menlove, R.C. *et al.* (1994) Randomized clinical trial of pressure controlled inverse ratio ventilation and extracorporeal cabon dioxide removal for ARDS. *Am. Rev. Respir. Dis.*, **149**, 295–305.

69. Shoemaker, W.C., Appel, P.L., Kram, H.B. *et al.* (1988) Prospective trial of supranormal values of survivors as therapeutic goals in high risk surgical patients. *Chest*, **94**, 1176–86.

70. Creamer, J.E., Edwards, J.D. and Nightingale, P. (1990) Hemodynamic and oxygen transport variables in cardiogenic shock secondary to acute myocardial infarction, and response to vasoactive therapy. *Am. J. Cardiol.*, **65**, 1297–300.

71. Boyd, O., Grounds, M. and Bennett, D. (1993) A randomized clinical trial of the effect of deliberate perioperative increase of oxygen delivery on mortality in high-risk surgical patients. *JAMA*, **270**, 2699–707.

72. Moore, E.E. and Jones, T.N. (1986) Benefits of feeding after major abdominal trauma – a prospective randomized study. *J. Trauma*, **26**, 874–81.

Jean-Louis Vincent and Daniel De Backer

Although initial studies of the syndrome of acute respiratory distress in adults (ARDS) focused on alterations in lung structure and function and specific means of supporting the lung, recent concepts have emphasized the importance of global alterations in physiology, involving the entire body (Chapter 18). Several factors can explain this evolution. Firstly, although ARDS may be associated with a primary lung injury such as aspiration, smoke inhalation or neardrowning, it often develops in the context of severe sepsis originating from other organs. Furthermore, when death occurs, it is more commonly related to sepsis and multiple organ failure than to refractory hypoxemia. Important information in this regard was provided by Montgomery et al. [1], who observed that only 16% (5 of 32) of patients with ARDS died from irreversible respiratory failure (Chapter 2).

Secondly, a better understanding of the inflammatory response to a number of injuries has identified a series of cellular elements (leukocytes, macrophages, endothelial cells) and inflammatory mediators, such as tumor necrosis factor (TNF), that are simultaneously involved in the development of ARDS and the failure of other organs. Thirdly, ARDS is associated with alterations in peripheral gas exchange, characterized by an abnormal relationship between oxygen consumption (V_{O_2}) and oxygen delivery (D_{O_2}). Since tissue hypoxia may be involved in the development of ARDS like other forms of organ failure, these developments may have important clinical implications. This chapter summarizes these concepts, presents some of the controversies surrounding them and evaluates some of the implications in the management of these patients.

CONCEPT OF V_{O_2}/D_{O_2} DEPENDENCY

In physiological conditions, V_{O_2} is independent of D_{O_2}. If D_{O_2} decreases, oxygen extraction (O_2ER) by the tissues increases to maintain a constant V_{O_2} to equal oxygen demand. It is only when D_{O_2} is reduced below a very low value (D_{O_2}crit) that this compensatory increase in O_2ER becomes insufficient and V_{O_2} starts to decline. In these conditions, V_{O_2} becomes dependent on D_{O_2}. O_2ER at D_{O_2}-crit (O_2ERcrit) is usually around 70–75%. Below D_{O_2}crit, the development of tissue hypoxia is reflected in an increase in blood lactate levels [2–6] and a significant widening of the venoarterial P_{CO_2} gradient [7,8] (Figure 19.1). These physiological changes, well described initially by Cain [2], were subsequently further documented by other groups of investigators [3–9]. A similar scheme has been established on various models where D_{O_2} is reduced by a reduction in blood flow, hemoglobin levels or Pa_{O_2} [2–9].

Some of these experimental studies have reproduced the alterations in extraction capabilities by administration of endotoxin or

ARDS Acute Respiratory Distress in Adults. Edited by Timothy W. Evans and Christopher Haslett. Published in 1996 by Chapman & Hall, London. ISBN 0 412 56910 8

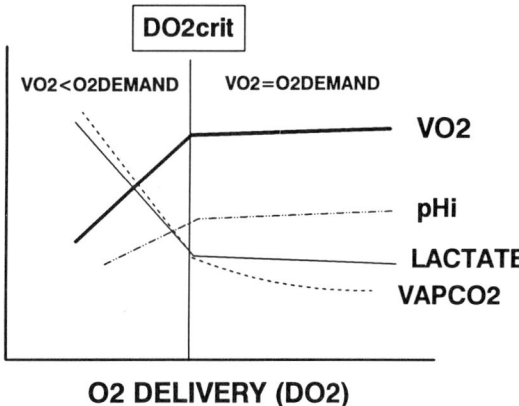

Figure 19.1 Relationship between oxygen consumption (V_{O_2}) and oxygen delivery (D_{O_2}) in animal studies where D_{O_2} is progressively reduced. Critical D_{O_2} levels can be determined from V_{O_2} levels, from lactate levels or from venoarterial CO_2 gradients.

bacteria to animals. In a model of hemorrhagic shock [3] the administration of endotoxin was shown to result in an increase in D_{O_2}crit from 6.8 to 12.8 ml/kg/min, reflecting the alterations in extraction capabilities during sepsis. Similarly, in a model of cardiac tamponade [6] an increase in D_{O_2}crit was deducted from 9.6 to 12.1 ml/kg/min and a simultaneous reduction of o_2ERcrit from 60.3 to 47.2% (Figure 19.2). Thus, animal experiments clearly demonstrate that sepsis can acutely alter oxygen extraction capabilities, although these may not be related specifically to the presence of respiratory failure. In particular, neither the development of acute lung injury induced by oleic acid administration [10] nor the application of positive end expiratory pressure (PEEP) [10,11] alter the V_{O_2}/D_{O_2} relationship.

If oxygen demand is simultaneously increased by the inflammatory response to infection, these alterations may account for what has been called pathological V_{O_2}/D_{O_2} dependency, whereby V_{O_2} remains dependent on D_{O_2} above the value of D_{O_2}crit found under control conditions. It is noteworthy

that differences in D_{O_2}crit and o_2ERcrit observed in acute experimental studies are significant and large enough to allow the documentation of the beneficial effects of some therapeutic interventions [12,13].

Decreased oxygen extraction could be induced in earlier studies in experimental models using microembolization with microspheres [14,15]. Furthermore, alterations in oxygen extraction are primarily attributed to microvascular disturbances associated with the release of various mediators, leukocyte plugging, endothelial swelling, alterations in the control of vascular tone and formation of edema. Alterations in oxygen convection therefore seem to predominate over alterations in diffusion, since an increase in Pa_{O_2} does not improve the extraction capabilities [16].

In anesthetized men undergoing surgery involving cardiopulmonary bypass [17] a reduction in D_{O_2} below 330 ml/min/m^2 was associated with a fall in V_{O_2} and a simultaneous rise in blood lactate levels. More recently [18], serial measurements of V_{O_2} when D_{O_2} was progressively reduced during terminal discontinuation of lifesupport showed a very low D_{O_2}crit (3.8–4.5 ml/min/m^2) and a critical o_2ER of approximately 60%.

PATHOLOGICAL V_{O_2}/D_{O_2} DEPENDENCY

The idea of pathological V_{O_2}/D_{O_2} dependency in patients with ARDS was proposed more than 20 years ago [19] when changes in V_{O_2} and D_{O_2} were measured during the application of PEEP, and a strong positive correlation was detected between the two variables. In 1980 [20], V_{O_2} was shown to vary directly and linearly with changes in D_{O_2} in patients with ARDS, but not in another group of mechanically ventilated patients. In both studies, the observations were made when D_{O_2} was well within the normal range, suggesting that oxygen extraction capabilities were markedly altered in these patients. Such observations may have important clinical

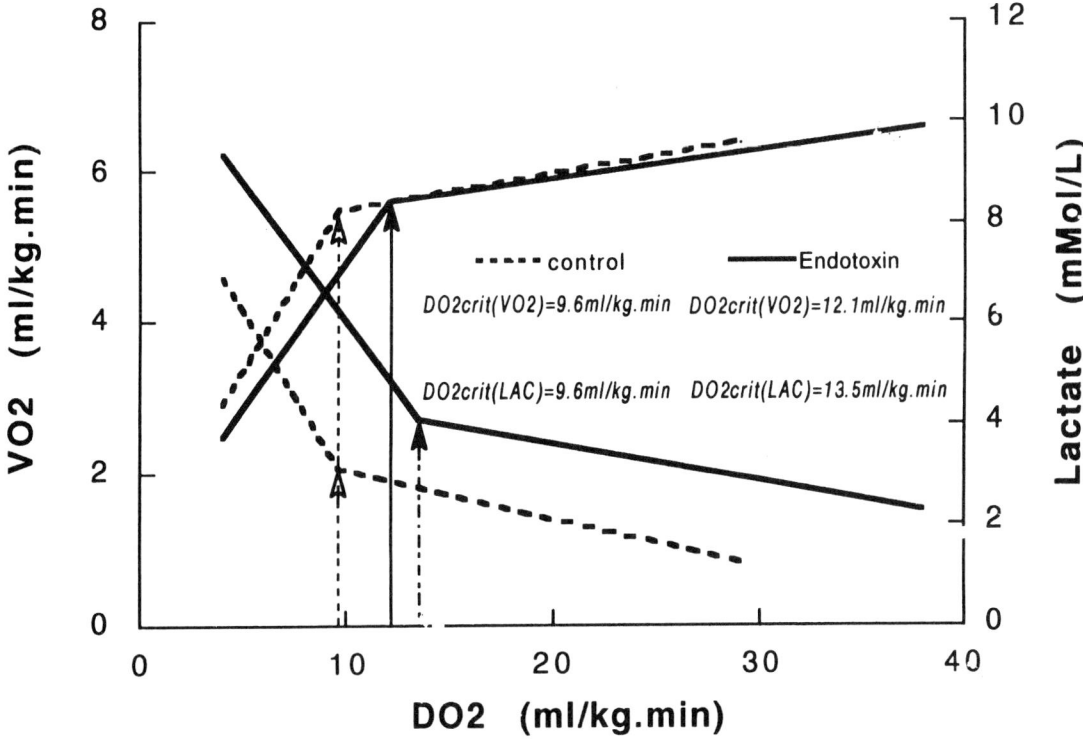

Figure 19.2 Effects of endotoxin on the relation between oxygen uptake and oxygen delivery when cardiac output is progressively reduced by tamponade. (Reproduced with permission from Zhang and Vincent [6]).

implications, since in the absence of effective methods to increase V_O^2, a further increase in D_{O_2} may represent a valuable therapeutic option to correct underlying cellular hypoxia.

Similar observations were extended to patients with severe sepsis with or without ARDS. Thus [21], an increase in D_{O_2} induced by prostacyclin was thought to reveal pathological V_{O_2}/D_{O_2} dependency characteristic of nonsurvivors. In survivors and normal volunteers, prostacyclin infusion increased D_{O_2} to the same degree, but failed to increase V_{O_2}. A number of investigators have subsequently confirmed the presence of a pathological V_{O_2}/D_{O_2} dependency in some patients but with one possible exception [22], they have failed to relate it to mortality. However, several studies [23–26] related the presence of patho-

logical V_{O_2}/D_{O_2} dependency to the presence of increased blood lactate levels, suggesting that V_{O_2}/D_{O_2} dependency is a hallmark of acute circulatory failure, reflecting the presence of tissue hypoxia.

CHALLENGES TO THE V_{O_2}/D_{O_2} DEPENDENCY THEORY

Several challenges have been presented to the existence of pathological V_{O_2}/D_{O_2} dependency. Five major questions have been raised.

Could changes in oxygen demand account for the observed alterations in the V_{O_2}/D_{O_2} relationship?

It is quite obvious that oxygen demand can vary substantially in critically ill patients under the effects of stress, sedation or paralysis [27]; the various modes of ventilation and other interventions at the bedside [28]. Hence, a single plot of V_{O_2}/D_{O_2} showing a significant relationship between the two variables may indicate a normal response to changes in oxygen demand (the independent variable) rather than pathological V_{O_2}/D_{O_2} dependency. Similar observations can be made in surgical patients during the early postoperative phase [29] or even in healthy humans, whose cardiac output can be lower during the night but higher during exercise. However, most recent studies have reported changes in V_{O_2} during an acute increase in D_{O_2} when all other factors were otherwise maintained stable, so that oxygen demand can be assumed to have remained constant.

Could pathological V_{O_2}/D_{O_2} dependency be artifactual?

A problem of mathematical coupling arises when a variable is included in the two components of a regression analysis. The effect of any error of this variable is thereby enhanced, so that it may force an association between two otherwise independent variables [30]. Many studies describing pathological V_{O_2}/D_{O_2} relations were exposed to this problem of mathematical coupling of data, since both V_{O_2} and D_{O_2} were calculated from the same measurements of cardiac output, hemoglobin concentration and arterial oxygen saturation. While errors in the last two parameters are likely to be relatively small, inaccuracies in the thermodilution technique may be as high as 5–10% [31]. This thesis was supported by several studies in which no change in V_{O_2} was observed during acute interventions resulting in changes in D_{O_2} [32–35]. Several arguments can be advanced to refute these criticisms.

Firstly, the problem of mathematical coupling of data is particularly significant when simple plots of V_{O_2} and D_{O_2} are used, but can hardly explain the pathological V_{O_2}/D_{O_2} relationship found during an acute intervention that increases D_{O_2}. Indeed, if any measurement of cardiac output is associated with a relative error, the value obtained after the acute intervention might be erroneously

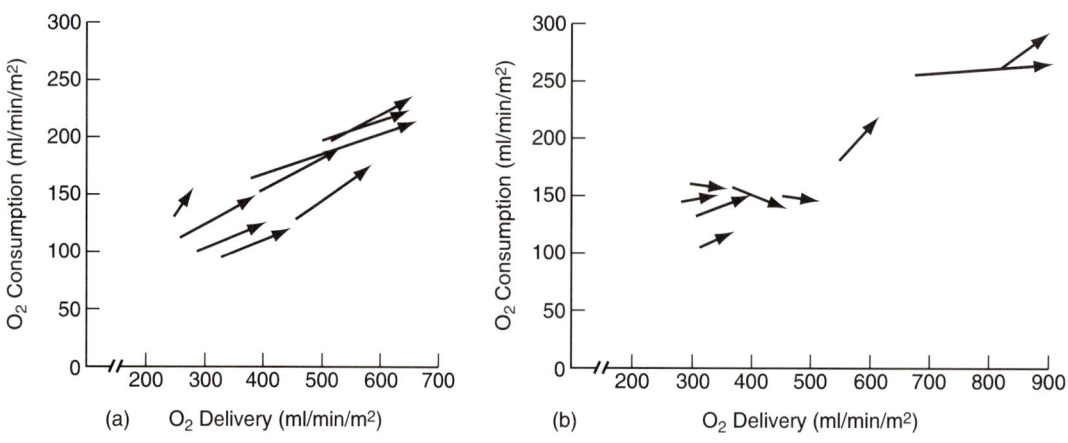

Figure 19.3 Effects of a limited dose (5 μg/kg/min) of dobutamine on the relation between oxygen uptake (V_{O_2}) and oxygen delivery (D_{O_2}) in patients with ARDS (a) with ($n = 9$, increased lactate) and (b) without ($n = 9$, normal lactate) acute circulatory failure (as reflected by blood lactate levels). (Reproduced with permission from Vincent *et al.* [25].)

higher **or** lower than the actual value. Hence, this problem would mask rather than enhance any V_{O_2}/D_{O_2} dependency. Nevertheless, Ronco *et al.* [35] implied that the thermodilution technique may significantly overestimate a high cardiac output. Such an overestimation should be highly significant, but this is not supported by the many studies validating the thermodilution technique [31]. Secondly, the mathematical problem has been studied in depth [36] and is probably small, provided that the error in measurement is reasonable, and the increase in D_{O_2} large enough. Thirdly, several studies have observed V_{O_2}/D_{O_2} dependency in some groups of patients but not in others. In particular, the presence or absence of elevated blood lactate levels was used to separate these groups [4,23–26] (Figure 19.3). Since the degree of change in V_{O_2} and D_{O_2} was similar between these groups, it is difficult to explain how the problem of mathematical coupling may take place in one group of patients and not in the other. Fourthly, a number of studies has shown a good agreement between direct and indirect determinations of V_{O_2} [37–40] and, in our experience, the two methods usually correlate well [41]. Fifthly, the problem of mathematical coupling of data can be avoided by considering the relationship between cardiac output and the arteriovenous oxygen difference or oxygen extraction, and such an analysis yields the same type of conclusion [9,42,43]. This is the approach that we prefer today, because it is also the simplest one. Finally, those who challenge the determination of V_{O_2} from the reverse Fick equation,

can be challenged themselves for the very stable V_{O_2} consistently observed in all their critically ill patients. In one study, V_{O_2} remained quite stable, even during the administration of large doses (15 µg/kg/min) of dobutamine [33]. In a second, blood transfusion increased D_{O_2} through an increase in arterial oxygen content, but the thermodilution cardiac output remained unchanged [35], while the arteriovenous oxygen difference increased. The V_{O_2} estimated indirectly increased, whereas that estimated directly remained stable, so that the authors incriminated the thermodilution cardiac output measurements in a spurious pathological V_{O_2}/D_{O_2} phenomenon. There are only two possible explanations for these findings. One is that the direct V_{O_2} determinations were correct, in which case the increase in arteriovenous oxygen difference implied a reduced cardiac output. In these circumstances, D_{O_2} would not have increased during blood transfusion, thereby invalidating the study. Alternatively, cardiac output remained unchanged, so that V_{O_2} increased and the direct measurement of V_{O_2} was erroneous. Indeed, the authors admitted that they did not trust the thermodilution measurements when they were included in one equation (indirect V_{O_2}), but found them to be accurate when they were used in the other (D_{O_2}).

One should underline that any measurement has an inherent degree of inaccuracy, and that even an expensive instrument is not devoid of such problems. Some investigators find that the calculation of V_{O_2} by indirect (Fick derived) methods involves too many

Table 19.1 Formulas involved in indirect and direct V_{O_2} determinations

$V_{O_2}\text{indir} = CO \times (Ca_{O_2} - Cv_{O_2}) \cong CO \times Hb \times (Sa_{O_2} - Sv_{O_2})$

$V_{O_2}\text{dir} = V_E ((F_{IO_2}[(1 - F_{ECO_2} - F_{EO_2})/(1 - F_{IO_2})]) - F_{EO_2})$

CO = cardiac output; Ca_{O_2} = arterial oxygen content; Cv_{O_2} = venous oxygen content; Hb = hemoglobin saturation; Sa_{O_2} = arterial oxygen saturation; Sv_{O_2} = mixed venous oxygen saturation; V_E = expired minute volume; F_{IO_2} = inspired oxygen fraction; F_{EO_2} = expired oxygen fraction; F_{ECO_2} = expired carbon dioxide fraction.

sources of error. However, the direct method involves approximations in the measurements of expired minute volume, inspired and expired oxygen fractions and expired carbon dioxide fraction (Table 19.1). What is true is that V_{O_2} is usually found to be higher when determined from direct gas analysis than from indirect calculation [41] because oxygen consumption by the lungs is not included in the latter analysis [44].

Could the administration of adrenergic agents increase V_{O_2} by a thermogenic effect?

It has been recognized for many years that catecholamines can stimulate cellular metabolism and induce a thermogenic effect in the tissues [45,46]. This observation was taken into account when dobutamine was used as an inotropic agent to increase D_{O_2} acutely [25]. Two more recent studies have shown that dobutamine can also increase V_{O_2} in normal volunteers [47,48]. In critically ill patients, it was hypothesized that the thermogenic effect of dobutamine would be less significant as they are already under stress and often under the influence of elevated levels of endogenous catecholamines. Indeed, previous studies suggested that V_{O_2} remained stable during the administration of dobutamine in patients with congestive heart failure [49,50]. The experience showed that dobutamine induced a significantly greater increase in V_{O_2} in patients with hemodynamic instability, as reflected by elevated blood lactate levels, than it did in those who were hemodynamically stable, with normal blood lactate levels [25]. Other studies confirmed that limited doses of dobutamine do not increase V_{O_2} in the critically ill [9,33,41,51–53]. The different effects of dobutamine on V_{O_2} in volunteers and in critically ill patients under stress are illustrated by a recent study by Uusaro *et al.* in volunteers showing that the thermogenic effects of dobutamine are reduced by stress induced by a triple hor-

mone infusion [54]. Hence, a thermogenic effect of catecholamines cannot account for spurious V_{O_2}/D_{O_2} dependency.

Do blood lactate levels represent good markers of cellular hypoxia?

Experimental studies have consistently detected an abrupt increase in blood lactate as soon as D_{O_2} falls below D_{O_2}crit [2–6]. The recent report of dying patients in whom D_{O_2} decreased during withdrawal of cardio-respiratory support showed the same observations [18]. The suggestion that V_{O_2}/D_{O_2} dependency is observed in the presence of increased blood lactate levels has been challenged by investigators who found no such dependency, even in patients with normal blood lactate levels [33,35]. This controversy stems from a misinterpretation of the former studies, in which patients with sepsis or heart failure with acute circulatory failure were compared with those without evidence of circulatory impairment. Blood lactate levels were used only as a marker of cellular hypoxia: Ronco and colleagues [33,35] acknowledged that they studied patients who were hemodynamically stable, in whom increased blood lactate levels may reflect previous rather than ongoing hypoxia, or altered liver failure could account for a delayed clearance of lactate.

Unfortunately, evaluation of tissue oxygen status cannot be based only on blood lactate levels. If this were true, the monitoring of cardiac output and mixed venous oxygen saturation ($S_{V_{O_2}}$) would no longer be necessary because treatment could be guided by blood lactate levels only. This is obviously an oversimplification.

Can the experimental observations be reproduced in patients?

A fundamental difference between the experimental and clinical studies investigating the relation between V_{O_2} and D_{O_2} is that the former [2–8] have usually investigated changes in V_{O_2} during an acute reduction in D_{O_2}. By contrast, most clinical studies (with the exception of some studies applying PEEP to decrease cardiac output [32,55]) employed acute increases in D_{O_2} because these are safer to apply. In addition, experimental studies allow the collection of numerous data points, whereas clinical studies are often limited to two or three measurements. An exception is the investigation of Ronco *et al.* [18], which studied V_{O_2} consequent upon the reduction in D_{O_2} associated with the withdrawal of cardiorespiratory support, with very similar findings to those seen in experimental studies.

PRACTICAL IMPLICATIONS

Despite these controversies, the importance of maintaining adequate oxygen delivery in patients with ARDS is now accepted. There are several ways to increase D_{O_2} (Table 19.2). Respiratory support should be provided to maintain Pa_{O_2} close to the normal range, and in any case above 60 mmHg to avoid the brisk fall in Sa_{O_2} associated with lower values of Pa_{O_2}. Nevertheless, attempts to maintain a high D_{O_2} by supranormal Pa_{O_2} cannot be recommended for two reasons. Firstly, the impact on D_{O_2} of an increase in Sa_{O_2} would be minimal and the increase in dissolved oxygen negligible, such that the risk to the patient in terms of oxygen toxicity and PEEP may far outweigh the minimal gain. Secondly, hyperoxia induced vasoconstriction may limit oxygen supply to the periphery, rather than increasing it.

The problem of optimal hematocrit is also complex, as large vessel hematocrit can be higher than that measurable in the capillaries. Furthermore, there is an inverse relationship between cardiac output and hematocrit, so that an increase in hemoglobin is not always associated with an increase in D_{O_2} and a lower hematocrit may improve the oxygen extraction capabilities of the body [5]. Hence, a hematocrit between 30 and 33% is considered optimal in patients with ARDS.

A third problem concerns the adequacy of cardiac output. There are good reasons to maintain D_{O_2} by increasing blood flow rather than arterial oxygen content. Firstly, the oxygen extraction capabilities are limited less by problems of diffusion than by oxygen convection [16]. Thus, increasing Pa_{O_2} is unlikely to increase cellular oxygen availability when D_{O_2} has fallen below D_{O_2}crit. Secondly, the organism can compensate for a fall in arterial content by increasing cardiac output, but the reverse is not true, at least in acute conditions. Thirdly, the development of diaphragm fatigue is retarded by an increase in blood flow, but not by an increase in arterial oxygen content [56]. Fourthly, an increase in V_{O_2} may be more consistently obtained with dobutamine than with blood transfusion [57]. Finally, recent studies have indicated that a higher blood flow may limit the cellular damage consequent upon the inflammatory reaction [58].

Table 19.2 The three levels of oxygen delivery, with their components and the possible interventions

Level	Component	Intervention
Global (aortic)	Pa_{O_2}	Oxygen, PEEP
	Hemoglobin	Blood transfusion
	Cardiac output	Fluids/dobutamine/vasodilators
Regional (interorgan)	Blood flow	Dopamine?
	Distribution	Dopexamine?
Microvascular (intraorgan)	Arteriolar tone	Crystalloids versus colloids
	Capillary surface	N-acetylcysteine, pentoxiphylline, prostaglandin E_1, etc.

WHAT ARE THE GUIDES TO THERAPY?

There are basically three possible approaches to therapy: the global, 'nonbeliever' and titrated approaches.

GLOBAL APPROACH: MAINTENANCE OF Do_2 AT SUPRANORMAL LEVELS IN ALL PATIENTS AT RISK

This approach, proposed by Shoemaker and colleagues [59], and followed by others [60], is based on the observation that among patients with ARDS, survivors have a higher Do_2 than nonsurvivors [61,62]. Furthermore, the maintenance of Do_2 at supranormal levels (above $600\,ml/min/m^2$) in surgical patients at risk may reduce morbidity and mortality rates [59] and has been proposed as a means of avoiding ARDS in trauma patients [63]. However, employing the same approach in patients with septic shock was not associated with a significant increase in survival, although patients with a higher Do_2 may have a better outcome, regardless of whether the supranormal value was part of the protocol or not [60]. Others [64,65] have extended these observations by showing that patients with higher Do_2 values may have a better chance of survival because they have greater physiological reserves than other patients.

More importantly, the patient at risk of complications, in whom tissue hypoxia may still be present, must be identified. The maintenance of supranormal Do_2 values in a large number of at risk patients may lead to overzealous administration of fluid and adrenergic agents in patients who may not need this form of therapy, and which may worsen gas exchange and myocardial ischemia, and even increase mortality rate [66].

'NONBELIEVER' APPROACH

In view of the controversies raised above, the inherent risk of increasing Do_2 to supranormal values in all at risk patients, and the difficulties in assessing the oxygen status of the tissues, some clinicians still prefer to adopt a conservative approach, relying more on their clinical examination, repeated chest radiographs and arterial blood gas analyses to guide therapy. These clinicians still focus their management on the maintenance of 'dry' lungs by fluid restriction, generous diuretic therapy and perhaps infusion of low doses of dopamine or use of hemofiltration techniques. Even though the use of the pulmonary artery catheter has been criticized [67], this attitude becomes increasingly difficult to defend in the presence of accumulating data to support the view that ARDS is part of a global disease process and that hypoxia and hypoxemia are not synonymous (Chapter 18).

TITRATED APPROACH

Other investigators base their management on the fact that tissue hypoxia may play a role in the development and worsening of ARDS. Although overhydration should be avoided, the maintenance of hypovolemia is also undesirable because it can compromise cardiac output, Do_2 and tissue function. It is only when the hemodynamic status is stable and provided that it remains stable that prudent fluid restriction can be applied. Fluid administration should be carefully monitored under the guidance of invasive hemodynamic monitoring. Even monitoring of lung water has been recommended [68] (Chapter 28).

It is only when blood volume has been restored that vasopressors may be indicated to sustain tissue perfusion pressure in the presence of circulatory shock. Vasoconstriction should be avoided by all means, so that the use of dobutamine as an inotropic agent may be indicated to increase blood flow and Do_2 to the tissues [69]. This therapeutic option is further supported by the observation that myocardial depression is an early event in severe sepsis, especially in nonsurvivors [70]. In addition to the monitoring of cardiac filling pressures, therapy with fluids and vasoactive agents can be guided by repeated measurements of cardiac output and blood oxygen content. Several monitoring sytems can be considered.

Cardiac index/o₂ER diagram

It is evident that the first management step is to correct hypoxemia and anemia. Once this has been achieved, cardiac output becomes the primary determinant of Do_2 and must therefore be adapted to the oxygen needs of the tissues. Rather than trying to maintain a supranormal cardiac output in all critically ill patients, it is more reasonable to take oxygen demand into account. For instance, a low cardiac output may be appropriate in a sedated, paralyzed patient with ARDS undergoing mechanical ventilation, and without evidence of infection. By contrast, it may be inappropriate in another patient treated with continuous positive airway pressure, with underlying sepsis and some degree of anxiety. The measurement of Svo_2 can be very useful in interpreting the adequacy or otherwise of cardiac output. A relationship between cardiac output and Svo_2 may be considered useful [71,72], but the relationship between cardiac index and o_2ER is more advisable for three reasons.

Firstly, Svo_2 is directly influenced by arterial oxygen saturation (Sao_2), and Sao_2 can still vary by up to 10% (e.g. between 90 and 98%) in the patient with ARDS. Secondly, the relationship between cardiac index and Svo_2 is curvilinear, rendering the interpretation of data quite difficult [72,73]. However, in the relationship between cardiac index and o_2ER, Vo_2 is represented by curvilinear isopleths, so that patients with low Vo_2 will be found closer to the origin and those with either high Vo_2 or anemia will be in the zone far from the origin (Figure 19.4). Furthermore, the diagram allows the introduction of a line of reference which is derived from observations in exercising individuals. During exercise, the increase in Vo_2 is obtained by equal contribu-

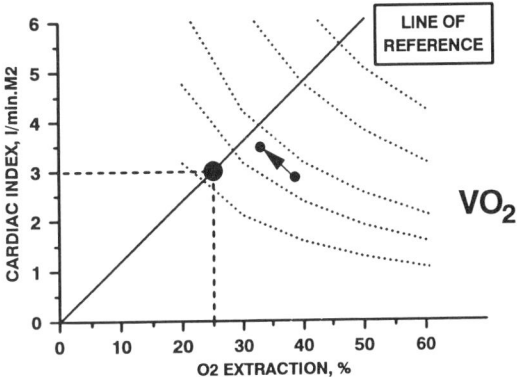

Figure 19.4 Cardiac index/oxygen extraction diagram to interpret hemodynamic data. The line of reference to exercise starts from the origin and passes through normal values of cardiac index (3 l/min/m²) and o_2ER (25%), respectively. The figure shows the hemodynamic response of a patient with ARDS to an infusion of 5 μg/kg/min of dobutamine. Initially, the cardiac index was normal but the o_2ER was increased (the data points were below the line of reference). The movement along the Vo_2 isopleths during the dobutamine infusion indicates Vo_2/Do_2 independence.

tions of an increase in cardiac output and an increase in o_2ER [74]. Thus, the distance between the data points of an individual and the linc of reference will reflect the degree of cardiac dysfunction. This type of cardiac index/o_2ER diagram reflects the relationship between central (cardiac output) and peripheral (how the tissues adapt to their blood flow) parameters, but does not produce any information about the distribution of blood flow or the presence of tissue hypoxia.

Blood lactate levels

In experimental studies where Do_2 is progressively reduced by an acute intervention, the coincidence of a reduction in Vo_2 and an increase in blood lactate levels is striking (Figure 19.1), to the extent that Do_2crit can be determined from either Vo_2 or lactate measurements, the two results being superposable [2–6]. However, the clinical interpretation of increased blood lactate levels is much more complex. Specifically, they reflect not only lactate production, but also lactate elimination, which can be protracted in the presence of liver dysfunction. In addition, pyruvate metabolism can be altered in the presence of sepsis, so that lactate levels may be increased in the absence of established tissue hypoxia [75]. Nevertheless, the V_{O_2}/D_{O_2} dependency phenomenon is usually associated with hyperlactatemia, provided that this is related to the presence of acute circulatory failure [23–26]. Hyperlactatemia has been shown to correlate with mortality and organ failure in septic shock [41,76].

Gastric intramucosal pH

Tonometric measurements of gastric intramucosal pH (pHi) are supposed to reflect the adequacy of perfusion of the gastric mucosa. In addition, the gut mucosa may be particularly at risk of ischemia during hypoperfusion states [77]. The presence of a persistently low pHi has been correlated with a poor outcome in critically ill patients [78,79]. A low pHi has also been related to the presence of V_{O_2}/D_{O_2} dependency [52].

Increased venoarterial P_{CO_2} gradients

In animal studies the onset of tissue hypoxia (i.e. below D_{O_2}crit) is also associated with a brisk increase in the venoarterial P_{CO_2} gradient (VAP_{CO_2}), reflecting the development of cellular acidosis [8]. Again, several factors can influence VAP_{CO_2} in critically ill patients. Nevertheless, VAP_{CO_2} has been reported to be higher in nonsurvivors from septic shock [80,81], and a trend analysis of VAP_{CO_2} may be helpful.

V_{O_2} challenge

If the question of whether or not tissue oxygenation is adequate remains unanswered, a simple test can be performed to evaluate whether V_{O_2} is influenced by a transient increase in cardiac output. This 'V_{O_2} challenge' can be accomplished via the administration of fluids or blood, although a fluid challenge is not always indicated in ARDS. Alternatively, Bihari *et al.* [21] showed that a given dose of 5 ng/kg/min of prostacyclin could disclose the V_{O_2}/D_{O_2} dependency in patients with sepsis or acute respiratory failure. They called this an 'O_2 flux test', implying that microcirculatory effects of prostacyclin could play a role in increasing V_{O_2}. Unfortunately, although prostaglandins may improve tissue oxygen extraction capabilities in sepsis [12], prostacyclin is not always well tolerated in these patients. We have found it particularly convenient to use a limited dose of 5 µg/kg/min of dobutamine, which has significant effects on cardiac output and thus D_{O_2}, but is well tolerated even in the presence of circulatory shock [69]. When compared with dobutamine, prostacyclin can reduce arterial pressure and impair gas exchange [42]. Note that a larger dose of dobutamine is associated with an increase in V_{O_2} in all individuals by a thermogenic effect, and should be avoided for the purposes of this test. As this V_{O_2} challenge requires that the oxygen demand of the patient remains stable during the procedure, it should not take more than 20 – 30 minutes and should be performed in a stable, quiet environment. Particular care must be taken to measure cardiac output accurately and to determine Sv_{O_2} simultaneously.

Using the cardiac index/O_2ER diagram, avoids cumbersome calculations of D_{O_2} and V_{O_2}, since one can assume that hemoglobin level does not change. Therefore, the increase in cardiac index should be matched by a corresponding reduction in O_2ER, and the data points should move along the isopleths drawn on the diagram (Figure 19.4). If, on the other hand, the V_{O_2} increases significantly, as indicated by a movement which is no longer parallel to the V_{O_2} isopleths, cardiac output would probably not be adequate to meet the oxygen demand, so that some form of ther-

Table 19.3 The four steps in the interpretation of a cardiac output value

---

1. Refer to patient's size
   Body surface area
2. Refer to oxygen delivery
   Sa_{O_2}
   Hb
3. Refer to oxygen consumption
   Sv_{O_2} or o_2ER
4. Refer to oxygen demand
   Lactate
   pHi
   VAP_{CO_2}
   Vo_2 challenge

---

apy aimed at increasing cardiac output would be rational. This could consist of the administration of intravenous fluids or a vasoactive agent, such as dobutamine, but this time for therapeutic rather than diagnostic purposes.

CONCLUSION

A pathological Vo_2/Do_2 dependency state can be found in some patients with ARDS, in whom it reflects the presence of underlying tissue hypoxia. Since tissue hypoxia can lead to organ failure and increased mortality, the identification of tissue hypoxia and its correction whenever present is a reasonable therapeutic goal. Instead of aiming at attaining supranormal Do_2 values in all patients with ARDS, it is probably more desirable to tailor therapy according to the patient's needs at any given time. After correction of hypoxemia and anemia, a careful interpretation of the cardiac output in relation to o_2ER is warranted and should be complemented by monitoring other indices of hypoxia, such as blood lactate levels, gastric intramucosal pH and venoarterial Pco_2 gradients. Table 19.3 summarizes our four steps in the interpretation of values of cardiac output. The combination of these elements can help in recognizing the persistence of underlying tissue hypoxia and correcting it rapidly by the most appropriate therapy. This approach is likely to increase survival from ARDS.

REFERENCES

1. Montgomery, B.A., Stager, M.A., Carrico, J. *et al.* (1985) Causes of mortality in patients with the adult respiratory distress syndrome. *American Review of Respiratory Disease*, **132**, 485–91.
2. Cain, S.M. (1965) Appearance of excess lactate in anesthetized dogs during anemic and hypoxic hypoxia. *American Journal of Physiology*, **209**, 604–8.
3. Nelson, D.P., Samsel, R.W., Wood, L.D. *et al.* (1988) Pathological supply dependency of systemic and intestinal O_2 uptake during endotoxemia. *Journal of Applied Physiology*, **64**, 2410–19.
4. Bakker, J. and Vincent, J.L. (1991) The oxygen supply dependency phenomenon is associated with increased blood lactate levels. *Journal of Critical Care*, **6**, 152–9.
5. Van der Linden, P., Gilbert, E., Paques, P. *et al.* (1993) Influence of hematocrit on tissue O_2 extraction capabilities in anesthetized dogs during acute hemorrhage. *American Journal of Physiology*, **264**, H1942–7.
6. Zhang, H. and Vincent, J.L. (1993) Oxygen extraction is altered by endotoxin during tamponade-induced stagnant hypoxia in the dog. *Circulatory Shock*, **40**, 168–76.
7. Bowles, S.A., Schlichtig, R., Kramer, D.J. *et al.* (1992) Arteriovenous pH and partial pressure of carbon dioxide detect critical oxygen delivery during progressive hemorrhage in dogs. *Journal of Critical Care*, **7**, 95–105.
8. Zhang, H. and Vincent, J.L. (1993) Arteriovenous differences in Pco_2 and pH are good indicators of critical hypoperfusion. *American Review of Respiratory Disease*, **148**, 867–71.
9. De Backer, D., Roman, A., Van der Linden, P. *et al.* (1992) The effects of balloon filling into the inferior vena cava on the Vo_2/Do_2 relationship. *Journal of Critical Care*, **7**, 167–73.
10. Long, G.R., Nelson, D.P., Sznajder, J.I. *et al.* (1988) Systemic oxygen delivery and consumption during acute lung injury in dogs. *Journal of Critical Care*, **3**, 249–55.
11. Pepe, P.E. and Culver, B.H. (1985) Independently measured oxygen consumption during reduction of oxygen delivery by positive end-expiratory pressure. *American Review of Respiratory Disease*, **132**, 788–92.
12. Zhang, H., Benlabed, M., Spapen, H. *et al.* (1994) Prostaglandin E1 increases oxygen extraction capabilities in experimental sepsis. *Journal of Surgical Research*, **57**, 470–9.

13. Zhang, H., Spapen, H., Nguyen, D.N. *et al.* (1994) Protective effects of *N*-acetylcysteine in endotoxemia. *American Journal of Physiology*, **266**, H1746–54.

14. Landau, S.E., Alexander, R.S., Powers, S.R. *et al.* (1982) Tissue oxygen exchange and reactive hyperemia following microembolization. *Journal of Surgical Research*, **32**, 38–43.

15. Cain, S.M., King, C.E. and Chapler, C.K. (1988) Effects of time and microembolization on O_2 extraction by dog hindlimb in hypoxia. *Journal of Critical Care*, **3**, 89–95.

16. Bredle, D.L., Samsel, R.W., Schumacker, P.T. *et al.* (1989) Critical O_2 delivery to skeletal muscle at high and low Po_2 in endotoxemic dogs. *Journal of Applied Physiology*, **66**, 2553–8.

17. Shibutani, K., Komatsu, T., Kubai, K. *et al.* (1983) Critical level of oxygen delivery in anesthetized man. *Critical Care Medicine*, **11**, 640–3.

18. Ronco, J.J., Fenwick, J.C., Tweeddale, M.G. *et al.* (1993) Identification of the critical oxygen delivery for anaerobic metabolism in critically ill septic and nonseptic humans. *JAMA*, **270**, 1724–30.

19. Powers, S.R., Shah, D., Ryon, D. *et al.* (1977) Hypertonic mannitol in the therapy of the acute respiratory distress syndrome. *Annals of Surgery*, **185**, 619–25.

20. Danek, S., Lynch, J.P., Weg, J.G. *et al.* (1980) The dependence of oxygen uptake on oxygen delivery in the adult respiratory distress syndrome. *American Review of Respiratory Disease*, **122**, 387–95.

21. Bihari, D., Smithies, M., Gimson, A. *et al.* (1987) The effects of vasodilation with prostacyclin on oxygen delivery and uptake in critically ill patients. *New England Journal of Medicine*, **317**, 397–403.

22. Gutierrez, G. and Pohil, R.J. (1986) Oxygen consumption is linearly related to O_2 supply in critically ill patients. *Journal of Critical Care*, **1**, 45–53.

23. Haupt, M.T., Gilbert, E.M. and Carlson, R.W. (1985) Fluid loading increases oxygen consumption in septic patients with lactic acidosis. *American Review of Respiratory Disease*, **131**, 912–6.

24. Gilbert, E.M., Haupt, M.T., Mandanas, R.Y. *et al.* (1986) The effect of fluid loading, blood transfusion and catecholamine infusion on oxygen delivery and consumption in patients with sepsis. *American Review of Respiratory Disease*, **134**, 873–8.

25. Vincent, J.L., Roman, A., DeBacker, D. *et al.* (1990) Oxygen uptake/supply dependency: effects of short-term dobutamine infusion. *American Review of Respiratory Disease*, **142**, 2–8.

26. Kruse, J.A., Haupt, M.T., Puri, V.K. *et al.* (1990) Lactate levels as predictors of the relationship between oxygen delivery and consumption in ARDS. *Chest*, **98**, 959–62.

27. Boyd, O., Grounds, M. and Bennett, D. (1992) The dependency of oxygen consumption on oxygen delivery in critically ill postoperative patients is mimicked by variations in sedation. *Chest*, **101**, 1619–24.

28. Weissman, C. and Kemper, M. (1991) The oxygen uptake/oxygen delivery relationship during ICU interventions. *Chest*, **99**, 430–5.

29. Routsi, C., Vincent, J.L., Bakker, J. *et al.* (1993) Relation between oxygen consumption and oxygen delivery in patients after cardiac surgery. *Anesthesia and Analgesia*, **77**, 1104–10.

30. Archie, J. (1981) Mathematic coupling of data: a common source of error. *Annals of Surgery*, **193**, 296–303.

31. Vincent, J.L. (1994) How stable is a 'stable' cardiac output? [Editorial.] *Critical Care Medicine*, **22**, 5–6.

32. Annat, G., Viale, J.P., Percival, C. *et al.* (1986) Oxygen delivery and uptake in the adult respiratory distress syndrome: lack of relationship when measured independently in patients with normal blood lactate concentrations. *American Review of Respiratory Disease*, **133**, 999–1001.

33. Ronco, J.J., Fenwick, J.C., Wiggs, B.R. *et al.* (1993) Oxygen consumption is independent of increases in oxygen delivery by dobutamine in septic patients who have normal or increased plasma lactate. *American Review of Respiratory Disease*, **147**, 25–31.

34. Vermeij, C.G., Feenstra, B.W.A. and Bruining, H.A. (1990) Oxygen delivery and oxygen uptake in postoperative and septic patients. *Chest*, **98**, 415–20.

35. Ronco, J.J., Phang, P.T., Walley, K.R. *et al.* (1991) Oxygen consumption is independent of changes in oxygen delivery in severe adult respiratory distress syndrome. *American Review of Respiratory Disease*, **143**, 1267–73.

36. Stratton, H.H., Feustel, P.J. and Newell, J.C. (1987) Regression of calculated variables in the presence of shared measurement error. *Journal of Applied Physiology*, **62**, 2083–93.

37. Chappell, T.R., Rubin, L.J., Markham, R.V. *et al.* (1983) Independence of oxygen consumption and systemic oxygen transport in patients with either stable pulmonary hypertension or refractory left ventricular failure. *American Review of Respiratory Disease*, **128**, 30–3.

38. Keinanen, O., Takala, J. and Kari, A. (1992) Continuous measurement of cardiac output by the Fick principle: clinical validation in intensive care. *Intensive Care Medicine*, **20**, 360–5.

39. Lipkin, D. and Poole–Wilson, P.A. (1985) Measurement of cardiac output during exercise by the thermodilution and direct Fick techniques in patients with chronic congestive heart failure. *American Journal of Cardiology*, **56**, 321–4.

40. Iparraguirre, H.P., Finiger, R., Garber, V.A. *et al.* (1988) Comparison between measured and Fick-derived values of hemodynamic and oxymetric variables in patients with acute myocardial infarction. *American Journal of Medicine*, **85**, 349–52.

41. De Backer, D., Moraine, J.J., Berre, J. *et al.* (1994) Effects of dobutamine on oxygen consumption in septic patients: direct vs indirect determinations. *American Review of Respiratory and Critical Care Medicine*, **150**, 95–100.

42. De Backer, D., Berré, J., Zhang, H. *et al.* (1993) Relationship between oxygen uptake and oxygen delivery in septic patients: effects of prostacyclin vs dobutamine. *Critical Care Medicine*, **21**, 1658–64.

43. Silance, P.G., Simon, C. and Vincent, J.L. (1994) The relation between cardiac index and oxygen extraction in acutely ill patients. *Chest*, **105**, 1190–7.

44. Light, R. (1988) Intrapulmonary oxygen consumption in experimental pneumococcal pneumonia. *Journal of Applied Physiology*, **64**, 2490–5.

45. Klocke, F., Kaiser, G., Ross, J. *et al.* (1965) Mechanism of increase of myocardial oxygen uptake produced by catecholamines. *American Journal of Physiology*, **209**, 913–8.

46. Wolfe, R., Herndon, D., Jahoor, F. *et al.* (1987) Effect of severe burn injury on substrate cycling by glucose and fatty acids. *New England Journal of Medicine*, **317**, 403–8.

47. Bhatt, S.B., Hutchinson, R.C., Tomlinson, B. *et al.* (1992) Effect of dobutamine on oxygen supply and uptake in healthy volunteers. *British Journal of Anaesthesiolog*, **69**, 298–303.

48. Green, C., Frazer, R., Underhill, S. *et al.* (1992) Metabolic effects of dobutamine in normal man. *Clinical Science*, **82**, 77–83.

49. Liang, C., Sherman, L., Doherty, J. *et al.* (1984) Sustained improvement of cardiac function in patients with congestive heart failure after short-term infusion of dobutamine. *Circulation*, **69**, 113–9.

50. Maskin, C., Forman, R., Sonneblick, E. *et al.* (1983) Failure of dobutamine to increase exercise capacity despite hemodynamic improvement in severe chronic heart failure. *American Journal of Cardiology*, **51**, 177–82.

51. Teboul, J.L., Annane, D., Thuillez, C. *et al.* (1992) Effects of cardiovascular drugs on oxygen consumption/oxygen delivery relationship in patients with congestive heart failure. *Chest*, **101**, 1582–7.

52. Silverman, H. and Tuma, P. (1992) Gastric tonometry in patients with sepsis: Effects of dobutamine infusions and packed red blood cell transfusions. *Chest*, **102**, 184–8.

53. Mathru, M., Dries, D.J., Kanuri, D. *et al.* (1990) Effect of Cardiac output on gas exchange in one-lung atelectasis. *Chest*, **97**, 1121–4.

54. Uusaro, A., Hartikainen, J., Parviainen, M. *et al.* (1995) Metabolic stress modifies the thermogenic effect of dobutamine in man. *Critical Care Medicine*, **23**, 674–80.

55. Wysocki, M., Besbes, M., Roupie, E. *et al.* (1992) Modification of oxygen extraction ratio by change in oxygen transport in septic shock. *Chest*, **102**, 221–6.

56. Ward, M.E., Magder, S.A. and Hussain, S.N.A. (1992) Oxygen delivery-independent effect of blood flow on diaphragm fatigue. *American Review of Respiratory Disease*, **145**, 1058–63.

57. Lorente, J.A., Landin, L., De Pablo, R. *et al.* (1994) Effects of blood transfusion on oxygen transport variables in severe sepsis. *Critical Care Medicine*, **21**, 1312–8.

58. Walman, A., Parker, S., Traystman, R. *et al.* (1984) Isoproterenol protects against pulmonary edema in endotoxin lung injury. *Anesthesiology*, **61**, 3–8.

59. Shoemaker, W.C., Appel, P.L., Kram, H.B. *et al.* (1988) Prospective trial of supranormal values of survivors as therapeutic goals in high-risk surgical patients. *Chest*, **94**, 1176–86.

60. Tuchschmidt, J., Fried, J., Astiz, M. *et al.* (1992) Elevation of cardiac output and oxygen delivery improves outcome in in septic shock. *Chest*, **102**, 216–20.

61. Boyd, O., Grounds, M. and Bennett, E.D. (1993)

A randomized clinical trial of the effect of deliberate perioperative increase of oxygen delivery on mortality in high-risk surgical patients. *JAMA*, **270**, 2699–707.

62. Russell, J.A., Ronco, J.J., Lockhat, D. *et al.* (1990) Oxygen delivery and consumption and ventricular preload are greater in survivors than in nonsurvivors of the adult respiratory distress syndrome. *American Review of Respiratory Disease*, **141**, 659–65.

63. Fleming, A., Bishop, M., Shoemaker, W.C. *et al.* (1992) Prospective trial of supranormal values as goals of resuscitation in severe trauma. *Archives of Surgery*, **127**, 1175–81.

64. Hayes, M.A., Yau, E.H., Timmins, A.C. *et al.* (1993) Response of critically ill patients to treatment aimed at achieving supranormal oxygen delivery and consumption. *Chest*, **103**, 886–95.

65. Yu, M., Levy, M.M., Smith, P. *et al.* (1993) Effect of maximizing oxygen delivery on morbidity and mortality rates in critically ill patients: a prospective, randomized, controlled study. *Critical Care Medicine*, **21**, 830–8.

66. Hayes, M.A., Timmins, A.C., Yau, E.H. *et al.* (1994) Elevation of systemic oxygen delivery in the treatment of critically ill patients. *New England Journal of Medicine*, **330**, 1717–22.

67. Robin, E.D. (1987) Death by pulmonary artery flow-directed catheter: time for a memorandum? *Chest*, **92**, 727–31.

68. Mitchell, J.P., Schuller, D., Calandrino, F.S. *et al.* (1992) Improved outcome based on fluid management in critically ill patients requiring pulmonary artery catheterization. *American Review of Respiratory Disease*, **145**, 990–8.

69. Vincent, J.L., Roman, A. and Kahn, R.J. (1990) Dobutamine administration in septic shock: addition to a standard protocol. *Critical Care Medicine*, **18**, 689–93.

70. Vincent, J.L., Gris, P., Coffernils, M. *et al.* (1992) Myocardial depression characterizes the fatal course of septic shock. *Surgery*, **111**, 660–7.

71. Weber, K.T., Janicki, J. and Maskin, C. (1985) Pathophysiology of cardiac failure. *American Journal of Cardiology*, **56**, 3b–6b.

72. Vincent, J.L. (1991) Advances in the concepts of intensive care. *American Heart Journal*, **121**, 1859–65.

73. Jain, A., Shroff, S.G., Janicki, J.S. *et al.* (1991) Relation between mixed venous oxygen saturation and cardiac index. *Chest*, **99**, 1403–9.

74. Sutton, J.R., Reeves, J.T., Wagner, P.D. *et al.* (1988) Operation Everest II: oxygen transport during exercise at extreme simulated altitude. *Journal of Applied Physiology*, **64**, 1309–21.

75. Vary, T.C., Siegel, J.H., Tall, B.D. *et al.* (1988) Metabolic effects of partial reversal of pyruvate dehydrogenase activity by dichloroacetate in sepsis. *Circulatory Shock*, **24**, 3–18.

76. Bakker, J., Coffernils, M., Leon, M. *et al.* (1991) Blood lactate levels are superior to oxygen derived variables in predicting outcome in human septic shock. *Chest*, **99**, 956–62.

77. Fiddian-Green, R.G. (1993) Associations between intramucosal acidosis in the gut and organ failure. *Critical Care Medicine*, **21**, 103–7.

78. Gutierrez, G., Palizas, F., Doglio, G. *et al.* (1992) Gastric intramucosal pH as a therapeutic index of tissue oxygenation in critically ill patients. *Lancet*, **339**, 195–9.

79. Maynard, N., Bihari, D., Beale, R. *et al.* (1993) Assessment of splanchnic oxygenation by gastric tonometry in patients with acute circulatory failure. *JAMA* **270**, 1203–10.

80. Bakker, J., Vincent, J.L., Gris, P. *et al.* (1992) Veno-arterial carbon dioxide gradient in human septic shock. *Chest*, **101**, 509–15.

81. Mecher, C.E., Rackow, E.C., Astiz, M.E. *et al.* (1990) Venous hypercarbia associated with severe sepsis and systemic hypoperfusion. *Critical Care Medicine*, **18**, 585–9.

CRITICAL ROLE OF THE ALVEOLAR EPITHELIAL BARRIER

Michael A. Matthay

The overall objective of this chapter is to consider the role of the alveolar epithelial barrier in the development and the resolution of acute lung injury. The chapter is divided into five sections. The first examines the role of the alveolar epithelial barrier in maintaining lung fluid balance in the uninjured lung, with an emphasis on the role of sodium transport and the recently discovered water channels for regulating fluid transport across the alveolar epithelial barrier. The second section focuses on the central role of the alveolar epithelial barrier in acute lung injury and includes a discussion of the concept that the degree of alveolar barrier disruption is a major determinant of the severity of experimental and clinical acute lung injury. The third section discusses the function of the alveolar barrier in acute lung injury, emphasizing that the degree of damage ranges from mild to severe. This section also briefly reviews some of the mechanisms that may be important in causing injury to the alveolar epithelial barrier. The fourth section reviews data on the effects of endogenous and exogenous catecholamines on the function of the alveolar epithelial barrier under pathological conditions, a topic with several important clinical implications. The final section considers new strategies for attenuating or preventing lung endothelial and epithelial injury

in adult patients with the syndrome of acute respiratory distress (ARDS).

ROLE IN LUNG FLUID BALANCE

Until approximately mid-1980s, fluid movement across the alveolar epithelial barrier was thought to depend entirely on passive hydrostatic forces [1]. Both experimental and clinical work demonstrated that alveolar flooding in hydrostatic or increased permeability pulmonary edema occurred when the quantity of edema fluid in the lung interstitium exceeded the capacity of the interstitial space, resulting in bulk flow of the interstitial fluid into the air spaces of the lung [2–4] (Chapter 16). It was recognized that the epithelial barrier offered a much greater resistance to the passive movement of protein and solutes than the lung endothelial barrier [5,6], but the ability of the alveolar epithelial barrier to regulate transepithelial fluid movement by active ion transport was not appreciated for several reasons. Firstly, some early experimental studies were carried out at 25°C [1], a temperature that inhibits active ion transport across the alveolar epithelial barrier [7]. Secondly, direct access to the distal pulmonary epithelium was difficult and methods for culturing and studying isolated alveolar epithelial type II cells were not then developed. Therefore, the

ARDS Acute Respiratory Distress in Adults. Edited by Timothy W. Evans and Christopher Haslett. Published in 1996 by Chapman & Hall, London. ISBN 0 412 56910 8

mechanism for reabsorption of alveolar edema fluid was not understood.

Our initial experimental studies were designed to determine how excess alveolar fluid and protein could be removed from the alveoli. We hypothesized that an intact alveolar epithelial barrier would be necessary for the reabsorption of alveolar edema fluid. Initially, we tried to answer this question by instilling a protein solution (autologous serum) into the distal air spaces of one lung in anesthetized sheep. We then measured the clearance of both the liquid volume and the protein fraction of the serum from the alveoli of the lung. Those studies provided the first *in vivo* evidence that there was differential clearance of liquid and protein across the alveolar epithelial barrier [8]. In 4 hours, approximately 33% of the alveolar liquid volume was removed, but only 2–4% of the instilled protein was cleared from the air spaces. Further studies in sheep and dogs over 4, 12 and 24 hours demonstrated that the clearance of alveolar liquid continued across the alveolar epithelial barrier even though there was a progressive concentration of protein in the air spaces of the lung, sometimes to levels that were twice the protein concentration of the circulating bloodstream (Figure 20.1) [10,11]. These findings provided strong evidence to support the hypothesis that an active ion transport system was driving the reabsorption of excess alveolar fluid and that the mechanism depended at least in part on sodium transport because amiloride, an apical sodium channel inhibitor, blocked a significant fraction of the reabsorption in sheep [12]. Also, concurrent work on alveolar epithelial type II cells *in vitro* demonstrated that these cells were capable of transporting sodium from the apical to the basal surface in cultured monolayers [13,14]. Thus, these results from both *in vivo* and *in vitro* studies provided further evidence that removal of alveolar fluid across the epithelial barrier depended primarily on a sodium transport system.

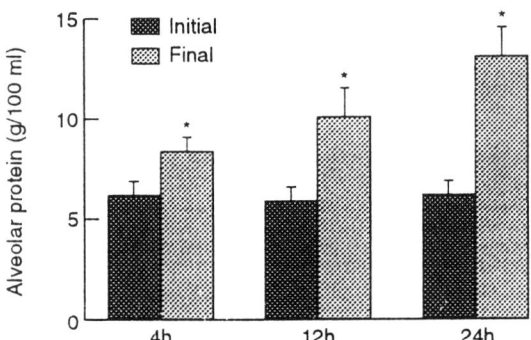

Figure 20.1 Data (mean ±SD) from experiments in unanesthetized sheep in which 100 ml of autologous serum was instilled into one lower lobe. After 4, 12 or 24 hours a final alveolar sample was obtained for total protein concentration. The data in this figure shows the initial protein concentration in the instilled serum and the final protein concentration aspirated from the distal air spaces of the lung. There was a progressive concentration of alveolar proteins at each time period, indicating a progressive removal of alveolar liquid from the air spaces of the lung. At the final time (24 hours), approximately 80% of the alveolar liquid had been removed from the air spaces of the lung based on the progressive concentration of protein over this time period (see text for explanation of calculation of alveolar liquid clearance based on alveolar protein concentration). Independent measurement of total lung liquid clearance using gravimetric techniques indicated that 76% of the instilled volume had been removed from the lung as a whole. (Reproduced with permission from Matthay [9].)

Ten years later, it is now widely accepted by investigators in this field that the primary mechanism driving reabsoption of alveolar fluid is sodium transport [15–25]. Work from our laboratory has established that there are significant differences in the basal rate of alveolar liquid clearance in different species, ranging from dogs (low), to sheep and goats (intermediate) to rats and rabbits, which have a fast basal rate of alveolar liquid clearance [10,11,26,27] (Figure 20.2). Interestingly, our estimates of alveolar liquid clearance in man, based on studies in patients [21,28] and in recently excised human lungs [25] indicate that the rate of alveolar liquid clearance in the

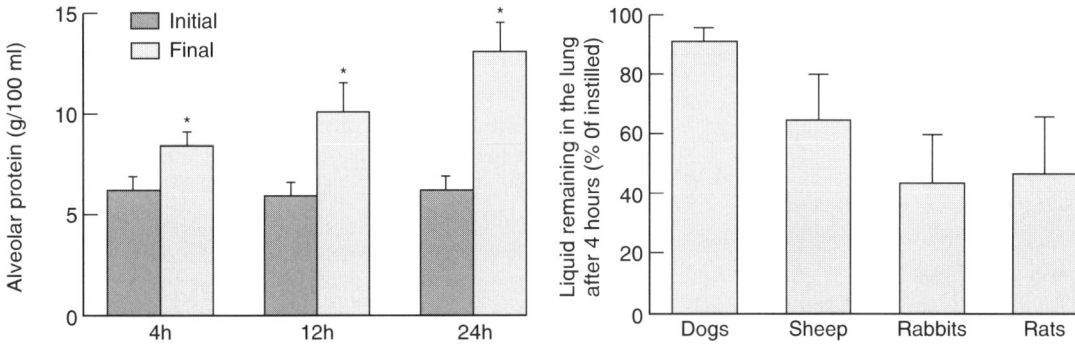

Figure 20.2 Residual lung water 4 hours after instillation of 3 ml/kg of a protein solution into the distal air spaces of one lung in four different species. Note that clearance is slowest in dogs, intermediate in sheep (similar to goats, as in Serikov *et al.* [7]), and fastest in rabbits and rats. Note that our estimate of our alveolar liquid clearance in humans (based on Matthay and Wiener-Kronish [21]) is similar to the faster clearance rates in rabbits and rats. (Reproduced with permission from Matthay and Wiener-Kronish [21].)

human lung may be fast, similar to the rates found in rabbits and rats. Currently, there is no good explanation for these differences among species, which do not apparently depend on differences in surface area or the way in which the experiments were done.

Furthermore, our *in vivo* work has established that β adrenergic agonists are capable of accelerating alveolar liquid clearance in sheep, dogs and rats, but not in rabbits. Other investigators have also found that β adrenergic agonists had no effect on alveolar liquid clearance in rabbits [29] or hamsters [30]. Because of these species differences, we thought it important to determine whether the human lung responds to β adrenergic stimulation. In a recently completed study of the excised human lung, we discovered that these agents markedly accelerate alveolar liquid clearance [25], a finding consistent with a prior study that used autoradiographic techniques to demonstrate a number of β receptors in the alveoli of the human lung [31]. As will be discussed in the last section of this article, this finding may have important therapeutic implications.

Our current understanding of the mechanisms regulating alveolar fluid reabsorption can be summarized as follows. The first step in the removal of excess alveolar fluid depends on sodium uptake by the apical surface of alveolar type II cells [22]. Once the sodium has entered the alveolar epithelial cell, it is then extruded into the lung interstitium by the Na^+,K^+-ATPase system along the basolateral surface of alveolar type II cells [23,24,32]. The active movement of sodium is followed by chloride through transcellular pathways that have not been identified. The water fraction appears to move through specific transcellular water channels [33]. We have established that there is a functional water channel, CHIP28, in isolated alveolar type II cells from rats, as well as possibly in both type I and type II cells in the alveolar epithelium in the human, the sheep and the rat lung [34]. In addition, more recent studies have indicated that there is another water channel in the lung [35]. Over the next few years, detailed morphologic and physiological studies will be carried out to better understand how the regulation and expression of these channels is involved in net alveolar fluid clearance in the lung. A summary of our current understanding of solute

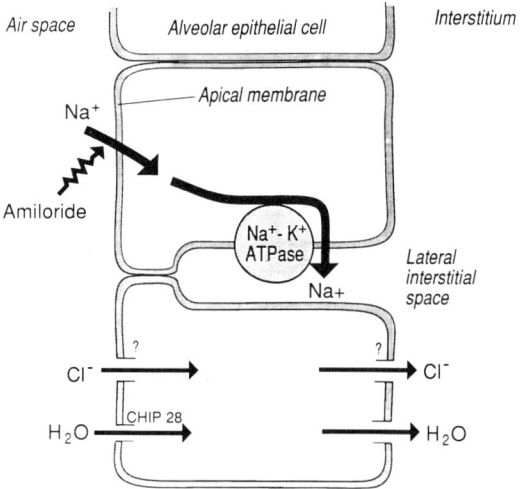

Figure 20.3 A model of alveolar liquid reabsorption which depends on sodium uptake across the alveolar epithelial cell membrane (a process which can be partially blocked by amiloride). The sodium is eventually pumped across the basolateral surface of the alveolar epithelial cell into the interstitial space by the Na^+,K^+-ATPase pump. In order to maintain electrical neutrality, chloride follows, probably by a transcellular route that has not been completely characterized. In order to maintain isomolar reabsorption, water is transported by specific transmembrane water pathways which include CHIP28. (Reproduced with permission from Matthay *et al.* [36].)

and water clearance pathways across the alveolar epithelium is presented in Figure 20.3.

One of the important findings of all our experimental studies has been that an intact alveolar epithelial barrier is required for net alveolar liquid clearance to take place. In other words, in order for the active ion transport system to work optimally, there needs to be a sufficiently tight alveolar epithelial barrier so that passive movement between the two spaces is minimal. As will be discussed in the next section, the epithelial barrier under some pathological conditions can still remove some excess alveolar fluid, but the rate of clearance is usually slower.

EVIDENCE FOR DAMAGE IN ACUTE LUNG INJURY

The best morphologic evidence for injury to the alveolar epithelial barrier derives from the ultrastructural studies of Bachofen and Weibel [37,38] in the mid-1970s on patients who died with acute lung injury. These classic investigations established that there was evidence of both endothelial and epithelial injury in the first few days following acute lung injury, often with denuding of type I alveolar epithelial cells with vacuolization and evidence of injury to alveolar type II cells as well (Figure 20.4). In the subacute phase (day 5 to 10), there was still evidence of alveolar epithelial barrier injury in many patients, particularly those with sepsis, but there was also proliferation of alveolar epithelial type II cells in an apparent attempt to form a new epithelial barrier following the necrosis of type I cells.

The epithelial barrier is clearly breached in most patients with acute lung injury, as evidenced by the presence of alveolar edema, both radiographically and clinically. Direct evidence for an increase in alveolar epithelial barrier permeability was derived from studies at our institution in which it was demonstrated that patients with acute lung injury had an initial alveolar edema protein concentration that was higher (75% or greater) than that of plasma [4]. Furthermore, experimental studies demonstrated that in the presence of acute lung injury there was flooding of the air spaces with protein-rich pulmonary edema fluid [2,3,39]. Thus, both morphological and physiological evidence suggests that the clinical syndrome of acute lung injury or ARDS includes flooding of the air spaces with protein-rich edema fluid and a loss of a primary protective function of the alveolar epithelial barrier.

Much early experimental work on the pathogenesis of acute lung injury focused on mechanisms of endothelial damage, partly because experimental models were available,

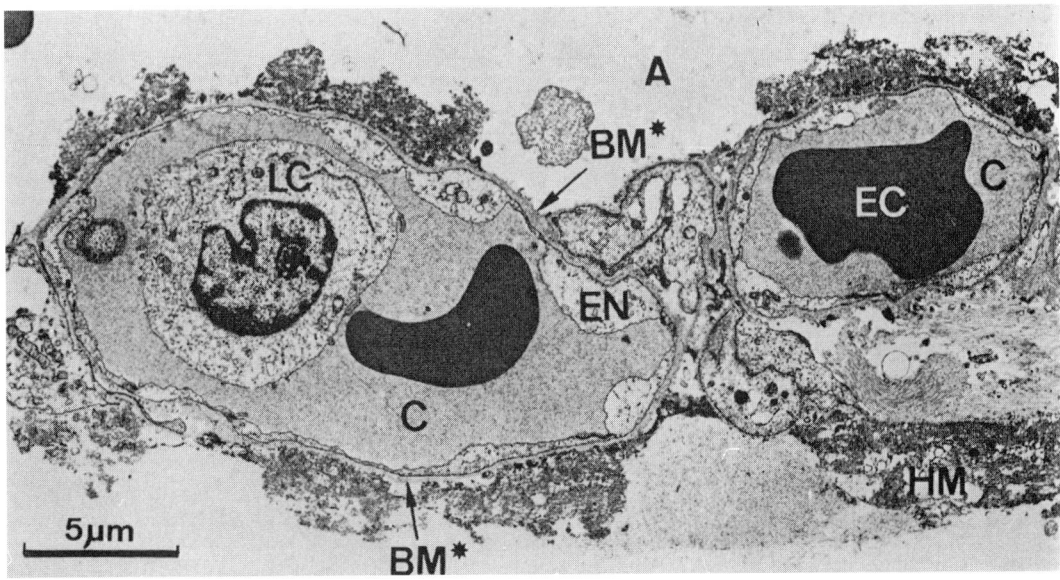

Figure 20.4 Electron microscopic section of an alveolar septum in a lung from a patient who died 4 days after developing acute lung injury from sepsis. Note there is injury to both the endothelial and epithelial barriers with vacuolization of endothelial (EN) cells and frank denuding and loss of alveolar epithelial cells. The epithelial barrier is covered only by barely visible basement membrane (BM) and cellular debris including hyaline membrane (HM), a sign of protein exudation and precipitation in the alveoli. LC = leukocyte; C = capillary; A = alveolus; EC = intravascular erythrocyte. (Reproduced with permission from Bachofen and Weibel [38].)

and especially as lung lymph flow could be sampled in sheep and goats [40]. Also, it was possible to study the early phase of acute lung injury by using the isolated perfused lung preparation, in which net weight gain could be used as an index of endothelial damage. Furthermore, the injection of a vascular protein tracer could be used as a marker of pulmonary endothelial injury by measuring its escape from the circulation as well as its accumulation in the lung. Considerable work has been done on both neutrophil dependent [41] and neutrophil independent [42] mechanisms of acute lung endothelial injury using these models. Until recently, little work had been done on the role of the alveolar epithelial barrier in acute lung injury nor the mechanisms by which it is injured.

It is important to appreciate the factors that are associated with alveolar flooding, both in hydrostatic and high permeability pulmonary edema. Firstly, if there is a sufficient increase in lung interstitial edema from any cause, a rise in lung interstitial pressure alone will lead to alveolar flooding. In experimental and clinical studies of cardiogenic pulmonary edema, alveolar flooding occurs because there is sufficient accumulation of edema in the lung interstitium to cause at least a temporary decrease in epithelial barrier resistance with flooding of the air space of the lung [43,44]. The exact site for movement of edema fluid from the interstitium into the air spaces has not been identified clearly, although some evidence suggests that there may be flooding in terminal or respiratory bronchioles, where epithelial junctions might not be as tight as they are in the alveolar epithelial barrier [45]. In this model, pulmonary edema fluid would fill the alveoli in a retrograde fashion. After interstitial edema has flooded the air spaces of the lung and the increase in lung microvascular pressure has returned towards normal, the alveolar epithelial barrier rapidly regains its tight barrier properties, allowing reabsorption of excess alveolar fluid. Thus, when hydrostatic pulmonary edema results in alveolar flooding, it is associated with an increase in alveolar epithelial barrier permeability, probably from a transient opening of tight junctions in the distal pulmonary epithelium. This concept of alveolar flooding from high pressure pulmonary edema may also be relevant to some forms of increased permeability pulmonary edema, in which the acute lung injury may be primarily confined to the lung endothelial barrier. In these cases, there may be a rapid accumulation of protein-rich edema fluid in the lung interstitium, which then results in alveolar flooding if there is a sufficient increase in the total quantity of lung interstitial edema fluid, as in uncomplicated hydrostatic pulmonary edema. In this case, the injury may be confined primarily to the lung endothelium without any actual injury to the epithelial barrier. We have clinical evidence for this pattern of acute lung injury in some patients who rapidly reabsorb some of their protein-rich alveolar edema within a short time [21,28]. This kind of acute lung injury, which may be more typical of transient lung endothelial injury, seems to be associated with blood product reactions, surgery involving cardiopulmonary bypass, and high altitude or neurogenic pulmonary edema, in which there may be a combination of both increased pressure and increased permeability primarily affecting the lung endothelial barrier. By contrast, those clinical conditions in which there is injury to both lung endothelial and epithelial barriers, such as bloodborne sepsis, primary lung infection and gastric aspiration, morphological and physio-logical evidence for injury to both the endothelial and epithelial barriers of the lung is present [21,37,46] (Figure 20.4). It has been suggested that barotrauma in patients with acute lung injury may be primarily a function of the extent of lung injury and the damage to the alveolar epithelial barrier [47].

INJURY MAY BE MILD, MODERATE OR SEVERE IN ACUTE LUNG INJURY

It should be appreciated conceptually that injury to the alveolar epithelial barrier is a dynamic process. In other words, there may be alveolar flooding and accumulation of protein-rich edema fluid in the air spaces of the lung initially, followed by either a sustained injury to the epithelial barrier with persistent flooding of the air spaces, or a return to a more normal alveolar epithelial barrier with gradual resolution and reabsorption of some of the excess alveolar fluid. Thus, we have reported that some patients with acute lung injury, especially associated with sepsis, have persistent alveolar flooding and persistently poor arterial oxygenation. These patients characteristically have little evidence of reabsorption of alveolar edema, at least within 12 – 24 hours of the development of acute lung injury [21]. Experimentally, we have found a similar pattern of injury in rabbits in whom fluids of low pH were instilled into the distal air spaces of the lung [48]. There was no evidence of reabsorption of alveolar fluid and physiologically there was good evidence of injury to both the endothelial and epithelial barriers. By contrast, in some of our clinical studies, after an initial phase of severe alveolar flooding with protein-rich edema fluid, some patients begin to reabsorb some excess alveolar fluid within 6–12 hours [21,28]. This phase of alveolar reabsorption is associated with a decrease in edema fluid on the chest radiograph and an improvement in arterial oxygenation.

Experimentally, we have reported these same phenomena in different models. In sheep, severe acute lung injury that was induced with intravenous oleic acid caused severe pulmonary edema with protein-rich edema fluid that was associated with a major increase in extravascular lung water in the first 2–3 hours [39]. However, after 4–5 hours, there was evidence of some reabsorption of the excess alveolar fluid such that after 8 hours the extravascular lung water declined by 20–30% from its peak (4 hours) value. There was a parallel increase in alveolar edema fluid protein concentration, indicating that the alveolar epithelial barrier was sufficiently functional to remove some of the excess fluid. In our experimental studies of sepsis or bacterial pneumonia in sheep and rabbits, we have also observed that the alveolar barrier was capable of resisting injury or recovering from endothelial and epithelial injury within several hours [49–51]. As already mentioned, in a model of severe experimental injury from acid aspiration, there was no evidence of recovery of alveolar barrier function [46].

Both experimental and clinical evidence therefore favor the conclusion that injury to the alveolar epithelial barrier may be mild, moderate or severe. In fact, our clinical studies have supported the hypothesis that the ability to reabsorb some alveolar edema fluid in the first 12 hours after the development of acute lung injury is a favorable prognostic finding, associated with a mortality of only 20%. By contrast, the inability to reabsorb alveolar edema fluid early in the course of acute lung injury is associated with a mortality of nearly 80% [21] (Figure 20.5). Thus, the function of the alveolar epithelial barrier early in the course of acute lung injury may be a useful prognostic index, perhaps because of the central importance of damage to the alveolar epithelial barrier in acute lung injury [36].

What mechanisms have been identified to date that may be responsible for injury to the alveolar epithelial barrier? In studies of *Pseudomonas aeruginosa* induced acute lung

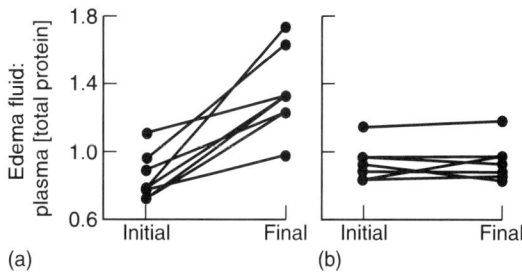

Figure 20.5 Individual data points are shown for the initial and final alveolar edema fluid to plasma total protein concentration ratio in (a) the nine group A patients with ARDS who improved clinically, compared with (b) the seven group B patients with ARDS who did not improve clinically. The time between the initial and final alveolar fluid sample was similar between the group A (6.8 ± 5.1 hours; $P < 0.01$) compared with group B (5.4 ± 4.1 hours; P not significant) patients. (Reproduced with permission from Matthay and Wiener-Kronish [21]).

injury we have found bacterial products to be a major cause of epithelial barrier injury, such as the specific exoproduct, exoenzyme S [50]. It is possible that inflammatory cells also contribute to the barrier injury in pneumonia, although it appears that neutrophils are primarily protective in this setting. Other investigators have provided evidence that oxygen radicals may be important mediators of injury under certain conditions, such as oxygen toxicity or noxious gases, including nitrogen dioxide [52,53]. Neutrophils may play a role in injuring the epithelial barrier in certain types of acute lung injury, such as gastric aspiration [46] or even septicemia, although further work on this hypothesis is required.

ENDOGENOUS AND EXOGENOUS CATECHOLAMINES AND ACUTE LUNG INJURY

Studies in the fetal lung have indicated that elevated plasma levels of epinephrine may be important in hastening reabsorption of fetal lung fluid at the time of birth [15]. Our own experimental studies have demonstrated that exogenous administration of β adrenergic agonists, either intravenously or directly into the distal air spaces, markedly increased alveolar liquid clearance in several species including sheep, dogs and rats [11,17,27] and most recently in the human lung [25]. We recently extended these observations to study the possible effect of catecholamines under pathological conditions, examining the effects of both endogenous as well as exogenously administered catecholamines [9,54].

ENDOGENOUS CATECHOLAMINES IN SHORT TERM EXPERIMENTAL SPETIC SHOCK

Pathological conditions which were associated with a marked increase in circulating catecholamine levels might be associated with an acceleration in alveolar fluid clearance. To test this possibility, we induced septic shock and metabolic acidosis with a bolus dose of intravenous *P. aeruginosa* in anesthetized, ventilated rats. As expected, there were markedly elevated levels of epinephrine detectable in the circulating plasma. Over 4 hours, the rats developed lung endothelial injury with interstitial pulmonary edema but no evidence of alveolar edema. Using our standard experimental protocol, we instilled a test solution of 3 ml/kg of a protein solution into one lung and found that the rate of alveolar fluid clearance was nearly doubled in the rats who were in septic shock compared with the normotensive, control rats. This marked increase in clearance was inhibited by administration into the alveoli of either amiloride, an apical sodium channel inhibitor, or propranolol, a β adrenergic antagonist. To further confirm that the accelerated alveolar fluid clearance was due to the increased circulating levels of epinephrine, we carried out similar studies in rabbits which which are unresponsive to β adrenergic agonists in terms of alveolar fluid clearance [26,29]. Septic shock in rabbits resulted in marked elevations of plasma catecholamines, but there was no change in alveolar fluid clearance. These experimental

studies may have major implications for the potential role of circulating catecholamines under some pathological conditions [54]. Firstly, it has been clearly documented in our clinical studies, as well as from work at other centres, that only 30–35% of patients with septic shock develop clinical acute lung injury with alveolar flooding [55]. Elevated levels of circulating catecholamines may help to protect against flooding, providing that the epithelial barrier is sufficiently intact, particularly in patients with shock from sepsis, hypovolemia, trauma or cardiac failure. Further studies are needed to define in more detail the clinical conditions under which this mechanism may function.

EXOGENOUS CATECHOLAMINES AS A METHOD FOR ACCELERATING ALVEOLAR FLUID CLEARANCE IN THE PRESENCE OF ACUTE LUNG INJURY

Some of our studies have suggested that alveolar fluid clearance might be accelerated in the presence of mild to moderate lung injury. In rats exposed to 100% oxygen for 40 hours with gravimetric evidence of moderate pulmonary edema, β adrenergic agonist therapy was effective in increasing the rate of alveolar fluid clearance [56]. Further studies are needed to determine experimentally if alveolar fluid clearance in acute lung injury can be accelerated with β adrenergic agonists. These agents might be beneficial because they have been shown to increase surfactant secretion from alveolar type II cells [57] and to decrease endothelial injury in some experimental models [58]. Thirdly, they might be useful in reversing some of the increase in airway resistance that has been reported in some patients with acute lung injury [59]. Finally, their mild vasodilating properties might reduce lung microvascular pressures, thus reducing the accumulation of pulmonary edema fluid in the lung [60].

PREVENTION AND TREATMENT OF ALVEOLAR EPITHELIAL AND ENDOTHELIAL BARRIER INJURY IN PATIENTS WITH ACUTE LUNG INJURY

All studies of outcome in patients with acute lung injury have concluded that pulmonary and non-pulmonary infections are the major cause of death [61,62]. Nosocomial pneumonia complicates the clinical course of many patients with ARDS, and primary bacterial pneumonia is an important cause of acute lung injury.

Therefore, part of our work on the role of the alveolar epithelial barrier in acute lung injury has been to study the mechanisms of bacterial induced epithelial injury and to identify novel approaches to reduce the injury. In a recently published study, we found that a type specific antibody to *P. aeruginosa* was successful in preventing alveolar epithelial barrier injury in sheep when given 24 hours before or at the same time as the instillation of live *P. aeruginosa* organisms in the lung [63]. Interestingly, a high level of type specific antibody in the circulation (achieved by vaccination) was not effective in preventing the alveolar epithelial injury, although it did attenuate the lung endothelial injury. The effectiveness of type specific antibody in the air spaces was reflected in the total excess water that accumulated in the lung and the adjacent pleural space (Figure 20.6). In the presence of elevated levels of circulating type specific antibody to *P. aeruginosa*, the excess water was similar in the lung and pleura to the sheep instilled with *P. aeruginosa*. However, when type specific antibody was present in the distal air spaces, the excess lung and pleural water was in the same range as control sheep (Figure 20.6).

Thus, these studies raise the intriguing possibility that delivery of type specific antibody to Gram-negative organisms in the distal air spaces of the lung might be an effective method for preventing nosocomial Gram-negative pneumonia in patients with ARDS

or at high risk of developing ARDS. This therapy could conceivably be given by aerosolization. In the future, it is clear that adjunctive therapy will be needed to prevent and treat pulmonary infections in ARDS because antibiotics alone have not been successful in significantly reducing mortality [61,62].

SUMMARY

New knowledge regarding the role of the alveolar epithelial barrier in regulating lung fluid balance (sodium and water transport) under normal and pathological conditions has made it possible to appreciate the critical role of the alveolar barrier in patients with acute lung injury. The function of the barrier appears to be a major prognostic factor in clinical acute lung injury. Recent studies have provided some new insights into neutrophil dependent and neutrophil independent mechanisms responsible for alveolar barrier injury. There are at least three promising future directions for therapeutic interventions directed specifically at the alveolar barrier. Firstly, aerosolized β adrenergic agonists might be of value in some patients because of their potential to accelerate alveolar fluid clearance and increase surfactant production. Secondly, in the future, prevention or treatment of nosocomial bacterial pneumonia in patients with ARDS might be possible with aersolized delivery of type specific antibodies against Gram-negative organisms. This approach would serve both to protect the alveolar epithelial barrier and also to provide a much needed additional treatment for pulmonary infections in ARDS.

Finally, there is evidence that the fibrosing alveolitis that occurs in many patients with acute lung injury may be a function, in part, of the initial severity of injury to the endothelial and epithelial barriers of the lung [64]. Both *in vivo* and *in vitro* studies have established the critical role of alveolar epithelial

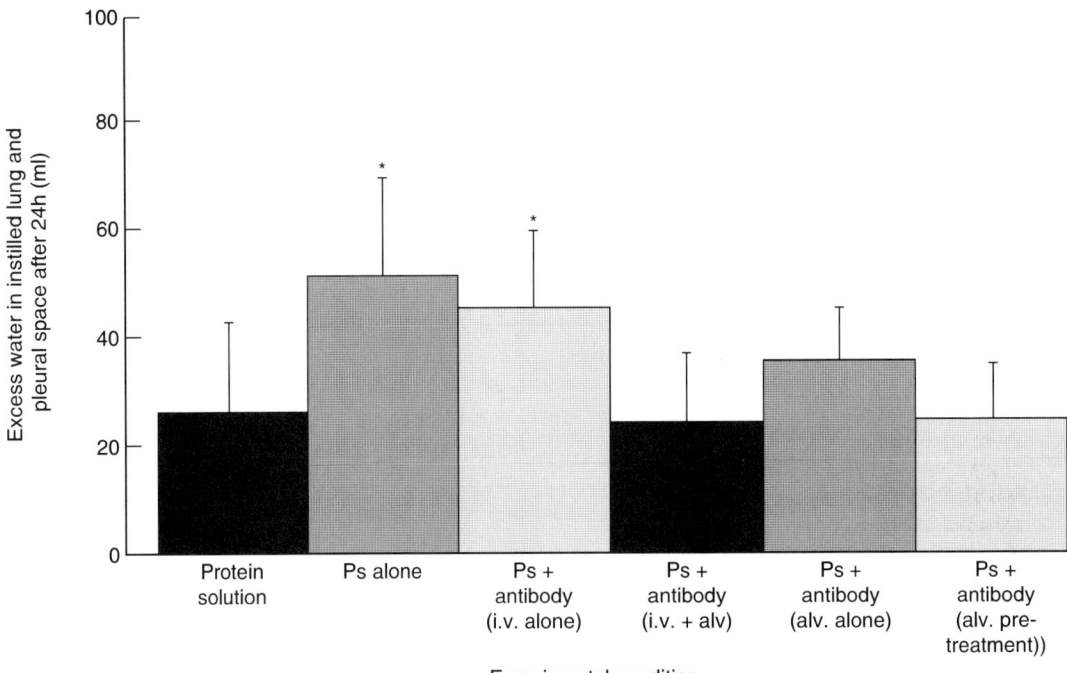

Figure 20.6 Extravascular water content of the instilled lung and the adjacent pleura space (mean ± SD) is shown for all experimental groups. The quantity of excess water in the instilled lung and the pleural space 24 hours after instillation of *P. aeruginosa* (Ps) (group 1B) was significantly increased compared with the control studies (group 1A). The sheep with circulating IgG antibody to *P. aeruginosa* alone (group 2) had a similar increase in excess water in the lung and pleural space after 24 hours. In contrast, concurrent instillation of IgG antibody to *P. aeruginosa* into the air spaces (groups 3 and 4) or pretreatment with IgG antibody (group 5) prevented any significant increase in excess water in the lung and pleural space. (Reproduced with permission from Pittet *et al.* [63].)

type II cells in providing a new epithelial barrier after denuding and necrosis of alveolar epithelial type I cells in acute lung injury [65]. The proliferation of alveolar epithelial type II cells also may increase the rate of alveolar epithelial sodium and fluid transport, thus facilitating the resolution of alveolar edema [66].

ACKNOWLEDGMENTS

I appreciate the help of Jill Richardson in preparing this manuscript. The work was supported in part by NIH HL 19155 and HL 51854.

REFERENCES

1. Taylor, A.E., Guyton, A.C. and Bishop, V.S. (1965) Permeability of the alveolar membrane to solutes. *Circulatory Research*, **16**, 353–62.
2. Vreim, C.F., Snashall, P.D., Demling, R.H. *et al.* (1976) Lung lymph and free interstitial fluid protein composition in sheep with edema. *Journal of Applied Physiology*, **230**, 1650–3.
3. Vreim, C.F., and Staub, N.C. (1976) Protein composition of lung fluids in acute alloxan edema in dogs. *American Journal of Physiology*, **230**, 376–9.
4. Fein, A., Grossmann R.F., Jones J.G. *et al.* (1979) The value of edema fluid protein measurements in patients with pulmonary edema. *American Journal of Medicine* **67**, 32–39.
5. Schneeberger, E.E. and Karnovsky, M.J. (1971)

The influence of intravascular fluid volume on the permeability of newborn and adult mouse lungs to ultrastructural protein tracers. *Journal of Cell Biology*, **49**, 319–25.

6. Gorin, A.B. and Stewart, P.A. (1979) Differential permeability of the endothelial and epithelial barriers to albumin flux. *Journal of Applied Physiology*, **47**, 1315–24.

7. Serikov, V.B., Grady, M. and Matthay, M.A. (1993) Effect of temperature on alveolar liquid and protein clearance in an *in situ* perfused goat lung. *Journal of Applied Physiology*, **75**, 940–7.

8. Matthay, M.A., Landolt, C.C. and Staub, N.C. (1982) Differential liquid and protein clearance from the alveoli of anesthetized sheep. *Journal of Applied Physiology*, **53**, 96–104.

9. Matthay, M.A. (1994) The function of the alveolar epithelial barrier under pathological conditions. *Chest*, **105**, 67S–74S.

10. Matthay, M.A., Berthiaume, Y. and Staub, N.C. (1985) Long-term clearance of liquid and protein from the lungs of unanesthetized sheep. *Journal of Applied Physiology*, **59**, 928–34.

11. Berthiaume, Y., Broaddus, V.C., Gropper, M.A. *et al.* (1988) Alveolar liquid and protein clearance from normal dog lungs. *Journal of Applied Physiology*, **65**, 585–93.

12. Matthay, M.A. (1985) Resolution on pulmonary edema: mechanisms of liquid, protein, and cellular clearance from the lung. *Clinics in Chest Medicine*, **6**, 521–45.

13. Mason, R.J., William, M.C., Widdicombe, J.H. *et al.* (1982) Transepthelial transport by pulmonary alveolar type II cells in primary culture. *Proceedings of the National Academy of Sciences of the USA*, **79**, 6033–37.

14. Goodman, B.E., Fleischer, R.S. and Crandall, E.D. (1983) Evidence for active sodium transport by cultured monolayers of pulmonary alveolar epithelial cells. *American Journal of Physiology*, **245**, C79–83.

15. Olver, R.E., Ramsden, C.A., Strang, L.B. and Walters, V. (1986) The role of amiloride-blockable sodium transport in adrenaline-induced lung liquid absorption in the fetal lamb. *Journal of Physiology*, **376**, 321–340.

16. Crandall, E., Heming, R.A., Palomb, R.L. and Goodman, B.E. (1986) Effects of terbutaline on sodium transport in isolated perfused rat lung. *Journal of Applied Physiology*, **60**, 289–94.

17. Berthiaume, Y., Staub, N.C. and Matthay, M.A. (1987) Beta-adrenergic agonists increase lung liquid clearance in anesthetized sheep. *Journal of Clinical Investigation*, **79**, 335–43.

18. Effros, R.M., Mason, G.R., Hukkanen, J. and Silverman, P. (1989) New evidence for active sodium transport in fluid-filled rat lungs. *Journal of Applied Physiology*, **66**, 906–19.

19. Cheek, K., Kim, K.J. and Crandall, E.D. (1989) Tight monolayers of rat alveolar epithelial cells: bioelectric properties and active sodium transport. *American Journal of Physiology*, **256**, C688–93.

20. O'Brodovich, H., Hannam, V., Seear, M. and Mullen, J.B. (1990) Amiloride impairs lung water clearance in newborn guinea pigs. *Journal of Applied Physiology*, **68**, 1758–62.

21. Matthay M.A. and Wiener-Kronish, J.P. (1990) Intact epithelial barrier function is critical for the resolution of alveolar edema in humans. *American Review of Respiratory Disease*, **142**, 1250–7.

22. Matalon, S. (1991) Mechanisms and regulation of ion transport in adult mammalian alveolar type II pneumocytes. *American Journal Physiology*, **261**, C1–12.

23. Saumon, G and Basset, G. (1993) Electrolyte and fluid transport across the mature alveolar epithelium. *Journal of Applied Physiology*, **74**, 1–15.

24. Sakuma, T., Pittet, J.F., Jayr, C. *et al.* (1993) Alveolar liquid and protein clearance in the absence of blood flow or ventilation in sheep. *Journal of Applied Physiology*, **74**, 176–85.

25. Sakuma, T., Okaniwa G, Nakada, T. *et al.* (1994) Alveolar fluid clearance in the resected human lung. *American Journal of Respiratory and Critical Care Medicine*, 150, 305–10.

26. Smedira, N., Gates, L., Hastings, R. *et al.* (1991) Alveolar liquid clearance in anesthetized rabbits. *Journal of Applied Physiology*, **70**, 1827–35.

27. Jayr, C., Garat, C., Meignan, C. *et al.* (1994) Alveolar liquid and protein clearance in anesthetized, ventilated rats. *Journal of Applied Physiology*, **76**, 2636–42.

28. Hastings, R.H., Grady, M., Sakuma, T. and Matthay, M.A. (1992) Clearance of different-sized proteins from the alveolar space in humans and rabbits. *Journal of Applied Physiology*, **73**, 1310–6.

29. Effros, R.M., Mason, G., Hukkanen, J. and Silverman, P. (1987) Reabsorption of solutes and water from fluid-filled rabbit lungs. *American Review of Respiratory Disease*, **6**, 669–76.

30. Goodman, B.E. and Waltz, W.F. (1993) Species

differences in regulation of sodium transport, in *Fluid and Solute Transport in the Airspaces of the Lungs* (eds R.M. Effros and H.K. Chang), Marcel Dekker, New York, pp. 489–504.

31. Carstairs, J.R., Nimmo, A.J. and Barnes, P. (1985) Autoradiographic visualization of beta-adrenergic receptor subtypes in human lung. *American Review of Respiratory Disease*, **132**, 541–7.

32. Nici, L., Dowin, R., Gilmore-Hebert, M. *et al.* (1991) Upregulation of rat lung Na, K-ATPase hypoxic lung injury. *American Journal of Physiology*, **261**, L307–14.

33. Verkman, A.S. (1992) Water channels in cell membranes. *Annual Review of Physiology*, **54**, 97–108.

34. Folkesson, H.G., Matthay, M.A., Hasegawa, H. *et al.* (1994) Transcellular water transport in lung alveolar epithelium through mercurial-sensitive water channels. *Proceedings of the National Academy of Science of the USA*, **91**, 4970–4.

35. Hasegawa, H., Ma, T., Skach, W. *et al.* (1994) Molecular cloning of a mercurial-insensitive water channel expressed in selected water transporting epithelia. *Journal of Biological Chemistry*, **269**, 5497–500.

36. Matthay, M.A., Folkesson, G., Campagna, A. and Kheradmand, F. (1993) Alveolar epithelial barrier and acute lung injury. *New Horizons*, **1**, 613–22.

37. Bachofen, M. and Weibel, E.R. (1977) Alterations of the gas exchange apparatus in adult respiratory insufficiency associated with septicemia. *American Review of Respiratory Disease*, **116**, 589–615.

38. Bachofen, M. and Weibel, E.R. (1982) Structural alteration of lung parenchyma in the adult respiratory distress syndrome. *Clinics in Chest Medicine*, **3**, 35–56.

39. Wiener-Kronish, J.P., Broaddus, V.C., Albertine, K.H. *et al.* (1988) Pleural effusions are associated with increased permeability pulmonary edema in anesthetized sheep. *Journal of Clinical Investigation*, **82**, 1422–9.

40. Ohkuda, K., Nakahara, K., Binder, A. *et al.* (1981) Venous air emboli in sheep: reversible increase in lung vascular permeability. *Journal of Applied Physiology*, **51**, 887–94.

41. Wortel, C.H. and Doerschut, C.M. (1993) Neutrophil and neutrophil-endothelial cell adhesion in adult respiratory distress syndrome. *New Horizons*, **1**, 631–7.

42. Ognibene, F.C., Martin, S.E. and Parker, M.M. (1986) Adult respiratory distress syndrome in patients with severe neutropenia. *New England Journal of Medicine*, **315**, 547–51.

43. Zumsteg, T.A., Havill, A.M. and Gee, M.H. (1982) Relationships among lung extravascular fluid compartments with alveolar flooding. *Journal of Applied Physiology*, **67**, 2234–42.

44. Bhattacharya, J., Gropper, M.A. and Staub, N.C. (1984) Interstitial fluid pressure gradient measured by micropuncture in excised dog lung. *Journal of Applied Physiology*, **56**, 271–7.

45. Conhaim, R.L. (1989) Airway level at which edema liquid enters the airspace of isolated dog lungs. *Journal of Applied Physiology*, **67**, 2234–42

46. Folkesson, H.G., Matthay, M.A., Hébert, C. and Broaddus, V.C. (1995) Acid aspiration-induced lung injury in rabbits is mediated by interleukin-8-dependent mechanism. *Journal of Clinical Investigation*, **96**, 107–16.

47. Schnapp, L.M., Chin, D.P., Szaflarski, N. and Matthay, M.A. (1995) Frequency and importance of barotrauma in 100 patients with acute lung injury. *Critical Care Medicine*, **23**, 272–8.

48. Folkesson, H., Kheradmand, F. and Matthay, M.A. (1993) A new method for sequential measurement of alveolar epithelial barrier function during the course of acute lung injury in anesthetized ventilated rabbits. *FASEB Journal*, **7**, A191.

49. Wiener-Kronish, J.P., Albertine, K.H. and Matthay, M.A. (1991) Differential effects of *E. coli* endotoxin on the lung endothelial and epithelial barriers of the lung. *Journal of Clinical Investigation*, **88**, 864–75.

50. Wiener-Kronish J.P., Sakuma, T., Kudoh, I. *et al.* (1993) Alveolar epithelial injury and pleural empyema in acute *P. aeruginosa* pneumonia in anesthetized rabbits. *Journal of Applied Physiology*, **75**, 1661–9.

51. Pittet, J.F., Wiener-Kronish, J.P., Serikov, V. and Matthay, M.A. (1995) Resistance of the alveolar epithelium to injury from septic shock in sheep. *American Journal of Respiratory and Critical Care Medicine*, **151**, 1093–100.

52. Bauer, M.L., Beckman, J.S., Bridges, R.J. *et al.* (1992) Peroxynitrite inhibits sodium uptake in rat colonic membrane vesicles. *Biochimica et Biophysica Acta*, **1104**, 87–94.

53. Kim, K.J. and Suh, D.J. (1993) Asymmetric effects of H_2O_2 on alveolar epithelial barrier

properties. *American Journal of Physiology*, **264**, L308–15.

54. Pittet, J.F., Wiener-Kronish, J.P., McElroy, M.C. *et al.* (1994) Stimulation of alveolar epithelial liquid clearance by endogenous release of catecholamines in septic shock. *Journal of Clinical Investigation*, **94**, 663–71.

55. Rubin, D.B., Wiener-Kronish, J.P., Murray, J.F. *et al.* (1990) Elevated von Willebrand factor-antigen is an early plasma predictor of impending of acute lung injury and death in non-pulmonary sepsis syndrome. *Journal of Clinical Investigation*, **86**, 474–80.

56. Garat, C., Meignan, M., Harf, A. *et al.* (1993) Effect of exposure to 100% oxygen for 40 hours on alveolar and lung liquid clearance in rats. *American Review of Respiratory Disease*, **147**, A43.

57. Brown, L.A.S. and Longmore, W.J. (1981) Adrenergic and cholinergic regulation of lung surfactant secretion in the isolated perfused rat lung and in the alveolar type II cell in culture (1981). *Journal of Biological Chemistry*, **256**, 66–72.

58. Minnear, F.L., Johnson, A. and Malik, A.B. (1986) [P101]-Adrenergic modulation of pulmonary transvascular fluid and protein exchange. *Journal of Applied Physiology*, **60**, 266–274.

59. Tantucci, C., Corbeil, C., Chasse, M. *et al.* (1992) Flow and volume dependent of respiratory system flow resistance in patients with the adult respiratory distress syndrome. *American Review of Respiratory Disease*, **145**, 355–60.

60. Prewitt, R.M., McCarthy, J. and L.D.H. Wood (1981) Treatment of acute low pressure pulmonary edema in dogs. *Journal of Clinical Investigation*, **67**, 409–418.

61. Bell, R.C., Coalson, J., Smith, J.D. and Johanson, W.G. (1983) Multiple organ failure and infection in adult respiratory distress syndrome. *Annals of Internal Medicine*, **99**, 293–8.

62. Montgomery, A.B., Stager, M.A., Carrico, C.J. *et al.* (1985) Causes of mortality in patients with the adult respiratory distress syndrome. *American Review of Respiratory Disease*, **132**, 485–9.

63. Pittet, J.F., Matthay, M.A., Pier, G. *et al.* (1993) *Pseudomonas aeruginosa*-induced lung and pleural injury in sheep. *Journal of Clinical Investigation*, **92**, 1221–8.

64. Matthay, M.A. (1995) Fibrosing alveolitis in the adult respiratory distress syndrome. *Annals of Internal Medicine*, **122**, 65–66.

65. Kheradmand, F., Folkesson, H.G., Shum. L. *et al.* (1994) Transforming growth factor-[P100] enhances alveolar epithelial cell repair in a new *in vitro* model. *American Journal of Physiology*, **267**, L728–38.

66. Nitenberg, G. Folkesson, H.G., Osorio, O. *et al.* (1995) Alveolar epithelial liquid clearance is markedly increased 10 days following acute lung injury from bleomycin. *American Journal of Respiratory and Critical Care Medicine*, **151**, A620.

PART FOUR

CLINICAL ASSESSMENT AND MANAGEMENT

David M. Hansell

Since the first clinical description of the syndrome of acute respiratory distress in adults (ARDS), an abnormal chest radiograph has come to be regarded as a *sine qua non* for the diagnosis of the established condition [1]. However, at the time of the initiation of lung injury and shortly afterwards, the chest radiograph is frequently normal. The poor sensitivity of chest radiography in the early stages of ARDS is compounded by the limited specificity of the radiographic abnormalities as the disease becomes established: widespread ground-glass opacification and pulmonary consolidation is seen in many other conditions, including severe pulmonary infection, aspiration pneumonia, pulmonary edema, drug toxicity, pulmonary contusion and fat embolism [2,3]. Despite these limitations, there are many insights to be gained from serial chest radiographs in patients with ARDS, always bearing in mind the technical drawbacks of portable radiography.

A significant limitation of the chest radiograph in the assessment of any diffuse lung pathology is the two dimensional representation of a volume of disease. Because of this, regional inhomogeneity in the distribution of disease is often invisible. Cross-sectional imaging techniques lend greater precision to the depiction of disease distribution [4] and, in particular, high resolution computed tomography (CT) shows morphological abnormalities at the level of the secondary pulmonary lobule [5]. However, CT (or any

other technique which requires moving a critically ill patient from the intensive care unit) cannot, unlike the ubiquitous chest radiograph, be used for monitoring serial change.

CHEST RADIOGRAPHY

TECHNICAL CONSIDERATIONS

Mobile or portable chest radiography has the very real advantage that it can be performed without moving the patient from the intensive care unit, but has many shortcomings compared with its departmental counterpart, the erect posteroanterior chest radiograph. The maximum milliamperage output of portable X-ray machines is severely limited, so that relatively long exposure times are needed, with the attendant risk of blurring of the image due to patient movement. Similarly, a high kilovoltage technique is not possible with portable machines. Furthermore, the use of grids (which reduce scattered radiation and improve image quality) is limited by difficulties in aligning them with the X-ray beam.

The short X-ray tube to film distance, inherent in portable radiography, results in undesirable magnification, most obviously of the cardiac silhouette, and is further exacerbated by the anteroposterior projection used for most supine or semirecumbent patients. The supine position of most patients also

ARDS Acute Respiratory Distress in Adults. Edited by Timothy W. Evans and Christopher Haslett. Published in 1996 by Chapman & Hall, London. ISBN 0 412 56910 8

allows the liver and abdominal contents to gravitate into the thorax, reducing lung volume and producing a ground-glass pattern which convincingly mimics diffuse lung pathology. Similarly, changes in the state of inflation of the lungs or the method of ventilation can cause errors of interpretation on serial films.

The exposure of a portable chest radiograph is not controlled by a phototimer and the chosen exposure is a matter of judgment, based mainly on the patient's body habitus. However, even an experienced radiographer cannot take into account the extent of intrathoracic pathology, which will dictate the need for a greater or lesser exposure to produce a diagnostic radiograph. The narrow latitude of conventional radiographic film (which makes it sensitive to under- or over-exposure) means that exactly comparable radiographs, in terms of overall optical density, are difficult to obtain. The result is serial radiographs that are often difficult to compare. As the diagnosis and monitoring of patients with ARDS depends largely on the appearance of serial changes in the radiographic density of the lungs, non-comparable films represent a considerable disadvantage. Consequently, any method of improving the quality of portable chest radiography would represent a significant advance. In this sense, digital chest radiography has proved valuable.

DIGITAL CHEST RADIOGRAPHY

Digital technology is an integral part of techniques such as CT, magnetic resonance imaging (MRI) and ultrasonography. It has long been recognized that conventional film as a means of image capture, storage and display represents something of a compromise [6], and it has become apparent that digital image acquisition, transmission, display and storage can be applied to chest radiography with advantage. Most commercially available digital systems have a reusable photostimulable phosphor plate (europium-doped barium fluorohalide) [7] instead of a conventional film–screen combination. Phosphor plate digital radiography has now been installed in many institutions, particularly as a substitute for portable film radiography. The phosphor plate is a large area detector which is housed in a 'filmless' cassette. On scanning the plate with a focused laser beam, the stored energy is emitted as light, which is detected by a photomultiplier and converted to a digital signal. The digital information can then be manipulated, displayed and stored in whatever format is desired (Figure 21.1).

An unequivocal advantage of phosphor plate computed radiography over conventional techniques is the exactly linear photoluminescence dose response, which is a full order of magnitude greater than that of conventional film. This extremely wide latitude coupled with the facility for image processing [8] produces diagnostically acceptable images over a wide range of exposures. The ability to retrieve an image of diagnostic quality from a suboptimal exposure, which with conventional film would result in an uninterpretable radiograph, has led to the increasing use of such systems for portable chest radiography.

RADIOGRAPHIC ABNORMALITIES AND THEIR EVOLUTION

The radiographic features of ARDS and their subsequent changes correlate well with pathological findings at postmortem examination [2,9,10] (Chapter 4). Many systems have been devised to divide the course of ARDS into different stages by either clinical or pathological criteria. There is broad concordance between the phases described, whether they are based on clinical, radiographic or pathological changes (Figure 21.2).

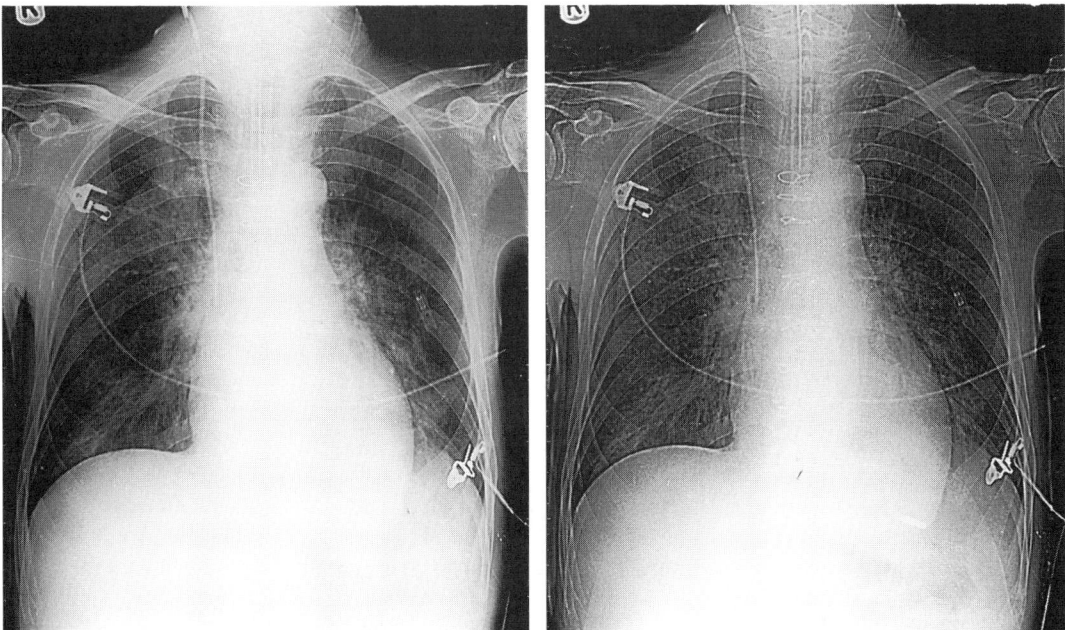

Figure 21.1 Digital chest radiograph of a mechanically ventilated patient. The left hand image is analogous to a conventional film radiograph. The right hand image has been manipulated to improve visualization in the low contrast areas (e.g. the mediastinum), edge enhancement increases the conspicuity of central lines.

0–24 hours

There is typically a delay of at least 12 hours between the precipitating event and the appearance of ARDS related radiographic abnormalities [10,11]. This cryptic phase of the disease may be as long as 24 hours; in general, the more devastating the lung injury, the shorter the latent period. Any radiographic abnormality of the lungs within the first day raises the possibility, usually in retrospect, that the abnormality represents either the precipitating cause itself or some complicating factor, such as aspiration pneumonia or fluid overload, respectively.

The first definite radiographic abnormality that occurs at around 24 hours is ill-defined opacification of the lungs, usually extending from the hila. This so-called 'ground-glass' opacification obscures the underlying pulmonary vasculature and may be indistinguishable from interstitial pulmonary edema (Figure 21.2a). A confounding factor in identifying this abnormality is that lung volumes are often reduced, possibly reflecting diffuse microatelectasis [10,12] (Chapter 16). Thus, the contribution of extravascular water in the interstitium [13] and relative under-inflation of the lungs to the diffuse pulmonary opacification is usually unclear.

As the leakage of fluid into the interstitium continues, peribronchovascular thickening, a relatively subjective sign, may become apparent. The generalized ground-glass opacification, which appears relatively uniform when first appears, rapidly progresses to patchy areas of frank consolidation (Figure 21.2b), the hallmark of increased permeability pulmonary edema. It has been observed that this type of edema tends to have a peripheral distribution [14–16]. Other features that mil-

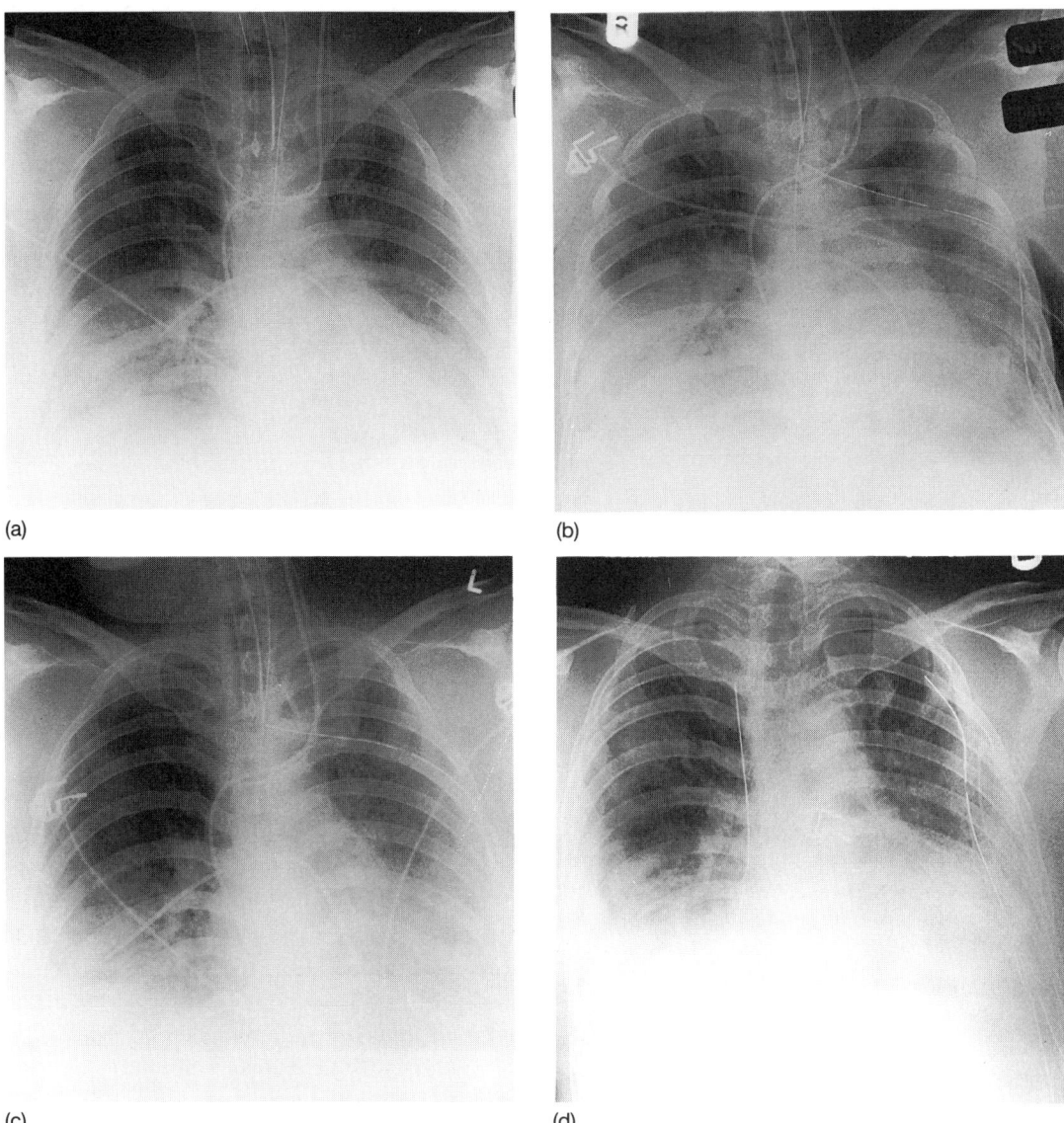

(a)   (b)

(c)   (d)

Figure 21.2 Typical radiographic sequence in a patient with ARDS: (a) 30 hours after the initial insult, there is ground-glass opacification of the mid- and lower lung zones; (b) 36 hours after the first radiograph there is dense consolidation, particularly in the lower lobes, with an air bronchogram in the right lower zone; (c) 24 hours later the patient was turned prone for a few hours, resulting in some re-expansion of the lower lobes; (d) 3 weeks after the initial injury, some collapse and consolidation persists in the lower lobes and a faint reticulonodular pattern has developed in the mid- and upper zones.

itate against a cardiogenic cause for the pulmonary edema are a normal heart size and vascular pedicle. The upper zone vessels are usually distended (in common with all patients radiographed in the supine position), so that this cannot be used as a reliable indicator of cardiac failure. The outpouring of hemorrhagic proteinaceous fluid into the air spaces and hyaline membrane formation result in a pattern of dense air space consolidation within which air bronchograms are strikingly conspicuous.

2–3 days

The patchy areas of consolidation soon coalesce to form widespread air space shadowing throughout both lungs. The distribution is usually diffuse with no particular predilection for the upper or lower zones. Furthermore, the perihilar and peripheral regions of the lungs are equally involved, rarely the case with cardiogenic pulmonary edema. The two dimensional nature of chest radiography tends to exaggerate the homogeneity of the distribution of the diffuse lung shadowing in ARDS (the axial distribution of disease is discussed in more detail in the section on CT). Although lung involvement is generally symmetrical, marked asymmetry between these zones and between the right and left lung may occur.

In the critically ill patient it is easy to overlook pre-existing lung disease which may be responsible for modifying the appearances of developing ARDS. The most obvious example is emphysema, which influences the development and texture of air space consolidation. In some patients, severe upper zone emphysema may give the spurious impression that the upper zones are relatively disease-free. Any diffuse lung disease, particularly one resulting in cystic air spaces and lung destruction, will affect the appearance of the lungs (Figure 21.3).

Within the first 2 days there is histopathological evidence of injury to both the alveolar epithelium and capillary endothelium [17,18]. Angiographic and pathological features suggest that the endovascular damage results in thrombosis in segmental and subsegmental arteries [19,22]. The signs of the generalized small vessel thrombosis seen on angiography are unlike the appearances of filling defects in larger vessels seen in classical pulmonary

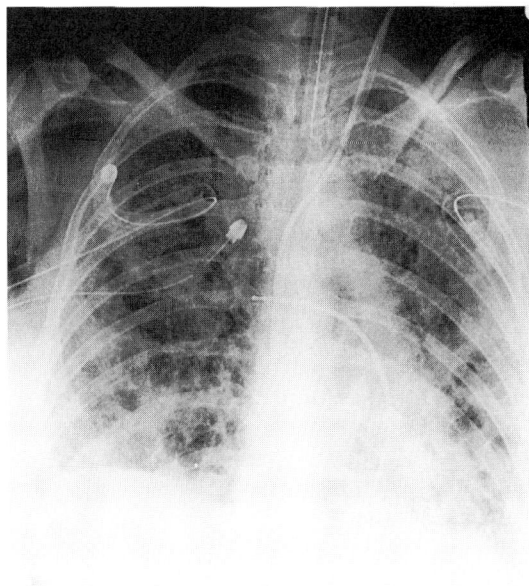

Figure 21.3 A patient with ARDS as a result of a fulminant staphylococcal pneumonia. The development of numerous pneumatoceles has modified the usual pattern of homogeneous ground-glass opacification and patchy consolidation.

thromboembolism. Areas of underperfused lung, whether due to primary or secondary microthrombosis, further aggravate endothelial injury. As a result, cardiac output may be diminished, and in the more severe cases of ARDS radiographic evidence of right and left sided heart failure may become apparent at this stage.

Although an infrequent accompaniment, pleural effusions have been reported in clinical practice [23] and in an animal model of ARDS [24]. In the animal study, approximately 20% of the excess lung water (which was of high protein content similar to that of serum) accumulated in the pleural space. It is probable that the pleural effusions of patients with ARDS are similarly exudative in nature. Effusions are seen more commonly when a large volume of lung is consolidated and suggest that movement of extravascular pulmonary fluid into the pleural space acts as an important means of drainage. When pleural collections develop it is difficult to be certain of their etiology. It is conceivable that they represent a combination of pleural reaction to subpleural hemorrhagic or infarcted/infected lung, fluid overload or concurrent cardiac failure.

4–7 days

After the first 36 hours few radiographic changes occur for a variable period in patients with uncomplicated ARDS. Any focal progression of lung shadowing at this stage suggests supervening infection or pulmonary infarction. A more widespread increase in lung shadowing should raise the possibility of fluid overload.

Pulmonary infection is a frequent complication, which may be difficult to distinguish from ARDS related consolidation that is progressing asymmetrically. The radiographic diagnosis of supervening pulmonary infec-

tion in mechanically ventilated patients has been shown to be poor due to high false-negative and false-positive readings. By contrast, the diagnosis of uncomplicated ARDS from chest radiographs is relatively high [25].

Even with meticulous radiographic technique serial changes in the appearances of the lungs during this phase may be both under- or over-interpreted. The most potent cause of apparent changes of widespread lung shadowing is the state of inflation of the lungs, determined by the type of mechanical ventilation. In particular, the application of positive end expiratory pressure (PEEP) results in dramatic and rapid variations in the overall opacification of the lungs [26,27]. Thus, any interpretation of overall appearances of the lung shadowing must take into account the type of ventilation and phase of inflation of the lungs at which the radiograph was taken (Figure 21.4). Continuous positive pressure ventilation can also lead to a confusing radiographic appearance of diffuse interstitial

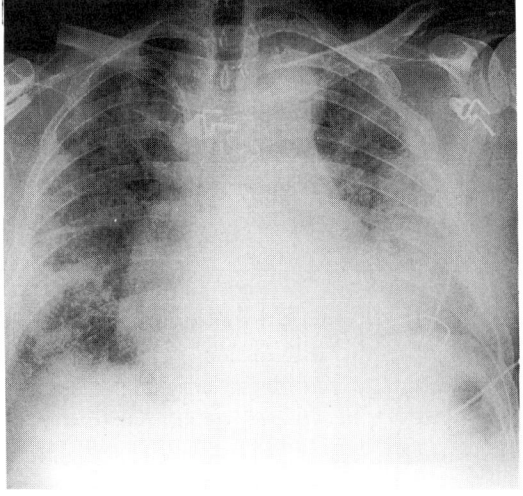
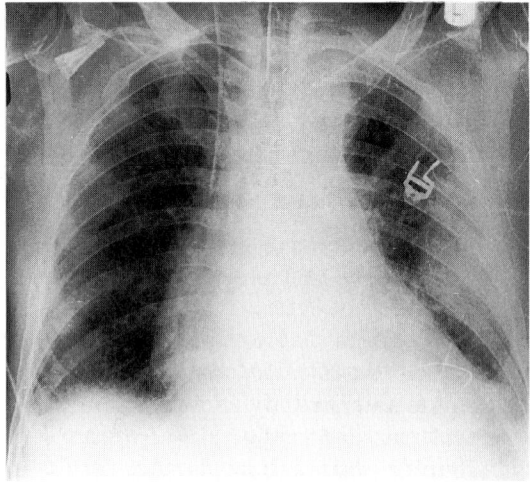

(a)   (b)

Figure 21.4 (a) Radiograph of a patient with ARDS shortly after extubation; (b) after reintubation and the commencement of ventilation there is apparent clearing of the generalized opacification of the lungs. The dense area in the periphery of the left mid-zone was due to an extrapleural hematoma.

emphysema, which may be particularly conspicuous against the background of extensive air space consolidation. The lungs take on a curious texture: small linear transradiancies, tracking towards the hila, are characteristic of ventilator induced interstitial air. This radiographic sign often presages a pneumomediastinum and/or pneumothorax.

The development of interstitial emphysema is clearly related to the intra-alveolar pressures generated by ventilation and its duration [28,29]. Although lucent streaking due to the perivascular dissection of air along the interstitium of bronchopulmonary bundles is typical, a more subtle stippling or 'salt and pepper' appearance superimposed on the background consolidation may be the only manifestation of interstitial air [30]. The recognition of pulmonary interstitial emphysema is important because its physiological effect of pulmonary vascular compression may compromise cardiac output and reduce the capillary surface area available for gas exchange. Furthermore, it is another cause for the radiographic appearance of increased lung volumes and decreased lung density which spuriously suggest improvement, despite the fact that the patient shows poor arterial oxygenation and worsening static compliance.

Apparent radiographic improvement of the lungs, shown by asymmetric increasing transradiancy of one lung, should always raise the possibility of the development of a pneumothorax: in the supine patient, air in the pleural space collects anteriorly and a visceral pleural edge parallel to the lateral chest wall may not be present despite a considerable volume of air in the anterior (nondependent) part of the pleural space. The radiographic manifestation of a supine pneumothorax is thus often subtle and may merely result in slightly increased transradiancy of the hemithorax (Figure 21.5). A variety of radiographic projections have been recommended, including a lateral shoot-through view using a horizontal X-ray beam

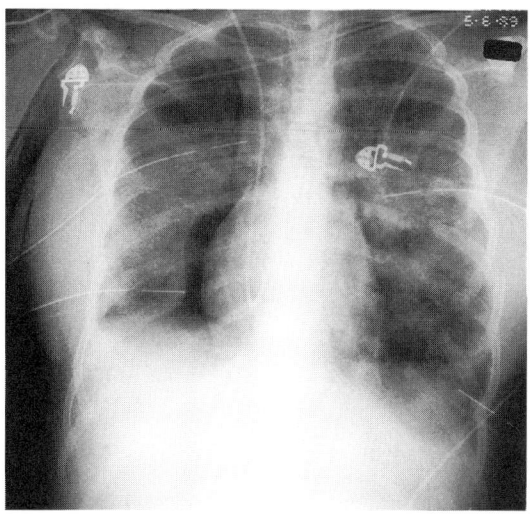

Figure 21.5 Bilateral pneumothoraces in a patient with ARDS. The visceral pleural edge adjacent to the right heart border is obvious. By contrast, there is no pleural edge associated with the left sided pneumothorax which has collected in the pleural space anteriorly: this is shown as an area of increased transradiancy over the lower zone.

to show the retrosternal visceral pleural edge [31].

After a variable period, of at least 4 days, radiographic improvement in the appearances of widespread pulmonary consolidation begins (Figure 21.6). Many patients do not survive past this radiographic phase of the disease and succumb to multi-organ system failure or overwhelming sepsis [32]. The first radiographic signs of resolution are almost imperceptible and may be concealed by inconsistent radiographic technique. The inhomogeneous clearing of the pulmonary consolidation represents regression of the high permeability edema.

In those patients in whom radiographic resolution becomes apparent, it is important to recognize that there may be considerable disjunction of the radiographic-pathological picture: at this stage there is hyperplasia of the type II pneumocytes with increased fibroblast activity and deposition of connective tissue [1]. As a result, there may be consider-

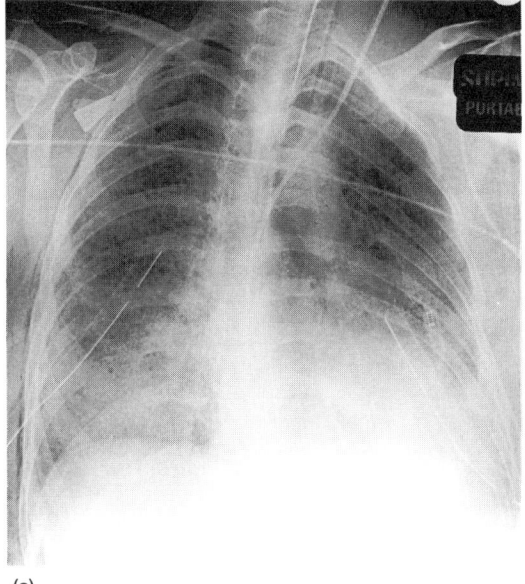

(a)

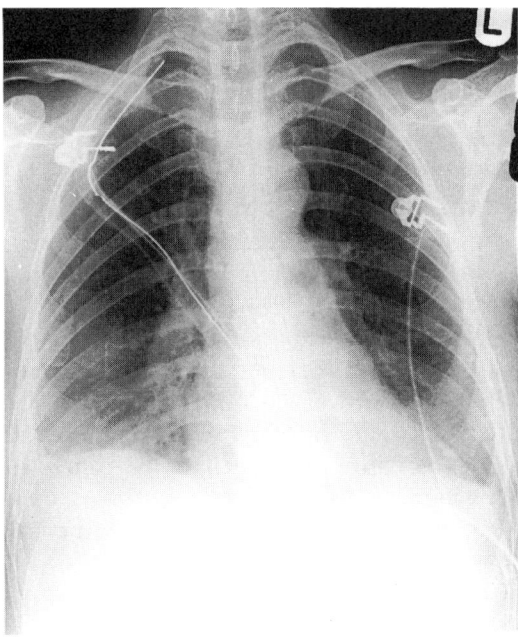

(b)

Figure 21.6 (a) Radiograph of a patient with established ARDS, 8 days after the initial lung injury; (b) 15 days after the preceding radiograph, the patient is extubated and there has been considerable clearing of the ground-glass opacification and basal consolidation.

able and progressive functional impairment, despite the apparent radiographic improvement.

7 days

While there is clearing of the consolidation, the lungs tend to remain diffusely abnormal and show linear, reticular or ground-glass patterns [9,33]. It is therefore often difficult to categorize the radiographic shadowing into one particular morphological pattern. At this stage the radiographic pattern probably represents variable proportions of diffuse interstitial and air space fibrosis.

Long term survivors of ARDS may have remarkably few radiographic changes, but careful analysis often reveals linear opacities and areas of relative transradiancy in areas formerly densely consolidated, particularly in the lung periphery [10]. These transradiant regions may correspond to ischemic or infarcted areas of lung distal to occluded pulmonary arteries and are at risk of becoming cystic air spaces, particularly if positive pressure ventilation has been aggressive. The air filled cysts may resemble pneumatoceles and tend to be in a subpleural location [28,29,34]. Histologically, the cysts have no epithelial lining, but have a wall consisting of compressed or destroyed lung and fibrous tissue. When large they may mimic a loculated pneumothorax.

The laying down of collagen may start within 2 weeks of the initial insult. It is likely that there is active remodeling in the reparative process of ARDS and it has been postulated that different types of collagen are deposited in the early and later stages of ARDS, thereby determining the degree of long term respiratory deficit seen in survivors [35]. Obvious radiographic features of scarring is seen in some ARDS survivors (Figure 21.7], although the exact prevalence of these radiographic abnormalities in long term survivors is unknown.

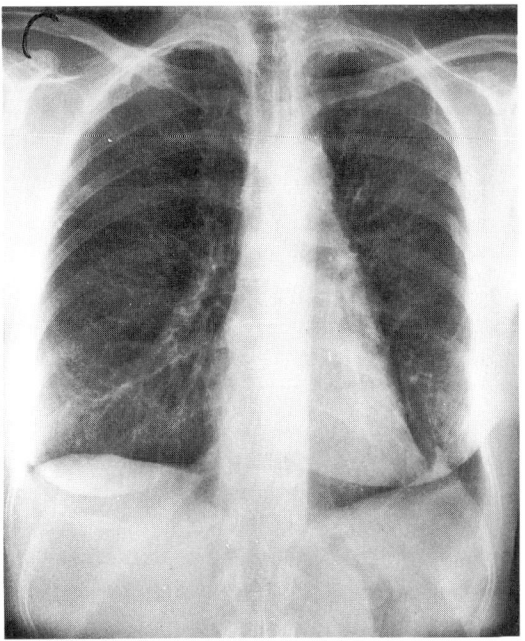

Figure 21.7 Linear opacities in the upper lobes with associated loss of volume, particularly on the left, indicating pulmonary fibrosis in a long term ARDS survivor.

SPECIFICITY OF RADIOGRAPHIC APPEARANCES OF INCREASED PERMEABILITY PULMONARY EDEMA VERSUS HYDROSTATIC EDEMA

The common radiographic picture of increased permeability pulmonary edema (typified by ARDS) and hydrostatic pulmonary edema (most commonly due to left ventricular failure) is of widespread shadowing representing lung consolidated by fluid. While distinguishing between the two causes is therapeutically relevant, particularly in the context of the critically ill patient, the chances of making a clear cut distinction on radiographic grounds alone (in isolation of other more reliable parameters, such as the pulmonary arterial occlusion pressure) should not be overestimated. Furthermore, increased permeability and hydrostatic edema often coexist in critically ill patients, making radiographic differentiation even more fraught.

The specificity of three major and six minor radiographic features was evaluated in 119 patients all with overt pulmonary edema (28 with ARDS, 30 with renal failure or volume overload and 61 with cardiac disease) [14]. The highest level of discrimination using these radiographic signs was between ARDS and the other two causes of edema. The differentiating radiographic features of the two types of pulmonary edema are summarized in Table 21.1. The most discriminatory features were the distribution of pulmonary blood flow, the pulmonary edema itself and the width of the vascular pedicle (taken as the width of the superior mediastinum just above the aortic arch). Only 10% of patients with ARDS showed inversion of the normal distribution of blood flow (in contrast to 50% of patients with cardiogenic pulmonary edema). A further 40% of patients with cardiogenic pulmonary edema showed a balanced distribution. In broad terms, the distribution of shadowing in the non cardiogenic pulmonary edema of ARDS was more often peripheral (45% of patients) and patchy with small intervening areas of unaffected lung, whereas cardiogenic pulmonary edema showed a more even distribution and was more or less homogeneous from the heart borders to the chest wall.

The width of the superior mediastinal vascular pedicle (which may be regarded as a crude manometer) was widened in 60% of patients with cardiogenic pulmonary edema (and of normal width in 40%), in contrast to the ARDS group, in whom a third had a narrow vascular pedicle and a further third a normal pedicle. Clearly, account has to be taken of the position of the patient because these radiographic signs are influenced strongly by gravity [36].

Starting with the premise that these features can be used to categorize pulmonary edema into non cardiogenic and cardiogenic causes, Miniati *et al.* [37] showed that two observers were able to suggest the correct category in 86 and 90% of cases respectively.

Table 21.1 Radiographic features distinguishing cardiogenic pulmonary edema from ARDS (noncardiogenic)

Feature	Cardiogenic	Noncardiogenic
Heart size	Enlarged	Not enlarged
Vascular pedicle	Normal/enlarged	Normal/reduced
Pulmonary blood flow distribution	Inverted	Normal/balanced
Pulmonary blood volume	Normal/increased	Normal
Septal lines	Not common	Absent
Peribronchial cuffs	Very common	Not common
Air bronchogram	Not common	Very common
Regional distribution of edema (horizontal axis)	Even	Peripheral
Pleural effusions	Very common	Not common

A later study [38] achieved an accuracy of 83% on the basis of heart size and the presence or absence of septal lines. However, these workers were unable to provide a radiographic strategy to differentiate cardiogenic from renal/fluid overload edema or increased permeability pulmonary edema from renal/fluid overload edema. Importantly, because of the severity of the pulmonary edema, an accurate assessment of the pulmonary vasculature could not be made. Furthermore, the width of the vascular pedicle did not distinguish between the three groups in this study [38].

Different conclusions were reached from an analysis of 45 patients with severe pulmonary edema of either hydrostatic or permeability types. Three observers classified chest radiographs as showing patterns indicating hydrostatic, increased permeability or mixed pulmonary edema, without knowledge of the clinical diagnosis: 87% patients with hydrostatic edema were correctly identified but only 60% of those with permeability edema were correctly characterized. The single most discriminatory criterion was a patchy, peripheral distribution, which occurred in 50% of patients with permeability edema, but only 13% of those with hydrostatic oedema [15]. More predictably, an increased heart size and septal lines were more common in patients with hydrostatic edema. In agreement with the study of Smith *et al.* [38], neither distribu-

tion of blood flow nor the width of the vascular pedicle reliably distinguished between the two types of pulmonary edema.

In conclusion, although some generalizations can be made about the differences in radiographic pattern observed between populations of patients with hydrostatic (or cardiogenic) and permeability pulmonary edema, the application of these rules to individual patients should be guarded and modified in the light of the rest of the clinical jigsaw.

SCORING OF CHEST RADIOGRAPHS

There have been many attempts to standardize the reading of chest radiographs of patients with ARDS to give a reproducible and objective measure of the severity of lung involvement. Chest radiography has been shown to correlate reasonably well with other measures of the extent of pulmonary edema [39,40], and in the face of a normal chest radiograph, estimations of extravascular lung water using thermodilution techniques are within normal limits [41–43]. A detailed scoring system [44] (derived from earlier work [45,46]) that analyzes both the presence and 'intensity' of radiographic signs, ranging from enlargement of the main pulmonary artery to the distribution of hazy or patchy lung shadowing, has been devised. When this scoring system was compared to arterial oxygen tension (with PEEP suspended at the time of sampling) and the measured Pa_{O_2} standardized to a Pa_{CO_2} of 40 Torr (5.3 kPa), a highly significant curvilinear correlation was found ($r = 0.87$, $P < 0.001$), consistent with the concept that Pa_{O_2} may be significantly reduced in the early stages of ARDS when radiographic changes are minimal, and again in the recovery phase when the radiograph is relatively normal (despite the presence of fine interstitial fibrosis). These findings reinforce the maxim that the chest radiograph should never be interpreted in isolation.

The validity of this type of scoring system has been confirmed more recently by correlation with densitometric analysis of the lungs using CT [47]. A significant correlation was found between the extent of lung injury as reflected by the mean CT number (the density of the lung measured in Hounsfield units) and the radiographic score ($r = 0.71$, $P < 0.01$). These studies lend support to the use of chest radiography as a readily available and effective means of estimating the extent of lung involvement in established ARDS.

COMPUTED TOMOGRAPHY

CLINICAL APPLICATION OF CT

Computed tomography has a major role in the evaluation of patients with diffuse infiltrative lung disease [48–51]. The images of high resolution CT, (HRCT) closely match the macroscopic appearances of pathological specimens of inflated lung [52,53]. The improved sensitivity and specificity of HRCT over chest radiography in the context of diffuse lung disease is now well established [54–56] and in some conditions, notably fibrosing alveolitis, the HRCT pattern is virtually pathognomonic [57]. To date, most clinical evaluations of HRCT have concentrated on chronic diffuse infiltrative lung disease. Although experience in the assessment of acute diffuse lung disease with HRCT is increasing [58,59], it is probably the inaccess-

ibility of CT in the acute situation that has prevented HRCT from reaching its potential in this area. As a result, few studies have been published on the application of CT in patients with acute lung injury, particularly in its early phase.

Clinical experience with CT in patients with ARDS is largely confined to the identification of complications that are otherwise radiographically occult: for example, the detection of a focus for infection, such as lung abscesses within densely consolidated lung; the evaluation of a complex, loculated pneumothorax [60,61]. In the recovery phase of ARDS, CT may help to define the extent and severity of supervening interstitial fibrosis, particularly if there is a discrepancy between radiographic and functional indices.

Small cystic air spaces, which probably represent a combination of loculated interstitial emphysema and frank destruction of small areas of lung, can be identified in some ventilated patients with ARDS. Confluence of these cysts leads to the formation of larger, thin walled, often subpleural air spaces [62]. Patients who develop these lung cysts tend to have a higher mortality (13/16, 81.2% versus an overall mortality of 22/28, 78.6%) [59].

MORPHOLOGICAL AND FUNCTIONAL CORRELATIONS USING CT

CT evaluation of the lungs in ARDS in the early stages of the disease has been limited to a few centers but has produced important new insights about the evolution, distribution and behavior of the disease [63–68].

The cross-sectional images of CT have shown that, in contrast to appearances on chest radiography, the distribution of disease in ARDS is far from homogeneous, particularly in patients scanned in the early phases of the disease [4,69,70]. Areas of relatively normal lung are interspersed between patches of densely consolidated and collapsed lung [4,63] (Figure 21.8). The distribution of densely consolidated lung tends to be

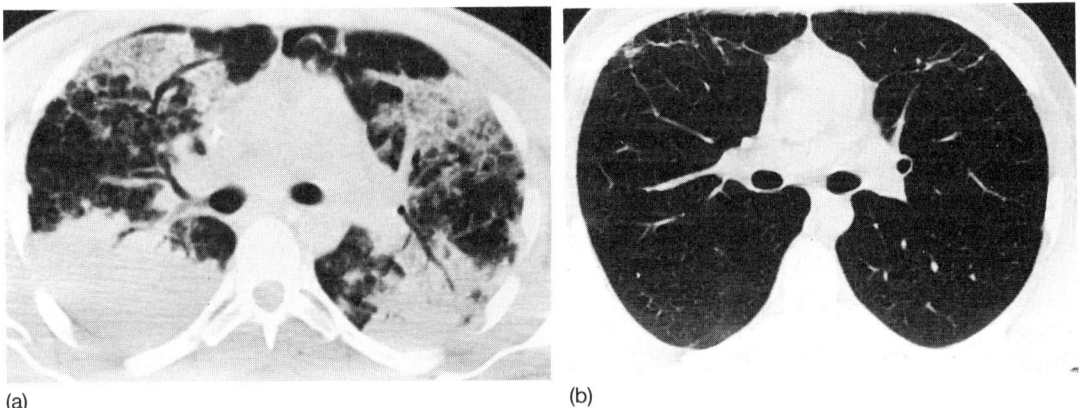

(a)   (b)

Figure 21.8 (a) CT through the upper lobes of a patient with ARDS. Multifocal areas of consolidation interspersed with relatively normal areas of lung. There are small pleural effusions posteriorly. (b) Residual linear and reticular opacities representing fibrosis in the anterior segments of the upper lobes on a follow up CT, 7 months later.

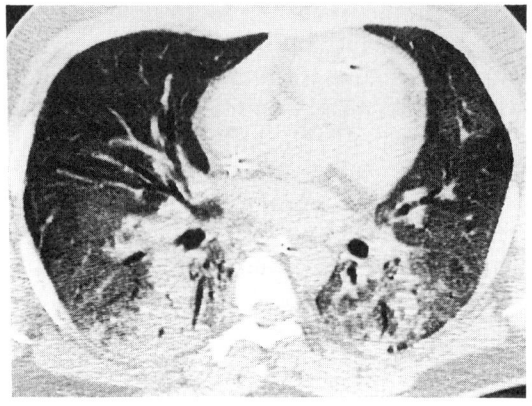

Figure 21.9 Thin section CT through the lower lobes showing volume loss and dense consolidation in the dependent posterobasal segment of the lower lobes. There is ground-glass opacification in other parts of the lungs.

gravity dependent and is thought to be due to compression by the generalized increase in weight of the overlying lung (Chapter 16). Thus in the supine patient, the greatest volume of dense parenchymal opacification is seen in the posterobasal segments of the lower lobes (Figure 21.9). Away from areas of dense consolidation, the lung is often of increased attenuation giving a ground-glass pattern (Figure 21.10). This hazy opacification

of the lung parenchyma can be regarded as reflecting a decrease in the overall air content within in the slice volume: this may be the result of an outpouring of cells or exudate into the air spaces (short of causing frank pulmonary consolidation), interstitial thickening or merely underinflation of the lung. As a general rule, a ground-glass pattern, although diagnostically nonspecific, usually denotes a reversible process [71,72].

Deciding which of the many pathological processes is responsible for the pattern of ground-glass opacification is not easy, and in the case of acute lung injury there are many variables at play (for example, the method of ventilation, fluid balance status and phase of the disease). For this reason, although the overall lung weight can be precisely measured from analysis of CT density of the lung parenchyma (with an error of about 1%) [63], interpretation of regional density measurements in isolation must be guarded. Nevertheless, using estimates of the lung weight and frequency distribution of CT measures of lung density, fractions of normally aerated, poorly aerated and unaerated lung can be calculated [63,65]. Comparing these data with functional measurements of static lung compliance, shunt fraction and Pa_{O_2} can produce

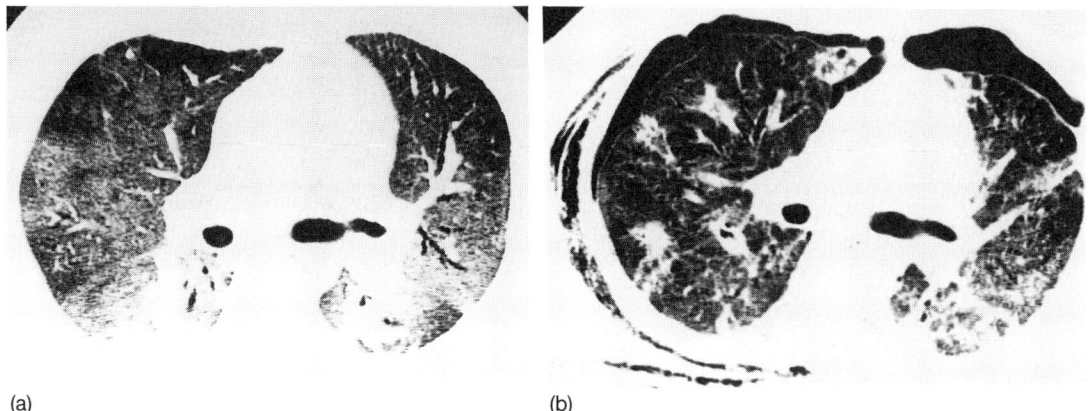

(a)   (b)

Figure 21.10 Widespread ground-glass opacification of the lung parenchyma 6 days after the initial lung injury; (b) two weeks later there are bilateral pneumothoraces and the generalized increase in density has resolved but there are numerous focal opacities, possibly representing areas of infarcted lung.

informative correlations between structure and function of the injured lung. Such data from CT indicate that static lung compliance correlates well with the amount of normally aerated lung, but not with the proportion of poorly or unaerated lung, and is thus a useful indicator of the fraction of residual healthy lung in ARDS. Not surprisingly, both Pao_2 and shunt fraction are inversely correlated to the fraction of unaerated lung tissue quantified by CT. Increasing the level of PEEP from 5 to 15 cmH$_2$O increases the fraction of normally aerated lung 'as quantified by CT' showing that recruitment of previously collapsed alveoli occurs with this maneuver. Accompanying this phenomenon is a decrease in shunt fraction, indicating that improved arterial oxygenation is due to recruitment of otherwise nonventilated, but still perfused, alveolar units.

The redistribution of apparently densely consolidated lung on repositioning the patient with ARDS has been well documented [67,73,74]. These observations suggest that the injured lung behaves as a sponge-like body of diffusely increased weight due to its water content, the dependent part of which is compressed by the weight of the overlying lung. This phenomenon is seen, to a lesser extent, in normal individuals [75]. The

increased density of atelectatic lung in the dependent posterobasal segments can be abolished by turning the patient prone (Figure 21.11).

In the latest of increasingly sophisticated analyses of morphological changes in relation to differing methods of ventilation, Gattinoni *et al.* have shown with CT densitometry that increased hydrostatic pressure superimposed on an area of lung is responsible for atelectasis and that this maybe prevented when the PEEP is equal to or greater than this pressure [68,76]. Predictably, if PEEP is able to inflate the most dependent atelectatic parts of the lung, the nondependent, relatively normal lung becomes markedly overdistended (Chapter 15).

Objective assessment of the extent of abnormal lung on CT in both the acute and convalescent phases of the disease has shown that there is a significant correlation between the lung injury score [1] and volume of lung involvement on CT ($r = 0.75$, $P < 0.01$). Furthermore, the extent and type of pulmonary abnormalities in long term survivors of ARDS are more precisely characterized by HRCT [77] than chest radiography, and some patients with apparently normal chest radiographs will have CT evidence of interstitial fibrosis (Figure 21.2).

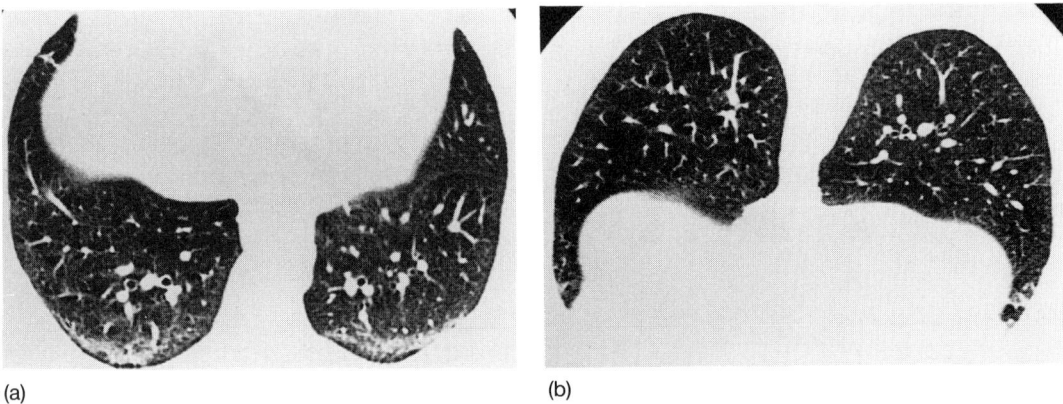

(a)   (b)

Figure 21.11 (a) Normal individual scanned in the supine position. Note the increased density in the dependent part of the lower lobes due to gravity-induced atelectasis. (b) The patient has been turned prone and rescanned a few minutes later: the density in the posterobasal segments has disappeared.

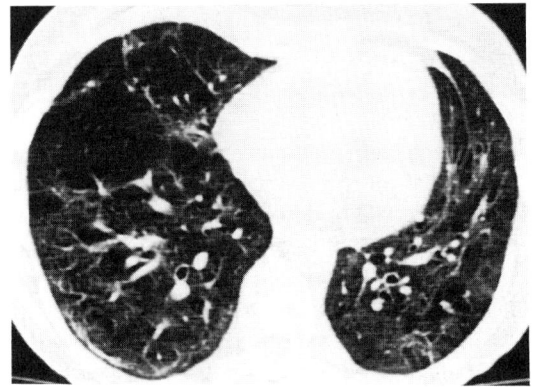

Figure 21.12 Distortion of the pulmonary parenchyma with a reticular pattern and several linear opacities traversing the lung representing established fibrosis. The CT was performed 11 months after discharge from the intensive care unit. At the time of the CT scan, the patient was mildly dyspneic, with a chest radiograph which was questionably abnormal.

MAGNETIC RESONANCE IMAGING

The clinical application of MRI to the assessment of critically ill patients remains limited because of the prolonged examination time and difficulties of monitoring patients, with nonmagnetic equipment, within the magnet's bore.

Since protons (in abundance in water) are responsible for the signal, MRI has the poten-tial to detect increased lung water content. Thus, although MRI in its current state of development, has considerably less spatial resolution than CT, the sensitivity of MRI for the detection of lung water is of great interest [78,79]. Early studies showed the ability of MRI to map the distribution of water in both normal and edematous lung [80,81], although more sophisticated analyses of T1 and T2 weighted images have not shown that it can consistently discriminate cardiogenic from noncardiogenic forms of pulmonary edema [82,83]. However, other animal work has suggested that MRI can, in the absence of variations in lung water content, detect and monitor experimental lung injury [84].

Discrimination between increased pulmonary capillary permeability and hydrostatic pulmonary edema using the timing and distribution of lung enhancement on MRI after the administration of a macromolecular paramagnetic contrast agent has been described in an experimental model [85]. However, there are simpler and less cumbersome methods of determining pulmonary vascular permeability, including the clearance of inhaled tracer particles or transvascular protein flux techniques [86] (Chapter 16).

The attractions of magnetic resonance imaging of the injured lung are the acquisition of both morphological information (although of lower resolution than CT) and physiological data (particularly quantitation of lung water) in a single examination. Continuing improvements in imaging sequences and reductions in scanning times may lead to the more widespread use of MRI in this context.

POSITRON EMISSION TOMOGRAPHY

Positron emission tomography (PET) is based on the detection of the annihilation radiation (two 511 keV γ rays emitted at 180° to one another) that results from the collision of a positron with an electron. The positron arises from the nucleus of an unstable isotope and travels only a few millimeters in soft tissues before the interaction with an electron occurs [87,88]. Positron emitting isotopes have been shown to be suitable for the radioactive labeling of agents which allow measurements of extravascular and intravascular water to be made. For example, water itself can be labeled with the positron-emitting isotope oxygen-15.

Not only can PET quantitate the amount of extravascular water, it can also, because of its tomographic nature, map the distribution of water in the lungs [89]. The specific application of PET to the evaluation of pulmonary vascular permeability in patients with ARDS, using transferrin labeled with gallium-68, has shown that the index of permeability is elevated in the early phase of the disease and, despite measures of extravascular lung water returning to normal, pulmonary vascular permeability remains high for at least 2 weeks after onset [90]. Secondly, PET measurements of extravascular water in areas of radiographic abnormality in patients with ARDS, congestive heart failure and pneumonia are raised compared with normal subjects [91]. The index of vascular permeability (using the transcapillary escape rate of ^{68}Ga-labeled transferrin) was abnormal only in ARDS and pneumonia patients. Furthermore, vascular permeability was abnormal in areas of lung away from the radiographically visible pulmonary consolidation, suggesting that PET is a highly sensitive (although nonspecific) technique for identifying increased vascular permeablility.

CONCLUSION

The advent of digital radiography has improved the quality and reproducibility of portable chest radiographs. As a result, evaluation of serial changes in patients with ARDS using digital radiography can be made more reliably. While the chest radiograph remains the most common imaging investigation of the critically ill patient, cross-sectional techniques provide superior information about the precise extent and distribution of disease. CT, in particular, has an important role in the identification of radiographically cryptic complications of ARDS. Correlations between the detailed images of HRCT and physiological parameters are likely to produce further insights into the natural history and effects of therapeutic maneuvers in ARDS. The greater availability and quicker examination times of MRI (and to a lesser extent PET) scanning should ensure that these powerful tools are increasingly employed to unravel the pathophysiology of ARDS.

REFERENCES

1. Murray, J.F., Matthay, M.A., Luce, J.M. *et al.* (1988) An expanded definition of the adult respiratory distress syndrome. *Am. Rev. Respir. Dis.*, **138**, 720–3.
2. Joffe, N. (1974) The adult respiratory distress syndrome. *AJR*, **122**, 719–32.
3. Putman, C.E. (1992) Cardiac and non-cardiac edema: radiologic approach, In *Critical Care Imaging*, 3rd edn. (eds L.R. Goodman and C.E. Putman), W.B. Saunders, Philadelphia, pp. 107–27.
4. Maunder, R.J., Shuman, W.P., McHugh, J.W. *et al.* (1986) Preservation of normal lung

regions in the adult respiratory distress syndrome: analysis by computed tomography. *JAMA*, **255**, 463–5.

5. Müller, N.L. and Ostrow, D.N. (1991) High-resolution computed tomography of chronic interstitial lung disease. *Clin. Chest Med.* **12**, 97–114.

6. Goodman, L.R., Wilson, C.R. and Foley, W.D. (1988) Digital radiography of the chest: promises and problems. *AJR*, **150**, 1241–52.

7. Sonoda, M., Takano, M., Miyahara, J. and Kato, H. (1983) Computed radiography utilizing scanning laser stimulated luminescence. *Radiology*, **148**, 833–8.

8. Jennings, P., Padley, S.P.G. and Hansell, D.M. (1992) Portable chest radiography in intensive care: a comparison of computed and conventional radiography. *Br. J. Radiol.*, **65**, 852–6.

9. Ostendorf, P., Birzle, H. and Vogel, W. (1975) Pulmonary radiographic abnormalities in shock. Roentgen-clinical pathological correlation. *Radiology*, **115**, 257–63.

10. Greene, R. (1987) Adult respiratory distress syndrome: acute alveolar damage. *Radiology*, **163**, 57–66.

11. Newell, J.D., Underwood, G.H. and Kelley, M.J. (1983) The ICU chest film: cardiac versus pulmonary disease. *Cardiol. Clin.*, **1**, 729–43.

12. Hallman, M., Spragg, R., Harrell, J.H. *et al.* (1982) Evidence of lung surfactant abnormality in respiratory failure. *J. Clin. Invest.*, **70**, 673–83.

13. Goodman, L.R. and Putman, C.E. (1984) Diagnostic imaging in acute cardiopulmonary disease. *Clin. Chest Med.*, **5**, 247–64.

14. Milne, E.N.C., Pistolesi, M., Miniati, M. *et al.* (1985) The radiologic distinction of cardiogenic and noncardiogenic edema. *AJR*, **144**, 879–94.

15. Aberle, D.R., Wiener-Kronish, J.P., Webb, W.R. *et al.* (1988) Hydrostatic versus increased permeablity pulmonary edema: diagnosis based on radiographic criteria in critically ill patients. *Radiology*, **168**, 73–9.

16. Fraser, R.G., Pare, J.A.P., Pare, P.D. *et al.* (eds) (1990) Pulmonary hypertension and edema, in *Diagnosis of Diseases of the Chest*, 3rd edn, W. B. Saunders, Philadelphia, pp. 1823–1968.

17. Albertine, K.H. (1985) Ultrastructural abnormalities in increased-permeability pulmonary edema. *Clin. Chest Med.*, **6**, 345–69.

18. Bachofen, H., Bachofen, M. and Weibel, E.R. (1988) Ultrastructural aspects of pulmonary edema. *J. Thorac. Imaging*, **3**, 1–7.

19. Greene, R., Zapol, W.M., Snider, M.T. *et al.* (1981) Early bedside detection of pulmonary vascular occlusion during acute respiratory failure. *Am. Rev. Respir. Dis.*, **124**, 593–601.

20. Greene, R., Jantsch, H., Boggis, C. *et al.* (1983) Respiratory distress syndrome with new considerations. *Radiol. Clin. North. Am.*, **21**, 699–708.

21. Greene, R. (1986) Pulmonary vascular obstruction in the adult respiratory distress syndrome. *J. Thorac. Imaging*, **1**, 31–8.

22. Vesconi, S., Rossi, G.P., Pesenti, A. (1988) Pulmonary microthrombosis in severe adult respiratory distress syndrome. *Crit. Care Med.*, **16**, 111–3.

23. Wiener-Kronish, J.P. and Matthay, M.A. (1988) Pleural effusions associated with hydrostatic and increased permeablity pulmonary edema. *Chest*, **93**, 852–8.

24. Wiener-Kronish, J.P., Broaddus, V.C., Albertine, K.H. *et al.* (1988) Pleural effusions are associated with increased permeability pulmonary edema in anesthetized sheep. *J. Clin. Invest.*, **82**, 1422–9.

25. Winer-Muram, H.T., Rubin, S.A., Ellis, J.V. *et al.* (1993) Pneumonia and ARDS in patients receiving mechanical ventilation: diagnostic accuracy of chest radiography. *Radiology*, **188**, 479–85.

26. Zimmerman, J.E., Goodman, L.R. and Shahvari, M.B.G. (1979) Effect of mechanical ventilation and positive end-expiratory pressure (PEEP) on chest radiograph. *AJR*, **133**, 811–5.

27. Johnson, T.H., Altman, A.R., McCaffree, R.D. *et al.* (1982) Radiologic considerations in the adult respiratory distress syndrome treated with positive end expiratory pressure (PEEP). *Clin. Chest Med.*, **3**, 89–100.

28. Woodring, J.H. (1985) Pulmonary interstitial emphysema in the adult respiratory distress syndrome. *Crit. Care Med.*, **13**, 786–91.

29. Unger, J.M., England, D.M. and Bogust, G.A. (1989) Interstitial emphysema in adults: recognition and prognostic implications. *J. Thorac. Imaging*, **4**, 86–94.

30. Aberle, D.R. and Brown, K. (1990) Radiologic considerations in the adult respiratory distress syndrome. *Clin. Chest Med.*, **11**, 737–54.

31. Morgan, R.A., Owens, C.M., Collins, C.D. *et al.* (1993) The improved detection of pneumo-

thoraces in critically ill patients with lateral shoot-through digital radiography. *Clin. Radiol.*, **48**, 249–52.

32. Bell, R.C., Coalson, J.J., Smith, J.D. *et al.* (1983) Multiple organ system failure and infection in adult respiratory distress syndrome. *Ann. Intern. Med.*, **99**, 293–8.

33. Dyck, D.R. and Zylak, C.J. (1973) Acute respiratory distress in adults. *Radiology*, **106**, 497–501.

34. Hert, R. and Albert, R.K. (1994) Sequelae of the adult respiratory distress syndrome. *Thorax*, **49**, 8–13.

35. Pingleton, S.K. (1988) Complications of acute respiratory failure. *Am. Rev. Respir. Dis.*, **137**, 1463–93.

36. Pistolesi, M., Milene, ENC, Miniati, M. *et al.* (1984) The vascular pedicle of the heart and the vena azygos. Part II: acquired heart disease. *Radiology*, **152**, 9.

37. Miniati, M., Pistolesi, M., Paoletti, P. *et al.* (1988) Objective radiographic criteria to differentiate cardiac, renal, and injury lung edema. *Invest. Radiol.*, **23**, 433–40.

38. Smith, R.C., Mann, H., Greenspan, R.H. *et al.* (1987) Radiographic differentiation between different etiologies of pulmonary edema. *Invest. Radiol.*, **22**, 859–63.

39. Pistolesi, M., Milne, ENC, Miniati, M. *et al.* (1986) Detection and measurement of pulmonary oedema: the chest radiographic approach. *Intensive Crit. Care Dig.*, **5**, 34–6.

40. Miniati, M., Pistolesi, M., Milne, ENC. *et al.* (1987) Detection of lung edema. *Crit. Care. Med.*, **15**, 1146–55.

41. Baudendistel, L., Shields, J.B. and Kaminski, D.L. (1982) Comparison of double indicator thermodilution measurements of extravascular lung water (EVLW) with radiographic estimation of lung water in trauma patients. *J. Trauma*, **22**, 983–8.

42. Sibbald, W.J., Warshawski, F.J., Short, A.K. *et al.* (1983) Clinical studies of measuring extravascular lung water by the thermal dye technique in critically ill patients. *Chest*, **83**, 25–31.

43. Laggner, A., Kleinberger, G., Haller, J. *et al.* (1984) Bedside estimation of extravascular lung water in critically ill patients: comparison of the chest radiograph and the thermal dye technique. *Intensive Care Med.*, **10** 309–13.

44. Pistolesi, M., Miniati, M. and Giuntini C. (1988) A radiographic score for clinical use in the adult respiratory distress syndrome. *Intensive Crit. Care Dig.*, **7**, 2–4.

45. Halperin, B.D. Feeley, T.W., Mihm, F.G. *et al.* (1985) Evaluation of the portable chest roentgenogram for quantitating extravascular lung water in critically ill adults. *Chest*, **88**, 649–52.

46. Pistolesi, M., Milne, ENC. *et al.* (1985) The chest roentgenogram in pulmonary edema. *Clin. Chest Med.*, **6**, 315–44.

47. Bombino, M., Gattinoni, L., Pesenti, A. *et al.* (1991) The value of portable chest roentgenography in adult respiratory distress syndrome. Comparison with computed tomography. *Chest*, **100**, 762–9.

48. Müller, N.L. and Miller, R.R. (1990) Computed tomography of chronic diffuse infiltrative lung disease (part 1). *Am. Rev. Respir. Dis.*, **142**, 1206–15.

49. Müller, N.L. and Miller, R.R. (1990) Computed tomography of chronic diffuse infiltrative lung disease (part 2). *Am. Rev. Respir. Dis.*, **142**, 1440–8.

50. Hansell, D.M. and Kerr, I.H. (1991) The role of high resolution computed tomography in the diagnosis of interstitial lung disease. *Thorax*, **46**, 77–84.

51. Müller, N.L. (1991) Clinical value of high resolution CT in chronic diffuse lung disease. *AJR*, **157**, 1163–70.

52. Hruban, R.H., Meziane, M.A., Zerhouni, E.A. *et al.* (1987) High resolution computed tomography of inflation-fixed lungs. *Am. Rev. Respir. Dis.*, **136**, 935–40.

53. Itoh, H., Murata, K., Konishi, J., *et al.* (1993) Diffuse lung disease: pathologic basis for the high-resolution computed tomography findings. *J. Thorac. Imaging*, **8**, 176–88.

54. Mathieson, J.R., Mayo, J.R., Staples, C.A. and Müller, N.L. (1989) Chronic diffuse infiltrative lung disease: comparison of diagnostic accuracy of CT and chest radiography. *Radiology*, **171**, 111–16.

55. Padley, SPG, Hansell, D.M., Flower, CDR and Jennings, P., (1991) Comparative accuracy of high resolution computed tomography and chest radiography in the diagnosis of chronic diffuse infiltrative lung disease. *Clin. Radiol.*, **44**, 227–31.

56. Grenier, P., Valeyre, D., Cluzel, P. *et al.* (1991) Chronic diffuse interstitial lung disease: diagnostic value of chest radiography and high-resolution CT. *Radiology*, **179**, 123–32.

57. Tung, K.T., Wells, A.U., Rubens, M.B. *et al.* (1993) Accuracy of the typical computed tomographic appearances of fibrosing alveolitis. *Thorax* **48**, 334–8.

58. Aberle, D.R. (1993) HRCT in acute diffuse lung disease. *J. Thorac. Imaging*, **8**, 200–12.

59. Stark, P., Greene, R., Kott, M.M. et al. (1987) CT findings in ARDS. *Radiologie*, **27**, 367–9.

60. Snow, N., Bergin, K.T. and Horrigan, T.P. (1990) Thoracic CT in critically ill patients: information obtained frequently alters management. *Chest*, **97**, 1467–70.

61. Mirvis, S.E., Tobin, K.D., Kostrubiak, I. and Belzberg, H. (1987) Thoracic CT in detecting occult disease in critically ill patients. *AJR*, **148**, 685–9.

62. Stark, P., and Jasmine, J., (1989) CT of pulmonary edema. *Crit. Rev. Diagn. Imaging*, **29**, 245–55.

63. Gattinoni, L., Presenti, A., Torresin, A. *et al.* (1986) Adult respiratory distress syndrome profiles by computed tomography. *J. Thorac. Imaging*, **1**, 25–30.

64. Gattinoni, L., Mascheroni, D., Torresin A. *et al.* (1986) Morphological response to positive end-expiratory pressure in acute respiratory failure: computerized tomography study. *Intensive Care Med.*, **12**, 137–42.

65. Gattinoni, L., Pesenti, A., Avalli, L. *et al.* (1987) Pressure–volume curve of total respiratory system in acute respiratory failure. Computed tomographic scan study. *Am. Rev. Respir. Dis.*, **136**, 730–6.

66. Gattinoni, L., Pesenti, A., Bombino, M. *et al.* (1988) Relationships between lung computed tomography density, gas exchange, and PEEP in acute respiratory failure. *Anesthesiology*, **69**, 824–32.

67. Gattinoni, L., Pelosi, P., Pesenti, A. *et al.* (1991) CT scan in ARDS: clinical and physiopathological insights. *Acta Anaesthesiol. Scand.*, **35** (suppl. 95), 87–96.

68. Gattinoni, L., D'Andrea, L., Pelosi, P. et al. (1993) Regional effects and mechanism of positive end-expiratory pressure in early adult respiratory distress syndrome. *JAMA*, **269**, 2122–7.

69. Marini, J.J. (1990) Lung mechanics in the adult respiratory distress syndrome: recent conceptual advances and implications for management. *Clin. Chest Med.*, **11**, 673–90.

70. Marini J.J. (1992) New approaches to the ventilatory management of the adult respiratory distress syndrome. *J. Crit. Care*, **7**, 256–67.

71. Remy-Jardin, M., Remy, J., Giraud, F. *et al.* (1993) Computed tomography (CT) assessment of ground-glass opacity: semiology and significance. *J. Thorac. Imaging*, **8**, 249–64.

72. Leung, A.N., Miller, R.R. and Müller, N.L. (1993) Parenchymal opacification in chronic infiltrative lung diseases: CT-pathologic correlation. *Radiology*, **188**, 209–14.

73. Langer, M., Mascheroni, D., Marcolin, R. and Gattinoni, L. (1988) The prone position in ARDS patients. *Chest*, **94**, 103–7.

74. Gattinoni, L., Pelosi, P., Vitale, G., *et al.* (1991) Body position changes redistribute lung computed-tomographic density in patients with acute respiratory failure. *Anesthesiology*, **74**, 15–23.

75. Morimoto, S., Takeuchi, N., Imanaka, H. *et al.* (1989) Gravity-dependent atelectasis: radiologic, physiologic and pathologic correlation in rabbits on high-frequency oscillation ventilation. *Invest. Radiol.*, **24**, 522–33.

76. Bone, R.C. (1993) The ARDS lung. New insights from computed tomography. *JAMA*, **269**, 2134–5.

77. Owens, C.M., Evans, T.W., Keogh, B.F. and Hansell, D.M. (1994) The natural history of adult respiratory distress syndrome assessed with high resolution computed tomography. *Chest*, **106**, 1815–21.

78. Cutillo, A.G., Morris, A.H., Ailion, D.C. *et al.* (1986) Determination of lung water content and distribution by nuclear magnetic resonance imaging. *J. Thorac. Imaging*, **1** 39–51.

79. Cutillo, A.G., Morris, A.H., Ailion, D.C. *et al.* (1988) Quantitative assessment of pulmonary edema by nuclear magnetic resonance methods. *J. Thorac. Imaging*, **3**, 51–8.

80. Carroll, F.E., Loyd, T.E., Nolop, K.B. *et al.* (1985) MR imaging parameter in the study of lung water: a preliminary study. *Invest. Radiol.*, **20**, 381–7.

81. Wexler, H.R., Nicholson, R.L., Prato, F.S. *et al.* (1985) Quantitation of lung water by nuclear magnetic resonance imaging: a preliminary study. *Invest. Radiol.*, **20**, 583–90.

82. Podgorski, G.T., Carroll, F.E. and Parker, R.E. (1986) NMR evaluation of pulmonary interstitial and intravascular fluids. *Invest. Radiol.*, **21**, 478–83.

83. Vinitski, S., Steiner, R.M., Wexler, H.R. and

Rifkin, M. (1988) Assessment of lung water by magnetic resonance in three types of pulmonary edema. *Heart Vessels*, **4**, 88–93.

84. Shioya, S., Christman, R., Ailion, D.C., *et al.* (1993) Nuclear magnetic resonance Hahn spin-echo decay (T2) in live rats with endotoxin lung injury. *Magn. Reson. Med.*, **29**, 4411–5.

85. Berthezene, Y., Vexler, V., Jerome, H. et al. (1991) Differentiation of capillary leak and hydrostatic pulmonary edema with a macromolecular MR imaging contrast agent. *Radiology*, **181**, 773–7.

86. Miniati, M. and Pistolesi, M. (1993) Imaging strategies in the detection and evaluation of ARDS. *Schweiz. Med. Wochenschr.*, **123**, 464–72.

87. Hughes, J.M.B., Brudin, L.H., Valind, S.O. *et al.* (1985) Positron emission tomography in the lung. *J. Thorac. Imaging*, **1**, 79–88.

88. Wollmer, P. and Rhodes, C.G. (1988) Positron emission tomography in pulmonary edema. *J. Thorac. Imaging*, **3**, 44–50.

89. Wollmer, P., Rhodes, C.G., Deanfield, J. *et al.* (1987) Regional extra-vascular density of the lung in patients with acute pulmonary edema. *J. Appl. Physiol.*, **63**, 1890–6.

90. Calandrino, F.S., Dixie, J.A., Mintun, M.A. and Schuster, D.P. (1988) Pulmonary vascular permeability during the adult respiratory distress syndrome: a positron emission tomographic study. *Am. Rev. Respir. Dis.*, **138**, 421–8.

91. Kaplan, J.D., Calandrino, F.S. and Schuster, D.P. (1991) A positron emission tomographic comparison of pulmonary vascular permeability during the adult respiratory distress syndrome and pneumonia. *Am. Rev. Respir. Dis.*, **143**, 150–4.

SEVERITY SCORING

John S. Turner and Peter D. Potgieter

PHILOSOPHY

The art of clinical prediction has assumed major importance in critical care medicine; patients and their families increasingly expecting absolute accuracy in this regard, even though modern life support technology is sometimes more successful in delaying death than restoring health. The cost of medical care has also increased, with much of the expenditure occurring in the intensive care unit (ICU) setting and in the last few weeks or months of life. More recently, cost has been highlighted by the development of new and expensive drugs and life support devices, such as monoclonal antibodies for sepsis, and artificial surfactant and intravenacaval oxygenation (IVOX) for the syndrome of acute respiratory distress in adults (ARDS) (Chapters 26, 29 and 30). These developments have emphasized the need for accurate prediction of the severity of disease, to optimize both patient care and resource utilization in an era of shrinking medical care funding, and also for acceptable scientific evaluation of these new therapeutic modalities. Severity scoring systems are now regarded by many as prognostic indicators and there has inevitably been much confusion and unrealistic expectation about their capacity in this regard, which has led in many instances to their inappropriate application.

HISTORY

APACHE

The forerunner of current severity of illness scoring systems was APACHE (acronym for Acute Physiology And Chronic Health Evaluation), introduced in 1981 and impractical for routine use as it required a total of 34 physiological measurements [1]. It never gained acceptance and two years later the simplified acute physiological score (SAPS) was introduced, using only 14 easily obtained and readily available physiological variables [2]. However, it was the APACHE II score, published in 1985 [3], that rapidly gained widespread acceptance and that has become extremely widely used in general ICUs, including general surgical ICUs, throughout the world. The larger studies of its efficacy include those from the USA [3–6], the Middle East [7], Africa [8,9], Europe [10], the Far East [11], and the UK [12]. It has also been reported in a comparative study between New Zealand and the USA of patient selection for intensive care [13]. All of these studies showed that in general terms APACHE II was applicable worldwide [14], although the UK study, which evaluated 8796 admissions to 26 general ICUs in Britain and Ireland, showed that the predicted and actual mortality rates were significantly different in some units. It was felt that the (USA derived) APACHE II predictive equation did not fit all

ARDS Acute Respiratory Distress in Adults. Edited by Timothy W. Evans and Christopher Haslett. Published in 1996 by Chapman & Hall, London. ISBN 0 412 56910 8

the local data and might need modification for use in the UK [12]. APACHE II has also been used in ICUs dealing with specific clinical problems. These include outcome in hematological malignancy [15,16], abdominal sepsis [17], hemodialysis [18], cardiogenic pulmonary edema [19], patients receiving total parenteral nutrition [20], pancreatitis [21,22], acute renal failure [23], acute myocardial infarction [24], upper gastrointestinal hemorrhage [25], trauma [26], malignancy [27], after cardiac arrest [28], coronary care [29], cardiothoracic surgery [30], breast cancer [31] and asthma [32]. It has also been used in predicting organ failure and mortality in postoperative surgical patients [33], cost containment and quality assurance [34] and in predicting the usefulness of total parenteral nutrition [35].

Some of the APACHE II mortality predictions in specific groups of patients have been perceived to be successful; for example in pancreatitis [21,22], abdominal sepsis [17], and trauma [26]. Other clinical conditions have proved less amenable to this approach, as in postoperative surgical patients [33] and cardiogenic pulmonary edema [19]. However, this may simply reflect differences in the expectations of the users and observer bias. Nevertheless, in no study has APACHE II been accurate enough to predict confidently outcome in individuals, even though it has been refined by the ability to calculate a disease specific risk of dying [3] for the individual patient. This allows a comparison between predicted deaths and actual deaths to be made, enabling the performance of different hospitals to be compared, while taking into account the severity of illness of their respective populations [36].

The APACHE II scoring system evaluates the deviation from normal of 11 physiological variables, each scoring from 0 to 4 points as the deviation increases; it also includes the Glasgow coma scale, and allocates points for age and chronic health. It is easy to use, needing only simple physiological measure-ments and routinely performed blood tests, and all the information needed to perform scoring is published [3]. A refinement of APACHE II, using the trend of daily scores and integrating a coefficient for organ system failure [37], has shown promise in predicting outcome, but has not gained as wide acceptance as the original version. The most recent release is the APACHE III prognostic system [38], designed to be capable of delivering objective probability estimates. The predictions from the original database are most impressive [38]. However, APACHE III requires a greater amount of clinical and biochemical data and uses complicated score algorithms which remain copyright material; it is marketed as a hardware and software package by APACHE Medical Systems (Washington, USA).

Both APACHE II and III have been subjected to comparison with clinical judgment. Mortality predictions by clinicians were better than APACHE II in two studies [39,40] and there was no significant difference in a third [41]. However, APACHE III was slightly better at predicting mortality than clinicians and was also more consistently accurate at all levels of mortality [42].

Other scoring systems

The Mortality Prediction Model [43] employs 11 binary clinical variables selected by multiple logistic regression; although it compares well with APACHE II and SAPS [44], its use has not been as widely reported in the literature. Recently, Mortality Probability Model II [45] and SAPS II [46] have been published, both based on very large numbers of patients and both potentially powerful predictors of mortality. The organ system failure score [47], developed in parallel with APACHE, has tight definitions for organ failure, providing a very accurate predictive value for death. Thus, the failure of three or more organ systems on the fourth day of any organ failure carries a 96% mortality [47]. Other scoring

Table 22.1 Mortality in ARDS

First author	Year published	Patients	Mortality (%)
Pepe [52]	1982	46	41
Bell [53]	1983	141	74
Montgomery [54]	1985	47	68
Fowler [55]	1985	88	65
Seidenfeld [56]	1986	129	71
Mancebo [57]	1987	35	69
Maunder [58]	1989	136	65
Villar [59]	1989	104	56
Artigas [60]	1992	583	59
Suchyta [61]	1992	215	53
Kraus [62]	1993	83	45

systems for more specific disorders include the injury severity score [48] and the TISS method [49] for trauma; and the pediatric risk of mortality (PRISM) score [50] for infants and children. The therapeutic intervention scoring system (TISS) scores monitoring and therapeutic tasks [51] and may show variations in score according to different treatment philosophies and availability of resources, thereby reflecting the level of medical and nursing intervention rather than the severity of illness.

MORTALITY

OVERALL MORTALITY

Overall mortality in ARDS varies between 41 and 74% in 11 separate major clinical studies [52–62] published from 1982 to 1993 (Table 22.1) with no discernible trend towards improvement in the more recent studies. Unfortunately, as both the definition of ARDS and the demographics vary between the studies, strict comparison is difficult (Chapter 2).

INFLUENCE OF THERAPEUTIC INTERVENTIONS

Mortality is highest in patients with severe ARDS, with a 91% mortality reported for randomized patients in the extracorporeal membrane oxygenation study [63], although more recent mortality figures for patients with the same blood gas criteria are lower at 55% [64]. Although other new and exciting supportive techniques have been developed, no single treatment has been critically shown to have influenced mortality. Some have been tested in well conducted clinical studies including positive end expiratory pressure (PEEP) for the prevention of ARDS [65], extracorporeal membrane oxygenation [63], high frequency jet ventilation [66], extracorporeal carbon dioxide removal [67], and non ventilatory therapies such as corticosteroids [68], prostaglandin E_1 [69], and *N*-acetylcysteine [70]. Nevertheless, survival figures from uncontrolled studies on pressure controlled inverse ratio ventilation [71,72] (Chapter 23), extracorporeal carbon dioxide removal [73] (Chapter 25 and 27), permissive hypercapnia [74] (Chapter 23), careful fluid restriction [75,76] (Chapter 28) and more recently intravenacaval oxygenation [77,78] have proved encouraging when compared with historical controls, as has initial experience with inhaled nitric oxide [79], (Chapter 29).

CAUSE OF DEATH

Because these new therapies have failed to meet expectations in influencing mortality, examining both the actual cause of death and predictors of mortality (which may be interdependent) is highly relevant, especially when considering severity scoring systems. Even this approach provides conflicting results. Most early deaths (in the first 3 days) are said to be related to the underlying disorder, while 73% of late deaths were related to the sepsis syndrome [54]. By contrast, others have found that only 28% of patients die of sepsis, while 40% succumb to respiratory failure and 19% to cardiac dysfunction [61]. The differences between these studies are not easily explained but have relevance in that no scoring system currently classifies patients with ARDS by underlying pathology (Chapter 2).

PREDICTORS OF MORTALITY

The predictors of mortality in ARDS are no less inconsistent. They can be broadly divided into etiology, and the degree of disordered physiology produced. Although much data exists from a number of large clinical studies [52–62], strictly comparable data may be hard to find and much of it is contradictory.

Etiology

The etiology of ARDS has a major bearing on mortality. In the European Collaborative Study of 583 patients from 38 centers [59], mortality ranged from 38% (trauma) through 68% (intra-abdominal sepsis) to 86% (opportunistic pneumonia). More recently, an even wider range was reported, with mortality of 17% from fat embolism compared with 54% for sepsis and 75% for pancreatitis [62]. It is impossible to establish the effects of age and previous health status on these figures. Infection emerges consistently as an important factor; in addition its nature, site and severity may be significant. A 75% mortality has been reported in patients whose risk for ARDS was sepsis, compared with 54% for trauma and 44% for aspiration or overdose [58]. Elsewhere it has been shown not only that survival was significantly affected by the presence of sepsis (mortality 79% with sepsis, 33% without) but that the site of infection was important; mortality in pulmonary infection was 87% and in abdominal infection was 41% [56]. Furthermore, there were no survivors if blood cultures were positive and the site of infection was unknown [53,56]. However, in one recent study only aspiration pneumonia was associated with a significantly lower mortality [61]; in another there was no significant difference between infectious and noninfectious etiologies [57].

Indices of disordered physiology

Direct and indirect indices of disordered physiology have been identified as predictors of mortality in the major clinical studies; significant factors include increasing age [53,57,58,61], the number of complications occurring [57], less than 10% band forms on peripheral blood smear, arterial pH less than 7.4, serum bicarbonate of less than 20 mg/ml [55], Pao_2/Fio_2 ratio at 3 days [58], response of oxygenation indices to therapy [53,80], compliance [58,61], positive fluid balance [58], presence of sepsis [53,56,61], development of multiple organ failure [53,61,81], and calculated indices such as ratio of respiratory index to pulmonary shunt and right ventricular to left ventricular stroke work [82]. In contrast to the above, Fowler *et al.* found age not to be significant [55], and Mancebo and Artigas found neither sepsis nor indices of oxygenation to be predictive of mortality [57]. In addition, a variety of putative biochemical prognostic indicators [83,84] have been identified but these have little clinical significance at present. Despite this confusion, some of these disparate factors might be used in a prognostic and severity score for ARDS.

GENERAL SCORING SYSTEMS

Only 65 patients with ARDS (designated non-operative, noncardiogenic pulmonary edema) were included in the original APACHE II data base of 5030 patients [3]. The mortality of this group was 37% and the diagnostic category was heavily weighted (i.e. giving a high risk of death for a given APACHE II score) for the performance of the calculation of risk of death [3]. The APACHE III data base has included 107 such patients out of a total of 17 440 patients with a remarkably similar mortality rate of 37.4% [38]. The precise definition of ARDS in these studies is not clear. Other studies using APACHE II in general ICU settings have not expressly evaluated the predictive ability of severity scoring in ARDS [4–7,9–12], although a comparison has been

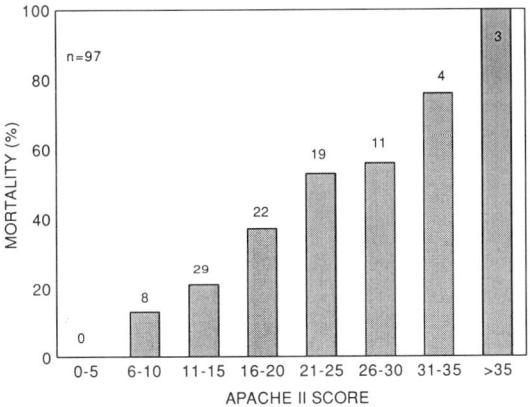

Figure 22.1 Mortality (%) versus APACHE II scores for patients with pneumonia. (Reproduced with permission from Turner *et al.*, [8].)

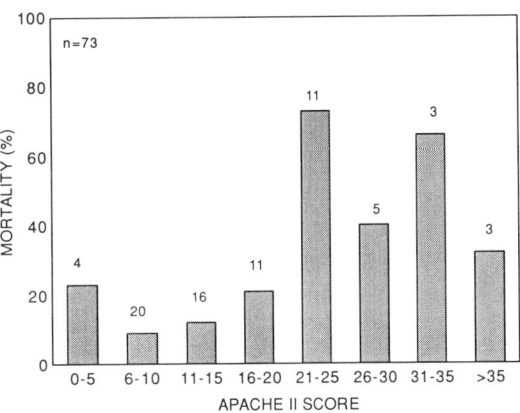

Figure 22.2 Mortality (%) versus APACHE II scores for patients with ARDS. (Reproduced with permission from Turner *et al.* [8].)

made of APACHE II scoring in ARDS and pneumonia [8]. ARDS in this study was defined as $Pa_{O_2} < 8\,kPa$ on $F_{I_{O_2}} \geqslant 0.4$, diffuse radiological infiltrates, wedge pressure $< 18\,mmHg$ (or no clinical evidence of heart failure) and an identifiable cause. Patients with pneumonia were diagnosed clinically on history and clinical and radiological features even if they subsequently developed ARDS. The mortality in 97 patients with pneumonia rose linearly with increasing APACHE II score (Figure 22.1) but in 73 patients with ARDS there was no correlation at all (Figure 22.2). It was hypothesized that this was due to heterogeneous causative factors for ARDS and the development of late and unpredictable complications in such patients [8]. Clinical studies of ARDS have also investigated severity scoring. Both APACHE II scoring for nontrauma cases and the injury severity score for trauma have been shown to have significant predictive power for mortality [54]. Although SAPS on admission has been shown to be not significantly different between survivors and nonsurvivors, it improved in survivors and got worse in nonsurvivors [57]. This has apparently been confirmed in the European Collaborative Study [59]. Finally, the admission APACHE II

score has been shown to correlate poorly with outcome in two studies of ARDS patients. It significantly underestimated mortality in one study, with predicted mortality being 39% and actual mortality 45% [62], a discrepancy possibly due to the presence of other coexistent organ failure, or to the development of ARDS after ICU admission (the mortality in 36 such patients was 58%). In the other study APACHE II significantly overestimated mortality: predicted mortality was 39.6% and actual mortality 16% [74].

SPECIFIC SCORING SYSTEMS

Thus ARDS is not only difficult to define, with different criteria appearing in different studies [52–63,69], but also difficult to quantify. This makes interpretation and comparison of studies difficult and less meaningful and has almost certainly contributed to the marked paucity of scoring systems for use in ARDS. Consequently, the introduction of an expanded definition of ARDS [85] was welcomed as a measure to quantify the presence, severity and evolution of ARDS. It consists of three parts: the course (acute or chronic), the severity (the lung injury score, Table 1.2), and the cause or associated disorder. All the com-

Table 22.2 Pulmonary failure scoring system

Score	Chest radiograph	A-aD$_{O_2}$/F$_{IO_2}$[a]	Compliance (ml/cmH$_2$O)	Mean PAP (mmHg)
0	Normal	< 300	> 80	< 20
1	Moderately increased interstitial marking	300–375	70–80	20–25
2	Markedly increased interstitial marking	375–450	50–70	25–30
3	Patchy air space consolidation	450–525	30–50	30–35
4	Extensive air space consolidation	> 525	< 30	> 35

PAP = pulmonary artery pressure.
[a] A-aD$_{O_2}$ is the alveolar–arterial gradient, measured in mmHg; continuous positive airway pressure (CPAP) or PEEP of more than 5 cmH$_2$O increases the score by 1 point.
The final score consists of the mean of all the individual score values.
Source: Morel *et al.* [84].

ponents of these parts should be easily available. The full extent of its use is not known as it has only recently been validated and correlated with mortality [62]. However, in a separate study there was no significant difference in lung injury score between survivors and nonsurvivors [74]. In addition, the lung injury score has been criticized on three (radiology, PEEP and compliance) of its four constituent parts. Many factors affect the perception of chest radiographs [86], and since inverse ratio ventilation has become widely used it has been difficult to know how to score the values for PEEP and compliance. A similar system (Table 22.2) was proposed some years earlier by Morel *et al.* [84] but did not gain widespread acceptance, although it was used in the multicenter European Collaborative Study, in which it was significantly correlated with mortality [59].

Another scoring system for ARDS is the ventilator score [87]. This was derived from a small retrospective study of 30 patients with ARDS, 15 of whom died. An equation was obtained (the method is not described) that separated survivors from nonsurvivors. The equation read as follows:

$$\text{ventilator score} = 0.5 \times \text{age} + 0.6 \times \text{A-aD}_{O_2} + 1.2 \times \Delta P\text{aw},$$

where age is in years, A-aD$_{O_2}$ represents the alveolar–arterial oxygen gradient in kilopascals, and ΔPaw is the difference between the mean peak airway pressure over 24 hours and a control pressure derived from people with normal lungs, measured in centimeters of water. In this study, all patients with a score of more than 80 died [87], but in separate studies the score had poor predictive power [88] and there was no significant difference between survivors and nonsurvivors [74].

FUTURE TRENDS

THE IDEAL SCORING SYSTEM

For any scoring system to be useful it must utilize easily available and directly measured (not derived) parameters. It must be reproducible both locally and abroad; the outcome must be clearly measurable (for example death); and its uses and limitations need to be established and adhered to. With all the above scoring systems available to them, which are investigators currently using? In the multicenter study of artificial surfactant (Exosurf) in acute respiratory failure (Chapter 16), the APACHE III score [38] was used, while the investigators of IVOX used the lung injury score of Murray *et al.* [85]. As noted previously, there is as yet no ideal general or specific scoring system for ARDS. From our present knowledge of scoring systems, causes of mortality and predictors of outcome, it would seem that the ideal scoring system in ARDS would consider a combination of the

Table 22.3 Proposed scoring system for ARDS

1. Cause rated 1–3 points

1 point	**2 points**	**3 points**
Trauma	Abdominal sepsis	Sepsis (unknown site)
Fat embolism	Pneumonia (community acquired)	Pneumonia (all other)
Aspiration	Cardiac bypass	Pancreatitis
Overdose		
Toxic gas inhalation		

2. Alveolar–arterial gradient (A-aD_{O_2}) in kPa (according to the formula A-a$D_{O_2} = 0.95 \times F_{I_{O_2}}$ (%) – $Pa_{O_2} - Pa_{CO_2}$)
3. APACHE II score (3)
4. Organ failure as described by Montgomery *et al.* (52). One organ failure would give a ratio (by which to multiply the APACHE II score) of 1.1, two organ failure 1.2, etc.
5. Age points as allocated in the APACHE II methodology (3)

The final formula for the score would appear as follows:
score = cause points × 20 + APACHE × OSF ratio + A-aD_{O_2} + age points ×3.

OSF = organ system failure.

cause of ARDS, the extent and severity of lung injury, the degree of disordered physiology (including organ system failure) and associated features such as age. To derive such a score by mathematical methods would require hundreds if not thousands of comparable patients; this will never be feasible. In addition, scores derived in this fashion usually have complicated equations, often involving logarithmic functions. We would therefore propose a simply calculated system (Table 22.3), based on the most easily available and definable of the above factors and taking into account the literature reviewed above.

This scoring system could be calculated from readily available data either locally or over the telephone when considering a referral. As it takes into account both severity and prognostic indicators, it could be used to make decisions about the need for nonconventional ventilatory management as well as survival estimates. Retrospective logistic regression analysis of predictive factors in 42 patients in the ARDS database at the Royal Brompton Hospital in London showed the cause of ARDS to be significantly related to mortality in both univariate and multivariate analyses, while APACHE II score was sig-

nificant in the univariate analysis only. In addition, our proposed scoring system was significantly correlated with mortality ($P = 0.04$, Fisher's exact test) when a score of 100 was used as a cut off; moreover, no patient with a score of less than 100 died. A note of caution: the numbers used to derive this scoring system are small and the patient spectrum may have been relatively narrow. Systems such as this one, for scoring severity of illness or making a prognostic estimate in ARDS, will need further refinement and validation.

REFERENCES

1. Knaus, W.A,, Zimmerman, J.E., Wagner, D.P. *et al.* (1981) APACHE – acute physiology and chronic health evaluation: a physiologically based classification system. *Critical Care Medicine*, **9**, 591–7.
2. Le Gall, J.R., Loirat, P., Alperovitch, A. *et al.* (1984) A simplified acute physiology score for ICU patients. *Critical Care Medicine*, **12**, 975–7.
3. Knaus, W.A., Draper, E.A., Wagner, D.P. and Zimmerman, J.E. (1985) APACHE II: a severity of disease classification system. *Critical Care Medicine*, **13**, 818–29.
4. Marsh, H.M., Krishan, I., Naessens, J.M. *et al.* (1990) Assessment of prediction of mortality by using the APACHE II scoring system in inten-

sive-care units. *Mayo Clinic Proceedings*, **65**, 1549–57.

5. Lockrem, J.D., Lopez, E., Gallagher, J. *et al.* (1991) Severity of illness: APACHE II analysis of an ICU population. *Cleveland Clinic Journal of Medicine*, **58**, 477–86.

6. Rutledge, R., Fakhry, S.M., Rutherford, E.J. *et al.* (1991) Acute physiology and chronic health evaluation (APACHE II) score and outcome in the surgical intensive care unit: an analysis of multiple intervention and outcome variables in 1238 patients. *Critical Care Medicine*, **19**, 1048–53.

7. Jacobs, S., Chang, R.W.S., Lee, B. and Lee, B. (1988) Audit of intensive care: a 30 month experience using the APACHE II severity of disease classification system. *Intensive Care Medicine*, **14**, 567–74.

8. Turner, J.S., Potgieter, P.D. and Linton, D.M. (1989) Systems for scoring severity of illness in intensive care. *South African Medical Journal*, **76**, 17–20.

9. Joshua, N., Jena, G.P. and Mletelwa, N.V. (1989) Multidisciplinary intensive care unit at Cecelia Makiwane Hospital, Mdantsane, Ciskei. *South African Medical Journal*, **75**, 286–9.

10. Giangiuliani, G., Mancini, A. and Gui, D. (1989) Validation of a severity of illness score (APACHE II) in a surgical intensive care unit. *Intensive Care Medicine*, **15**, 519–22.

11. Oh, T.E., Hutchinson, R., Short, S. *et al.* (1993) Verification of the acute physiology and chronic health evaluation scoring system in a Hong Kong intensive care unit. *Critical Care Medicine*, **21**, 698–705.

12. Rowan, K.M., Kerr, J.H., Major, E. *et al.* (1993) Intensive Care Society's APACHE II study in Britain and Ireland-II: outcome comparisons of intensive care units after adjustment for case mix by the American APACHE II method. *BMJ*, **307**, 977–81.

13. Zimmerman, J.E., Knaus, W.A., Judson, J.A. *et al.* (1988) Patient selection for intensive care: a comparison of New Zealand and United States hospitals. *Critical Care Medicine*, **16**, 318–26.

14. Kruse, J.A. and Carlson, R.W. (1993) Severity of illness scoring: East meets West. [Editorial.] *Critical Care Medicine*, **21**, 647–8.

15. Johnson, M.H., Gordon, P.W. and Fitzgerald, F.T. (1986) Stratification of prognosis in granulocytopenic patients with hematologic malig-

nancies using the APACHE II severity of illness score. *Critical Care Medicine*, **14**, 693–7.

16. Lloyd-Thomas, A.R., Wright, I., Lister, T.A. and Hinds, C.J. (1988) Prognosis of patients receiving intensive care for lifethreatening medical complications of haematological malignancy. *BMJ*, **296**, 1025–9.

17. Bohnen, J.M.A., Mustard, R.A., Oxholm, S.E. and Schouten, D. (1988) APACHE II score and abdominal sepsis. *Archives of Surgery*, **123**, 225–9.

18. Dobkin, J.E. and Cutler, R.E. (1988) Use of APACHE II classification to evaluate outcome of patients receiving hemodialysis in an intensive care unit. *Western Journal of Medicine*, **149**, 547–50.

19. Fedullo, A.J., Swinburne, A.J., Wahl, G.W. *et al.* (1988) APACHE II score and mortality in respiratory failure due to cardiogenic pulmonary oedema. *Critical Care Medicine*, **16**, 1218–21.

20. Hopefl, A.W., Taaffe, C.L. and Herrmann, V.M. (1989) Failure of APACHE II alone as a predictor of mortality in patients receiving total parenteral nutrition. *Critical Care Medicine*, **17**, 414–7.

21. Larvin, M. and McMahon, M.J. (1989) APACHE II score for assessment and monitoring of acute pancreatitis. *Lancet*, **ii**, 201–4.

22. Wilson, C., Heath, D.I. and Imrie, C.W. (1990) Prediction of outcome in acute pancreatitis: a comparative study of APACHE II, clinical assessment and multiple factor scoring systems. *British Journal of Surgery*, **77**, 1260–4.

23. Maher, E.R., Robinson, K.N., Scoble, J.E. *et al.* (1989) Prognosis of critically-ill patients with acute renal failure: APACHE II score and other predictive factors. *Quarterly Journal of Medicine*, **72**, 857–66.

24. Moreau, R., Soupison, T., Vauquelin, P. *et al.* (1989) Comparison of two simplified severity scores (SAPS and APACHE II) for patients with acute myocardial infarction. *Critical Care Medicine*, **17**, 409–13.

25. Schein, M. and Gecelter, G. (1989) APACHE II score in massive upper gastrointestinal haemorrhage from peptic ulcer: prognostic value and potential clinical applications. *British Journal of Surgery*, **76**, 733–6.

26. Rhee, K.J., Baxt, W.G., Mackenzie, J.R. *et al.* (1990) APACHE II scoring in the injured patient. *Critical Care Medicine*, **18**, 827–30.

27. Dart, R., Patel, B., Perez-Alard, J. *et al.* (1991) Prognosis of oncology patients receiving

intensive care using the APACHE II scoring system. *Maryland Medical Journal*, **40**, 273–6.

28. Niskanen, M., Kari, A., Nikki, P. (1991) Acute physiology and chronic health evaluation (APACHE II) and Glasgow Coma Scores as predictors of outcome from intensive care after cardiac arrest. *Critical Care Medicine*, **19**, 1465–73.

29. Teskey, R.J., Calvin, J.E. and McPhail, I (1991) Disease severity in the coronary care unit. *Chest*, **100**, 1637–42.

30. Turner, J.S., Mudaliar, Y.M., Chang, R.W.S. and Morgan C.J. (1991) Acute physiology and chronic health evaluation (APACHE II) scoring in a cardiothoracic intensive care unit. *Critical Care Medicine*, **19**, 1266–9.

31. Headley, J., Theriault, R and Smith, T.L. (1992) Independent validation of APACHE II severity of illness score for predicting mortality in patients with breast cancer admitted to the intensive care unit. *Cancer*, **70**, 497–503.

32. Day, A.C., Rankin, A.P.N. and Judson, J.A. (1993) Grading asthma severity: using the APS component of the APACHE II system. *Intensive Care Medicine*, **19**, 221–6.

33. Cerra, F.B., Negro, F. and Abrams, J. (1990) APACHE II score does not predict multiple organ failure or mortality in postoperative surgical patients. *Archives of Surgery*, **125**, 519–22.

34. Civetta, J.M., Hudson-Civetta, J.A. and Nelson, L.D. (1990) Evaluation of APACHE II for cost containment and quality assurance. *Annals of Surgery*, **212**, 266–74.

35. Chang, R.W.S., Jacobs, S. and Lee, B. (1986) Use of APACHE II severity of disease classification to identify intensive-care-unit patients who would not benefit from total parenteral nutrition. *Lancet*, **i**, 1483–7.

36. Knaus, W.A., Draper, E.A., Wagner, D.P., *et al.* (1986) An evaluation of outcome from intensive care in major medical centers. *Annals of Internal Medicine*, **104**, 410–8.

37. Chang, R.W.S., Jacobs, S. and Lee, B. (1988) Predicting outcome among intensive care unit patients using computerised trend analysis of daily APACHE II scores corrected for organ system failure. *Intensive Care Medicine*, **14**, 558–66.

38. Knaus, W.A., Wagner, D.P. Draper, E.A. *et al.* (1991) The APACHE III prognostic system. *Chest*, **100**, 1619–36.

39. Brannen, A.L., Godfrey, L.J. and Goetter W.E. (1989) Prediction of outcome from critical ill-

ness. A comparison of clinical judgement with a prediction rule. *Archives of Internal Medicine*, **149**, 1083–6.

40. Marks, R.J., Simons, R.S., Blizzard, R.A. and Brown DRG (1991) Predicting outcome in intensive therapy units – a comparison of APACHE II with subjective assessments. *Intensive Care Medicine*, **17**, 159–63.

41. Kruse, J.A., Thill-Baharozian, M.C. and Carlson, R.W. (1988) Comparison of clinical assessment with APACHE II for predicting mortality risk in patients admitted to a medical intensive care unit. *JAMA*, **260**, 1739–42.

42. Knaus, W.A., Wagner, D.P. and Lynn J (1991) Short-term mortality predictions for critically ill hospitalized adults: science and ethics. *Science*, **254**, 389–94.

43. Lemeshow, S., Teres, D., Avrunin, J.S. and Gage, R.W. (1988) Refining intensive care unit outcome prediction by using changing probabilities of mortality. *Critical Care Medicine*, **16**, 470–7.

44. Lemeshow, S., Teres, D., Avrunin, J.S. and Pastides, H. (1987) A comparison of methods to predict mortality of intensive care unit patients. *Critical Care Medicine*, **15**, 715–22.

45. Lemeshow, S., Teres, D., Klar, J. *et al.* (1993) Mortality probability models (MPM II) based on an international cohort of intensive care unit patients. *JAMA*, **270**, 2478–86.

46. Le Gall, J.R., Lemeshow, S. and Saulnier, F. (1993) A new simplified acute physiology score (SAPS II) based on a European/North American multicenter study. *JAMA*, **270**, 2957–63.

47. Knaus, W.A., Draper, E.A., Wagner, D.P. and Zimmerman, J.E. (1985) Prognosis in acute organ-system failure. *Annals of Surgery*, **202**, 685–93.

48. Baker, S.P., O'Neill, B., Hadden, W. and Long, W.B. (1974) The injury severity score: a method for describing patients with multiple injuries and evaluating emergency care. *Journal of Trauma*, **14**, 187–96.

49. Boyd, C.R., Tolson, M.A. and Copes, W.S. (1987) Evaluating trauma care: the TRISS method. *Journal of Trauma*, **27**, 370–8.

50. Pollack, M.M., Ruttimann, U.E. and Getson, P.R. (1988) Pediatric risk of mortality (PRISM) score. *Critical Care Medicine*, **16**, 1110–6.

51. Keene, A.R. and Cullen, D.J. (1983) Therapeutic intervention scoring system: update 1983 *Critical Care Medicine*, **11**, 1–3.

52. Pepe, P.E., Potkin, R.T., Reus, D.H., *et al* (1982)

Clinical predictors of the adult respiratory distress syndrome. *American Journal of Surgery*, **144**, 124–30.

53. Bell, R.C., Coalson, J.J., Smith, J.D. and Johanson, W.G. (1983) Multiple organ system failure and infection in adult respiratory distress syndrome. *Annals of Internal Medicine*, **99**, 293–8.

54. Montgomery, A.B., Stager, M.A., Carrico, C.J. and Hudson, L.D. (1985) Causes of mortality in patients with the adult respiratory distress syndrome. *American Review of Respiratory Disease*, **132**, 485–9.

55. Fowler, A.A., Hamman, R.F., Zerbe, G.O. *et al.* (1985) Adult respiratory distress syndrome. Prognosis after onset. *American Review of Respiratory Disease*, **132**, 472–8.

56. Seidenfeld, J.J., Pohl, D.F., Bell, R.C. *et al.* (1986) Incidence, site, and outcome of infections in patients with the adult respiratory distress syndrome. *American Review of Respiratory Disease*, **134**, 12–6.

57. Mancebo, J. and Artigas, A (1987) A clinical study of the adult respiratory distress syndrome. *Critical Care Medicine*, **15**, 243–6.

58. Maunder, R.J., Kublis, P.S., Anardi, D.M. and Hudson, L.D. (1989) Determinants of survival in the adult respiratory distress syndrome (ARDS). *American Review of Respiratory Disease*, **139**, A220.

59. Villar, J. and Slutsky, A.S. (1989) The incidence of the adult respiratory distress syndrome. *American Review of Respiratory Disease*, **140**, 814–6.

60. Artigas, A., Carlet, J., Chastang, C., *et al.* (1992) Adult respiratory distress syndrome: clinical presentation, prognostic factors and outcome, in *Adult Respiratory Distress Syndrome* (eds A. Artigas, F. Lemaire, P.M. Suter and W.M. Zapol), Churchill Livingstone, Edinburgh, pp. 509–25.

61. Suchyta, M.R., Clemmer, T.P. and Elliott, C.G., *et al.* (1992) The adult respiratory distress syndrome. A report of survival and modifying factors. *Chest*, **101**, 1074–9.

62. Kraus, P.A., Lipman, J., Lee, C.C.J. *et al.* (1993) Acute lung injury at Baragwanath ICU. An eight-month audit and call for consensus for other organ failure in the adult respiratory distress syndrome. *Chest*, **103**, 1832–6.

63. Zapol, W.M., Snider, M.T., Hill, J.D. *et al.* (1979) Extracorporeal membrane oxygenation in severe acute respiratory failure. A randomized prospective study. *JAMA*, **242**, 2193–6.

64. Suchyta, M.R., Clemmer, T.P., Orme, J.F. *et al.* (1991) Increased survival of ARDS patients with severe hypoxemia (ECMO criteria). *Chest*, **99**, 951–5.

65. Pepe, P.E., Hudson, L.D. and Carrico, C.J. (1984) Early application of positive end-expiratory pressure in patients at risk for the adult respiratory distress syndrome. *New England Journal of Medicine*, **311**, 281–6.

66. Carlon, G.C., Howland, W.S., Ray, C. *et al.* (1983) High frequency jet ventilation. A prospective randomised evaluation. *Chest*, **84**, 551–9.

67. Clemmer, T., Morris, A., Suchyta, M. *et al.* (1992) Extracorporeal support does not improve ARDS survival. *Critical Care Medicine*, **20**, S61.

68. Bernard, G.R., Luce, J.M., Sprung, C.L. *et al.* (1987) High-dose corticosteroids in patients with the adult respiratory distress syndrome. *New England Journal of Medicine*, **317**, 1565–70.

69. Bone, R.C., Slotman, G., Maunder, R. *et al.* (1989) Randomized double-blind, multicenter study of postaglandin E1 in patients with the adult respiratory distress syndrome. *Chest*, **96**, 114–9.

70. Jepsen, S., Herlevsen, P., Knudsen, P., *et al.* (1992) Antioxidant treatment with N-acetylcysteine during adult respiratory distress syndrome: a prospective, randomized, placebo-controlled study. *Critical Care Medicine*, **20**, 918–23.

71. Lain, D.C., DiBenedetto, R., Morris, S.L., *et al.* (1989) Pressure control inverse ratio ventilation as a method to reduce peak inspiratory pressure and provide adequate ventilation and oxygenation. *Chest*, **95**, 1081–8.

72. Tharratt, RS, Allen, R.P. and Albertson, T.E. (1988) Pressure controlled inverse ratio ventilation in severe adult respiratory failure. *Chest*, **94**, 755–62.

73. Gattinoni, L., Pesenti, A., Mascheroni, D. *et al.* (1986) Low frequency positive pressure ventilation with extracorporeal CO_2 removal in severe acute respiratory failure. *JAMA*, **256**, 881–6.

74. Hickling, K.G., Henderson, S.J. and Jackson, R. (1990) Low mortality associated with low volume pressure limited ventilation with permissive hypercapnia in severe adult respiratory distress syndrome. *Intensive Care Medicine*, **16**, 372–7.

75. Humphrey, H., Hall, J., Sznajder, I., *et al.* (1990)

Improved survival in ARDS patients associated with a reduction in pulmonary capillary wedge pressure. *Chest*, **97**, 1176–80.

76. Mitchell, J.P. (1992) Improved survival based on fluid management in critically-ill patients requiring pulmonary artery catheterization. *American Review of Respiratory Disease*, **145**, 990–8.

77. Conrad, S.A., Eggerstedt, J.M., Morris, V.F. and Romero, M.D. (1993) Prolonged intracorporeal support of gas exchange with an intravenacaval oxygenator. *Chest*, **103**, 158–61.

78. High, K.M., Snider, M.T., Richard, R. *et al* (1992) Clinical trials of an intravenous oxygenator in patients with adult respiratory distress syndrome. *Anesthesiology*, **77**, 856–63.

79. Rossaint, R., Falke, K.J., Lopez, F., *et al.* (1993) Inhaled nitric oxide for the adult respiratory distress syndrome. *New England Journal of Medicine*, **328**, 399–405.

80. Bone, R.C., Maunder, R., Slotman, G. *et al.* (1989) An early test of survival in patients with the adult respiratory distress syndrome. *Chest*, **96**, 849–51.

81. Bone, R.C., Balk, R., Slotman, G., *et al.* (1992) Adult respiratory distress syndrome. Sequence and importance of development of multiple organ failure. *Chest*, **101**, 320–6.

82. Laghi, F., Siegel, J.M., Rivkind, A.I. *et al.* (1989) Respiratory index/pulmonary shunt relationship: quantification of severity and prognosis in the post-traumatic adult respiratory distress syndrome. *Critical Care Medicine*, **17**, 1121–8.

83. Fontcuberta, J., Artigas, A. Sala, N. *et al.* (1986) Inhibitors of blood coagulation (protein C, antithrombin III and A2 macroglobulin) in adult respiratory distress syndrome. *Intensive Care Medicine*, **12**, 224.

84. Morel, D.R., Dargent, F., Bachmann, M. *et al.* (1985) Pulmonary extraction of serotonin and propanolol in patients with adult respiratory distress syndrome. *American Review of Respiratory Disease*, **132**, 479–84.

85. Murray, J.F., Matthay, M.A., Luce, J.M. and Flick, M.R. (1988) An expanded definition of the adult respiratory distress syndrome. *American Review of Respiratory Disease*, **138**, 720–3.

86. Brogdon, B.G., Kelsey, C.A. and Moseley, R.D. (1983) Factors affecting perception of pulmonary lesions. *Radiologic Clinics of North America*, **21**, 633–54.

87. Smith, P.E.M. and Gordon, I.J. (1986) An index to predict outcome in adult respiratory distress syndrome. *Intensive Care Medicine*, **12**, 86–9.

88. Jacobs, S., Chang, R.W.S. and Lee, B. (1991) Prognosis in the adult respiratory distress syndrome: comparison of a ventilatory index with the Riyadh intensive care programme. *Clinical Intensive Care*, **2**, 81–5.

A PRESSURE TARGETED APPROACH TO VENTILATING

John J. Marini

Recent interest in techniques for ventilating patients with acute lung injury has been driven by an evolving knowledge of respiratory mechanics (Chapter 15) and by recognition of the potential for iatrogenic lung damage. The need for protracted mechanical ventilation is associated with infection, multisystem organ dysfunction and increased mortality. Even when overt alveolar rupture does not occur, excessive stretching forces applied repeatedly to normal lungs increase capillary permeability and initiate hemorrhage or inflammation [1,2]. In view of this, investigators and clinicians have begun to reconsider the fundamental objectives of mechanical ventilation and to design ventilatory modes to accomplish these revised goals more effectively.

TRADITIONAL APPROACH TO MECHANICAL VENTILATION

The basic principles of managing acute lung injury (ALI) are well known, and within broad limits, remain valid. The primary objective is to accomplish effective gas exchange at the least inspired oxygen fraction (F_{IO2}) and pressure cost. The purpose of this discussion is to review briefly the basis for concern regarding the traditional approach to ventilatory support in ALI and, drawing from this evidence, to suggest a ventilatory strategy consistent with the lessons emerging from the admittedly incomplete data base currently at hand (Table 23.1). It should be understood from the outset that however rational newer approaches might appear, and however consistent the experimental evi-

Table 23.1 Alternative ventilatory strategies for acute lung injury (ARDS)

	Traditional	*Revised*
Objectives	Normal arterial blood gases	Adequate arterial blood gases Prevent alveolar injury Facilitate healing
Ventilation mode	Volume cycled ventilation	Pressure targeted ventilation
Settings		
PEEP	As needed for adequate Pa_{O_2}/F_{IO_2}	Sufficient to prevent tidal recruitment cycle and achieve adequate Pa_{O_2}/F_{IO_2} ratio
V_T	Preset (10–15 ml/kg)	> 5–8 ml/kg
Peak alveolar pressure	As required for PEEP and V_T	No higher than a transalveolar pressure of 30–35 cmH$_2$O

ARDS Acute Respiratory Distress in Adults. Edited by Timothy W. Evans and Christopher Haslett. Published in 1996 by Chapman & Hall, London. ISBN 0 412 56910 8

dence may seem to be, the benefit of altering the traditional strategy has not yet been rigorously demonstrated in the clinical setting.

Most traditional ventilatory strategies for intensive care evolved from anesthetic practice. When the lungs are uninjured and their capacity to expand is relatively normal, as is commonly true in the perioperative period, large tidal volumes (V_T) of 10–15 ml/kg are appropriate to prevent the microatelectasis that accompanies monotonous shallow breathing. Respiratory rate is usually adjusted to 'normalize' pH and/or Pa_{CO_2} [3], and sufficient positive end expiratory pressure (PEEP) is used to achieve acceptable O_2 delivery at what are assumed to be nontoxic concentrations of inspired oxygen (F_{IO_2}). As a rule, airway pressures are monitored but not rigidly specified or constrained. With few modifications, this high tidal volume, normoxic, normocapnic ventilation paradigm has become the standard approach to supporting most critically ill patients, including those with ALI. Consequently, V_T exceeding 800 ml and peak tidal (plateau) alveolar pressures exceeding 50 cmH$_2$O are commonplace in many intensive care units. How best to select 'optimal' PEEP remains controversial, but many practitioners advocate using the **least** PEEP consistent with accomplishing acceptable arterial oxygenation [4].

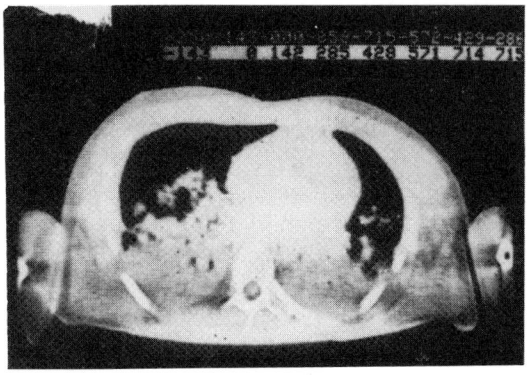

(a)

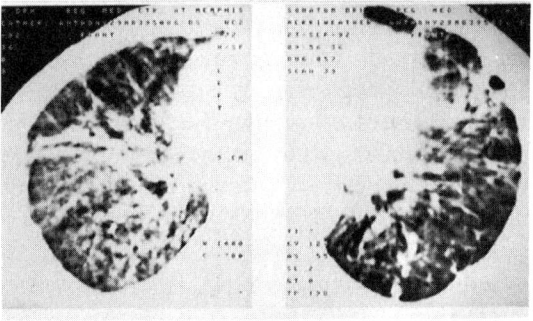

(b)

Figure 23.1 Computed tomographic scans of (a) early and (b) late phases of ARDS. Note dependency of infiltration during the earliest phase of ARDS and more homogenous interstitial changes (including cystic regions) in the late phase. (Reproduced with permission from (a) Gattinoni [5] and (b) Meduri, G. (1993) *New Horizons*, **1**, 563–77.)

VENTILATOR INDUCED LUNG DAMAGE

The pathology evolves continuously (but nonhomogenously) over the course of ALI (Figure 23.1) (Chapters 4 and 21). It is a reasonable assumption that all regions of the lung sustain injury more or less simultaneously, and that proliferation, organization, remodeling and fibrosis sequentially follow an initial phase of edema and atelectasis in most severe cases [6]. Although parenchymal damage is widespread, the nature, severity and perhaps even phase of injury vary from site to site within the lung.

Pressures which do not produce overt alveolar rupture early in the course may produce pneumothorax in the later stages. Although the reason for this is unclear, it seems reasonable to assume that the strong type IV collagen framework of the normal lung remains relatively intact during the first days of injury. After the disease is well established, however, the same stresses can result in alveolar disruption as inflammatory enzymes degrade the structural proteins and nonuniformly remodel the lung's architecture. This may explain the tendency for radiographic barotrauma to occur late in the course of the disease [7].

MICROMECHANICS IN ALI

Several previously unreported forms of radiographically evident, ventilator induced lung damage are now known to appear during the management of ALI (Table 23.2). Furthermore, clinical observations, as well as disturbing experimental data, strongly suggest that the conventional approach may put some regions of the injured lung at risk for retarded healing or further damage that is not manifest as extraalveolar gas. Even though the initial injury may be uniform, regional mechanics are quite different, even in the earliest phase of the process. Gravitationally dependent areas appear edematous and atelectatic, whereas nondependent regions tend to aerate better, at least early in the course [5]. Changes of position may alter some of these early radiographic changes, and hypoxemia may improve as well [8,9]. During the early phase of the syndrome of acute respiratory distress in adults (ARDS) at least 50% of patients respond to prone positioning by improving Pa_{O_2} (10). Only a fraction of the injured lung is accessible to gas; in severe cases, no more than one third of all alveoli remain patent. Given that ventilated lung units may retain nearly normal elastance and fragility, the apparent 'stiffness' of the lung in the early phase of ALI is better explained by the availability of fewer functioning alveoli than by a generalized increase in recoil tension [5,11]. (Increased recoil contributes more to reduced compliance later on, when cellular infiltration is intense, edema has been resorbed or organized, and atelectasis has been reversed.) Because the lung's functional compartment has a reduced capacity to expand but must receive the entire tidal volume, large (conventional) tidal volumes may subject it to overdistension, local hyperventilation, and inhibition or depletion of surfactant (Chapter 16) [1]. Particularly intense shearing forces may develop at the junctions of structures that are mobile (aerated alveoli) with those that are immobile (collapsed or consolidated alveoli, conducting airways) during rapid inflation to high transalveolar pressures. Indeed, in such a heterogeneous lung, junctional alveolar wall **tensions** may be severalfold greater than is suggested by the end inspiratory alveolar pressure itself [12]. Any tendency for damage is likely to be accentuated by increases in cycling frequency and duration of exposure.

Adhesed walls of collapsed bronchi often require high pressures to separate and may exhibit time-dependency of opening [13]. Once opened, however, much lower pressures preserve patency. If the terminal airways remain closed, their unsupported walls may be subjected to forces that approach the dynamic pressures applied to more central airways, which are girded by cartilage. Damage to the small bronchi may result much more frequently than is generally appreciated (Figure 23.2). A recent autopsy study, for example, detected bronchiolar dilatation, lung cyst formation, and/or microabscesses in the large majority of patients with ALI ventilated for lengthy periods with peak airway pressures considered modest by traditional clinical standards [14].

Damage resulting from overdistension of the alveolar-capillary membrane has been documented in excised lungs by a number of investigators [15,16]. In diverse animal models, **transalveolar** cycling pressures approximating those corresponding to total lung capacity ($\approx 35\,cmH_2O$) can diffusely injure previously normal alveoli over 15–60 minute periods, whether produced by positive or negative pressure [2,7,17]. When sustained for several days, even lower peak airway pressures ($\leq 30\,cmH_2O$) can damage normal lung

Table 23.2 Newly recognized forms of radiographic barotrauma in ARDS

Interstitial emphysema
Gas cysts
Intraparenchymal tension cavities
Bronchopulmonary damage
Systemic gas embolism

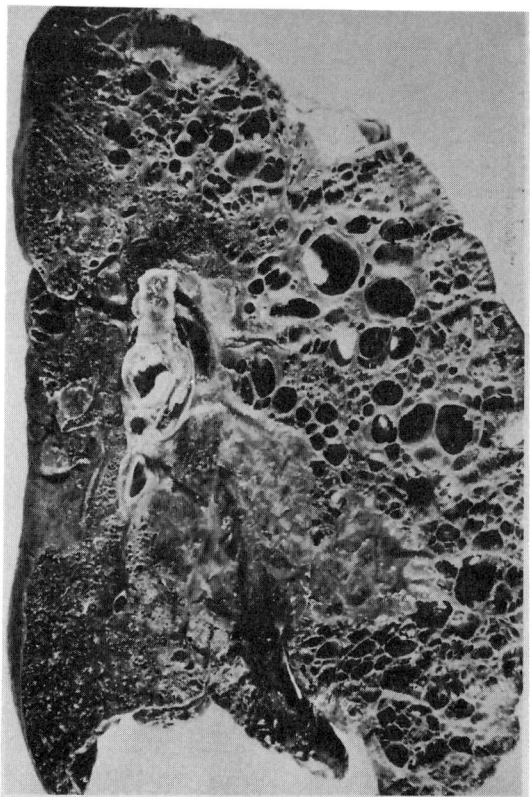

Figure 23.2 Pressure induced damage to bronchial airways produced cystic changes and other features compatible with bronchopulmonary injury ('dysplasia') in this previously normal patient with ARDS. (Reproduced with permission from Churg, A., Golden, J., Fligiel, S. and Hogg, J.C. (1983) *Am. Rev. Respir. Dis.*, **127**, 117–20.)

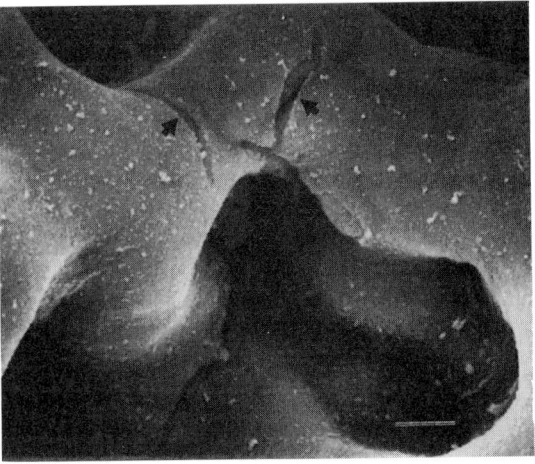

Figure 23.3 Scanning electron micrographic evidence of capillary stress fractures transverse to the longitudinal capillary axis. Such breaks can result in alveolar hemorrhage and gross protein leakage into the alveolar spaces. (Reproduced with permission from Fu *et al.* [21].)

tissues [18]. Recent data collected in patients with ARDS suggest that an upper inflection point of the pressure – volume curve of the respiratory system, an indicator of regional overdistension, can be detected in many patients at peak alveolar pressures ≤ 28 cmH$_2$O [19]. Moreover, certain noxious factors (e.g. alveolar pressure, inflammatory stimuli and increased F_{IO_2}) may well be additive; at least one study suggests that two factors acting in combination may produce injury that neither alone could inflict [20]. Microscopic injury to the endothelial membrane may be modulated by factors that influ-

ence transmural capillary pressure [21] (Chapter 20). Electron microscopic evidence strongly suggests that physical breaks in the gas–blood interface – capillary stress failure – can occur when **transmural** capillary pressures exceed ≈ 70 mmHg (Figure 23.3). Although **intravascular** pressures of this magnitude are seldom achieved in the clinical setting, **extramural** tensions surrounding vascular channels at the junction of collapsed and expanding lung units may well rise into this injurious range [12].

'BAROTRAUMA' VERSUS 'VOLUTRAUMA'

Because chest binding experiments have clearly shown that the absolute value of peak inflation pressure is not the variable of primary importance [22,23], 'volutrauma' may be a more appropriate term than 'barotrauma' [24]. In a certain sense, this newer terminology is more descriptive, so long as the 'volume' referenced is understood to be the volume of the individual alveolus, whose only measurable clinical correlate is **trans-**

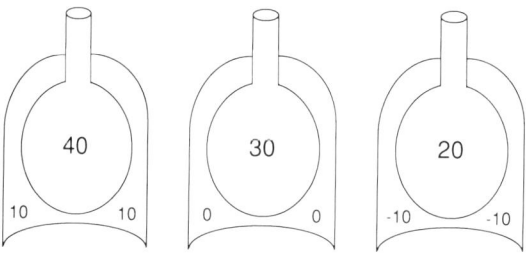

Figure 23.4 Concept of transalveolar pressure. A transalveolar pressure of 30 cmH$_2$O can be produced by any of the combinations shown.

alveolar pressure, (Figure 23.4). (Transalveolar pressure is roughly approximated by the difference between alveolar and pleural pressures.) One possibility is that it is more important to restrict the ventilatory pressure **excursion** of the alveolus (the end inspiratory minus end expiratory transalveolar pressure difference) [1,25]. In a given patient, this pressure excursion correlates with V_T. The impact of any specific V_T, however, depends on the aeratable capacity (and compliance) of the lung in question. Consequently, it may be misleading to formulate strict guidelines for V_T on the basis of milliliters per kilogram body weight. A growing body of evidence suggests that the end expiratory pressure and V_T selections are best made empirically by selecting a ventilation pattern that avoids the lower and upper inflexion points of the pressure–volume curve of the respiratory system [24–27].

IMPORTANCE OF MAINTAINING ADEQUATE END EXPIRATORY LUNG VOLUME

Alveolar overdistension is not the only factor of interest; failure to maintain a certain **minimum** alveolar volume in the setting of either pre-existing ALI or an excessive stretching force may also induce or accentuate lung damage, at least early in the time course [1,26,28,29] (Figure 23.5). One explanation suggests that at low lung volumes surfactant

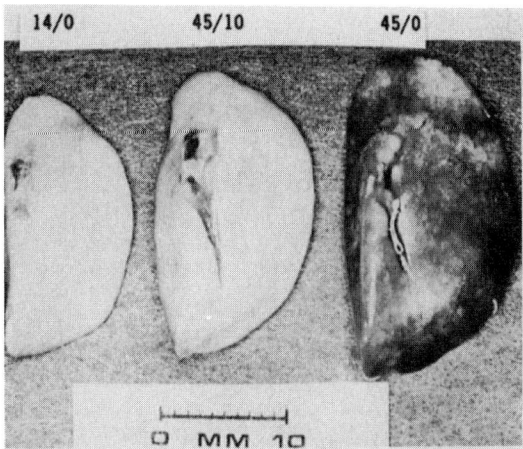

Figure 23.5 Protection afforded by PEEP in preventing pressure induced diffuse alveolar damage. Normal rats were ventilated for 1 hour periods with the indicated pressures and PEEP levels. Gross hemorrhagic pulmonary edema was produced by a pressure of 45 cmH$_2$O without PEEP. A similar peak pressure produced marginal damage when 10 cm H$_2$O PEEP was applied, despite a much higher mean airway pressure. (Reproduced with permission from Webb and Tierney [1].)

is depleted by the 'milking' action of tidal alveolar deflation or collapse (Chapter 16). When alveolar volume is too low, each tidal cycle may express surfactant into the terminal airways, where it is either inactivated or transported mouthward. High surface tension then predisposes the surfactant-poor alveolus to flood. A second possibility is that certain collapsible alveoli, unsupported by PEEP, wink open with every tidal cycle, producing damaging shearing stresses within junctional tissues of the type already outlined. Such a tidal recruitment cycle is implied by data that demonstrate optimal compliance at PEEP levels which vary inversely with V_T (Figure 23.6). Very recent computed tomographic scan/densitometry data appear to confirm this possibility [30] (Chapter 21).

A definite inflection region on the static pressure–volume curve of the passive respiratory system may indicate a population of alveoli at risk for such tidal stresses (Figure

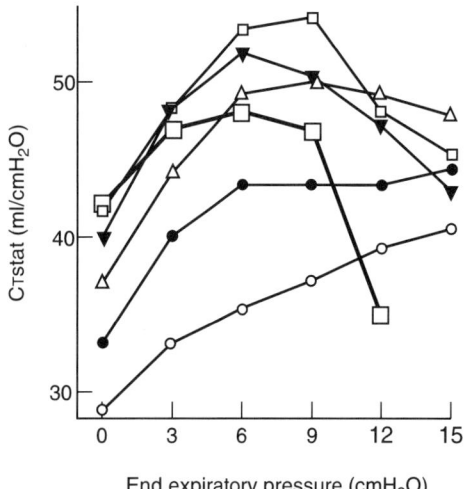

Figure 23.6 Family of curves demonstrating compliance as a function of both tidal volume and PEEP. With high tidal volumes, optimal recruitment and compliance occurs at PEEP levels that are much lower than those for small tidal volumes. Tidal volumes (ml/kg): ○ = 5; ● = 7, △ = 10, □ = 12, ▼ = 15, ☐ = 20. (Reproduced with permission from Suter, P.M., Fairley, H.B. and Isenberg, M.D. (1978) *Chest*, **73**, 158–62.)

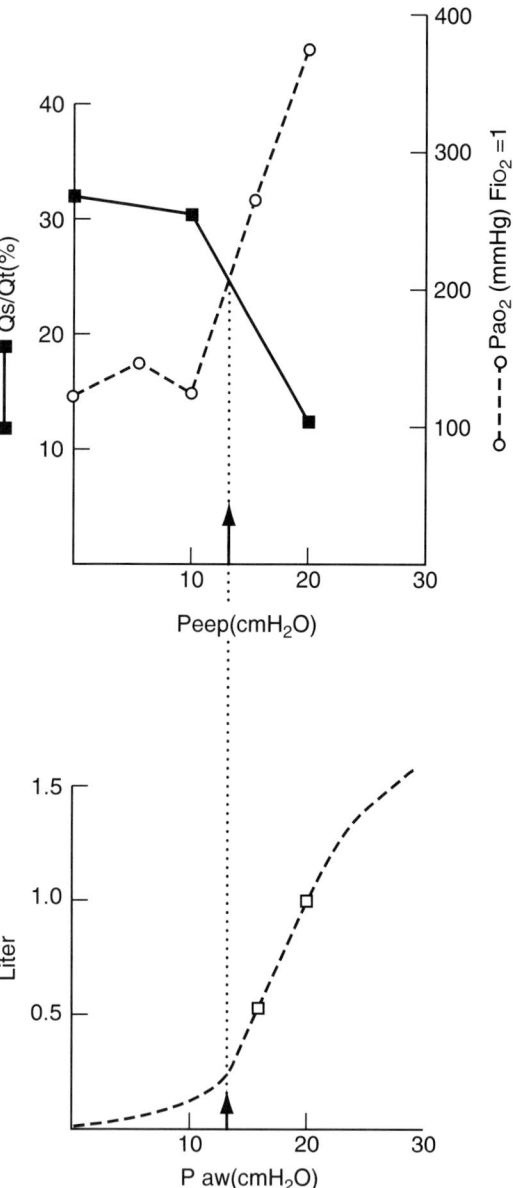

23.7). The point at which the slope of the pressure–volume curve stops rapidly improving (mathematically, when second derivative of volume with respect to pressure becomes zero) is known as the *P*flex point. Indeed, arterial oxygenation often improves markedly as the pressure range immediately spanning *P*flex is exceeded [27]. Many investigators currently believe that tidal ventilation that spans such an inflexion range must be avoided. Provision of sufficient PEEP and the progression of disease over time obliterate the 'Pflex point' [31]. When constant inspiratory flow is used under passive conditions and no 'auto-PEEP' is present, the pressure–volume contour may be readily deduced under dynamic conditions, facilitating measurement [32]. The efficacy of PEEP in improving oxygen exchange relates directly to the reversal of atelectasis and redistribution of lung water. It is not surprising, therefore that the effect-

Figure 23.7 Passive pressure–volume relationship of the respiratory system in early phase of ARDS. Note the sigmoidal shape of this curve, with a clear inflection range in the lower segment ('*P*flex', arrow). Note also that oxygen exchange improves markedly once static Paw exceeds *P*flex. (Reproduced with permission from Matamis *et al.* [27].)

iveness of PEEP tends to decline with the passage of time. Experimentally, relatively high inflation pressures can be used without serious damage, provided that enough PEEP is added to obliterate the lower inflection range. In fact, this observation may help to account for the recently reported tolerance of certain surgical patients to 'super-PEEP' ($> 20 \, cmH_2O$).

ALTERNATIVE VENTILATORY STRATEGIES

Recognition of the potential for subtle as well as radiographically overt 'volutrauma' has stimulated interest in less hazardous alternatives to accomplish ventilation. Several modes of mechanical ventilation (including pressure controlled ventilation (PCV) [33], airway pressure release ventilation [34,35] and inverse ratio ventilation (IRV) [36,37]) can be considered variants of a unifying '**pressure targeted**' approach in which the clinician selects only four variables other than F_{IO_2}: maximum airway pressure (Pset), PEEP, frequency (f), and inspiratory time fraction (duty cycle, T_I/T_T). Acceptance of upper and lower limits for alveolar pressure confines the practitioner to a maximum ventilating (or preset) pressure – the difference between maximum (Pmax) and end expiratory airway pressures.

In previous work, we developed [38] and validated [39,40] a clinically oriented, unicompartment, biexponential model for the dynamics of pressure preset ventilation that accounts for interactions between the inspiratory and expiratory phases of the ventilatory cycle. Several implications of that modeling project may bear relevance to managing ALI. Minute ventilation ($\dot{V}_E$) and V_T become curvilinear functions of frequency when maximum and minimum values for alveolar pressure are fixed by the selections of Pset and PEEP. As f rises, the lung neither fills nor empties to its equilibrium volumes, auto-PEEP adds to PEEP, and V_T falls. Consequently, total minute ventilation (the $f * V_T$ product) (pressure preset $V_T + V_D/V_T + \dot{V}_E$) approaches a precise upper limit determined by lung impedance characteristics, the applied pressure gradient (Pmax – total PEEP), and T_I/T_T. An optimum value for **alveolar** ventilation ($\dot{V}_A$) tends to occur at a finite and clinically relevant cycling frequency. This peak occurs because as V_T falls, the physiological dead space fraction (V_D/V_T) of each tidal breath rises, owing to the growing importance of a **relatively** fixed series ('anatomic') dead space. Our simplified model of pressure preset ventilation illustrates that CO_2 retention may be an inevitable consequence of a 'lung protective' strategy that tightly restricts applied pressure and maintains a certain minimum lung volume.

PERMISSIVE HYPERCAPNIA

Traditional guidelines suggest the maintenance of nearly normal values for arterial blood gases, adjusting the ventilator settings for F_{IO_2}, PEEP, and $\dot{V}_E$ to achieve these goals. For the great majority of patients, however, the need to maintain normocapnia has not been unequivocally demonstrated, particularly when CO_2 is retained gradually ($< 1 \, mmHg$ (0.13 kPa) per hour), and/or abrupt changes in pH are avoided. It can be effectively argued that maintaining normocapnia may not be appropriate if the cost is impaired lung healing and a heightened risk of barotrauma [40,41]. In uncontrolled reports it has been suggested that improved survival may be achieved by approaches that limit alveolar pressure, even if normal arterial blood gases cannot be maintained [42,43]. Retrospective studies indicate that 'permissive hypercapnia', a strategy that allows $\dot{V}_A$ and peak ventilatory pressures to fall and Pa_{CO_2} to rise, may reduce lung injury and enhance survival in status asthmaticus [42] and ALI [43,44]. A recent prospective study also strongly suggests an advantage to compliance and gas exchange for a lung protective approach [45].

Table 23.3 Primary consequences of CO_2 retention

Acute problems
Intracellular acidosis
Nervous system dysfunction
Intracranial pressure increase
Muscle weakness
Cardiovascular dysfunction
Chronic problems
Depressed ventilatory drive

The physiologic effects of CO_2 retention are functions of the severity of hypercapnia and the rate of its build up (Table 23.3). **Chronic** hypercapnia appears to have few notable side effects, apart from the reduction in ventilatory drive attendant to compensatory metabolic alkalosis. Although gradual elevations of Pa_{CO_2} (≈ 1 mmHg (0.13 kPa) increase per hour) are often tolerated remarkably well [43–46], hypercapnia may not be advisable for all patients with ALI (e.g. patients with coexisting head injury, recent cerebral vascular accident or significant cardiovascular dysfunction, uncorrected hypoxemia or adrenergic blockade). **Acute** elevations in Pa_{CO_2} increase sympathetic activity, raise cardiac output, heighten pulmonary vascular resistance, alter bronchomotor tone, dilate cerebral vessels and disturb crucial functions of the central nervous system [46]. Over the short term, arterial pH may not closely reflect the pH of the intracellular environment. The magnitude of any resulting intracellular acidosis, however, is almost certain to be less than the profound intracellular pH changes observed during ischemia. Because CO_2 affects cardiac output and influences vascular and bronchomotor tone, it is uncertain if hypercapnia disturbs $\dot{V}/\dot{Q}$ matching or modulates the extent of lung injury and edema during the course of mechanical ventilatory support. Implementation of permissive hypercapnia often requires deep sedation and/or paralysis, a requirement that may be associated with serious side effects: residual muscle weakness, impaired secretion clear-

ance and fluid retention. Moreover, permissive hypercapnia may not be advisable (or even possible) in the setting of coexisting **metabolic** acidosis.

PRONE POSITIONING

The great majority of mammals ambulate in the prone position, where vital organs are maximally protected. Furthermore, position changes occur very frequently, even during sleep. Numerous studies of patients with ARDS demonstrate improved oxygenation in the prone as opposed to the supine or side-lying positions, especially in the earliest phase of disease [73]. The optimal duration of prone positioning and the impact of this maneuver on the outcome have not yet been convincingly determined. Nonetheless, when undertaken with appropriate caution, prone positioning would appear to be a useful and safe intervention.

APRESSURE TARGETED APPROACH TO VENTILATIN ALI

Although no definitive clinical data are currently available to confirm the wisdom of adopting a nontraditional 'pressure targeted' approach, a rational strategy for ventilating patients with ALI can be formulated which is based on firm theoretical and experimental grounds (Table 23.4). Such a strategy recognizes that several mechanically distinct alveolar populations coexist within the injured lung, and that the underlying pathophysiology changes over time. This approach gives higher priority to controlling maximal and minimal transalveolar pressures than to achieving normocapnia [41].

Assuming that oxygen demand has been minimized and cardiac function has been addressed, its essential elements are as follows. **First**, because alveolar subpopulations with nearly normal elastic properties may coexist alongside flooded or infiltrated ones, the clinician must avoid applying **transalveo-**

Table 23.4 A lung protective strategy for ventilating ARDS

1. Tailor ventilatory strategy to the phase of the disease. (PEEP in early stage; withdraw PEEP later)
2. Minimize oxygen demands
3. Control alveolar pressure, not Pa_{CO_2}
4. Maintain total end expiratory $Palv$ (PEEP + auto-PEEP) several cmH_2O above P_{flex}. In general, this will be more than 7 cmH_2O but less than 15 cm H_2O
5. Avoid large V_T and use least $Palv$ required to meet **unequivocal** therapeutic goals
6. Hold transalveolar pressure < 35 cmH_2O
7. Make necessary increases in mean Paw by changing T_I/T_T not by raising PEEP
8. Consider specialized adjunctive measures to improve gas exchange and O_2 delivery[a]

[a] In addition to such standard measurements as skillful management of pulmonary vascular pressure, repositioning and use of cardiotonic agents, specialized adjunctive measures might include (where available) such experimental methods as extracorporeal CO_2 removal (ECCO$_2$R) or intratracheal catheter assisted gas exchanged (TGI).

lar pressures greater than normal lung tissue is designed to sustain at its maximum capacity (30–35 cmH_2O). This pressure generally corresponds to end inspiratory static airway pressures ('plateau' pressures) of 35–50 cmH_2O, depending on the stiffness of the chest wall. Pressures in this range are generally sufficient to reopen closed airways [13,47]. Whatever the appropriate maximal pressure setting might be for an individual patients, it seems wise to avoid the **upper** inflexion range of the static pressure – volume curve whenever possible [47,48]. **Second,** sufficient end expiratory transalveolar pressure must be used to avert tissue damage resulting from surfactant depletion or stresses associated with repeated opening and closing of collapsible units during the tidal breathing cycle. The total PEEP applied (the sum of PEEP and auto-PEEP) should be sufficient to obliterate the **lower** inflection point of the pressure – volume curve of the respiratory system, which at tidal volumes of 7–8 ml/kg generally occurs at a pressure of 10–15 cmH_2O in the early phase of ARDS. In truth, there is an inflection **range** rather than a single inflection point, as dependent alveoli in the lower regions of the lung require a greater **end** expiratory alveolar pressure to maintain patency than those more superior [49]. Improved arterial oxygenation tends to parallel effective recruitment, and CO_2 retention is a consequence of alveolar overdistension. Although actual measurement of the pressure–volume curve (static or dynamic with constant flow) is most precise, in practice, PEEP can initially be set at 10 cmH_2O and increased in small (2 cmH_2O) steps, looking for markedly improved oxygenation that corresponds to obliterating the range of $Pflex$. (Under certain circumstances, a reasonable alternative to the empirical use of PEEP steps is to extend the inspiratory time fraction gradually to create auto-PEEP.) Relatively small tidal volumes often result from imposing these upper and the lower bounds on ventilatory pressure. Therefore, periodic recruitment of 'sigh' breaths of ≈ 12 ml/kg may be needed in some patients to maintain adequate lung volume and avoid hypoxemia. **Third**, under conditions of passive inflation (no spontaneous efforts), the practitioner should adjust mean airway opening pressure ($\bar{P}aw$) to achieve acceptable pulmonary O_2 exchange by extending the duty cycle (T_I/T_T), or by raising PEEP. Extending the duty cycle improves the distribution of ventilation and may help to recruit or hold open otherwise collapsible lung units. Raising PEEP (and preserving a well-tolerated (T_I/T_T) may be the preferred option, however, when the patient retains control of the breathing rhythm. **Fourth**, when not contraindicated, hypercapnia should be accepted from the onset of therapy (buffered, when necessary, by judiciously infused sodium bicarbonate or tromethamine [USP]) in preference to violating the guidelines of controlling alveolar pressure. Pharmacologic buffering may also be needed to implement hypercapnia when deep sedation and/or paralysis are not used. The strategy of permissive hypercapnia may be difficult to implement in the presence of metabolic acidosis, when other measures (e.g. dialysis) may be needed adjunctively.

DECREASING SERIES DEAD SPACE BY TRACHEAL GAS INSUFFLATION (TGI)

A possible alternative to allowing extreme or rapidly developing hypercapnia in ALI is to enhance the efficiency of CO_2 elimination at low V_T and cycling pressures. Techniques to improve the efficiency of cyclical ventilatory pressure would be highly desirable when hypercapnia must be minimized or when the pace with which hypercapnia develops must be slowed. Extracorporeal CO_2 removal is resource intensive, hazardous and best implemented by an expert team (50) (Chapter 25). Improved oxygenation, as well as reduced need for high ventilating pressures, may be the outcome when this technique is successfully employed [51]. A somewhat less invasive proposal is to accomplish supplemental intravenacaval gas exchange via a femoral (IVOX) catheter that is comprised of gas exchanging hollow fibers [52].

Another less invasive approach is to insufflate fresh gas into the trachea (TGI) to reduce the concentration of CO_2 in the series (anatomic) dead space. The idea of bypassing the anatomic dead space has been applied to **spontaneously** breathing patients for many years. For example, the tracheostomy used to help spontaneously breathing patients with severe emphysema and ventilatory failure is a variant of this technique [53]. In 1968, Stresemann demonstrated the potential utility of flushing the proximal anatomic dead space with oxygen in normal subjects and in two patients with obstructive lung disease [54,55]. More recently, forms of TGI have been shown to be effective in spontaneously breathing hypercapnic animals and patients with a

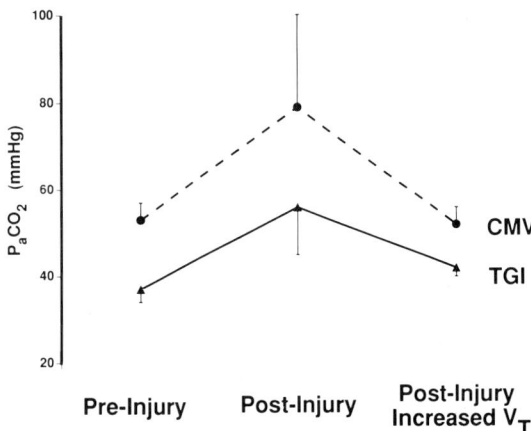

Figure 23.8 Effect of tracheal gas insufflation on alveolar ventilation in dogs with acute lung injury induced by oleic acid. At a fixed level of $\dot{V}_E$ provided by volume cycled ventilation (CMV), Pa_{CO_2} rises after injury. Relative effect of TGI is diminished by increasing tidal volume so as to match preinjury Pa_{CO_2} during CMV. (From A. Nahum, R. Shapiro, S.A. Ravenscraft and J.J. Marini, unpublished data.)

variety of forms of acute and chronic respiratory failure [56–60].

The effectiveness of TGI is undeniably compromised by the presence of a large **alveolar** dead space component. However, despite this undeniable limitation, TGI aided ventilation should be particularly effective in the lung protective ventilatory strategy just described for two important reasons: (1) small tidal volumes are associated with a higher percentage of series dead space; and (2) when Pa_{CO_2} is very elevated, small reductions in V_D/V_T are associated with large decreases of Pa_{CO_2} (Figure 23.8). During TGI aided ventilation, fresh gas delivery occurs either throughout the respiratory cycle (continuous catheter flow), or only during a segment of it (phasic catheter flow) [40,61–65]. During expiration, low to moderate continuous flows of fresh gas introduced near the carina dilute the proximal anatomic dead space (dead space flushing). During inspiration, catheter flow contributes to the total inspired V_T but also bypasses the anatomic dead space mouthward (proximal) of the gas jet. At high catheter flow rates, turbulence generated at the catheter tip can also enhance gas mixing in regions beyond its orifice, thereby contributing to CO_2 elimination [40,62,63,65].

The application of TGI as an **adjunct** to mechanical ventilation must be differentiated from techniques unassociated with conventional ventilation that inject fresh gas continuously in a valveless system [63–66] or use a shutter simply to regulate catheter flow [67–69]. High flow rates of fresh gas (30–60 l/min) delivered by continuous flow ventilation (CFV) during apnea can achieve adequate CO_2 elimination in dogs, but only if the catheter tips are positioned below the main carina [64,67]. During shuttered continuous flow ventilation, closure of an expiratory valve forces catheter flow to deliver all of the inspired V_T [67,68]. The catheter then acts as a miniventilator, whose circuit Y point is effectively positioned near the carina.

Sznajder and colleagues used a shutter that acts as an expiratory valve to deliver all the inspired V_T by catheter flow in dogs with oleic acid induced pulmonary edema [67]. Compared with conventional mechanical ventilation, the valved TGI catheter (which actually functioned as the ventilator in this setting) performed the same ventilatory task at 35% of the baseline V_T and with 70% of elastic end inspiratory pressure [67]. Using a similar strategy known as intratracheal pulmonary ventilation (ITPV), Kolobow and colleagues demonstrated that adequate ventilation can be accomplished in normal sheep with seven eighths of all lung tissue removed, without resorting to excessive V_E and airway pressures [68]. A mouth directed 'reverse thrust' injection catheter proved helpful in reducing alveolar pressure in those studies. Some encouraging preliminary experience with ITPV has now been gathered in infants as well.

TGI AS AN ADJUNCT TO CONVENTIONAL VENTILATION

Phasic TGI is delivered selectively during inspiration or expiration [61]. As already noted, **phasic inspiratory** TGI can be used as a source of fresh gas, with its contribution to total inspiratory flow (catheter plus ventilator) bypassing the anatomic dead space proximal to the catheter tip. During **phasic expiratory** TGI, catheter flow is timed to occur during all or part of expiration, augmenting $\dot{V}_A$ by flushing CO_2 from the tracheal and apparatus dead space [61,70]. Phasic dead space flushing by high frequency ventilation has also been applied as an adjunct to volume or pressure controlled mechanical ventilation in a limited number of experiments [70].

We have recently examined the efficacy of TGI as an adjunct to mechanical ventilation in a series of experiments involving normal dogs [40,61,62]. Our experiments were designed primarily to understand how TGI augments $\dot{V}_A$ and to define interactions between TGI settings and ventilatory parameters. In all of this work, TGI was used in conjunction with conventional mechanical ventilation. In our initial experiment [40], we established the feasibility of TGI (patient data with TGI) during pressure controlled ventilation. At a catheter flow rate of 14 l/min, TGI deceased P_aCO_2 and V_D/V_T by 41% and 75%, respectively, compared with PCV alone [40] (Figure 23.4). This effect was associated with only modest increases (1–2 cmH$_2$O) in the peak airway pressure recorded in the connecting tubing of the ventilator. These results are similar to those achieved by Boussignac and colleagues in normal pigs with a modified endotracheal tube that allows fresh gas injection [71]. Wolff and colleagues have used a similar technique in an experimental setting [60].

The ventilatory benefit which accrues from TGI is often modest in lungs with large alveolar dead space, and optimal usage and long term safety of this technique are yet to be fully defined. In experiments involving dogs with ALI, we have demonstrated a reduced efficacy of this method, partially offset by hypercapnia. The volume mouthward of the catheter tip can be considered pure dead space if its CO_2 concentration equals that of perfused alveoli. TGI becomes less effective during ALI as the CO_2 depleted gas from the alveolar dead space reduces the P_{aCO_2} concentration of the catheter flushable volume. In other words, the catheter flushes less **effective** dead space. Hypercapnia increases P_{ECO_2} as well as the number of CO_2 molecules flushed by the catheter. Unless the ventilator's delivered inspiratory volume is modified or pressure preset ventilation is used, TGI may raise mean alveolar pressure in direct proportion to the catheter flow rate and the percentage of the cycle during which the catheter flows. This may explain why TGI can sometimes improve oxygenation. The potential for TGI to cause mucosal damage, secretion retention and barotrauma remain to be determined. Nonetheless, the experience of workers using transtracheal ventilation in patients with chronic obstructive pulmonary disease and other stable conditions [56,57,59], as well as our own preliminary results with TGI in critically ill patients [72], indicate that it may eventually prove helpful in a variety of acute and chronic settings. Because of its potential to moderate the rate and extent of CO_2 retention, TGI would appear well suited as an adjunct to a pressure targeted, lung protective ventilatory support for ALI.

REFERENCES

1. Webb, H.H. and Tierney, D.F. (1974) Experimental pulmonary edema due to intermittent positive pressure ventilation with high inflation pressures. Protection by positive end-expiratory pressure. *Am. Rev. Respir. Dis.*, **110**, 556–65.
2. Dreyfuss, D., Basset, G., Soler, P.S. and Saumon, G. (1985) Intermittent positive-pressure hyperventilation with high inflation pressures produces pulmonary microvascular injury in rats. *Am. Rev. Respir. Dis.*, **132**, 880–4.
3. Gong, H.J. (1982) Positive pressure ventilation in the adult respiratory distress syndrome. *Clin. Chest Med.*, **3**, 69–88.
4. Carroll, G.C., Tuman, K.J., Braverman, B. *et al.* (1988) Minimal positive end-expiratory pressure (PEEP) may be 'best PEEP'. *Chest*, **93**, 1031–5.
5. Gattinoni, L., Pesenti, A. and Bombino, M. (1988) Relationships between lung computed tomographic density, gas exchange, and PEEP in acute respiratory failure. *Anesthesiology*, **69**, 824–32.
6. Meduri, G.U., Belenchia, J.M., Estes, R.J. *et al.* (1991) Fibroproliferation phase of ARDS: clinical findings and effects of corticosteroids. *Chest*, **100**, 943–52.
7. Gammon, B.R., Shin, M.S. and Buchalter, S.E. (1992) Pulmonary barotrauma in mechanical ventilation: patterns and risk factors. *Chest*, **102**, 568–72.
8. Gattinoni, L., Pelosi, P., Vitale, G. *et al.* (1991) Body position changes redistribute lung computed tomographic density in patients with acute respiratory failure. *Anesthesiology*, **74**, 15–23.
9. Albert, R.K., Leasa, D., Sanderson, M. *et al.* (1987) The prone position improves arterial oxygenation and reduced shunt in oleic acid-induced acute lung injury. *Am. Rev. Respir. Dis.*, **135**, 628–33.
10. Pappert, D., Rossaint, R., Lopez, F. *et al.* (1993) Merker G. Gerlach H., Falke K. pcCMV The prone position – ventilation/perfusion distribution and continuous blood gas measurement (abstract). *Proceedings of the International Conference on Recent Advances in the Treatment of the Adult Respiratory Distress Syndrome*, July 5–8, 1993, Tutzing, Germany.
11. Marini, J.J. (1990) Lung mechanics in adult respiratory distress syndrome. Recent conceptual advances and implications for management. *Clin. Chest Med.*, **11**, 673–90.
12. Mead, J., Takishima, T. and Leith, D. (1970) Stress distribution in lungs: a model of pulmonary elasticity. *J. Appl. Physiol.*, **28**, 596–608.
13. Gaver, D.P., Samsel, R.W. and Solway, J. (1990) Effects of surface tension and viscosity on airway opening. *J. Appl. Physiol.*, **69**, 74–85.
14. Rouby, J.J., Lherm, T., Martin de Lassale, E. *et al.* (1993) Histologic aspects of pulmonary

barotrauma in critically ill patients with acute respiratory failure. *Intensive Care Med.*, **19**, 383–9.

15. Egan, E.A. (1982) Lung inflation, lung solute permeability and alveolar edema. *J. Appl. Physiol.*, **53**, 121–25.

16. Carlton, D.P., Scherer, R.G., Cummings, J.S. *et al.* (1988) Lung overexpansion injures the pulmonary microcirculation in lambs. *Pediat. Res.*, **23**, 500 (abstract).

17. Kolobow, T., Moretti, M.P., Fumagalli, R. *et al.* (1987) Severe impairment of lung function induced by high peak airway pressure during mechanical ventilation. *Am. Rev. Respir. Dis.*, **135**, 312–5.

18. Tsuno, K., Prato, P. and Kolobow T. (1990) Acute lung injury from mechanical ventilation at moderately high airway pressures. *J. Appl. Physiol.*, **69**, 956–61.

19. Roupie, E., Dambrosio, M., Mentec, H. *et al.* (1993) Titration of tidal volume reduction and permissive hypercapnia in adult respiratory distress syndrome (ARDS). *Am. Rev. Respir. Dis.*, **147**, A351 (abstract).

20. Hernandez, L.A., Coker, P.J., May, S. *et al.* (1990) Mechanical ventilation increases microvascular permeability in oleic acid injured lungs. *J. Appl. Physiol.*, **69**, 2057–61.

21. Fu, Z., Costello, M.L., Tsukimoto, K. *et al.* (1992) High lung volume increases stress failure in pulmonary capillaries. *J. Appl. Physiol.*, **73**, 123–33.

22. Dreyfuss, D., Soler, P., Basset, G. *et al.* (1988) High inflation pressure pulmonary edema. Respective effects of high airway pressure, high tidal volume, and positive end expiratory pressure. *Am. Rev. Respir. Dis.*, **137**, 1159–64.

23. Hernandez, L.A., Peevy, K.J., Moise, A.A. *et al.* (1989) Chest wall restriction limits high airway pressure-induced lung injury in young rabbits. *J. Appl. Physiol.*, **66**, 2364–8.

24. Dreyfuss, D. and Saumon, G. (1992) Barotrauma is volutrauma, but which volume is the one responsible? *Intensive Care Med.* **18**, 139–41.

25. Slutsky, A.S. (1993) Barotrauma and alveolar recruitment (Editorial). *Intensive Care Med.*, **19**, 369–71.

26. Muscedere, J.G., Mullen, J.B.M., Gan, K. *et al.* (1992) Tidal volume at low airway pressures can cause pulmonary barotrauma. *Am. Rev. Respir. Dis.*, **145**, A454.

27. Matamis, D., Lemaire, F., Harf, A. *et al.* (1984) Total respiratory pressure volume curves in the adult respiratory distress syndrome. *Chest*, **86**, 58–66.

28. McCulloch, P.R., Forkert, P.G. and Froese, A.B. (1988) Lung volume maintenance prevents lung injury during high frequency oscillatory ventilation in surfactant-deficient rabbits. *Am. Rev. Respir. Dis.*, **137**, 1185–92.

29. Corbridge, T.C., Wood, L.D.H., Crawford, G.P. *et al.* (1990) Adverse effects of large tidal volumes and low PEEP in canine acid aspiration. *Am. Rev. Respir. Dis.*, **142**, 311–5.

30. Pelosi, P., Valenza, F., Crotti, S. *et al.* (1993) TAC study of barotrauma (abstract). *Proceedings of the International Conference on Recent Advances in the Treatment of the Adult Respiratory Distress Syndrome*, July 3–5, 1993, Tutzing, Germany.

31. Benito, S. and Lemaire, F. (1990) Pulmonary pressure–volume relationship in acute respiratory distress syndrome in adults: role of positive end expiratory pressure. *J. Crit. Care*, **5**, 27–34.

32. Ranieri, V.M., Giulani, R., Fiore, T. *et al.* (1994) Volume–pressure curve of the respiratory system predicts effects of PEEP in ARDS: 'occlusion' versus 'constant flow' technique. *Am. J. Respir. Crit. Care Med.*, **149**, 19–27.

33. Abraham, E. and Yoshihara, G. (1990) Cardiorespiratory effects of pressure controlled ventilation in severe respiratory failure. *Chest*, **98**, 1445–9.

34. Stock, M.C., Downs, J.B. and Frolichter, D.A. (1987) Airway pressure release ventilation. *Crit. Care Med.*, **15**, 462–6.

35. Rouby, J.J. (1990) Pressure release ventilation, in *Update in Intensive Care and Emergency Medicine* (ed. J.L. Vincent), Springer, Berlin, pp. 185–95.

36. Marcy, T.W. and Marini, J.J. (1991) Inverse ratio ventilation in ARDS: rationale and implementation. *Chest*, **100**, 494–504.

37. Cole, A., Weller, S. and Sykes, M. (1984) Inverse ratio ventilation compared with PEEP in adult respiratory failure. *Intensive Care Med.*, **10**, 227–32.

38. Marini, J.J., Crooke, P.S. and Truwit, J.D. (1989) Determinants and limits of pressure-preset ventilation: a mathematical model of pressure control. *J. Appl. Physiol.*, **67**, 1081–92.

39. Burke, W.C., Crooke, P.S., Marcy, T.W. *et al.* (1993) Comparison of mathematical and mechanical models of pressure controlled ventilation. *J. Appl. Physiol.*, **74**, 922–33.

40. Nahum, A., Burke, W.C., Ravenscraft, S.A. *et al.* (1992) Lung mechanics and gas exchange during pressure controlled ventilation in dogs: augmentation of CO_2 elimination by an intratracheal catheter. *Am. Rev. Respir. Dis.*, **146**, 965–73.

41. Marini, J.J. (1991) Controlled ventilation: targets, hazards and options, in *Ventilatory Failure* (eds J.J. Marini and C. Roussos), Springer, New York, pp. 269–92.

42. Darioli, R. and Perret, C. (1984) Mechanical controlled hypoventilation in status asthmaticus. *Am. Rev. Respir. Dis.*, **129**, 385–7.

43. Hickling, K.G., Henderson, S.J. and Jackson R. (1990) Low mortality associated with low volume, pressure limited ventilation with permissive hypercapnia in severe adult respiratory syndrome. *Intensive Care Med.* **16**, 372–7.

44. Lewandowski, K., Sama, K. and Falke, K.J. (1992) Approaches to improve survival in severe ARDS, in *Update in Intensive Care and Emergency Medicine*, vol. 16 (ed. J.L. Vincent), Springer, Berlin, pp. 372–83.

45. Amato, M.B.P., Barbas, C.S.V., Medeiros, D.M. *et al.* (1993) Improved lung mechanics and oxygenation achieved through a new approach to mechanical ventilation in ARDS. *Am. Rev. Respir. Dis.*, **147**, 890 (abstract).

46. Hickling, K.G. (1992) Low volume ventilation with permissive hypercapnia in the adult respiratory distress syndrome. *Clin. Intensive Care*, **3**, 67–78.

47. Lachmann, B. (1992) Open up the lung and keep the lung open. *Intensive Care Med.*, **18**, 319–21.

48. Mancebo, J. (1992) PEEP, ARDS, and alveolar recruitment. *Intensive Care Med.*, **18**, 383–5.

49. Gattinoni, L., D'Andrea, L., Pelosi, P. *et al.* (1993) Regional effects and mechanism of positive end-expiratory pressure in early adult respiratory distress syndrome. *JAMA*, **269**, 2122–7.

50. Gattinoni, L., Brazzi, L. and Pesenti, A. (1991) Extracorporeal carbon dioxide removal in ARDS, in *Ventilatory Failure* (eds J.J. Marini and C. Roussos), Springer, Berlin, pp. 308–317.

51. Gattinoni, L., Pesenti, A., Mascheroni, D. *et al.* (1986) Low frequency positive pressure ventilation with extracorporeal CO_2 removal in severe acute respiratory failure. *JAMA*, **256**, 881–6.

52. Mortensen, J.D. (1991) Augmentation of blood gas transfer by means of an intravascular blood gas exchanger (IVOX), in *Ventilatory Failure* (eds J.J. Marini and C. Roussos), Springer, Berlin, pp. 318–46.

53. Cullen, J.H. (1963) An evaluation of tracheostomy in pulmonary emphysema. *Ann. Intern. Med.*, **58**, 953–60.

54. Stresemann, E. (1968) Washout of anatomical dead space. Design of a method and experimental study using an external dead space. *Respiration*, **25**, 281–91.

55. Stresemann, E., Votteri, B.A. and Sattler, F.P. (1969) Washout of anatomical dead space for alveolar hypoventilation. *Respiration*, **26**, 425–34.

56. Hurewitz, A., Bergofsky, E. and Vomero, E. (1991) Airway insufflation: increasing flow rates progressively reduce dead space in respiratory failure. *Am. Rev. Respir. Dis.*, **144**, 1229–33.

57. Bergofsky, E.H. and Hurewitz, A.N. (1989) Airway insufflation: physiologic effects on acute and chronic gas exchange in humans. *Am. Rev. Respir. Dis.*, **140**, 885–90.

58. Long, S.E., Menon, A.S., Kato, H. *et al.* (1988) Constant oxygen insufflation (COI) in a ventilatory failure model. *Am. Rev. Respir. Dis.*, **138**, 630–5.

59. Benditt, J., Pollock, M., Roa, J. and Celli, B. (1993) Transtracheal delivery of gas decreases the oxygen cost of breathing. *Am. Rev. Respir. Dis.*, **147**, 1207–10.

60. Wolff, G., Brunner, J.X. and Troillet, J.L. (1987) Disturbances of gas exchange in adult respiratory distress syndrome. *Atemw. Lungenkrkb.*, **13**, 236–43.

61. Burke, W.C., Nahum, A., Ravenscraft, S.A. *et al.* (1993) Modes of tracheal gas insufflation: comparison of continuous and phase specific gas injection in normal dogs. *Am. Rev. Respir. Dis.*, **148**, 562–8.

62. Nahum, A., Ravenscraft, S.A., Nakos, G. *et al.* (1992) Tracheal gas insufflation during pressure controlled ventilation: effect of catheter position, diameter, and flow rate. *Am. Rev. Respir. Dis.*, **146**, 1411–8.

63. Slutsky, A.S., Watson, J., Leith, D.E. and Brown, R. (1985) Tracheal insufflation O_2 (TRIO) at low flow rates sustains life for several hours. *Anesthesiology*, **63**, 278–86.

64. Isabey, D., Boussignac, G. and Harf, A. (1989) Effect of air entrainment on airway pressure during endotracheal gas injection. *J. Appl. Physiol.*, **67**, 771–9.

65. Slutsky, A.S. and Menon, A.S. (1987) Catheter position and blood gases during constant-flow ventilation. *J. Appl. Physiol.*, **62**, 513–9.

66. Sznajder, J.I., Nahum, A., Crawford, G.D. *et al.* (1989) Alveolar-pressure in homogeneity and gas exchange during constant flow ventilation in dogs. *J. Appl. Physiol.*, **67**, 1489–94.

67. Sznajder, J.I., Becker, C.J., Crawford, G.P. and Wood, L.D.H. (1989) Combination of constant-flow and continuous positive-pressure ventilation in canine pulmonary edema. *J. Appl. Physiol.*, **67**, 817–23.

68. Muller, E., Kolobow, T., Mandava, S. *et al.* (1991) On how to ventilate lungs as small as 12% of normal. Intratracheal pulmonary ventilation (ITPV). A new mode of pulmonary ventilation. *Am. Rev. Respir. Dis.*, **143**, A693 (abstract).

69. Gilbert, J., Larsson, A., Smith, R.B. and Bunegin, L. (1991) Intermittent-flow expiratory ventilation (IFEV): delivery technique and principles of action – a preliminary communication. *Biomed. Instrument Technol.*, **25**, 451–6.

70. Jonson, B., Similowski, T., Levy, P. *et al.* (1990) Expiratory flushing of airways: a method to reduce dead space ventilation. *Eur. Respir. J.*, **3**, 1202–5.

71. Boussignac, G., Bertrand, C., Huguerard, P. and Teissère B. (1989) Efficiency of a new endotracheal set up allowing a constant additional gas flow. *Urgences Med.*, **8**, 47–9.

72. Ravenscraft, S.A., Burke, W.C., Nahum, A. *et al.* (1993) Tracheal gas insufflation augments CO_2 clearance during mechanical ventilation. *Am. Rev. Respir. Dis.*, **148**, 345–51.

73. Pappert, D., Rossaint, R., Slama, K. *et al.* (1994) Influence of positioning on ventilation–perfusion relationships in severe adult respiratory distress syndrome. *Chest*, **106**, 1511–16.

Eric H. Gluck and Brian F. Keogh

High frequency ventilation (HFV) is a broad term applied by clinicians to those ventilatory modes that employ frequencies greater than four times the natural respiratory frequency of the ventilated subject [1]. In the adult patient, HFV therefore mandates a frequency of 60 breaths per minute or more and, under most circumstances, the tidal volume approximates to that of the anatomical dead space. Such techniques have generated substantial scientific interest, not the least because understanding of the associated physiology and fluid mechanics has remained tantalizingly obscure. Theoretical benefits for HFV in the syndrome of acute respiratory distress in adults (ARDS) have long been recognized [2], most particularly in view of the potential to achieve acceptable gas exchange whilst decreasing the pressure–volume cost of ventilation. Despite this, the use of HFV in ARDS has achieved limited acceptance and currently remains restricted to those intensive care units with both access to the appropriate technology and enthusiasm for the technique.

HISTORY AND DEFINITIONS

HFV is not new, having been employed clinically for approximately 30 years. Indeed, the ability to ventilate and oxygenate using tidal volumes less than the anatomical dead space was first anticipated in 1915 by Henderson and colleagues, who observed that air moving along a tube assumed a parabolic velocity profile [3]. Fresh air could therefore reach the alveolar area even when the anatomical dead space had not yet been filled by inspired gas. Subsequently, Briscoe and colleagues noted that with tidal volumes of 60 ml or less, adequate gas exchange could take place if the frequency was sufficiently increased [4].

Many different ways of applying HFV to human subjects have been described. Enthusiasm for this approach, particularly in the 1970s, led to the development of HFV technology with much diversity in system design and performance. It must be recognized that relatively minimal changes in design can lead to enormous differences in performance between different types of HFV equipment and within a particular device [5].

Between 1965 and 1970, Swedish investigators developed the first clinically applicable form of HFV, high frequency positive pressure ventilation (HFPPV), and demonstrated its ability to provide adequate ventilation without causing cardiovascular embarrassment [6]. HFPPV employed conventional-type ventilators with very small tidal volumes (3–4 ml/kg) at frequencies of 60–100 cycles/min. Although these systems represent the foundation on which HFV technology developed, their use has been restricted to anesthesia [7] and an application in ARDS has not been established.

High frequency jet ventilation (HFJV) has probably been scrutinized more than any

ARDS Acute Respiratory Distress in Adults. Edited by Timothy W. Evans and Christopher Haslett. Published in 1996 by Chapman & Hall, London. ISBN 0 412 56910 8

Table 24.1 Historical developments in HFV

Mode	Setting	Author	Frequency/min	Year	Reference
HFPPV	Animal	Sjostrand	60–100	1967	6
HFPPV	Clinical	Hiejman and Sjostrand	60–100	1972	7
HFJV	Clinical	Klain and Smith	100	1977	8
HFJV	Animal	Gluck	450	1988	9
HFJV	Clinical	Gluck	300	1989	10
HFO	Animal	Lunkenheimer	2400	1972	12
HFO	Clinical	Butler	900	1980	13

other technique of mechanical ventilation for the treatment of patients with ARDS. It is based on the principle of a jet injector through which gas is accelerated, thereby creating a negative lateral pressure and entraining additional gases along with the fresh inspired gas emanating from the nozzle. The nozzle can be placed either within the endotracheal tube or at its proximal end, the latter position providing the most effective entrainment of heated and humidified 'bias' gases. The technique was introduced to clinical anesthesia in 1977 [8] and typically employed frequencies of 60–150 breaths per minute. Ventilators of this type were used in ARDS in the late 1970s and early 1980s with mixed results. In the mid-1980s, our laboratory developed a high frequency jet ventilator which was capable of achieving effective gas exchange in ARDS at higher frequencies, typically 300 breaths per minute [9,10]. This machine, now called the Infrasonics Adult Star 1010 High Frequency Ventilator (Infrasonics, San Diego, USA), has recently received USA Food and Drug Administration approval for use in ARDS after undergoing a multicenter clinical trial [11], and has been designed to overcome many of the technical difficulties in HFJV application, namely ventilator potency, safety, monitoring of ventilator–patient interaction and the efficiency of humidification.

HFPPV and HFJV both rely on passive expiration of respiratory gases. A different technique, high frequency oscillation (HFO), first described by Lunkenheimer and col-

leagues in 1972 [12], was first used clinically in 1980 [13]. Oscillatory flow can be induced either by a piston pump or a large oscillating diaphragm similar to that of a loud speaker found in stereo sound systems. Uniquely, in this technique both positive and negative pressure are applied at the endotracheal tube and, therefore, inspiration and expiration are both active. A bias flow to the system provides fresh gas for ventilation and aids carbon dioxide removal during exhalation. Under these circumstances the tidal volumes are extremely small, usually in the range of 1–3 ml/kg. Emphasis in the application of HFO has been in neonatal respiratory distress where many studies have demonstrated its ability to improve clinical outcome, both as a prophylactic technique [14] and also when used as a salvage therapy [15]. With the exception of selected cases in pediatric patients [16], HFO has not thus far been widely applied in ARDS.

Table 24.1 summarizes historical developments in HFV.

GAS EXCHANGE IN HFV

A major difficulty in the introduction of HFV has been the inability of investigators to make *in vitro* measurements of, or even to describe mathematically, the characteristics of alveolar gas exchange. This has not, however, limited the number of theories about how gas exchange can be accomplished at tidal volumes less than the anatomical dead space.

Despite the uncertainty relating to the true nature of alveolar gas exchange in HFV, several components have been identified.

GAS MIXING

Ventilation frequency in the physiological range combines convection and diffusion. Convection occurs in the larger airways. Diffusion, where both CO_2 and oxygen move down their concentration gradients, occurs from respiratory bronchioles to the alveoli. In the smaller airways, where flow is said to be laminar, it has been suggested that it is possible to augment the diffusion process by increasing the energy of the gas molecules [17]. Increasing the diffusivity of the gases would enhance gas exchange at tidal volumes that were significantly smaller than the anatomical dead space. Empirical data have demonstrated that CO_2 elimination in HFV was proportional to the product of frequency and tidal volume [18]. Other investigators have suggested that CO_2 elimination is more closely related to the product of frequency multiplied by tidal volume raised to the second power ($f \times V_T^2$) [19].

In addition to the normal mixing that takes place along the length of the small airways, Taylor dispersion promotes movement of gas molecules in a lateral direction. This allows oxygen and CO_2 to move down concentration gradients at acute angles relative to the bulk flow that is being maintained in the lumen. Augmented diffusion had been demonstrated in a model of the adult airways suggesting that, under these circumstances, when tidal volume was held constant, CO_2 elimination would be enhanced at the resonant frequency of the lung [17]. In subsequent animal experiments, a specific frequency at or near the resonant frequency of the animal's lungs demonstrated enhanced CO_2 elimination when compared to frequencies above and below this point.

PENDELLUFT

An additional, and probably very important, mechanism for gas exchange during HFV is pendelluft; that is, the movement of gases back and forth from one alveolus to another. The pendelluft effect results when the time constant for an alveolar–respiratory bronchiolar unit is different from that of a neighbouring unit. After the unit with the shorter time constant is completely filled and starts to empty, that with the longer time constant has not yet filled. The pressure inside the alveolus with the short time constant is significantly higher than the other units in its vicinity and gas moves from this alveolus both out towards the trachea and towards neighboring alveoli. During the subsequent breath, the pressure in the alveolus with the long time constant is now higher than the one with the short time constant and gas moves back again to the original alveolus. This effect has significant potential for distributing oxygen and removing CO_2.

GAS DISTRIBUTION

Recent work on the distribution of inspired gas, utilizing oscillatory flows and radionucleotide imaging techniques, has demonstrated that at low ventilatory frequencies gas is distributed to the lower lobes in preference to the upper and middle lung zones [20]. As the ventilatory frequency is increased, however, gas distribution is more uniform with preferential filling of the central units in all three lobes. These data suggest that, at low frequencies, lung capacitance plays a major role in the distribution of gases at tidal volumes that are normally applied in conventional ventilation. As the frequency is increased, the distribution of gas is no longer related to the capacitance of the lung but more to the resistance of the airways and lung tissue. This has been shown to occur in normal lungs, in lungs with acute diffuse injury, and in nonhomogeneous lung injuries as well. The redistribution of gas flow into the lung at high frequencies could in part explain the improved gas exchange that has been demonstrated clinically in many different studies of the use of HFV.

In conclusion, there are many suppositions used to explain oxygenation and CO_2 elimination during HFV. There are also facts that can be clearly quantified. The most important is that gas flows through a cylinder in a parabolic profile and not in a square wave. Gas molecule kinetics due to Taylor dispersion and other phenomena have been clearly demonstrated in the laboratory and, in part, explain some of the gas exchange that takes place. Pendelluft effect has been demonstrated at both low and high frequencies under appropriate circumstances and certainly plays a role in gas exchange. Despite the lack of hard scientific data on respiratory gas disposition in HFV, there is abundant empirical data demonstrating how to manipulate HFV techniques in order to enhance or retard the elimination of carbon dioxide and to enhance oxygenation.

PRACTICAL ASPECTS OF HFJV TECHNOLOGY

High frequency jet ventilators are simple mechanical devices. At the heart is the mechanism by which high pressure gas is chopped into small pulses which provide the high frequency breaths. Most contemporary machines achieve this via a solenoid valve, regulated in terms of frequency and duty cycle (inspiratory time). The driving pressure (the third control), set by the operator, regulates the amount of flow that crosses the solenoid valve when open. Although the three control parameters seemingly conspire to provide a given tidal volume, each one may be used individually to regulate gas exchange in the patient.

Oxygenation in ARDS relies on the generation of mean airway pressure to maintain lung volume. Of the three variables in HFV, the inspiratory time (I-time) has the greatest

effect on mean airway pressure and hence oxygenation. At frequencies > 300 breaths per minute, an increase of 2% I-time has the same effect as an increment of positive end expiratory pressure (PEEP) of 5 cmH_2O. Increasing I-time also has a small effect on tidal volume but increasing driving pressure has the greatest effect. Theoretical and empirical data have demonstrated that CO_2 elimination is related to frequency and to tidal volume raised to the second power (V_{CO_2} is proportionate to the frequency times V_T^2) [19]. Therefore, any change in ventilator function that would increase tidal volume would have a significant effect on CO_2 elimination. The driving pressure is therefore used as the major control to augment CO_2 elimination and reduce Pa_{CO_2}. Frequency should also have a profound affect on both oxygen and CO_2 exchange, especially as, at the resonant frequency of the lung, ventilation and oxygenation are markedly enhanced [17]. Such a dramatic frequency effect has not, however, been noted in some clinical trials [11]. Frequency changes influence absolute inspiratory time and an increase in frequency therefore decreases tidal volume. If the anatomical and physiological dead space remain constant, a change in tidal volume would either increase or decrease CO_2 elimination. A common clinical dilemma is that of hypocarbia. Decreasing the driving pressure to prevent excessive CO_2 clearance also lowers mean airway pressure, with subsequent adverse effects on oxygenation. Changing the frequency, however, varies tidal volume without having a major effect on mean airway pressure. An increase in frequency, therefore, can limit CO_2 elimination and is the appropriate maneuver in ARDS patients who develop respiratory alkalosis but in whom oxygenation depends on the maintenance of mean airway pressure (Chapter 23). Thus, each of the three controls can be used independently to achieve the desired control of oxygenation and CO_2 elimination. We have evaluated over 1000 ventilator changes performed in over 150 patients and found that the above maneuvers will result in the expected changes in arterial gas tension in more than 95% of circumstances.

HUMIDIFICATION

One of the difficulties encountered with HFV in the past has been the effective humidification of inspired gases. Pathological changes can be seen within the trachea and upper airways in animals as early as 2 hours after humidification if HFV is disrupted. The ventilators of the late 1970s provided humidification by dripping fluid in front of the jet pulsations, which aerosolized it into the patient's airways. Small deviations of the jet gas flow or the water droplets could result in total absence of humidification. Jet nozzles were later modified to entrain water droplets at the point of air exit from the nozzle. This provided better and more reliable humid-

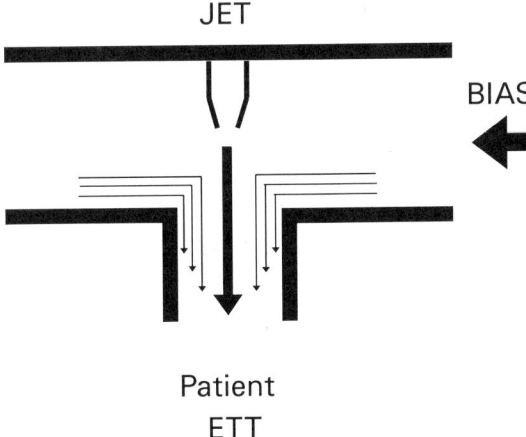

Figure 24.1 Jet nozzle and entrainment chamber. The jet nozzle sits within the entrainment chamber placed at the proximal end of the endotracheal tube (ETT). Proximal positioning provides an entrainment ratio of up to 200%. By contrast, distal positioning of the jet may provide an entrainment ratio as low as 25%. The bias gas of oxygen enriched air, heated to 42°C and fully saturated, represents the source of humidification and variation in F_{IO_2}.

ification but water still did not diffuse adequately into the interior of the jet gas stream. Recent developments have resulted in the design of a novel nozzle system (Figure 24.1) which results in very high entrainment ratios (up to 200%). A bias gas heated to 40–42°C and 100% humidified is entrained by the nozzle gas (dry at room temperature), providing fully humidified gas at body temperature after mixing occurs in the endotracheal tube. This system has been employed in more recently developed ventilators and has resulted in a significant diminution of airway inflammation and mucous desiccation.

NEW HFJV TECHNOLOGY

The major differences in HFJV of the 1990s to that available in the 1970s are the ability to monitor adequately and to protect the patient from potential barotrauma or 'runaway' ventilation. Early ventilators had poor alarm systems, mainly because adequate computer driven software was unavailable at the time. Recently developed HFJV ventilators are equipped with very rapid pressure and flow analyzing units capable of reacting to a change in ventilator function in less than 500 ms. This results in significant protection of the patient from ventilator and particularly solenoid valve malfunction. Additionally, such devices have substantially improved monitoring, with cathode ray tube screens capable of demonstrating airway pressure in real time. This provides the clinician with visual output with respect to ventilator–patient interactions.

Technological advance has also resulted in improved ventilatory capacity in newer devices. As the frequency of pulsations increases, the time that is required to open and close the solenoid valve can become significant. Slow responding valves degrade the square wave electronic signal into a pseudo sine wave mechanical output. The result is a loss of some volume per pulse and a reduction in the mean airway pressure attainable.

The latest generation of adult jet ventilators have incorporated technology which can improve valve response times and ensure maintenance of effective tidal volumes and desired mean airway pressure, even at frequencies above 5 Hz. Patients with very low compliance and severely disrupted alveolar and interstitial architecture can thus be adequately ventilated to acceptable goals of both oxygenation and CO_2.

The newer jet ventilators also contain most of the conveniences offered by conventional technology. Some have battery packs, which allow disconnection from an electrical outlet and hence movement of the patient from the intensive care unit to X-ray or operating room without disruption. Additionally, in the event of power failure, the ventilator would continue to operate normally without interference. Such machines also incorporate self-diagnostic equipment as well as their own bookkeeping system, whereby all the settings, pressure readings and alarms are downloaded automatically to floppy diskettes for archiving.

BAROTRAUMA

One of the major concerns in the therapy of ARDS is the role of mechanical ventilation in the causation of barotrauma. HFV theoretically provides a favorable profile in terms of pressure–volume changes at the alveolar level and has been advocated in ARDS for this reason. Barotrauma presents in various forms, the gross manifestation being bronchopleural fistula. Pulmonary interstitial emphysema, a more subtle form, is also recognized. Experimental studies in intact animals have clearly demonstrated a relationship between peak inspiratory pressure (PIP) and barotrauma [21] (Chapter 23). Two studies of HFV in ARDS which aimed to limit PIP have not, however, demonstrated a reduction in the incidence of barotrauma. Carlon and colleagues randomized patients with ARDS to receive HFV or conventional ventilation [22].

HFV was associated with PIP 10–20 cmH_2O below the conventionally ventilated group. Despite this reduction, the incidence of barotrauma was identical in both groups. In this instance, however, barotrauma was only defined as the formation of bronchopleural fistulae. A multicentre study by Gluck and colleagues, also using HFV, but at significantly higher frequencies, aimed to reduce PIP but at the same time maintain a mean airway pressure at the same level that the patients were receiving when on conventional ventilation. This study also demonstrated a similar incidence of barotrauma, as defined by interstitial emphysema, as well as bronchopleural fistulae, in the HFV group when compared with literature controls [11]. Thus, in two clinical investigations involving more than 300 patients, HFV-related reductions in PIP in patients with ARDS did not apparently reduce the incidence of barotrauma.

What then are the other contributory factors to the incidence of barotrauma in ARDS? The next most likely theory concerns inhomogeneous ventilation. Under these circumstances, alveolar–respiratory bronchiolar units with differing time constants fill and empty at different rates (i.e. asynchronously). Under the appropriate circumstances, significant pressure gradients can exist between one unit and another. If these become sufficiently high, alveolar rupture can occur, air dissipates into the interstitial space and eventually into the pleural space. Although several studies have demonstrated that HFV provides more uniform ventilation than conventional techniques, this is a macroscopic rather than microscopic observation. Therefore, even with improved distribution of ventilation with HFV, alveolar pressure gradients can still exist.

A third proposal for the mechanism by which barotrauma appears in ARDS is unrelated to the form of mechanical ventilation that the patient receives, but rather to the underlying pulmonary disease process. Patients with conditions associated with small areas of lung necrosis are more likely to develop barotrauma. In reviewing the subset of ARDS patients who developed barotrauma associated with mechanical ventilation, we saw a preponderance of patients with sepsis related ARDS. Primary infection of the lung has the highest incidence of barotrauma, an observation which implicates the underlying disease process as a major cause of barotrauma. If this is the case in a particular individual, the form of mechanical ventilation employed may be irrelevant; barotrauma will be inevitable and should be expected.

PULMONARY MICROVASCULAR INJURY

It has been demonstrated recently in animal models that high PIP [23], and even moderate PIP of 30 cmH$_2$O [24], results in an increased accumulation of interstitial lung water. It was subsequently demonstrated that the large volume excursions associated with such ventilation, rather than the high PIP applied, are primarily responsible for this phenomenon [25] (Chapters 20 and 23). Certainly, when applying any form of ventilatory support to patients with ARDS, who already exhibit increased capillary permeability, further fluid filtration into the interstitial pulmonary space would be of serious clinical significance. Data accumulated recently have suggested that smaller tidal volumes are associated with less lung water accumulation [26]. We have demonstrated clinically that lung water can be reduced by applying this concept to patients with ARDS, despite the maintenance of similar cardiac output, pulmonary artery occlusion pressure, vascular resistances and fluid balance. In six patients, HFJV significantly improved lung edema as gauged by radiographic estimation of lung water. In the preliminary results of a study in which the radiologists are blinded to the mode of ventilation, the initiation of HFJV resulted in significant clearance of lung water and subsequent reappearance of alveolar edema when HFJV was discontinued. Further studies are

necessary before any significant conclusions can be reached about the role of mechanical ventilation in the causation of increased lung water but this information is clearly of interest.

In animal models, Froese, McCulloch and colleagues have investigated the formation of hyaline membranes and small airway damage in the surfactant deficient lung [27]. This can be significantly reduced using ventilatory support with very small tidal volumes at oscillatory frequencies even when maintaining the same mean airway pressure. Indeed, when oscillatory frequencies were applied at various mean airway pressures, lower mean airway pressures resulted in an increased incidence of small airway damage and alveolar hyaline membrane formation. This suggests that there is a minimum threshold value of mean airway pressure that must be maintained. Further studies from this group [28] and others [29] suggest that volume recruitment maneuvers, in this case sustained inflation, should be incorporated into the ventilatory technique and would result in improved arterial oxygenation.

How should one evaluate the pressure burden that the patient receives from mechanical ventilation? Many intensivists believe that mean airway pressure is the best measure of the pressure burden caused by mechanical ventilation. Others suggest that PIP is a more reliable indicator. The animal data and clinical experience with HFV might suggest that a more precise measurement would be the product of the mean airway pressure and the tidal volume. This index would take into account the fact that large tidal volumes result in more inhomogeneous ventilation and increases edemagenesis. However, the work of Froese and colleagues suggests that mean airway pressure is a necessary 'evil' of mechanical ventilation, which at an appropriate level protects small airways and alveolae from damage, but when associated with large tidal volumes can, by itself, cause significant trauma to the small airways and alveoli. Thus an upper and a lower limit to the lung pressure burden exists, between which lies the least traumatic and most appropriate ventilatory form.

Much remains to be done to sort out the nuances of the role of mechanical ventilation in causing barotrauma. The lack of reasonable animal models that truly depict the changes in the lung of human subjects inflicted by ARDS has hindered work in the past. Fortunately, newer models are being developed which should guide the clinician on the ventilatory management of ARDS. The animal data that exist today are consistent with using smaller tidal volumes at high frequencies while maintaining the appropriate level of mean airway pressure. A clinical strategy, based on these studies, should result in adequate gas exchange while limiting ventilator induced damage to the patient's lungs.

CLINICAL TRIALS OF HFV IN ARDS

The introduction of HFJV into critical care prompted the first case reports [30] and small series [31] describing its use, which suggested potential advantages over conventional techniques in acute respiratory failure. Enthusiasm for the approach was somewhat dampened when, in 1983, Carlon and colleagues published their often quoted, prospective, randomized, crossover comparison in 309 patients of conventional ventilation versus HFJV at 100/min and inspiratory:expiratory ratio of 1:2 [22]. Identical survival rates of 38% were reported in both groups. Although HFJV was found to be a safe, reliable, predictable and effective method of mechanical ventilation, no substantial advantage over conventional techniques could be identified. Similar conclusions were drawn from a subsequent short (< 4 hours) crossover comparative study in 100 patients with respiratory failure [32].

Interpretation of the Carlon study must take into account the lack of volume recruitment techniques or attempts to maintain mean airway pressure and hence lung volume in either treatment arm. Indeed, changes in lung volume were poorly regulated by the ventilator manipulations designated by the study. Despite these potential deficiencies, the authors found no evidence that HFJV was harmful or less effective than conventional techniques, suggesting that ongoing investigation of HFJV in ARDS was appropriate.

A smaller, prospective, comparative study of HFJV versus conventional ventilation in patients at risk of ARDS revealed that HFJV treated patients who subsequently developed ARDS reached preset gas exchange end points at significantly lower airway pressures [33]. No obvious influence on clinical outcome was, however, identified.

In the mid-1980s Gluck and colleagues, recognizing deficiencies in the available HFJV technology, particularly when applied to poorly compliant ARDS patients, developed a new, potent HFJV ventilator specifically for use in this condition. Features of the device included improved monitoring and safety, a proximal jet entrainment chamber leading to enhanced ventilatory capacity and effective humidification, and a low inertia, rapid response solenoid switching valve. The ventilator frequency employed (5–7 Hz) was designed to harness potential advantages in gas exchange resulting from the use of frequencies near lung resonance. The term 'ultrahigh' frequency jet ventilation was coined to describe this concept. Animal studies showed that the amplitude of phasic changes in central airway pressure during the respiratory cycle was much attenuated and that in the 2 mm distal airway, airway pressure was virtually constant and approximated to the centrally measured mean airway pressure (Figure 24.2). This observation implied a favorable and limiting influence on the degree of alveolar volume changes associated with ventilation. An international multicenter feasibility study was established to assess the efficacy of this ventilator in severe ARDS. Entrance criteria (Table 24.2) included the

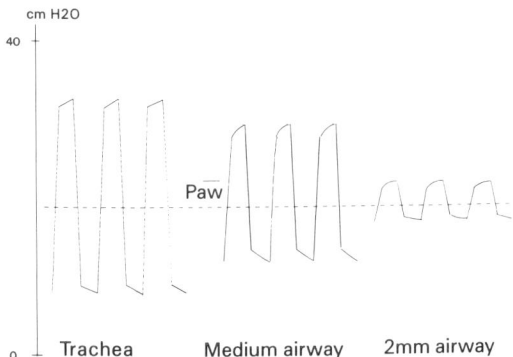

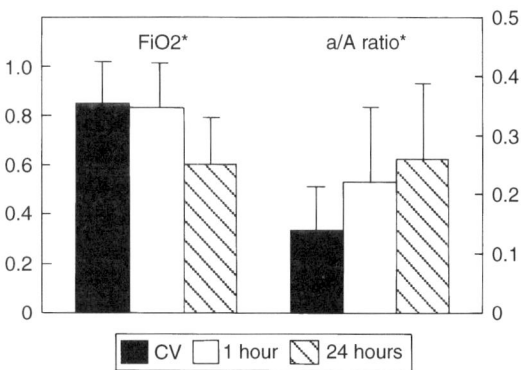

Figure 24.2 Amplitude of airway pressure fluctuations in respiratory tree with HFJV. Centrally measured airway pressure fluctuations with HFJV are markedly attenuated on passing down the respiratory tree. Maximum and minimum pressures converge to a value at the 2 mm airway which fluctuates at low amplitude (2–3 cmH$_2$O) around a value which approximates to the centrally measured mean pressure. (Data obtained with retrograde catheter technique in pig – E.H. Gluck.)

Figure 24.3 Oxygenation parameters from multi-center HFJV trial (11). Mean F_{IO_2} decreased from 0.85 on conventional ventilation (CV) to 0.6 after 24 hours of HFJV with corresponding improvement in a/A from 0.14 to 0.26. $* = P < 0.05$ at 24 hours. Total patient number = 90. Note: F_{IO_2} 0.9, Pa_{O_2} 6 kPa = a/A ratio approx 0.1; F_{IO_2} 0.6, Pa_{O_2} 9 kPa = a/A ratio approx 0.2. Reproduced with permission from data in Gluck *et al.*, Use of Ultrahigh Frequency Ventilation in Patients with ARDS (1993) *Chest*, **103**, 1413–20.

Table 24.2 Entry criteria for ultrahigh frequency ventilation multicenter feasibility study

Diagnosed ARDS from any cause
and
$Pa_{O_2} < 8.5$ kPa at $F_{IO_2} > 0.7$
or
$Pa_{O_2} < 8.5$ kPa at $F_{IO_2} = 0.7$
or
PEEP > 15 cmH$_2$O
or
Peak inspiratory pressure > 65 cmH$_2$O
and
Failing conventional ventilation

proviso that patients were considered to be failing conventional ventilatory support on the basis of the direction of cardiorespiratory vectors or the intensity of ventilatory support. A preliminary report of results from the first three USA centers, describing 90 patients, was published in 1993 [11].

The study was a prospective, nonrandomized assessment of the application of the new HFJV ventilator with each patient serving as his or her own control whilst receiving conventional ventilation. The basic philosophy in ventilator application was that smaller tidal volumes would result in reduced peak airway pressures. Additionally, while most of the prior clinical studies sought to reduce the mean airway pressure, a certain minimal mean airway pressure was assumed to be necessary to maintain small airway and alveolar distension. Thus, a definite aim was to reduce the peak airway pressures but not necessarily the mean pressure.

Results from the study showed a significant improvement in arterial oxygenation at 1 and 24 hours after the switch to HFJV (Figure 24.3), as well as statistically significant reductions in both peak and mean airway pressures (Figure 24.4). These changes were observed without adverse effects on hemodynamics. Carbon dioxide clearance was extremely

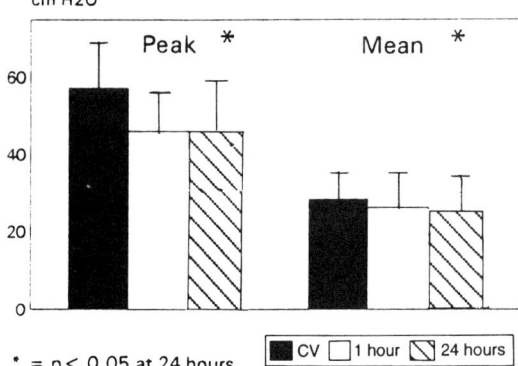

cm H2O

Peak *   Mean *

* = p< 0.05 at 24 hours

■ CV □ 1 hour ⧅ 24 hours

Figure 24.4 Airway pressure measurements from multicenter HFJV trial (11). Mean values of peak inspiratory pressure fell from 57 cmH$_2$O on conventional ventilation (CV) to 46 cmH$_2$O after 24 hours HFJV. Mean airway pressure fell from 28 to 25 cmH$_2$O which, in common with PIP observations, proved statistically significant. Reproduced with permission from data in Gluck *et al.*, Use of Ultrahigh Frequency Ventilation in Patients with ARDS (1993) *Chest*, **103**, 1413–20.

effective and frequently excessive, resulting in quite profound respiratory alkalosis and necessitating an increase in the ventilatory frequency. Adverse effects noted were pneumothorax (15%) (although half of these patients had pre-existing bronchopleural fistulae), mucous desiccation (15%) and tracheitis (1%). The episode of tracheitis was attributable to user error resulting in interruption of humidification.

The survival rate in the preliminary report was 58%. The addition of another 30 patients from other USA and one UK centre resulted in an overall survival of 53%. More compelling survival information was derived from the outcome observed in 25 patients who were switched to HFJV after less than 48 hours of conventional ventilation [34]. Despite similar severity of disturbances of gas exchange to the whole group, 19 (76%) of these patients survived, adding further credence to the view that the institution of appropriate HFJV support early in the disease process may limit the extent of ventilator induced lung damage and thus favorably influence disease outcome.

HFJV IN PEDIATRICS

A recent report of HFJV in 29 children with severe acute respiratory distress syndrome represents the largest reported series in the pediatric population [35]. Selection criteria included evidence of barotrauma associated with conventional ventilation. HFJV driving parameters were regulated to achieve a satisfactory arterial oxygen saturation (Sao$_2$ > 90%). Survival rate was 69%. Despite no identifiable difference in the degree of pulmonary dysfunction between survivors and nonsurvivors prior to HFJV, survivors demonstrated significantly improved oxygenation indices and lower mean airway pressures on HFJV. Survivors were also noted to have spent significantly less time on conventional ventilation (3.7 ± 2.1 days) compared to nonsurvivors (9.6 ± 4.5 days). On this basis the authors speculated that early application of HFJV limited the progression of ventilation induced damage to airways and lung parenchyma.

COMBINED HIGH FREQUENCY VENTILATION

Combined high frequency ventilation (CHFV) incorporates features of both conventional and high frequency techniques. It has been applied in ARDS since the early 1980s, and despite a paucity of related publications, CHFV has clearly gained popularity in selected European centres. CHFV techniques with a primary emphasis on each of the two basic components have been described.

The clinical use of CHFV was first reported in 1983 [36]. An integrated unit compatible with the Siemens Servo 900C ventilator was subsequently developed which superimposed small volume, high frequency pulsations (600–1200/min) on conventional volume or pressure controlled breaths. Two groups reported their experience in the use of CHFV in the salvage of patients with ARDS who were deemed to be failing conventional ventilation [37,38]. Both studies demonstrated improved arterial oxygenation, adequate CO_2 clearance and a favorable hemodynamic profile. The survival rate for the 73 patients in the two studies was only 16% but CHFV was only applied late in the clinical course (average 17 days after admission in one study) as an attempted salvage maneuver from catastrophic pulmonary failure.

A slightly different approach has been reported in which HFJV at 250–300/min was superimposed on conventional ventilation with small tidal volumes, and the degree of conventional ventilation decreased to the point where CO_2 retention occurred [39]. The need to maintain lung volume and mean airway pressure was recognized, but surprisingly a substantial decrease in centrally measured mean airway pressure was found, despite improved Pa_{O_2}, a phenomenon not yet fully explained. Survival figures of 66% were subsequently reported in a group of 22 adults and children with ARDS who had undergone CHFV for hypoxic salvage [40].

The advantages of CHFV should be assessed in the context of the ventilatory capacity of the HFJV ventilators used. The application of early HFJV technology was commonly associated with inadequate gas exchange, most particularly an inability to achieve coincident improvements in arterial oxygenation and CO_2 clearance. The addition of conventional ventilation, by enhancing lung volume and reintroducing tidal alveolar gas renewal, enhances the gas exchanging efficiency of the system. In addition, the combined system allows meaningful monitoring of ventilatory volumes, pulmonary mechanics and the incorporation of safety alarms.

The future for CHFV is uncertain. It represented a modification of a ventilatory system in which the properties of the HFJV component alone were insufficient to support gas exchange in severe ARDS. It remains to be seen whether its popularity in selected centers will persist as more potent and safer HFV devices, which prove capable of achieving desired ventilatory targets without the need for combined technology, become available.

HIGH FREQUENCY OSCILLATION

During the late 1980s HFO, delivered by various functionally similar ventilators, established a definite niche in the therapy of the infant respiratory distress syndrome (IRDS). Despite the equivocal results obtained from the large North American multicenter HIFI trial [41], the design of which was subsequently severely criticized for the lack of appropriate lung volume recruitment and maintenance techniques, HFO, especially when combined with surfactant therapy, has become the standard of care in many centers for IRDS.

Two recent publications reported a total of 19 pediatric patients with severe ARDS who underwent HFO (age range 1 month to 15 years) and of whom 13 survived [16,42]. As yet there is little other information on outcome in this rare patient group. Each series reported one 15 year old patient, both of whom survived, and both of whom presumably approached adult stature. Despite such isolated cases, and much research into the application of HFO in large animal models, it has not thus far proved possible to reliably apply HFO techniques to adult-size patients with ARDS. Problems encountered include noise, device bulk, the enormous heat generated in rapidly moving appropriate tidal volumes in systems with minimal compressible volume, adequate monitoring and safety. Specifically, HFO devices are usually closed system, volume preset or volume controlled ventilators. Patients with ARDS are known to exhibit variable degrees of airways resistance and auto-PEEP and this pathophysiological feature has enormous safety implications when applying HFO.

There are current projects in both Europe and Japan aimed at constructing an HFO device for application in adults. At this stage, however, progress is preliminary and it is likely to be some years before the clinical testing of such a device.

A recent case report detailed the successful management of a patient with atypical pneumonia during pregnancy who progressed to severe respiratory failure, refractory to conventional respiratory support [43]. HFO at 3000/min superimposed on conventional intermittent positive pressure ventilation afforded immediate improvement in gas exchange, a trend which continued. To the authors' knowledge, this is the only reported use of combined HFO in adult practice, a technique yet to be further investigated in patients with ARDS.

EXTERNAL HIGH FREQUENCY OSCILLATION

A fourth method of applying high frequency ventilation is via external oscillation of the chest wall. In this circumstance, a semirigid casing is placed around the chest and part of the abdomen. Oscillatory waves are applied from the outside of the chest wall, exciting the molecules within the chest and aiding in gas exchange. Frequencies in this technique usually vary between 3 and 10 Hz.

Externally applied high frequency oscillatory devices were reported in human studies in 1985 [44] and in patients with chronic obstructive pulmonary disease in 1987 [45]. The Hayek Oscillator (Flexco Medical Instruments AG, Zurich, Switzerland), a new external, cuirass-style ventilator which oscillates at frequencies of 8–999 cycles/min around a variable negative pressure baseline, has recently been introduced into clinical practice. Following validation in normal subjects [46], it is currently being investigated as a primary or adjunctive ventilatory therapy in a variety of respiratory conditions.

Theoretical advantages of the Hayek Oscil-

lator include lung volume maintenance at lower PIP and enhanced venous return with respect to positive pressure ventilation. Although PIP may be decreased, it is the transpulmonary pressure which is responsible for lung distension in this mode and high transpulmonary pressures remain capable of producing barotrauma/volotrauma despite low absolute PIP values [25]. Despite this note of caution, there have been encouraging results in the application of this ventilator early in the course of trauma induced ARDS in at least one center in the UK, the early results of which have been published in abstract form [47]. Improved oxygenation is undoubtedly secondary to effective lung volume recruitment and maintenance, and although the device appears effective under the relatively favorable conditions of early, trauma induced ARDS, it remains to be determined whether such responses will be a feature of its use later or in more advanced forms of the syndrome.

FUTURE DIRECTIONS FOR HFV

The development of HFV technology that is effective in the respiratory support of severe ARDS has occurred at a time of intense interest and activity in the field of adjuvant pharmacological respiratory therapy. It is inevitable that clinicians will require the HFV devices to incorporate the option of effective delivery of such agents, in particular nitric oxide (NO) (Chapter 29) and surfactant (Chapter 16).

NO is obviously used in conjunction with some form of mechanical ventilation and intuitively the combination with HFJV would seem reasonable. Since HFJV devices do not employ closed circuits some modifications will be necessary. Concentrations of the inspired gases will need to be measured after they enter the endotracheal tube and once mixing is complete. Most clinicians who use HFJV use endotracheal tubes that would permit gas concentration determination via sampling lumens sited near the distal end of the endotracheal tube, an appropriate site for NO determination. Expiratory scrubbing devices will also need to be incorporated to avoid unacceptable NO contamination of the patient environment.

Adult studies using exogenous surfactant replacement therapy in various forms have not resulted in the success observed in pediatric respiratory distress syndrome. Because of the expanded surface area and distance from trachea to alveolus in the adult, much of the medication never reaches its target. High frequency devices could be modified into air blast atomizers. Such devices direct high velocity gas jets at a liquid medium. The viscosity of the liquid, the velocity of the injected gas and the angle at which the two meet determine the size of the particles that are created. Surfactant, which is very viscous, could be dispersed in this manner into particles which are small enough to be carried by the jet stream to the distal lung. This could result in better distribution of the surfactant and a reduction in the quantity of the medication that would have to be delivered.

This atomizer technique could be used to deliver other medications as well, while adequate alveolar distension, lung volume and airway patency are maintained. The cost of delivering expensive medications such as prostacyclin, α_1-antitrypsin and even antibiotics could be reduced while therapeutic efficacy is maintained.

CONCLUSION

HFV holds a definite place in the ventilatory options for ARDS, but its exact niche has not yet been precisely determined. One of the difficulties associated with this technique is the understanding of its associated physiology, which lags behind the empirical clinical data. Multiple studies have demonstrated clear benefits in oxygenation and CO_2 elimination. Additionally, a reduction in peak airway pressures and even small reductions in mean airway pressures have been observed, in the context of hemodynamic stability and without adverse effects. Despite these findings, clinicians are waiting for data to demonstrate that this mode of ventilation will cause a favorable change in mortality. It is likely that this data will continue to prove very difficult to obtain since mechanical ventilation only plays a supportive role in patients with ARDS. The influence of appropriate ventilatory practice may be overwhelmed by a multitude of factors related to the ongoing pathophysiology of the condition, many of which play a more substantial role in determining outcome. Despite this dilemma, the theoretical advantages of HFV remain compelling and on this basis, and in the absence of identified adverse effects, the technique warrants more widespread application.

Of the HFV options available, HFJV remains the most promising. Clinical studies have suggested that certain patients with ARDS are more likely to benefit from HFJV, namely those who are switched to HFJV early in the course of the disease and those with lung injury secondary to trauma. Patients with ARDS following pulmonary infection or those who have undergone prolonged conventional ventilation are less likely to show specific benefits from this or any other ventilatory technique. Clinical studies designed to clarify these issues and further define benefits of HFJV in different subsets of patients with ARDS, especially trauma related, have commenced or are planned. In the meantime, the combination of theoretical benefit and the availability of new, clinically effective and safe HFJV technology should encourage both the further investigation and more widespread application of the technique.

REFERENCES

1. Slutsky, A.S., Brown, R., Lehr, J. *et al.* (1981) High frequency ventilation: a promising new approach to mechanical ventilation. *Med. Instrum.*, **15**, 229–33.

2. Lachmann, B., Danzmann, E., Haendley, B. and Jonson, B. (1982) Ventilator settings and gas exchange in respiratory distress syndrome, in Prakash O. (ed). *Applied Physiology in Clinical Respiratory Care* (ed. O. Prakash), Nijhoff, The Hague, pp. 141–76.

3. Henderson, Y., Chilingsworth, S.P. and Whitney, J.L. (1915) The respiratory dead space. *Am. J. Physiol.*, **38**, Pt 1.

4. Briscoe, W.A., Forster, R.E. and Comroe, J.H. (1954) Alveolar ventilation at very low tidal volumes. *J. Appl. Physiol.*, **7**, 27.

5. Froese, A.B. and Bryan, A.C. (1987) High frequency ventilation. *Am. Rev. Respir. Dis.*, **135**, 1363–74.

6. Sjostrand, U.H. and Eriksson, I.A. (1980) High rates and low volumes in mechanical ventilation – not just a matter of ventilatory frequency. *Anesth. Analg.*, **59**, 567–76.

7. Heijman, K., Heijman, L., Jonzon, A. *et al.* (1972) High frequency positive-pressure ventilation during anaesthesia and routine surgery in man. *Acta Anaesthesiol. Scand.*, **16**, 176–87.

8. Klain, M. and Smith, R.B. (1977) High frequency percutaneous transtracheal ventilation. *Crit. Care Med.*, **5**, 280–7.

9. Orlando, R., Gluck, E.H., Cohen, M. and Mesologites, C.G. (1988) Ultra-high-frequency jet ventilation in a bronchopleural fistula model. *Arch. Surg.*, **123**, 591–3.

10. Gluck, E., Heard, S. and Fahey, P. (1989) Ultra high frequency jet ventilation in ARDS – multicenter results. *Chest*, **96**, 175s.

11. Gluck, E., Heard, S., Patel, C. *et al.* (1993) Use of ultrahigh frequency ventilation in patients with ARDS. A preliminary report. *Chest*, **103**, 1413–20.

12. Lunkenheimer, P.P., Rafflenbeul, W., Keller, H.P. *et al.* (1972) Application of transtracheal pressure oscillation as modification of 'diffusion respiration'. *Br. J. Anaesth.*, **44**, 627.

13. Butler, W.J., Bohn, D.J., Bryan, A.C. and Froese, A.B. (1980) Ventilation by high frequency oscillation in humans. *Anesth. Analg.*, **59**, 577–84.

14. Octave Study Group (1991) Multicenter randomized controlled trial of high against low frequency positive pressure ventilation. *Arch. Dis. Child.*, **66**, 770–5.

15. Clark, R.H., Yoder, B.A. and Sell, M.S. (1994) Prospective randomised comparison of high frequency oscillation and conventional ventilation in candidates for extracorporeal oxygenation. *J. Pediatr.*, **124**, 447–54.

16. Arnold, J.H., Truog, R.D., Thompson, J.E. and Fackler J.C. (1993) High-frequency oscillatory ventilation in paediatric ventilatory failure. *Crit. Care Med.*, **21**, 272–78.

17. Fredberg, J.J. (1980) Augmented diffusion in the airways can support pulmonary gas exchange. *J. Appl. Physiol.*, **49**, 232–8.

18. Slutsky, A.S., Drazen, J.M. and Kamm, R.D. (1984) Alveolar ventilation at high frequency using tidal volumes less than anatomic dead space, in Engel L.A., Paica M., Linfant C. (Eds). *Lung Biology in Health Care* (eds L.A. Engel, M. Paica and C. Linfant), Marcel Dekker, New York, 137–76.

19. Banner, M.J. (1985) Technical aspects of high frequency ventilation. *Curr. Rev. Respir. Ther.*, **208**, 69–71.

20. Venegas, J.G., Yamada, Y., Custer, J. and Hales, C. (1988) Effects of respiratory variables on regional gas transport during HFV. *J. Appl. Physiol.*, **64**, 2108–18.

21. Kolobow, T., Moretti, M.P., Fumagalli, R. *et al.* (1987) Severe impairment in lung function induced by high peak airway pressure during mechanical ventilation: an experimental study. *Am. Rev. Respir. Dis.*, **135**, 312–15,

22. Carlon, G.C., Howland, W.S., Ray, C. *et al.* (1983) High-frequency jet ventilation. A prospective randomized evaluation. *Chest*, **84**, 551–9.

23. Dreyfuss, D., Basset, G., Soler, P. and Saumon, G. (1985) Intermittent positive pressure hyperventilation with high inflation pressures produces pulmonary microvascular injury in rats. *Am. Rev. Respir. Dis.*, **132**, 880–4.

24. Tsuno, K., Prato, P. and Kolobow, T. (1990) Acute lung injury from mechanical ventilation at moderately high airway pressures. *J. Appl. Physiol.*, **69**, 956–61.

25. Dreyfuss, D., Soler, P., Basset, G. and Saumon, G. (1988) High inflation pressure pulmonary edema: respective effects of high airway pressure, high tidal volume and positive end expiratory pressure. *Am. Rev. Respir. Dis.*, **137**, 1159–64.

26. Corbridge, T., Wood, L., Crawford, G. and Chudoba, M. (1990) Adverse effects of large tidal volumes and PEEP in canine aspiration. *Am. Rev. Respir. Dis.*, **142**, 311–5.

27. McCulloch, P.R., Forkert, P.G. and Froese, A.B. (1988) Lung volume maintenance prevents lung injury during high frequency oscillatory

ventilation in surfactant deficient rabbits. *Am. Rev. Respir. Dis.*, **137**, 1185–92.

28. Byford, L.J., Finkler, J.H. and Froese, A.B. (1988) Lung volume recruitment during high frequency oscillation in atelectasis-prone rabbits. *J. Appl. Physiol.*, **64**, 1604–17.

29. Walsh, M.C. and Carlo, W.A. (1988) Sustained inflation during HFOV improves pulmonary mechanics and oxygenation. *J. Appl. Physiol.*, **65**, 368–72.

30. Schuster, D.P., Snyder, J.V., Klain, M. *et al.* (1982) High frequency jet ventilation during the treatment of acute fulminant pulmonary edema. *Chest*, **80**, 682.

31. Schuster, D.P., Klain, M. and Snyder, J.V. (1982) Comparison of high frequency jet ventilation to conventional ventilation during severe acute respiratory failure in humans. *Crit. Care Med.*, **10**, 625.

32. Macintyre, N.R., Follett, J.V., Deitz, J.L. and Lawlor, B.R. (1986) Jet ventilation at 100 breaths per minute in adult respiratory failure. *Am. Rev. Respir. Dis.*, **134**, 897–901.

33. Hurst, J.M., Branson, R.D., Davis, K. *et al.* (1990) Comparison of conventional mechanical ventilation and high-frequency ventilation. *Ann. Surg.*, **211**, 486–91.

34. Keogh, B.F., Heard, S., Calkins, J. *et al.* (1991) Ultra high frequency ventilation: preliminary results from multicentre study. *Eur. Respir. J.*, **4** (suppl. 14), 176s (abstract).

35. Smith, D.W., Frankel, L.R., Derish, M.T. *et al.* (1993) High-frequency jet ventilation in children with the adult respiratory distress syndrome complicated by pulmonary barotrauma. *Pediatr. Pulmonol.*, **15**, 279–86.

36. El-Baz, N., Faber, L.P. and Doolas, A. (1983) Combined high-frequency ventilation for management of terminal respiratory failure: a new technique. *Anesth. Analg.*, **62**, 39.

37. Borg, U.R., Stoklosa, J.C., Siegel, J.H. *et al.* (1989) Prospective evaluation of combined high-frequency ventilation in post-traumatic patients with adult respiratory distress syndrome refractory to optimised conventional ventilatory management. *Crit. Care Med.*, **17**, 1129–42.

38. Andersen, J.B. (1989) Ventilatory strategy in catastrophic lung disease. Inverse ratio ventilation (IRV) and combined high-frequency ventilation (CHFV). *Acta Anesthesiol. Scand.*, **33** (suppl. 90), 145–8.

39. Berner, M.E., Rouge, J.C. and Suter, P.M. (1991) Combined high-frequency ventilation in children with severe adult respiratory distress syndrome. *Intensive Care Med.*, **17**, 209–14.

40. Suter, P.M. and Berner, M. (1991) HFJV combined with conventional ventilation in severe pulmonary failure, in *Proceedings of Third International Workshop on High Frequency Jet Ventilation* September, 1991, University of Bordeaux, France, (eds A.M. Cros and H. Guenard). University of Bordeaux, Bordeaux.

41. The HIFI Study Group (1989) High-frequency oscillatory ventilation compared with conventional mechanical ventilation in the treatment of respiratory failure in preterm infants. *N. Engl. J. Med.*, **320**, 88–93.

42. Rosenberg, R.B., Broner, C.W., Peters, K.J. and Anglin, D.L. (1993) High-frequency ventilation for acute pediatric respiratory failure. *Chest*, **104**, 1216–21.

43. Raphael, J.H. and Bexton, M.D.R. (1993) Combined high frequency ventilation in the management of respiratory failure in late pregnancy. *Anaesthesia*, **48**, 596–8.

44. Harf, A., Zidulka, A. and Chang, H.K. (1985) Nitrogen washout curves in humans during tidal breathing with superimposed oscillations of the chest wall. *Am. Rev. Respir. Dis.*, **132**, 350–3.

45. Piquet, J., Brochard, L., Isabey, D. *et al.* (1987) High frequency chest wall oscillation in patients with chronic airflow obstruction. *Am. Rev. Respir. Dis.*, **136**, 1355–9.

46. Petros, A.J., Fernando, S.S.D., Shenoy, V.S. and AL-Saady, N.M. (1995) The Hayek oscillator. Nomograms for tidal volume and minute ventilation using external high frequency oscillation. *Anaesthesia*, **50**, 601–6.

47. Campbell, J.M. and Nevin, M. (1993) Hayek oscillator; experience in intensive care. *Clin. Intensive Care*, **4** (suppl), 92.

EXTRACORPOREAL MEMBRANE OXYGENATION

Dirk Pappert, Rolf Rossaint, Herwig Gerlach and Konrad J. Falke

The development of silicon polymer membranes [1–4] for prolonged extracorporeal circulation stimulated the idea of using extracorporeal support systems in the treatment of the syndrome of acute respiratory distress in adults (ARDS). This disease is characterized primarily by severe impairment in pulmonary gas exchange, reduced compliance and radiological manifestation of interstitial and/or intra-alveolar edema. The clinical course of ARDS following the acute inflammatory phase is often complicated and prolonged by factors associated with therapeutic interventions such as mechanical ventilation. As ARDS progresses, high inspired oxygen concentrations as well as high mean airway pressures may be required to ensure adequate arterial oxygenation. Both factors are considered to be harmful to the lung [5,6], which may explain in part why the mortality rate has remained virtually unchanged since ARDS was first described in 1967 [7]. In this first clinical description mortality was 58% [7]. In the reduction of iatrogenic lung injury extracorporeal respiratory support may represent an alternative therapeutic strategy by which a reduced need for aggressive ventilatory strategies permits the lung to 'rest', allowing resolution of the disease process to occur [8].

Total circulatory support was the primary intention when extracorporeal cardiopulmonary support systems were developed in the 1930s for time-consuming cardiac surgical interventions; Gibbon's heart–lung machine permitting cardiocirculatory arrest for 1–2 hours [9,10]. After initial trials with bubble oxygenators, bypass-associated organ damage was recognized to be time-dependent and provoked by technical limitations in oxygenator design, tubing and pumps. Complications included thrombocytopenia, coagulopathy, generalized edema and severe hemolysis. Extracorporeal respiratory support for ARDS clearly requires oxygenators designed for long term use and the development of silicon polymer membrane lungs has allowed prolonged extracorporeal circulation to take place without the problems outlined above.

HISTORIC ASPECTS OF EXTRACORPOREAL GAS EXCHANGE

In the 1960s, Kolobow started to investigate the long term use of membrane oxygenators in severe ARDS. In animal models, up to 16 days of extracorporeal support were achieved, limited by technical problems, such as sepsis, platelet loss and coagulation disequilibrium over time [1,3,11]. After isolated, unsuccessful applications in patients, the first

ARDS Acute Respiratory Distress in Adults. Edited by Timothy W. Evans and Christopher Haslett. Published in 1996 by Chapman & Hall, London. ISBN 0 412 56910 8

Table 25.1 Abbreviations in use to describe extracorporeal support systems

ECMO	Extracorporeal membrane oxygenation
E(C)LA	Extracorporeal lung assist
ECCO$_2$R	Extracorporeal CO$_2$ removal
ECGE	Extracorporeal gas exchange
ECLS	Extracorporeal lung support

successful case of extracorporeal membrane oxygenation (ECMO) (Table 25.1) in patients was reported in 1972 in a 24 year old man suffering from traumatic disruption of the aorta and multiple fractures. Seventy-five hours of support were long enough for the lung to recover and re-establish its gas exchanging properties [12]. Soon other groups reported the successful use of extracorporeal support for patients with ARDS [13], achieving an overall 10–15% survival rate in 150 patients worldwide in 1974 [14].

US ECMO STUDY

Such isolated reports describing the successful application of ECMO in patients with ARDS formed the basis of a prospective, randomized multicenter US National study, comparing ECMO with conventional treatment. The study was initiated in 1974 and planned to recruit a total of 300 patients. The study was terminated in 1976 after 90 patients had been enrolled, when survival rates in both groups appeared to be less than 10% and unlikely to be significantly different at completion [8]. The final report confirmed the preliminary results and demonstrated a 90% mortality rate without any difference between the two groups [15]. The project was later accused of being poorly designed. Thus, the clinical and management approaches to ARDS concerning ventilator therapy, patient selection and other therapeutic strategies were not standardized and the participating centers were free to select the venoarterial bypass system and type of oxygenator employed (Kolobow, Lande-Edwards, Bramson and General Electric-Pierce) [16]. Some centers had very little experience with extracorporeal techniques. The inclusion criteria are summarized in Table 25.2. Venoarterial bypass was the preferrred route for vascular access, as at the time most survivors had been reported with this technique and experience with venovenous perfusion was limited. The reduction of pulmonary blood flow, resulting in a decrease in pulmonary artery pressures and shunt perfusion was thought to be advantageous for the recovery of the lung, but possibly increased the risk of pulmonary thrombosis. Extracorporeal support was allowed to be terminated after 5 days in patients in whom no improvement in pulmonary function was detectable. Later studies showed that an average bypass time of 20 days may be required for the lung to heal [17]. Lung rest during extracorporeal support, which was integral to the ECMO concept, was thought to be of no value or even detrimental, in that the decreased respiratory rate and tidal volumes caused a significant fall in pulmonary compliance [15]. The study results discouraged most researchers and clinicians to pursue the concept of ECMO further, although Bartlett and Kolobow suggested

Table 25.2 Inclusion criteria for patients enrolled in the US ECMO study [15]

Fast entry criteria
Pa_{O_2} < 50 mmHg for more than 2 hours at $F_{I_{O_2}}$ 1.0 and PEEP > 5 cmH$_2$O

Slow entry criteria
Maximal therapy for 48 hours
Pa_{O_2} < 50 mmHg for more than 12 hours at $F_{I_{O_2}}$ 0.6 and PEEP > 5 cmH$_2$O
Q_S/Q_T > 30% at $F_{I_{O_2}}$ 1.0 and PEEP > 5 cmH$_2$O

that the study was biased by the severity and irreversibility of the underlying diseases, mostly viral or bacterial pneumonia. At least the study had shown that the technique of ECMO itself was safe and reliable over an extended period of time.

ECMO IN NEONATAL RESPIRATORY FAILURE

As extracorporeal respiratory support was being evaluated in adults, the first clinical reports about its use in neonatal respiratory failure were published [18]. Immaturity of the lung or abnormal postnatal shunting are the underlying factors for the transient impairment in gas exchange that characterizes the neonatal respiratory distress syndrome. Extracorporeal support is employed to prevent the iatrogenic lung damage due to the hyperoxia and barotrauma associated with mechanical ventilation. Since the report about the first successful survivor in 1975 [19,20] by Bartlett and coworkers, extracorporeal life support in neonates has become an accepted and successful therapy established in many pediatric centers worldwide, confirmed in prospective studies [21,22].

EXTRACORPOREAL CO_2 REMOVAL

In 1977 Kolobow and colleagues first described the possible separation of gas exchange into oxygenation and decarboxylation and its therapeutic use. They hypothesized that ventilation is required principally for the removal of CO_2, which is a function of tidal volume and frequency of breathing. They demonstrated in lambs that oxygenation can be achieved by constant inflation and apneic ventilation alone, also called 'aventilatory mass flow' or 'diffusion respiration' [23] (Chapter 23). Under this assumption the purpose of a ventilator is mainly to remove carbon dioxide from the blood, rather than to oxygenate [17,24]. While the clinical application of ECMO was no longer pursued in the United States as a consequence of the dis-

couraging outcome of the National ECMO study, Gattinoni combined the concept of venovenous extracorporeal CO_2 removal (ECCO$_2$R) with a new ventilatory strategy. This consisted of a low ventilatory frequency (3–5 breaths/min) with a long expiratory phase, thereby reducing peak pressures ($<$ 45 cmH$_2$O); and the application of increased positive end expiratory pressure (PEEP) (15–25 cmH$_2$O) to keep mean airway pressures constant. An additional continuous flow of oxygen (1–2 l/min) was administered through a small catheter, placed proximal to the carina to compensate for oxygen consumption during the long expiratory phase. Low frequency, positive pressure ventilation with extracorporeal CO_2 removal (LFPPV-ECCO$_2$R) had several advantages over ECMO. The lung was allowed to rest, avoiding excessively high airway pressures. CO_2 removal was separated from the need for oxygenation and accomplished by the use of the extracorporeal membrane lung. Whereas the efficacy of oxygen uptake and delivery is mainly dependent on blood flow through the extracorporeal system, premembrane Sv_{O_2}, contact time of the erythrocytes and hemoglobin concentration; decarboxylation is mainly determined by the sweep gas flow through the oxygenator and its surface area [8]. ECCO$_2$R therefore allowed a reduction of blood flow, when compared with ECMO, resulting in increased safety through reduced systemic pressures in the extracorporeal system, extending the lifetime of the membrane lung and avoiding complications due to blood leaks or circuit disruption. Although imprecise from a technical point of view, the artificial lung for carbon dioxide removal, correctly described by Kolobow as a carbon dioxide membrane lung, was in general still named oxygenator.

Gattinoni chose venovenous vascular access, originally advocated by Kolobow [25] and restricted extracorporeal blood flow to 25–30% of total cardiac output [26]. As the net influx of blood from the extracorporal system to the low pressure part of the systemic circulation equals net outflux, cardiopulmonary blood flow is not compromised compared with venoarterial ECMO, where blood flow bypasses the heart and the lung and is returned to the high pressure part of the systemic circulation. Central venous pressures are not affected and exact monitoring of volume status is possible; cardiac output is completely dependent on myocardial performance and is not influenced by the amount of extracorporeal blood flow. Lung restitution may be enhanced by the prepulmonary oxygenation of blood. Arterial embolic complications with tissue loss or necrosis, as observed with venoarterial bypass techniques, may be avoided and the risk of pulmonary microthrombosis due to diminished blood flow reduced. Incomplete oxygenation, dependent on the placement of the cannulae, is absent. The first results of this technique by Gattinoni and colleagues [26–28], Falke and colleagues [29,30] and Lennartz and colleagues [31,32] were very promising, showing an improved survival rate of up to 52%, in patients selected according to the inclusion and exclusion criteria of the US ECMO study (Table 25.2). The major problems during this time were those of bleeding and coagulation disorders due to inactivation and destruction of thrombocytes, and activation of the coagulatory system by the surface of the extracorporeal system. Thrombocytopenia is common after initiation of the extracorporeal perfusion, possibly resulting from platelet trapping in the oxygenator [33]. Systemic heparinization, necessary to prevent the system from clotting and to avoid thromboembolic episodes, has been shown to induce thrombocytopenia and increase the risk of heparin-induced, uncontrollable hemorrhage [34]. Diffuse bleeding from the cannulation sites as well as spontaneous hemorrhage is common and can be catastrophic. In 58 patients undergoing extracorporeal respiratory support, Uziel and coworkers reported 11 patients with life threatening bleeding. Eight patients died,

accounting for a 13.8% mortality rate [35], exceeded only by a recent report demonstrating a 17.4% mortality rate [36].

HEPARIN COATED SYSTEMS

A solution to these problems was the development of a covalently bound heparin coating to the inner surface of extracorporeal circuitry, thus minimizing the activation of the coagulatory system (Carmeda, Sweden). Its clinical use was first described by Bindslev and coworkers [37,38]. Heparinized membrane oxygenators, connectors, cannulae and tubing theoretically allowed the extracorporeal system to run heparin-free [39]. Bleeding problems are reported to be reduced when compared to nonsurface heparinized systems and even major surgical interventions may be performed without an increased risk of uncontrolled hemorrhage [17,40,41].

THE BERLIN APPROACH TO EXTRACORPOREAL RESPIRATORY SUPPORT PROCEDURES

BYPASS AND CANNULATION TECHNIQUE

When the US ECMO study was designed, venoarterial bypass was chosen because this technique had previously been applied successfully [15]. Venovenous bypass techniques, as part of the concept described by Gattinoni, are now the most commonly used means of obtaining vascular access, except in neonatal ECMO, where venoarterial access may be preferred for therapeutic reasons [8,21]. Both techniques have in common the draining of blood via a cannula placed in the inferior vena cava proximal to the portocaval junction (Figure 25.1). In our institution, a second cannula is advanced via the femoral vein to the distal inferior vena cava. The blood is passively drained into a collapsible reservoir equipped with a servo switch, controlling the pump. From the reservoir it is pumped actively by a nearly occlusive roller

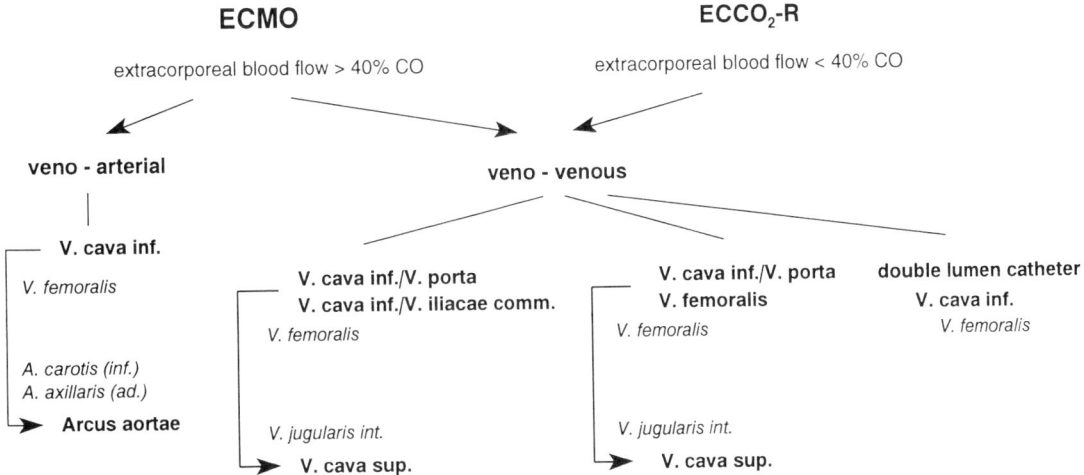

Figure 25.1 Possible bypass routes and cannulation sites for extracorporeal respiratory support systems. CO = cardiac output; V. = vein; A. = artery; inf. = inferior; sup. = superior; comm. = communis; ad. = adults; inf. = children; → = direction of blood flow, drainage and return, cannulation sites.

pump through the oxygenators back to the patient. For safety reasons and to facilitate membrane replacement, two roller pumps and membrane lungs may be used in parallel (Figure 25.2). The membrane oxygenators are ventilated with an oxygen/air sweep gas flow, controlled by a flowmeter and an oxygen blender. Thus oxygen delivery and CO_2 removal across the membrane lung can be adjusted to the patient's need. While the venous return route can be established easily by percutaneous cannulation techniques and placement of the tip of the cannula close to the right atrium can be achieved, arterial cannulation of the carotid artery requires surgical cutdown and ligation [8]. Hypoperfusion and selective oxygenation of the brain and right arm, dependent on the position of the cannula, represents a problem with the venoarterial perfusion route, obviated by the venovenous bypass technique. For safety reasons the venous return should be monitored by a bubble detector, preventing inadvertent air embolization in case of circuit disruption or leaks in negative pressure areas. Continuous monitoring of mixed venous oxygen saturation and oxygen saturation in the venous

tract of the bypass circuit gives precise information about the efficacy of the system.

During venovenous extracorporeal circulation, part of the venous return may recirculate through the system, depending on the ratio of extracorporeal to systemic blood flow and the position of the cannulae. Maximum extracorporeal lung assist can be achieved only when the return cannula is placed into the right ventricle.

Different types of cannula are commercially available, mostly spring wire reinforced and made of polyurethane. A double lumen cannula has been advocated to limit venous access to one site, thereby reducing cannulation related bleeding problems [42]. Due to its large diameter, surgical venous access is necessary. The relatively small internal diameter of the return limb limits blood flow and recirculation is likely when flow exceeds 3 l/min.

The original concept of $ECCO_2R$ with LFPPV has been modified by some groups, based on the experience that pulmonary oxygen transfer capability is so severely reduced in some patients that additional oxygen transfer across the membrane lung is necessary to

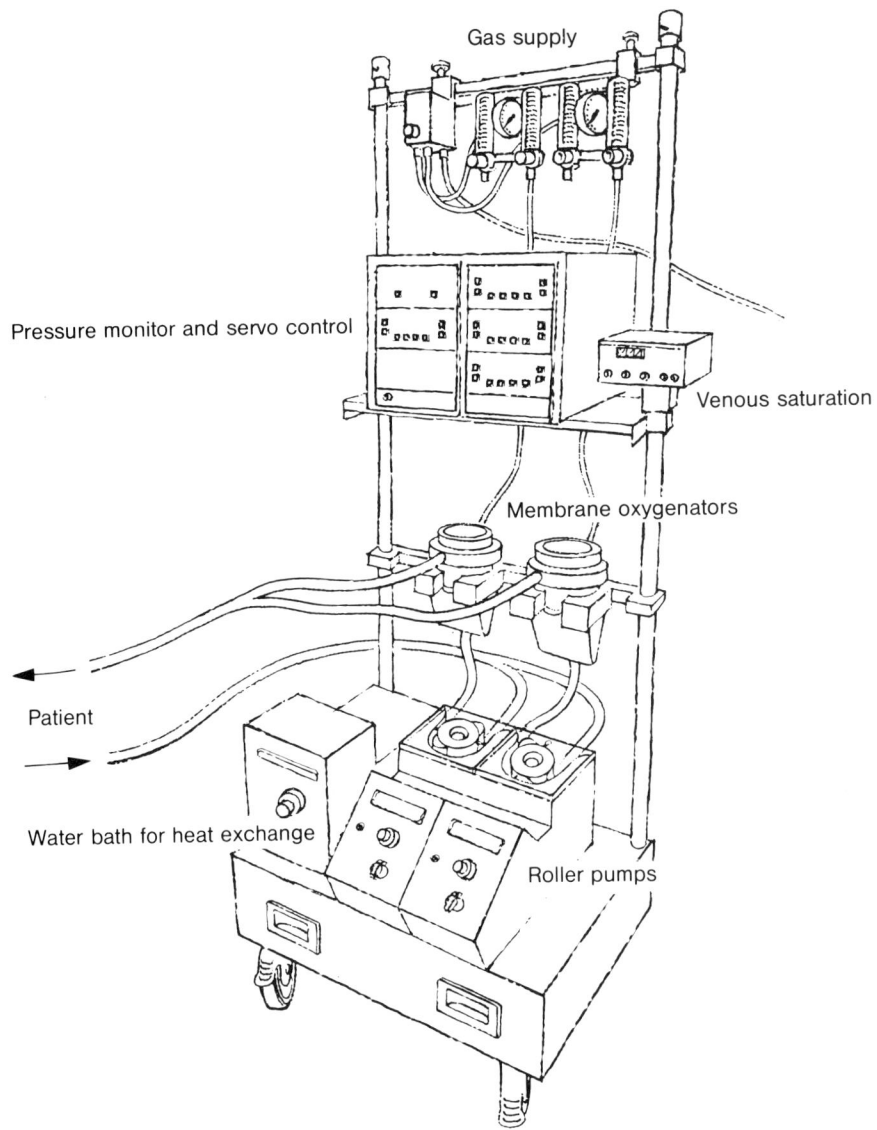

Gas supply

Pressure monitor and servo control

Venous saturation

Membrane oxygenators

Patient

Water bath for heat exchange

Roller pumps

Figure 25.2 Simplified setup of an extracorporeal respiratory support system with two roller pumps and membrane oxygenators in parallel.

maintain adequate blood oxygenation. To achieve optimal oxygen delivery with ECMO, extracorporeal blood flow is increased to the maximum possible. New cannulation techniques, using percutaneous venous access with spring wire enforced, thin walled cannulae, allow extracorporeal blood flows up to 60% of cardiac output (e.g. up to 4 l/min with a 21 Fr cannula: Biomedicus®) for the venous

return). To characterize the pressure flow relationships in cannulae with different design and diameter, the 'M number' was introduced [43,44].

Roller pumps are commonly used in most institutions, although they have drawbacks. The pump tubing is subject to wear and tear, which can be avoided by periodical transposition of the tubing segment. Clotting and the generation of emboli in the venous reservoir due to a reduction in blood flow and turbulence may occur, but are no longer a problem because modern pumps are equipped with a low pressure-controlled downregulation instead of a collapsible reservoir with a servo switch. Centrifugal pumps have been evaluated in some centers, but the tendency to accumulate clots near the rotor shaft and the increased risk of bubble formation following venous suction and degassing may cause hemolysis [8,17].

OXYGENATORS

With few exceptions, two types of membrane oxygenators are currently in use. The Sci-Med Kolobow oxygenator is a spiral silicone rubber membrane lung with an excellent performance, lasting in some instances for more than 3 weeks [17]. Microporous polypropylene hollow fiber oxygenators are now used most commonly since the development of surface heparinization by Carmeda (Medronic® Maxima) [37], although other internally coated systems are now available [45]. The long term use of hollow fiber oxygenators is often complicated by an increasing plasma leakage over time across the membrane pores and a consequent decrease in gas exchanging capability. How these problems are linked to the patient's condition has not been evaluated yet, but they may be related to the adsorption of phospholipids to the membrane surface [17,46]. Thus, coating the hydrophobic layer with hydrophilic components may facilitate the passage of plasma proteins across the membrane [47]. Anecdotally, we have experienced a reduced oxygenator life span in patients with severe sepsis or liver failure, requiring replacement every 24–48 hours, whereas in the same patient under nonseptic conditions the same type of oxygenator has been used for up to 3 weeks. A newly developed heparin coating (ECLA3®) for microporous hollow fiber oxygenators looks promising.

Although the life span of silicone rubber oxygenators is superior to other types, they are not yet commercially available with surface heparinization.

ANTICOAGULATION

The use of surface heparinized equipment permits the use of low dose systemic anticoagulation of 150–220 iu heparin/kg/24 h to avoid clotting in areas of reduced blood flow associated with diameter changes between connectors and tubing or the collapsible reservoir. Prolonged extracorporeal perfusion is associated with clot formation and emboli in such regions, and where surface properties are altered and flow is turbulent. In case of an inadvertent pump stop, heparinization prevents disastrous irreversible clotting of the oxygenators. Anticoagulation should be monitored every 4 hours and activated clotting time maintained around 120–150 s or activated partial thromboplastin time in the upper normal range. Antithrombin III levels should be kept at 80–100%. This approach allows even major surgical intervention without interruption of bypass. In our institution, 41 ECMO treated patients underwent 104 thoracotomies or sternotomies for chest tube insertion, lung surgery or cardiac tamponade. Four underwent laparotomy, and in four patients osteosynthesis of the pelvis and fixation of major fractures were necessary. None of the patients developed catastrophic bleeding [40].

In the US ECMO study, the requirement for blood replacement was 1000–1500 ml packed red cells or fresh frozen plasma per day. The use of surface heparinized devices and percutaneous cannulation should result in an overall reduction of blood replacement. A significantly reduced need for blood components has been demonstrated when comparing patients treated with surgical cannulation techniques versus percutaneous cannulation and heparinized equipment [17]. In our own study group, 41 patients treated with ECMO had a mean transfusion requirement of 1423 ml per day (3.0 units fresh frozen plasma/day and 2.7 units of packed red blood cells/day), not significantly different to historic controls. However, in the latter, blood loss is due to major coagulation problems, whereas most of the blood loss in our group is related to the leakage of the microporous polypropylene hollow fiber membrane lung. As the average life span of an oxygenator is 2.4 days and the extracorporeal system in our institution is equipped with two membrane lungs, each with a filling volume of 480 ml and running in parallel, about 400 ml of transfusion requirement per day is related to circuit volume replacement. Hemolysis results from the destruction of erythrocytes by shearing forces and other mechanical factors, including the roller pumps, and is reflected in raised carboxyhemoglobin levels. Despite unaltered transfusion requirements since the US ECMO study, the safety of the extracorporeal system is increased because uncontrollable bleeding is no longer a major problem.

VENTILATOR REGIMEN AND ADJUNCTIVE STRATEGIES

In our unit, during extracorporeal support, ventilator settings are adjusted to the decreased necessity of maintaining pulmonary gas exchange and to prevent further structural damage by high F_{IO_2}, large tidal volumes and/or high peak pressures. Patients are routinely ventilated in pressure control mode to increase mean airway pressure without affecting peak airway pressures (Chapter 23). This mode is also chosen for safety reasons because airway pressures cannot inadvertently increase as a result of reduced compliance. Respiratory rate is limited to $\leq$ 10/min, inspiratory/expiratory time (I/E) ratios from 1:2 to 1:1 and the pressure control is set to a maximum of 30–35 cmH$_2$O. Optimal PEEP is determined from periodically obtained pressure-volume curves if no bronchopleural fistula is present. In the

course of the disease, F_{IO_2} is adjusted to keep the Pa_{O_2} at 60–65 mmHg (8.0–8.6 kPa). Pulse oximetry and intra-arterial blood gas devices (Puritan Benett 3300 IABG System) have been found to be useful in monitoring for transient hypoxemic episodes during ECMO. Other adjunctive therapeutic measures like inhaled nitric oxide (Chapter 29), aggressive dehydration (Chapter 28), the prone position, permissive hypercapnia (Chapter 23) and physiotherapy can be applied simultaneously to accomplish a further improvement in gas exchange [48–55]. Fiberoptic bronchoscopy is performed frequently to clear mucous plugs or secretions producing atelectases.

INCLUSION CRITERIA

Our own inclusion criteria for ECMO still follow those of the US ECMO study (Table 25.3), but decisions are increasingly oriented towards the clinical trend and the progression of the disease, using ECMO as a 'last resort' life support therapy (Figure 25.3). Extended inclusion criteria are used in other institutions, oriented at the lung injury severity score by Morel (Chapter 22) [46,56] or including compliance and pulmonary shunt fraction [57]. Extracorporeal support is established when the pulmonary gas exchange deteriorates progressively despite maximum therapy – fast entry criteria, or when the patient's condition stabilizes under maximum therapy but further therapeutic measures are not available or iatrogenic lung damage is likely to occur – slow entry criteria. Fast entry criteria focus on the oxygenation index (Pa_{O_2}/F_{IO_2}), response to PEEP and efficiacy of supportive therapy and in our institution are mostly applied in patients shortly after transfer. Slow entry criteria are less strict in regards to oxygenation, but take into account physiologic parameters like compliance, shunt perfusion and extravascular lung water.

Patients with immunosuppression, cancer, end stage chronic pulmonary diseases, irreversible neurologic damage and diseases of

Table 25.3 Extended inclusion criteria for patients treated with ECMO at the Virchow-Klinikum, Berlin

---

Fast entry criteria are met, when despite maximal therapy for more than 2 hours:

$Pa_{O_2} < 50$ mmHg at F_{IO_2} 1.0

PEEP > 10 cmH$_2$O

Slow entry criteria are met, when three out of four of the following criteria are fulfilled after 24 – 120 hours of maximal therapy:

$Pa_{O_2}/F_{IO_2} < 150$ mmHg with PEEP > 10 cmH$_2$O

$Q_S/Q_T > 30\%$ at F_{IO_2} 1.0

extravascular lung water (EVLW) $\geq$ 15 ml/kg

total lung compliance $\leq$ 30 cmH$_2$O

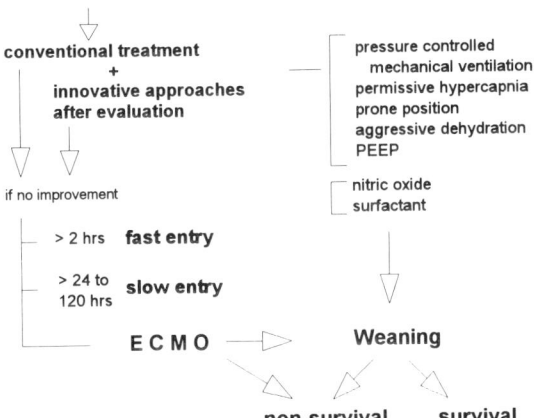

Figure 25.3 Therapeutic measures for patients enrolled for ECMO at the Virchow-Klinikum, Berlin.

the coagulation system are not treated with ECMO.

RESULTS

When ARDS was first described by Ashbaugh and coworkers, the mortality rate was 60% [7]. These results were verified by the Additional Data Collection (ADC) group of the US ECMO study [58] and exceeded by the 90% mortality rate quoted in the final report [15]. Newer studies have shown that the overall mortality rate for ARDS is between 59 and 65% without ECMO, despite major advances in therapy [59]. Outcome is clearly dependent upon the underlying disease: in one study mortality ranged from 38% in trauma patients to 86% in patients with opportunistic pneumonia [59,60] (Chapter 2). The time for a patient on extracorporeal support in the US ECMO study was frequently limited to 5 days, if no improvement occurred [15]. However, in studies reporting results using ECMO and ECCO$_2$R [61–63] obtained in the 1980s, mean bypass time was 5–6 days. It has became obvious over time that some patients require a much longer period of extracorporeal support before successful weaning is possible. Thus, mean bypass time of survivor groups treated between 1979–1988 and 1988–1992 has increased by more than 300%, from 153 $\pm$ 128 hours to 467 $\pm$ 321 hours, respectively. The bypass time for nonsurvivors has not changed significantly [17]. After the disappointing results from the US ECMO study and the dramatic reduction of mortality (Table 25.4) in patients undergoing ECCO$_2$R or ECMO treatment [61], efforts were made to find an explanation for the highly significant differences in survival rates. As most reports acknowledged that neither of the two studies showed any differences in patient selection criteria, differences in outcome have been attributed to advantages of the venovenous perfusion route and/or the use of additional supportive strategies. Historic comparison of

Table 25.4 ECMO survival rate for European centers (December 31, 1994) (ECMO treatment was stopped in mid-1993)

Centers	No. of cases	No. of survivors (%)
Marburg	165	97 (59)
Milan-Monza	98	43 (44)
Paris (31.12.1993)	64	27 (42)
Berlin	49	27 (55)
Freiburg	31	15 (48)
Stockholm[a]	26	9 (35)
Munich	21	17 (81)
Mannheim	9	4 (44)
Kuopio	6	1 (17)
Totals	469	240(51)

Values in parentheses are percentages.
[a] Personal communication.

actual results and those of the ECMO study is of questionable relevance. Knowledge and experience has accumulated since then and insight into the pathophysiology of ARDS has grown and influenced therapeutic concepts.

A major criticism of more recent results has been the lack of controls, and their non-prospective design. Only one study of a prospective randomized study has been published, comparing conventional therapy with ECCO₂R, showing no significant differences in the survival rate between groups [64,65]. However, shortcomings concerning patient population, bypass technique and ventilator strategy may have again influenced outcome [36].

PERSPECTIVES

We should not proceed on the fallacious assumption that where there is no randomization, there is no truth.

R.D. Truog [66]

Although a prospective randomized study may be desirable (Chapter 27), the current clinical results clearly justify the use of extracorporeal respiratory support as a last resort therapy. It may be difficult to conduct a trial of ECMO in a standardized fashion, because,

as a potentially life saving procedure, further technical and therapeutical improvements are constantly under evaluation. Nevertheless, a prospective observational type of study, at least for ECMO in neonates, should be considered [66]. Technical improvements are still subject to extensive research. Membrane lungs and other circuit components need to be improved in terms of safety, longevity and gas exchanging properties. The use of centrifugal pumps lowering the risk of hemolysis may improve flow characteristics in the extracorporeal system and allow increased blood flow.

After 20 years of increasing experience with venovenous extracorporeal respiratory support, mortality in more than 300 patients with severe acute respiratory distress syndrome has fallen to 54%, a superior outcome compared with the unchanged mortality rate of 38–86% for the same group of patients undergoing conventional treatment. These results underline the fact that extracorporeal lung assist techniques represent a last resort alternative to conventional therapy. When oxygenation is temporarily impossible, even with aggressive ventilator therapy using high inspiratory peak pressures, PEEP and a high F_{IO_2}, ECMO or CO_2 removal has the potential to reduce iatrogenic factors in the progression of ARDS and to buy time for the restitution of pulmonary gas exchange.

REFERENCES

1. Kolobow, T. Spragg, R.G., Pierce, and Zapol W.M. (1971). Extended term (to 16 days) partial extracorporeal blood gas exchange with the spiral membrane lung in unanesthetized lambs. *Trans. Am. Soc. Artif. Intern. Organs*, **17**, 350–4.
2. Kolobow, T., Tomlinson, T., Pierce, J. and Gattinoni, L. (1976) Platelet response to long-term spiral coiled membrane lung bypass without heparin using a carbon silicone rubber membrane. *Trans. Am. Soc. Artif. Intern. Organs*, **22**, 110–8.
3. Kolobow, T., Zapol, W. and Pierce, J. (1969) High survival and minimal blood damage in

lambs exposed to long term (1 week) veno-venous pumping with a polyurethane chamber roller pump with and without a membrane blood oxygenator. *Trans. Am. Soc. Artif. Intern. Organs*, **15**, 172–7.

4. Bramson, M.L., Osborn, J.J., Main, F.B. *et al.* (1965) A new disposable membrane oxygenator with integral heat exchanger. *J. Thorac. Cardiovasc. Surg.*, **50**, 391–5.

5. Kolobow, T., Moretti, M.P., Fumagalli, R. *et al.* (1987) Severe impairment in lung function induced by high peak airway pressure during mechanical ventilation. An experimental study. *Am. Rev. Respir. Dis.*, **135**, 312–5.

6. Tsuno, K., Miura, K., Takeya, M. *et al.* (1991) Histopathologic pulmonary changes from mechanical ventilation at high peak airway pressures. *Am. Rev. Respir. Dis.*, **143**, 1115–20.

7. Ashbaugh, D.G., Bigelow, B.D., Petty, T.L. and Levine, B.E. (1967) Acute respiratory distress in adults. *Lancet*, **ii**, 319–23.

8. Bartlett, R.H. (1990) Extracorporeal life support for cardiopulmonary failure. *Curr. Probl. Surg.*, **XXVII**(10).

9. Gibbon, J.H., Jr (1954) Application of a mechanical heart lung apparatus to cardiac surgery. *Minn. Med.*, **37**, 171.

10. Gibbon, J.H. Jr (1937) Artificial maintenance of circulation during experimental occlusion of pulmonary artery. *Arch. Surg.*, **34**, 1105–31.

11. Kolobow, T., Zapol, W., Pierce, J.E. *et al.* (1968) Partial extracorporeal gas exchange in alert newborn lambs with a membrane artificial lung perfused via an A-V shunt for periods up to 96 hours. *Trans. Am. Soc. Artif. Intern. Organs*, **14**, 328–34.

12. Hill, J.D., O'Brien, T.G., Murray, J.J. *et al.* (1972) Prolonged extracorporeal oxygenation for acute post-traumatic respiratory failure (shock-lung-syndrome). *N. Engl. J. Med.*, **286**, 629–34.

13. Schulte, H.D., Bircks, W. and Dudziak R. [Preliminary results with the Bramson membrane lung. (Also report of a successful, clinical long-term perfusion)]. *Thoraxchir. Vask. Chir.*, **20**, 54–9.

14. Gille, J.P. (1974) Respiratory support by extracorporeal circulation with a membrane artificial lung. *Bull. Physiopathol. Respir.*, **10**, 373–410.

15. Zapol, W.M., Snider, M.T., Hill, J.D., *et al.* (1979) Extracorporeal membrane oxygenation in severe acute respiratory failure. A randomized prospective study. *JAMA*, **242**, 2193–6.

16. Zapol, W.M., Snider, M.T. and Schneider, R.C. (1977) Extracorporeal membrane oxygenation for acute respiratory failure. *Anesthesiology*, **46**, 272–85.

17. Pesenti, A., Gattinoni, L. and Bombino, M. (1993) Long term extracorporeal respiratory support: 20 years of progress. *Intensive Care Crit. Care Dig.*, **12**, 15–7.

18. White, J.J. (1976) Membrane lung extracorporeal bypass for prolonged respiratory support in infants, in Zapol, W.M., Qvist, J., eds. *Artificial Lungs for Acute Respiratory Failure* (eds W.M. Zapol and J. Qvist), Academic Press, Washington, pp. 465–79.

19. Bartlett, R.H., Gazzaniga, A.B., Jeffries, M.R. *et al.* (1976) Extracorporeal membrane oxygenation (ECMO) cardiopulmonary support in infancy. *ASAIO Trans.*, **22**, 80–93.

20. Bartlett, R.H., Andrews, A.F. and Toomasian, J.M. (1982) Extracorporeal membrane oxygenation (ECMO) for newborn respiratory failure: 45 cases. *Surgery*, **92**, 425–33.

21. Bartlett, R.H., Roloff, D.W., Cornell, R.G. *et al.* (1985) Extracorporeal circulation in neonatal respiratory failure: a prospective randomized study. *Pediatrics*, **76**, 479–87.

22. O'Rourke, P.P., Crone, R., Vacanti, J. *et al.* (1989) Extracorporeal membrane oxygenation and conventional medical therapy in neonates with persistent pulmonary hypertension of the newborn: a prospective randomized study. *Pediatrics*, **84**, 957–63.

23. Kolobow, T., Gattinoni, L., Tomlinson, T. and Pierce, J.E. (1978) An alternative to breathing. *J. Thorac. Cardiovasc. Surg.*, **75**, 261–6.

24. Kolobow, T., Gattinoni, L., Tomlinson, T. *et al.* (1977) The carbon dioxide membrane lung (CDML): a new concept. *Trans. Am. Soc. Artif. Intern. Organs*, **23**, 17–21.

25. Kolobow, T., Stool, E., Sacks, K. and Vurek, G. (1975) Acute respiratory failure. Survival following ten days' support with a membrane lung. *J. Thorac. Cardiovasc. Surg.*, **69**, 947–53.

26. Pesenti, A., Pelizzola, A., Mascheroni, D. *et al.* (1981) Low frequency positive pressure ventilation with extracorporeal CO_2 removal (LFPPV – ECCO$_2$ R) in acute respiratory failure (ARF): technique. *Trans. Am. Soc. Artif. Intern. Organs*, **27**, 263–6.

27. Gattinoni, L., Agostoni, A., Pesenti, A. *et al.* (1980) Treatment of acute respiratory failure with low-frequency positive-pressure ventila-

tion and extracorporeal removal of CO_2. *Lancet*, ii, 292–4.

28. Gattinoni, L., Pesenti, A., Pelizzola, A *et al.* (1981) Reversal of terminal acute respiratory failure by low frequency positive pressure ventilation with extracorporeal removal of CO2 (LFPPV–ECCO2R). *Trans. Am. Soc. Artif. Intem. Organs*, **27**, 289–93.

29. Falke, K.J., Thies, W.R., Lenhsen, U *et al.* (1983) Improvement of lung function during clinical extracorporeal CO_2 elimination in severe adult respiratory distress syndrome. *Thorac. Cardiovasc. Surg.*, **31**, 1–40.

30. Schulte, H.D., Falke, K.J., Breulmann, M. *et al.* (1983) Clinical application of extracorporeal CO_2 removal in severe ARDS. *Progr. Artif. Organs*, 362–7.

31. Knoch, M., Müller, E., Höltermann, W. *et al.* (1987) Erfahrungen mit der extrakorporalen CO_2 Elimination. *Anaesthesist*, **36**, 210–6.

32. Knoch, M., Falke, K. and Lennartz, H. (1990) Extrakorporale CO_2 Elimination, in *Praktische Intensivmedizin – Trends und Entwicklungen* (eds F.L. Bertschat, K. Ibe and F. Martens), Zuckschwerdt, Munich, pp. 95–102.

33. Spragg, R.G., Hill, R.N., Wedel, M.K. *et al.* (1975) Platelet kinetics in venovenous membrane oxygenation. *Trans. Am. Soc. Artif. Intern. Organs*, **21**, 171.

34. Rhodes, G.R., Dixon, D. and Silver, D. (1973) Heparin induced thrombocytopenia with thrombotic and hemorrhagic manifestations. *Surg. Gynecol. Obstet.*, **136**, 409–16.

35. Uziel, L., Cugno, M., Fabrizi, I. *et al.* (1990) Physiopathology and management of coagulation during long-term extracorporeal respiratory assistance. *Int. J. Artif. Organs*, **13**, 280–7.

36. Brunet, F., Belghith, M., Mira, J. *et al.* (1993) Extracorporeal carbon dioxide removal and low-frequency positive-pressure ventilation. *Chest*, **104**, 889–98.

37. Bindslev, L., Gouda, I., Inacio, J. *et al.* (1986) Extracorporeal elimination of carbon dioxide using a surface-heparinized veno-venous bypass system. *ASAIO Trans.*, **32**, 530–3.

38. Bindslev, L., Eklund, J., Norlander, O. *et al.* (1987) Treatment of acute respiratory failure by extracorporeal carbon dioxide elimination performed with a surface heparinized artificial lung. *Anesthesiology*, **67**, 117–20.

39. Shanley, C.J., Hultquist, K.A., Rosenberg, D.M. *et al.* (1992) Prolonged extracorporeal circula-

40. Weidemann, H., Frey, D., Kaiser, D. *et al.* (1990) Major thoracic surgical procedure during $ECCO_2$ removal with heparin coated extracorporeal systems. *Thorac. Cardiovasc. Surg.*, **38** (I. suppl.), 129

41. Rossaint, R., Slama, K., Lewandowski, K. *et al.* (1992) Extracorporeal lung assist with heparin-coated systems. *Int. J. Artif. Organs*, **15**, 29–34.

42. Pesenti, A., Kolobow, T., Marcolin, R. *et al.* (1982) A double lumen catheter allowing single vessel cannulation for extracorporeal respiratory assistance. *Eur. Surg. Res.*, **14**, 119–23.

43. Montoya, J.P., Merz, S.I. and Bartlett, R.H. (1991) A standardized system for describing flow/pressure relationships in vascular access devices. *ASAIO Trans.*, **37**, 4–8.

44. Sinard, J.M., Merz, S.I., Hatcher, M.D. *et al.* (1991) Evaluation of extracorporeal perfusion catheters using a standardized measurement technique – the M-number. *ASAIO Trans.*, **37**, 60–4.

45. Toomasian, J.M., Hsu, L.C., Hirschl, R.B. *et al.* (1988) Evaluation of Duraflo II heparin coating in prolonged extracorporeal membrane oxygenation. *ASAIO Trans.*, **34**, 410–4.

46. Müller, E., Kolobow, T., Knoch, M. and Höltermann, W. (1992) Akutes Lungenversagen – Unterstützung des Gasaustausches mittels extrakorporaler oder implantierbarer Oxygenatoren – Gegenwärtiger Stand und zukünftige Entwicklung. *Anästhesiol. Intensivmed. Notfallmed. Schmerzther.*, **27**, 259–73.

47. Montoya, J.P., Shanley, C.J., Merz, S.I. and Bartlett, R.H. (1992) Plasma leakage through microporous membranes. Role of phospholipids. *ASAIO J.*, **38**, M399–405.

48. Rossaint, R., Slama, K. and Falke, K.J. (1991) Therapie des akuten Lungenversagens. *Dtsch. Med. Wochenschr.*, **116**, 1635–9.

49. Pappert, D., Rossaint, R., Lopez, F.A. *et al.* (1992) Prone position in severe ARDS influences ventilation/perfusion relationship of the lung. *Intensive Care Med.*, **18**(suppl. 2), S42

50. Rossaint, R., Falke, K.J., Lopez, F.A. *et al.* (1993) Inhaled nitric oxide for the adult respiratory distress syndrome. *N. Engl. J. Med.*, **328**, 399–405.

51. Rossaint, R., Pappert, D., Lewandowski, K. *et al.* (1992) A new therapeutic strategy to

reduce the mortality in severe ARDS. *Med. Care Int.*, **7–8**, 31–35.

52. Langer, M., Mascheroni, D., Marcolin, R. and Gattinoni, L. (1988) The prone position in ARDS patients. A clinical study. *Chest*, **94**, 103–7.

53. Lewandowski, K., Slama, K. and Falke, K.J. (1992) Approaches to improve survival in severe ARDS, in *1992 Yearbook of Intensive Care and Emergency Medicine* (ed. J.-L. Vincent), Springer, Berlin, pp. 372–83.

54. Lewandowski, K., Rossaint, R., Slama, K. *et al.* (1992) Aktueller Stand der Behandlung des schweren ARDS einschließlich der Verwendung des extrakorporalen Gasaustauschs. *Z. Herz-, Thorax- Gefäßchir.*, **6**, 300–5.

55. Lewandowski, K., Slama, K., Rossaint, R. *et al.* (1992) Algorithm for treatment of ARDS. *Chest*, **102**, S174.

56. Boutros, A.B. (1961) Anaesthesia and the thyroid gland. *Can. Anaesth. Soc. J.*, **8**, 586–615.

57. Gattinoni, L., Pesenti, A., Marcolin, R. *et al.* (1992) Extracorporeal support in acute respiratory failure, in *Adult Respiratory Distress Syndrome* (eds A. Artigas, F. Lemaire, P.M. Suter and W.M. Zapol), Churchill Livingstone, Edinburgh, pp. 469–75.

58. National Heart, Lung, and Blood Institute. (1979) *Extracorporeal Support for Respiratory Insufficiency*. US Department of Health, Education, and Welfare, National Institutes of Health, Washington.

59. Artigas, A., Carlet, J., Chastang, C. *et al.* (1992) Adult respiratory distress syndrome: clinical presentation, prognostic factors and outcome, in *Adult Respiratory Distress Syndrome* (eds A. Artigas, F. Lemaire, P.M. Suter and W.M. Zapol), Churchill Livingstone, Edinburgh, pp. 509–23.

60. Artigas, A., Carlet, J., Le Gall, J.R. *et al.* (1991) Clinical presentation, prognostic factors, and outcome of ARDS in the European Collaborative Study (1985–1987): a preliminary report, in *Adult Respiratory Distress Syndrome* (eds W.M. Zapol and F. Lemaire), Marcel Dekker, New York, pp. 37–63.

61. Gattinoni, L., Pesenti, A., Mascheroni, D. *et al.* (1986) Low-frequency positive-pressure ventilation with extracorporeal CO_2 removal. *JAMA*, **256**, 881–6.

62. Snider, M.T., Campbell, D.B., Kofke, W.A. *et al.* (1988) Venovenous perfusion of adults and children with severe acute respiratory distress syndrome. The Pennsylvania State University experience from 1982–1987. *ASAIO Trans.*, **34**, 1014–20.

63. Egan, T.H., Duffin, J., Glynn, MFX. *et al.* (1988) Ten-year experience with extracorporeal membrane oxygenation for severe respiratory failure. *Chest*, **94**, 681–7.

64. East, T.D., Böhm, S.H., Wallace, C.J. *et al.* (1992) A successful computerized protocol for clinical management of pressure control inverse ratio ventilation in ARDS patients. *Chest*, **101**, 697–710.

65. Morris, A.H., Wallace, C.J., Menlove, R.L. *et al.* (1994) Randomized clinical trial of pressure-controlled inverse ratio ventilation and extracorporeal CO_2 removal for adult respiratory distress syndrome. *Am. J. Respir. Crit. Care Med.*, **149**, 295–305.

66. Truog, R.D. (1992) Randomized controlled trials: lessons from ECMO. *Clin. Res.*, **40**, 519–27.

Brian F. Keogh and Kenneth M. Sim

Respiratory support in the syndrome of acute respiratory distress in adults (ARDS) remains a vexing clinical problem. Increased understanding of the complex and heterogeneous pulmonary pathophysiology of the syndrome has highlighted the deficiencies of conventional mechanical ventilation. The use of traditional tidal volumes applied to the reduced accessible alveolar volume in patients with ARDS risks gross regional hyperinflation and exposure of the residual functional lung to damaging shear forces [1,2] (Chapter 23). Ventilatory philosophy has recently concentrated on reducing the pressure and volume cost of ventilatory excursions. The widespread use of pressure controlled, and hence pressure limited, ventilation in ARDS is based on sound theoretical grounds [3] and has shown promise in small prospective series [4]. Even more novel approaches such as high frequency technology [5] (Chapter 24) and tracheal gas insufflation [6] have also been applied and share common aims with pressure limited ventilation; namely, improved efficiency of gas exchange at reduced cost. These options have evolved in concert with the widespread application of permissive hypercapnia in ARDS [7] and the acceptance of lower, and hence more realistic, levels of arterial oxygen saturation.

Extrapulmonary gas exchange may be considered in patients who are refractory to ventilatory support or in whom lung function can only be supported at the cost of further structural lung damage or severe hemodynamic compromise (Chapter 25). Until recently extracorporeal gas exchange (ECGE) was the sole option. The clinical application of ECGE is limited by technical complexity, resource implications and associated complications, and a failure to demonstrate outcome benefit in the few clinical trials reported has dampened enthusiasm for this intervention [8,9]. The debate surrounding the merits of ECGE is ongoing, spurred on by success in neonatal practice and reports of survival rates in refractory ARDS of around 50% in uncontrolled series from European centers [10,11]. In practical terms, however, effective ECGE can only be offered by a small number of appropriately resourced units and is therefore unlikely to be a realistic therapeutic option for the majority of patients with severe ARDS.

An alternative approach is that of intravascular gas exchange (IVGE), a recent development which offers the potential benefits of extrapulmonary gas exchange, but at reduced risk of complications and consuming fewer resources. IVGE is theoretically more widely applicable than ECGE and is particularly attractive to primary receiving critical care units, both in terms of long term support and in reducing the risk of transfer of patients to tertiary centers.

ARDS Acute Respiratory Distress in Adults. Edited by Timothy W. Evans and Christopher Haslett. Published in 1996 by Chapman & Hall, London. ISBN 0 412 56910 8

HISTORY

Hollow fiber membrane oxygenator technology was developed in the late 1970s – one of a number of parallel advances in the practice of cardiopulmonary bypass. Mortensen in Salt Lake City, Utah, USA recognized the gas transfer potential of an implantable hollow fiber bundle, and development of the first commercially available intravascular gas exchange device followed [12–15]. The name IVOX was coined to describe this device, an acronym for intravascular oxygenator. Testing of early laboratory prototypes during the 1980s confirmed that clinically significant volumes of respiratory gases could be transferred across the membrane in a configuration suitable for intravascular placement.

IVOX STRUCTURE AND DESIGN

In its current form the IVOX device is an elongated bundle of hollow fiber membranes, approximately 30–40 cm in length, mounted on central co-axial gas conduit tubing (Figure 26.1). Four sizes of device are available, comprising between 600 and 1100 microporous polypropylene fibers, each 240 μm in diameter. The device is surgically implanted into the venae cavae by common femoral or internal jugular venotomy. The fibers are tightly rolled or furled before insertion. Once positioned

within the inferior vena cava, right atrium and superior vena cava the fiber bundle is unfurled, enabling the device to occupy the entire cross-sectional area of the venae cavae loosely (Figure 26.2). Radiological guidance at insertion is essential to ensure correct positioning [16]. A vacuum source draws pure oxygen through the lumen of each hollow fiber at subatmospheric pressure (usually 45–50 kPa, obviating the possibility of gas embolization, and gas exchange with free-flowing venous blood takes place across the selectively permeable fiber walls. Oxygen diffuses into venous blood and carbon dioxide diffuses into the fiber lumen to be vented to atmosphere via the outflow limb of the co-axial gas conduit tubing. Blood flow patterns across the device are critical to its performance. Turbulent flow increases gas transfer capability and this is promoted by sinusoidal

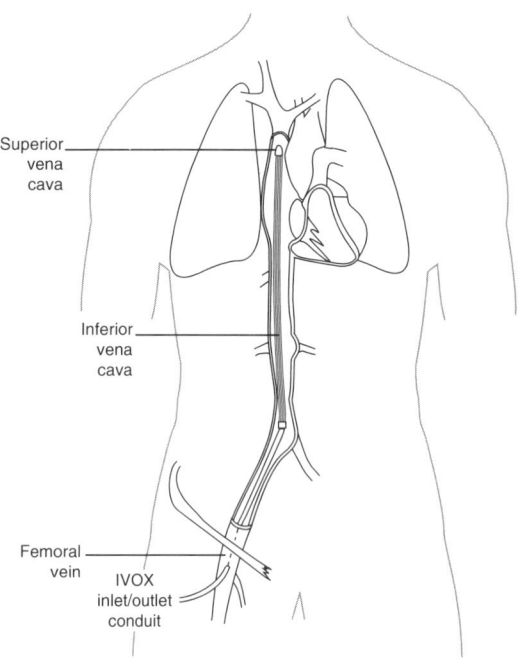

Figure 26.2 Placement of IVOX via a femoral venotomy.

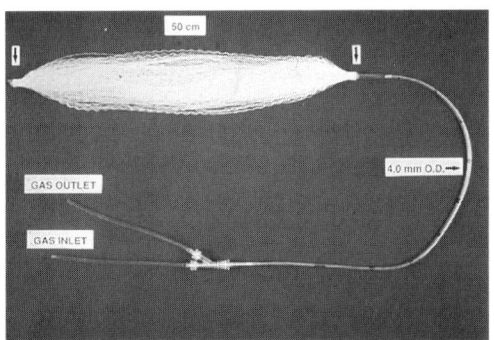

Figure 26.1 IVOX device in an unfurled state. Note that gas is drawn through the device under negative pressure to obviate the risk of air embolus.

Table 26.1 IVOX gas transfer: unspecified animal model, *in vivo* experiments, pooled results [18]

IVOX size (mm OD)	Oxygen transfer (ml/min)	CO_2 transfer (ml/min)
7	67	40
8	98	49
9	116	60
10	133	72

OD = outside diameter.

shaping of the fibers [17]. Design refinements to the fiber surface include an outer heparin bonded, siliconized coating which is ultrathin and continuous rather than porous. It is thus highly gas permeable, but impermeable to liquid, and nonthrombogenic, conferring a reduced requirement for systemic anticoagulation and increased functional longevity of the device.

LABORATORY EVALUATION OF IVOX PERFORMANCE (TABLE 26.1)

IVOX performance characteristics were studied extensively in laboratory animals and *in vitro* circulatory loops during the 1980s. Concerns were raised during trials using early models when even full heparinization failed to prevent rapid deposition of clot on the surface of the IVOX fibers, with resultant deterioration in gas exchange capacity over 3–4 days. This prompted the development of the new thromboresistant membrane surface which also markedly reduced systemic anticoagulation requirements.

Significant gas transfer capability was confirmed in the early animal implants, summarized in Table 26.1. Average oxygen uptake of 98 ml/min and CO_2 clearance of 40 ml/min were subsequently reported from several implants in an ovine smoke inhalation model [19]. IVOX was found to be safe when properly inserted and to provide approximately 25–30% of the animal's gas exchange require-

ments. Further *ex vivo* testing suggested that IVOX performance conformed to that of extracorporeal membrane oxygenators, with gas transfer correlating directly with blood flow and venous CO_2 partial pressure, and inversely with venous oxygen partial pressure [20]. Oxygen and CO_2 transfer rates rose significantly with increasing hemoglobin content of circulated blood. Subsequent implantation of IVOX by this group in a bovine hypoventilation model revealed that the device improved arterial blood gases, the degree of improvement being directly related to the severity of the pulmonary dysfunction [21].

Long term implants were investigated using the final prototype. No IVOX related morbidity or mortality was detected in standing, awake sheep after 19 days of implantation [13]; specifically, there were no significant changes in the hematological, bacteriological or biochemical profiles. No significant or irreversible damage to vascular structures was identified, nor was there any evidence of thromboembolic sequelae from prolonged IVOX use. Mechanical integrity of the device was confirmed by the absence of gas leaks, and gas exchanging capacity was well maintained throughout implantation periods.

In summary, laboratory investigations of IVOX in both artificial circuits and large animal models confirmed that significant gas transfer was possible, that the device was suitable for prolonged implantation and that this could be achieved safely and with apparently minimal adverse effects. These observations gave cause for considerable optimism in relation to application of the device in clinical practice.

CLINICAL APPLICATION OF IVOX

The first implantation of IVOX into a patient with acute respiratory failure was undertaken in 1990. Many individual case reports and reviews have subsequently highlighted the safety and simplicity of the devices, even during prolonged use [22–27]. Although IVOX insertion mandates surgical intervention to establish and control the introducing venotomy site, the simplicity in operation of the system once *in situ* has been confirmed. Maintenance of the implanted IVOX requires minimal supervision and logistical support, in marked contrast to currently available extracorporeal systems.

CLINICAL TRIAL DESIGN

IVOX clinical trials commenced with the recognition that performance would be limited by the membrane surface area available for gas exchange. The four sizes of device offered a surface area of between 0.2 and 0.5 square meters, compared with the 3.0 square meters of a typical extracorporeal membrane oxygenator. Animal experiments predicted that at best 30–50% of basal gas exchange requirements could be met using IVOX, requiring significant continuing contribution by natural lung function, in contrast to ECGE systems which have much greater potential to replace pulmonary gas exchange.

The USA Food and Drug Administration (FDA)-directed IVOX phase I trial recruited 20 patients with advanced respiratory failure. The objective was to determine the safety, risks and hazards associated with IVOX implantation. No major complications were recorded and favorable manipulations of ventilatory parameters were possible in 75% of patients [28]. Mean IVOX oxygen transfer of 68 ml/min and CO_2 elimination of 71 ml/min were reported. The subsequent phase 2 clinical trial was intended to recruit patients with acute, potentially reversible, respiratory failure who were receiving mechanical ventilatory support for at least 24 hours before trial entry (Table 26.2). Exclusion criteria included uncontrolled sepsis, recent major surgery or other contraindication to systemic anticoagulation and lack of suitable venous access.

Table 26.2 Inclusion criteria for phase 2 clinical trial

Trial entry threshold values of ventilatory parameters and arterial blood gas values. Ventilatory modes optimized but not standardized

1. F_{IO_2} of 0.50 to achieve Pa_{O_2} of 8 kPa or less

    and

    PEEP of 10 cmH_2O, or higher; or
    PIP of 45 cmH_2O, or higher; or
    MAP of 30 cmH_2O, or higher

    or

2. Minute volume > 150 ml/min/kg to achieve Pa_{CO_2} of 5.3 kPa

PEEP = positive end expiratory pressure; PIP = peak inspiratory pressures; MAP = mean airway pressure. Reproduced from Bagley *et al.*, Quantitative gas transfer into and out of circulating venous blood by means of an intravenacaval oxygenator. (1991) ASAIO Trans **37**, 413–415.

CLINICAL TRIAL RESULTS

Phase 2 trials recruited a further 140 patients between 1990 and 1993. Preliminary clinical findings in the total of 160 patients who underwent IVOX implantation have been published [29]. The patients were recruited from 35 participating trial centers, implying that few achieved any protracted experience with the device, rendering interpretation of the raw data difficult in view of the inevitable learning curve associated with the application of new and unique technology. Additionally, differing clinical management algorithms for severe lung injury are practised between US and European centers and between centers within these regions. In this feasibility study no attempt was made to standardize other aspects of critical care management. Furthermore, the etiology of respiratory failure in IVOX trial patients varied widely, resulting in the recruitment of a heterogeneous cohort whose individual prognosis for survival, prior to IVOX implantation, differed widely. In addition, the time from institution of mechanical ventilatory support to IVOX implantation varied from less than 48 hours to more than 14 days, with variation in the incidence of coexisting complications, such as barotrauma, systemic infection and organ system failure, at the time of trial entry. Finally, interpretation of IVOX performance in trial patients was further hampered by incomplete data sets in some 25% of those patients recruited. The intention to collect parallel data on patients meeting phase 2 entry criteria, but not subject to IVOX insertion, was not fully realized and this control data has not been published.

IVOX management protocols after the insertion procedure were not defined. It was recommended that moderate anticoagulation (activated clotting time of 180–200 seconds) should be maintained throughout the period of implantation, but other aspects of management, including decisions relating to the timing of explantation, were left to the discretion of participating clinicians. Interpretation of gas transfer data is difficult, as no attempt was made to standardize the approach of the study centres in order to maximize the benefit of IVOX. Construction of clinical protocols to include permissive hypercapnia, pressure limitation of ventilation and aggressive maintenance of lung volume may well have enhanced IVOX performance during the clinical trials. It is easy to be wise in retrospect and it must be remembered that these philosophies in patient management have really only been popularized within the time frame of IVOX clinical investigation, and certainly after a considerable number of implants had already been performed.

Clinical benefit to patients from IVOX use was reported recently, and showed quantitative improvement in blood gas tensions and a decrease in the intensity of mechanical ventilatory support [29]. The Pao_2/Fio_2 ratio increased by 25% or more in 70% of patients, although this statistical benefit was not related to clinical outcome. A similar proportion of patients had a favourable decrease in applied airway pressures and minute volume.

Table 26.3 IVOX gas transfer: clinical trial experience in patients (USA and international) [29]

IVOX size (mm OD)	CO_2 transfer (ml/min)	Oxygen transfer (ml/min)
7	40	44
8	46	60
9	54	60
10	73	71

OD = outside diameter.
Reproduced with permission from Conrad *et al.*, Major findings from the clinical trials of the intravascular oxygenation; published in *Artificial Organs*, **18**(11), by Blackwell Science.

The gas exchange performance for each size of the device is shown in Table 26.3.

Overall, survival to hospital discharge was reported in 37 patients, approximately 25% of the trial group. When analyzed according to severity of lung injury, 115 patients with a Murray score of 2.5 or greater (defined as severe) were entered into the trial (Chapter 22). Thirty-two of these, or 27%, survived. This figure does not improve upon recorded survival for patients with equivalent respiratory failure subjected to conventional management. Seventy-five patients survived IVOX utilization to reach the stage of explantation, although in some cases this was dictated by indications other than clinical improvement.

Postmortem examination was carried out in 68 patients who died during or after IVOX use. IVOX was directly implicated in the deaths of four of these patients, three through major bleeding complications and one by pulmonary embolus. A number of incidental IVOX-related pathological findings were recorded, including hematoma at the venotomy site, fibrin deposition on the intima of the vena cava and nonocclusive thrombus in the femoral or iliac veins. There was no evidence of trauma to the cavae or right atrium, or of obstruction to the venous return to the right heart.

Laboratory monitoring during IVOX implantation demonstrated that the platelet count fell shortly after insertion but reached a plateau after 3–4 days. There was no significant increase in plasma free hemoglobin, and no evidence of complement activation. A number of mechanical problems with device function, and technical problems during the insertion procedure, were recorded. Damage to some hollow fibers occurred in 12% of the devices and in half of these blood leaked into the gas outflow limb in sufficient volumes to warrant IVOX removal. The authors draw a number of conclusions from the clinical trials data relating to the perceived safety and efficacy of the device. Predictable gas exchange performance can be sustained for up to 29 days and mechanical ventilatory support can usually be decreased in intensity. IVOX related complications occurred in one quarter of the trial patients, although the clinical significance of these observations was variable. The authors concluded that IVOX utilization has a favourable risk/benefit ratio in patients with severe, acute reversible acute respiratory failure.

EXPERIENCE IN INDIVIDUAL CENTERS

A number of individual trial centers published their experiences in the form of case reports or short series, highlighting a number of issues distinct to, or expanding on, the data from the collective experience [30–32]. The largest UK series reported eight patients with IVOX implants lasting up to 12 days (median 4 days) of whom two survived [33]. Oxygen transfer of 68–140 ml/min and CO_2 removal of 40–106 ml/min were reported. Significant changes were reported in hemodynamic variables following insertion, and IVOX induced impaired venous return, neurogenic reflexes or mediator release from the caval endothelium were proposed as possible causes for these observations [34].

The largest published series from the USA, although not from the center with most implants, reported nine patients in whom IVOX implantation increased Pa_{O_2} and

reduced Pa_{CO_2}. However, the net effect did not allow a reduction in F_{IO_2} or ventilatory intensity [35]. IVOX insertion decreased cardiac index, with a resultant decrease in systemic oxygen delivery despite considerable fluid and inotropic support. Mortality was 80% and this group concluded that the current device was disappointing in its clinical efficacy, and adversely affected systemic oxygen transport. Another group reported six patients in whom significant reductions in peak and mean ventilatory pressures could be achieved, although their data also suggested that IVOX retarded systemic venous drainage [36]. IVOX used in a patient surviving ARDS secondary to multiple trauma resulted in improvements in gas exchange but coincident hepatic and renal dysfunction and iliac vein thrombosis [37]. These complications resolved on removal of the device. Interestingly, a diminishing return in terms of gas exchange from increasing IVOX size has been predicted by some investigators. Increased fiber volume and resistance to blood flow within the vena cava is likely to divert blood via the extra-caval azygous and hemiazygous systems [38]. Improved gas exchange might be expected if gas exchanging fibers were placed into the right atrium, right ventricle and pulmonary artery, although the hemodynamic effects of this approach are uncertain.

Few investigators have emphasized the primacy of CO_2 removal in the construction of ventilatory strategies for use in association with IVOX. Increased IVOX-mediated CO_2 removal as mixed venous CO_2 rose has been reported in experimental animals, resulting in a proposal for protocols involving more aggressive permissive hypercapnia in patients requiring IVOX [39–41]. This approach is based on the significant CO_2-clearing capacity of the device, which allows decreases in tidal and minute ventilation whilst permitting lung volume to be maintained with higher PEEP or longer inspiratory/expiratory time (I/E) ratios. Oxygenation therefore depends primarily on native pulmonary function, the efficiency of which is improved by more effective lung volume maintenance. The risk of high peak ventilatory pressures and resultant alveolar overdistension while maintaining this optimal lung volume is ameliorated by the decrease in ventilatory intensity which can be facilitated by IVOX-mediated extra-pulmonary CO_2 clearance.

EVOLVING IVGE TECHNOLOGIES

The limited clinical utility of removing only 25–30% of CO_2 production has led to the investigation of further design changes to IVOX, including an increase in the number of fibers, with a consequent decrease in their length and diameter, and increased fiber crimping. To date, only limited gas transfer data using these new prototypes are available: CO_2 removal was reported to have increased some 60–80% compared with the original model [42].

A new intravenous membrane oxygenator device (IMO) that actively promotes convective mixing of blood around hollow fibers has also been described [43,44]. The IMO incorporates a centrally located pulsatile balloon around which are mounted microporous hollow fibers. The rhythmic pulsations of the balloon induce changes in the fiber configuration, enhancing convective mixing and cross-flow of venous blood. Oxygen and CO_2 transfer rates with IMO increase with balloon frequency, and more effective oxygen transfer occurs in its shorter fibers. Gas flux has been progressively improved through six proto-types. The most recent prototype incorporates matted hollow fiber membranes arranged around a centrally placed tripartite balloon. Advantages include short gas flow paths, peristaltic motion to enhance venous return, and a 4–8-fold improvement in gas transfer related to balloon activation when the proto-type was tested in an *in vitro* circulatory loop. As yet, no results have been reported from intact animal models implanted with an IMO device. Consequently, although the device is

theoretically attractive, it would appear to be far from the stage of clinical investigation and its eventual application remains conjectural.

Whilst enthusiasm for new IVGE technology is understandable and can be supported on theoretical grounds, it is sobering to note that IVOX has undergone a long gestation period of more than 10 years and remains the only IVGE device to have undergone clinical trials. It therefore seems inappropriate to be more than speculative about the clinical application of modified IVOX or other IVGE technology.

PHYSIOLOGICAL DIFFICULTIES OF IVOX

Despite much enthusiasm for the potential applications of IVOX, its simplicity in application and favorable complication profile compared with other invasive support techniques, clinical experience until now suggests a disappointing gas exchange capability. More favorable clinical results will undoubtedly be obtained through better patient selection and ventilatory mode modifications based on a sound understanding of what IVOX can realistically be expected to achieve in the clinical setting.

Oxygenation transfer capacity is both limited and unpredictable due to the inherent inefficiency of a prepulmonary gas exchanger. Transfer rates reported from animal and clinical assessments involve measurement of prepulmonary oxygen diffusion, by the necessarily inexact method of measuring differences in mixed venous oxygen content obtained with on/off settings of IVOX. While such a measurement confers a numerical value on transfer performance, its clinical relevance is confounded by a fundamental inefficiency conferred by pulmonary physiology. Thus, although IVOX may result in an increase in mixed venous oxygen content, a considerable volume of IVOX oxygen enriched blood will subsequently perfuse ventilated alveoli. Such blood will be near to fully saturated when leaving the alveolus, regardless of its oxygen content on arrival; hence, only a certain percentage of calculated IVOX oxygen transfer, i.e. that which is subsequently diverted through regions of intrapulmonary shunt, will have relevance to the oxygen loading of arterial blood. Paradoxically, those patients with greater degrees of shunt will be less prone to this oxygenation inefficiency, but will obviously be in a more parlous clinical state. Similarly, the physiological hypoxic vasoconstriction reflex, manipulations of ventilatory mode which recruit or stabilize lung volume (and hence increase the population of effectively ventilated alveoli) or the use of selective pulmonary blood flow manipulation with agents such as nitric oxide (Chapter 29), all represent factors which will tend to exacerbate the inefficiency of IVOX oxygen transfer. In addition, the characteristics of the oxyhemoglobin dissociation curve mandate that the magnitude of the intrapulmonary shunt will be a far more powerful determinant of arterial oxygen saturation than any IVOX induced increase in the saturation of shunted mixed venous blood.

In addition, unfavorable oxygen transfer gradients are inherent in the IVOX design. Although 100% oxygen is drawn through the central fibers, the vacuum applied, which is mandatory in order to prevent gas embolism, results in an intraluminal partial pressure of oxygen of approximately 45 kPa. Since it is partial pressure and not oxygen concentration that determines transfer across the membrane, this represents a less favorable gradient than it first appears. Similarly, and particularly in ARDS, elevated mixed venous oxygen saturations in the region of 75–80% (with coincident slight elevation in venous partial pressure) are often encountered and the relevance of this apparently unfavorable influence on the oxygen gradient has not been assessed. No such physiological inefficiency exists with carbon dioxide clearance. Membranes are more permeable to CO_2 than to oxygen, and the transfer gradient remains favorable at intraluminal partial pressures of CO_2 varying between 0 kPa at the proximal fiber end to approximately 2 kPa at the exit port.

Clinical and experimental evidence confirms the potential for improving CO_2 clearance by the use of permissive hypercapnia to levels of 10–12 kPa. Clearance, easily measured as the product of the system gas flow and exhaust gas CO_2 content, is a net effect and depends on fiber mass and design, disposition of the fibers within the venae cavae, and hemodynamics and blood flow profiles around the fibers, and is little influenced directly by the distribution of ventilation and pulmonary blood flow.

Even if all the factors favoring IVOX oxygen transfer can be maximized, the physiology of gas carriage in blood dictates that the maximum achievable increase in the oxygen carrying capacity of blood remains limited by comparison to the potential for clearance of CO_2.

A CLINICIAN'S PERSPECTIVE OF IVOX

To date, clinical experience with IVOX has provided interesting but somewhat confusing data. The patient group exhibited heterogeneous pathology, and the number of centers participating in the study, differing management protocols and a lack of emphasis on the potential strengths of the device have led to difficulties in interpretation of somewhat disappointing data. Design changes are likely to provide a more potent device in terms of potential gas exchange, but suitable patient groups and adjunctive management protocols need to be more strictly defined in the application of future IVGE devices.

Our own experience with seven implants suggests that net oxygenation benefits with IVOX are unpredictable, but that the device has the potential to provide substantial and clinically relevant volumes of CO_2 clearance [45]. This would theoretically be most beneficial in conditions such as severe acute asthma and acute exacerbations of chronic obstructive pulmonary disease where a raised Pa_{CO_2} is likely to respond favorably to IVGE techniques. Insertion of IVOX by our unit in a young, severe asthmatic patient with life threatening cardiopulmonary compromise resulted in stabilization and successful treatment of this condition.

The role of IVOX in the support of patients with ARDS is not quite so clear. Acceptance of a limited oxygenator role allows construction of a ventilatory philosophy in which oxygenation depends primarily on native pulmonary function, while IVOX CO_2 clearance, in concert with the philosophy of permissive hypercapnia, would allow a considerable reduction of the pressure/volume cost of ventilation. Thus, lung volume would be maintained by manipulating mean airway pressure, but peak airway pressures could be considerably decreased and the amplitude of alveolar volume changes reduced by harnessing the potential contribution of IVOX to CO_2 clearance. Identification of those patients with ARDS most at risk of ventilation-induced damage, such as those with very low pulmonary compliance in the early phase of ARDS, could allow early and appropriate intervention with IVOX before the cycle of ventilation induced damage is established.

An appropriate philosophy to be applied along with IVOX implantation in ARDS would thus include pressure controlled ventilation to a limit of 35 cmH$_2$O or less, permissive hypercapnia to Pa_{CO_2} values of 10–12 kPa, manipulations of intrinsic and extrinsic PEEP and an I/E ratio to achieve the mean airway pressure, and hence lung volume, required to adequately oxygenate the patient, with the added goal of decreasing minute ventilation and particularly tidal volume to values in the order of 5–7 ml/kg. It is vital in the design of future clinical trials of IVOX or related devices that ventilatory protocols specifically designed for, and appropriate to, the condition being investigated be included in the study protocol.

Clearly, IVOX does not represent an alternative to extracorporeal support in the most catastrophic forms of ARDS. The current device is incapable of providing sufficient gas exchange to replace ECGE and is unlikely to ever achieve such a role due to the physiology associated with a prepulmonary gas exchanger. By contrast, even with venovenous cannulation, current ECGE systems can replace natural lung function because, at high flows, mixed venous blood can be much more effectively saturated, negating the effect of intrapulmonary shunt. The realistic aspiration remains, however, that IVOX or its successors will safely contribute to the successful management of a group of patients in whom IVOX facilitated ventilatory manipulation may avert the requirement to proceed to ECGE, or may allow safer and more effective ventilatory support of patients currently considered refractory to more conventional techniques.

SUMMARY

At the time of writing, IVOX has a favorable profile in terms of safety, simplicity of use and associated complications, but is limited in its gas transfer capability. Thus far, clinical trials suggest that it has potential in the management of ARDS as an adjunctive rather than a primary supportive measure. IVOX design modifications, and perhaps alternative IVGE devices, may provide enhanced gas exchange capacity and generate enthusiasm for further clinical investigation. Such trials should be undertaken after defining a patient population likely to respond to the favorable characteristics of IVOX, and with appropriate ventilatory modifications that are agreed and standardized throughout trial centers. Such an approach is vital to enhance our understanding of the merits of IVGE and to help define the role of this option in the support of acute respiratory failure.

ACKNOWLEDGEMENTS

Work supported by an anonymous donation to the Unit of Critical Care, National Heart of Lung Institute, Royal Brompton Hospital.

REFERENCES

1. Dreyfuss, D. and Saumon, G. (1992) Barotrauma is volotrauma, but which volume is the one responsible? *Intensive Care Med.*, 139–41.
2. Dreyfuss, D., Soler, P., Basset, G. and Saumon, G. (1988) Respective effects of high airway pressure, high tidal volume, and positive end-expiratory pressure. *Am. Rev. Respir. Dis.* **137**, 1159–64.
3. Lachmann, B. (1992) Open up the lung and keep the lung open. *Intensive Care Med.*, **18**, 319–21.
4. Rappaport, S.H., Shpiner, R., Yoshihara, G. *et al.* (1994) Randomised, prospective trial of pressure limited versus volume controlled ventilation in severe respiratory failure. *Crit. Care Med.*, **22**, 22–32.
5. Gluck, E., Head, S., Patel, *et al.* (1983) Use of ultra-high frequency ventilation in patients with ARDS. *Chest*, **84**, 551–9.
6. Marini, J.J. (1994) Pressure targeted, lung protective ventilatory support in acute lung injury. *Chest*, **105**, 109–15s.
7. Hickling, K.G., Henderson, S.J. and Jackson R. (1990) Low mortality associated with low volume pressure limited ventilation with permissive hypercapnia in severe adult respiratory distress syndrome. *Intensive Care Med.*, **16**, 372–7.
8. Zapol, W.M., Snider, M.T., Hill, J.D. *et al.* (1979) Extracorporeal membrane oxygenation in severe acute respiratory failure. A randomized prospective study. *JAMA*, **242**, 2193–6.
9. Morris, A.H., Wallace, C.J., Menlove, R.L. *et al.* (1994) Randomized clinical trial of pressure controlled inverse ratio ventilation and extracorporeal CO_2 removal for adult respiratory distress syndrome. *Am. J. Respir. Crit. Care Med.*, **149**, 295–305.
10. Pesenti, A., Gattinoni, L. and Bombino M. (1993) Long term extracorporeal respiratory support; 20 years of progress. *Intensive Crit. Care Digest*, **12**, 15–9.
11. Brunet, F., Belghith, M., Mira, J.P. *et al.* (1993) Extracorporeal carbon dioxide removal and low-frequency positive pressure ventilation. Improvement in arterial oxygenation with reduction of risk of pulmonary barotrauma in patients with adult respiratory distress syndrome. *Chest*, **104**, 889–98.
12. Mortensen, J.D. (1987) An intravenacaval blood gas exchange (IVCBGE) device: a preliminary report. *Trans. Am. Soc. Artif. Intern. Organs*, **33**, 570–3.
13. Mortensen, J.D. and Berry, G. (1989) Conceptual and design features of a practical, clinically effective intravenous mechanical blood oxygen/carbon dioxide exchange device (IVOX). *Int. J. Artif. Organs*, **12**, 384–9.
14. Mortensen, J.D., Berry, G. and Winters S. (1990) IVOX: an intracorporeal device for temporary augmentation of blood gas transfer in subjects with acute respiratory insufficiency. *Cardiac Chronicle*, **4**, 1–6.
15. Mortensen, J.D. (1992) Intravascular oxygenator: a new alternative method for augmenting blood gas transfer in patients with acute respiratory failure. *Artif. Organs*, **16**, 75–82.
16. Shukla, P.R., Snider, M.T., Hopper, K.D. *et al.* (1993) Radiologic evaluation of the intravenous oxygenator. *Radiology*, **187**, 783–6.
17. Bellhouse, B.J., Bellhouse, F.H., Curl, C.M. *et al.* (1973) A high efficiency membrane oxygenator and pulsatile pumping system, and its application to animal trials. *Trans. Am. Soc. Artif. Intern. Organs*, **19**, 72–9.
18. Bagley, B., Bagley, A., Henrie, J. *et al.* (1991) Quantitative gas transfer into and out of circulating venous blood by means of an intravenacaval oxygenator. *ASAIO Trans.*, **37**, M413–5.
19. Cox, C.S. Jr, Zwischenberger, J.B., Traber, L.D. *et al.* (1991) Use of an intravascular oxygenator/carbon dioxide removal device in an ovine smoke inhalation injury model. *ASAIO Trans.*, **37**, M411–3.
20. Tonz, M., von Segesser, L.K., Leskosek, B. and Turina, M.I. (1994) Quantitative gas transfer of an intravascular oxygenator. *Ann. Thorac. Surg.*, **57**, 146–50.
21. von Segesser, L.K., Weiss, B.M., Pasic, M. *et al.* (1992) Temporary lung support using an intravascular gas exchanger. *Thorac. Cardiovasc. Surg.*, **40**, 121–5.
22. Skoyles, J. and Pepperman, M. (1993) IVOX. [Editorial.] *Br. J. Anaesth.*, **70**, 603–4.
23. Kallis, P., al-Saady, N.M., Bennett, E.D. and Treasure, T. (1992) Intravascular oxygenation with the IVOX. *Br. J. Hosp. Med.*, **47**, 824–8.

24. Kirby, T.J. and Weidemann, H. (1992) Intravascular oxygenation: adjunct in acute respiratory failure. *Appl. Cardiopulmonary Pathophysiol.*, **4**, 287–91.

25. von Segesser, L.K., Schaffner, A., Stocker, R. *et al.* (1992) Extended (29 days) use of intravascular gas exchanger. *Lancet*, **339**, 1536.

26. Zapol, W.M. (1992) Volotrauma and the intravenous oxygenator in patients with adult respiratory distress syndrome. *Anesthesiology*, **77**, 847–9.

27. Shapiro, B. and Peruzzi, W. (1993) Intracorporeal respiratory support – a potential supplement to airway pressure therapy? *Chest*, **103**, 1–2.

28. Mortensen, J.D., Gaykowski, R. and Schaap, R.N. (1991) Results of phase 1 of the clinical trials of the intravenacaval oxygenator (IVOX). *Crit. Care Med.*, **19**, S91.

29. Conrad, S.A., Bagley, A., Bagley, B. *et al.* (1994) Major findings from the clinical trials of the intravascular oxygenator. *Artif. Organs*, **18**, 846–63.

30. Conrad, S.A., Eggerstedt, J.M., Morris, V.F. and Romero, M.D. (1993) Prolonged intracorporeal support of gas exchange with an intravenacaval oxygenator. *Chest*, **103**, 158–61.

31. Cockcroft, S., Kuo, J., Colvin, M.P. *et al.* (1992) Initial evaluation of an intracorporeal oxygenation device. *Anaesthesia*, **47**, 48–51.

32. Kallis, P., al-Saady, N., Bennett, D. and Treasure, T. (1991) Clinical use of intravascular oxygenation. *Lancet*, **337**, 549 (letter).

33. Kallis, P., al-Saady, N.M., Bennett, E.D. and Treasure, T. (1993) Early results of intravascular oxygenation. *Eur. J. Cardiothorac. Surg.*, **7**, 206–10.

34. Murdoch, L.J., Boyd, O.F., Mackay, J. *et al.* (1993) The peri-operative management of surgical insertion and removal of the intravenous oxygenator device (IVOX). A report of nine cases. *Anaesthesia*, **48**, 845–8.

35. Gentilello, L.M. Jurkovich, G.J., Gubler, K.D *et al.* (1993) The intravascular oxygenator (IVOX): preliminary results of a new means of performing extrapulmonary gas exchange. *J. Trauma*, **35**, 399–404.

36. Mira, J.P., Brunet, F. Belghith, M. *et al.* (1995) Reduction of ventilator settings allowed by intravenous oxygenator (IVOX) in ARDS patients. *Intensive Care Med.*, **21**, 11–7.

37. Gasche, Y. Romand, J.A. Pretre, R. and Suter, P.M. (1994) IVOX in ARDS: respiratory effects and serious complications. *Eur. Respir. J.*, **7**, 821–3.

38. High, K.M. Snider, M.T., Richard, R. *et al.* (1992) Clinical trials of an intravenous oxygenator in patients with adult respiratory distress syndrome. *Anesthesiology*, **77**, 856–63.

39. Cox, C.S. Jr, Zwischenberger, J.B., Graves, D.F. *et al.* (1993) Intracorporeal CO_2 removal and permissive hypercapnia to reduce airway pressure in acute respiratory failure. The theoretical basis for permissive hypercapnia with IVOX. *ASAIO J.*, **39**, 97–102.

40. Zwischenberger, J.B., Cox, C.S., Graves, D and Bidani, A. (1992) Intravascular membrane oxygenation and carbon dioxide removal – a new application for permissive hypercapnia? *Thorac. Cardiovasc. Surg.*, **40**, 115–20.

41. Brunet, F., Mira, J.P. Cerf, C. *et al.* (1994) Permissive hypercapnia and intravascular oxygenator in the treatment of patients with ARDS. *Artif. Organs*,

42. Nguyen, T.T., Zwischenberger, J.B., Tao, W. *et al.* (1993) Significant enhancement of carbon dioxide removal by a new prototype IVOX. *ASAIO J.*, **39**, M719–24.

43. Hattler, B., Reeder, G., Sawzik, P. *et al.* (1993) Toward the development of an intravenous membrane oxygenator (IMO). *Artif. Organs*, **17**, 510.

44. Hattler, B., Reeder, G., Sawzik, P. *et al.* (1994) Development of an intravenous membrane oxygenator: enhanced intravenous gas exchange through convective mixing of blood around hollow fibre membranes. *Artif. Organs*, **18**, 806–12.

45. Sim, K.M., Evans, T.W. and Keogh B.F. (1996) Clinical strategies in intravascular gas exchange. *Artif. Organs*, (in press).

Alan H. Morris

No overview or meta-analysis can substitute for a single randomized, controlled clinical trial of sufficient size and power to detect clinically important treatment effects. [1]

PROBLEMS WITH ARDS RESEARCH

BACKGROUND AND COMPLEXITY

Critical care accounts for about 30% of all acute care inpatient costs. The US national cost of intensive care unit (ICU) care is about $47 billion annually. There are 84 883 ICU beds in the United States [2]. The cost of a sophisticated modern ventilator is approximately $20 000. Despite the lack of conclusive evidence and the complexity of ICU care, mechanical ventilation techniques designed to minimize pressure applied across the chest are rapidly becoming standard in many hospitals. Pressure limited techniques, including pressure controlled inverse ratio ventilation (PCIRV), are being widely applied (Chapter 23). In Europe, low frequency positive pressure ventilation with extracorporeal carbon dioxide removal (LFPPV-ECCO$_2$R) has assumed an important clinical role (Chapter 25). However, it is difficult to justify the adoption of costly and complex new ICU therapies without clear proof of superior patient outcome [3].

The syndrome of acute respiratory distress in adults (ARDS) is associated with diffuse pathologic disturbance to the alveolar-capillary barrier [4] and profound alteration of the pulmonary vasculature [5]. Clinically, ARDS is a complicated spectrum resulting from the interaction of endothelial and epithelial cell dysfunction and biochemical events associated with lung tissue damage [6–11]. Polymorphonuclear leukocytes appear to enhance damage in experimental lung injury [12] and are altered in patients with ARDS [13]. Multiple cytokines have been implicated in lung inflammation and in ARDS [10,14]. Both blood and bronchoalveolar lavage fluid have provided evidence of the presence of tumor necrosis factor [10,15,16]. Leukotrienes have been recovered from lung edema and bronchoalveolar lavage fluid of patients with ARDS [17–19], as well as from their urine [20]. The metabolic activity of the ARDS lung is high. Lung metabolism can account for about 15% of the total body oxygen consumption ($\dot{V}O_2$) in dogs with unilobar bacterial pneumonia [21] and has been reported to account for up to 40% of the total body $\dot{V}O_2$ in patients with severe ARDS under extracorporeal support [22]. Much of this probably results from lung inflammation, including upregulation of polymorphonuclear leukocyte oxidative burst [23]. While recent evidence suggests that von Willebrand factor antigen (vWf-Ag) and endothelial cell leukocyte adhesion molecule (ELAM-1, E-selectin 1) may be early markers of endothelial cell injury and lung dysfunction [24,25], there are, to date, no good early markers of the syndrome. ARDS has not yet

ARDS Acute Respiratory Distress in Adults. Edited by Timothy W. Evans and Christopher Haslett. Published in 1996 by Chapman & Hall, London. ISBN 0 412 56910 8

been associated with a uniformly accepted definition [26,27]. This problem is currently being addressed, but much work needs to be done [28–30]. The problem is complex.

This complexity and the opportunity for great variation in medical practice is amply demonstrated by the large number of potential causes of decreased oxygenation in the mechanically ventilated patient [31]. Six major and 26 minor categories of such causes of impaired arterial oxygenation in critically ill mechanically ventilated patients are described. In addition to the potential harm that may be produced by application of high ventilatory rate (Ppeak) or delivery of large tidal volume (VT) to the chest [32,33], the therapeutic use of oxygen exposes the patient to additional risk. Oxygen is a well-defined pulmonary toxin [34–36] that produces endothelial cell damage and lung inflammation with microscopic changes indistinguishable from those associated with ARDS [37] (Chapter 11). Oxygen can potentiate inflammation in an already damaged lung [38] and may play an important role in the outcome of patients with ARDS [6,39]. This complexity has not been balanced by specific rules and executable guidelines for clinical care and for clinical research. Great variation in clinical practice has, in fact, characterized modern critical care. Some of this variation is undoubtedly clinically important. The complexity of ARDS mechanisms and the complexity and opportunity for large variation in medical practice impede the detection of important clinical outcome changes. This reduces our ability to recognize the effects of clinical interventions [40,41].

The lack of standardization of ARDS patient selection, treatment, process of care and techniques of data acquisition and evaluation makes comparison of many clinical results difficult [42–44]. The barrier to drawing credible inferences from published work plagued with nonuniform definitions and therapy is widely recognized [6,26,45–47]. In addition, the small number of patients enrolled in well designed randomized clinical trials reduces the power to detect confidently real differences in survival of patients supported with different therapies [48–51]. Stated another way, the confidence intervals for the observed survival rates are large. This precludes a compelling definition of desirable therapy for these patients and denies clinicians the guidance needed to aid them in difficult decisions for these complex clinical problems.

SURVIVAL VARIABILITY

Reported survival for patients with severe ARDS varies from 9 to 84% [52–57] (Chapters 2 and 22). Nevertheless, with mechanical ventilation support alone, survival appeared unchanged from the early 1970s to about 1988. From 1974 to 1988 in two of the nine original extracorporeal membrane oxygenation (ECMO) centers [53], the survival of patients with severe ARDS who met ECMO criteria, supported only with mechanical ventilation, ranged from none [58] to 15% [57]. The 13% average survival is not statistically significantly different from the 1974–77 ECMO clinical trial survival of 9% ($P = 0.15$) [59]. Less severely ill patients also appeared to have the same survival as in the 1970s [6,8,57,60,61]. It has been suggested that patients with ARDS are now more severely ill than those encountered in the past [62], but this is undocumented. In any case, the absence of definitive evidence that ARDS mortality has decreased is disappointing considering the technical advances in ICU care that have been made since the early 1980s [63–67].

More recent reports of mechanical ventilatory management have been associated with increased survival of patients with ARDS [52,68–70]. These have included patients at the LDS Hospital enrolled in the control group of the recent LFPPV-ECCO$_2$R clinical trial (control patients) [59,71] and patients not enrolled in that clinical trial [68]. However, none of the recent mechanical ventilator management techniques have been evaluated in controlled clinical trials. At present, there are no convincing data that any particular ventilatory support mode is superior for the support of patients with ARDS [72,73].

Inadequate signal-to-noise ratio for clinical outcomes

The detection of an association between an input signal of interest and an outcome measure requires that the signal of interest be capable of separation from other, unwanted, signals with which it may be confused or by which it may be obscured. A common measure of this capability is the signal-to-noise ratio. Unless the signal-to-noise ratio exeeds 1, the signal will be undetectable. The examples of auditory (Figure 27.1) and optical (Figure 27.2) signals and noise should help clarify this concept.

The focus in medicine for both clinical care and clinical research is patient outcome, the most important of which is survival with resumption of a productive life. Unfortunately, the signal-to-noise ratio associated with outcome differences in clinical trials for patients with ARDS is frequently very low. The noise in the clinical environment is both random and nonrandom (bias). Random noise can be reduced by increasing the number of

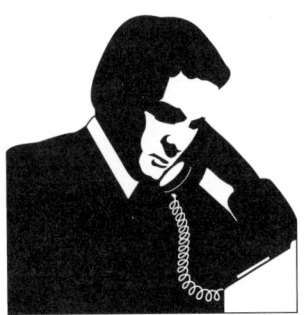

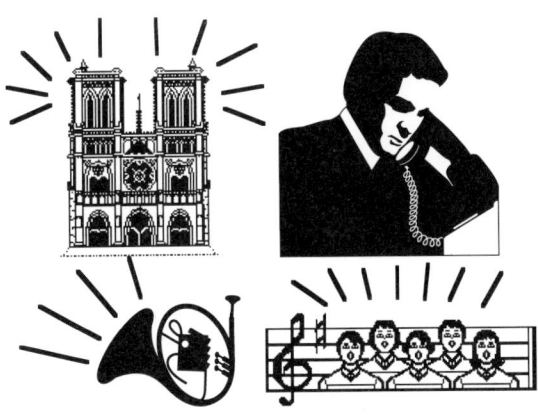

Figure 27.1 Auditory noise. (a) The auditory signal is easily heard in a quiet room because the signal-to-noise ratio is high. (b) The same auditory signal is difficult to distinguish from background sounds because the signal-to-noise ratio is now low.

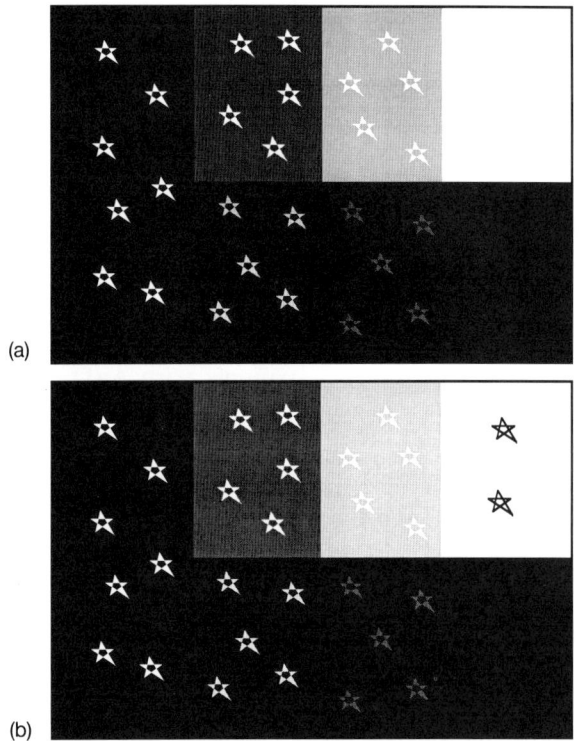

(a)

(b)

Figure 27.2 Visual noise. (a) The visual signals are the stars. They are easily seen on the black background at the left of the panel because the signal-to-noise ratio is high. As one moves the eye to the right the stars become more difficult to see, and finally disappear from view at the extreme right. In the upper half of panel a, the stars disappear because the background noise (light) is increasing from left to right until the signal-to-noise ratio is 1 (low) and the signals (stars), while present are invisible. In the lower half of panel a, The background noise is unchanged and remains 0. The stars disappear because the signals become faint and finally are 0, producing a signal-to-noise ratio of 0 at the extreme right. (b) The undetectable stars at the right in the upper half of panel b are outlined to indicate the presence of the signals even though they cannot be seen (detected). In the lower half of panel b the stars are actually missing because the signals are 0 at the extreme right.

observations (or number of patients) made in a clinical trial. Since the signal-to-noise ratio for random noise is proportional to the square root of the number of observations, increasing the number of observations (or patients) 100-fold would increase the signal-to-noise ratio by 10. This is a difficult challenge in critical care medicine because the acquisition of large numbers of patients in clinical trials is not only difficult but costly. In contrast, non-random noise (bias), quite common in clinical settings, is not influenced by increasing the

number of observations (or patients) and therefore must be reduced by other means.

Each of the major elements (the patient and the clinical caregiver) that determine the intensity of patient care and the patient outcome (Figure 27.3) is a source of random noise and of systematic noise (bias). The patient contributes noise because of uncontrollable host factors and because of disease etiology, severity, extent and duration. Local factors influence the patient's disease and spectrum of clinical problems. The patient

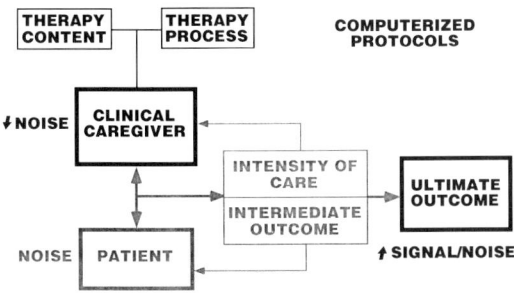

Figure 27.3 The major elements (patient and clinical caregiver) that interact in an iterative feedback manner to determine the intensity of care, the level of intermediate outcomes (e.g. Pao_2, Cth, etc.) and the ultimate outcome (e.g. survival). Both the patient and the clinical caregiver introduce random noise and nonrandom noise (bias) that decrease the signal-to-noise ratio for important outcome events. See text for discussion.

identification and selection process is quite imperfect and may incorporate much local bias due to the prejudices of individual clinicians and clinical investigators. This bias is the result of many factors, among which are characteristics of local clinical environments and failure of the medical community to establish broadly accepted specific definitions of many diseases, including ARDS [28–30]. The other major element, the clinical caregiver response to the patient, introduces both random noise and bias. Strong bias is injected into the response of clinical caregivers because of many factors that influence behavior, including general and local cultural factors, local technical abilities, background, training and experience.

The low probability of finding a striking effect in complex multifactorially determined clinical problems like ARDS probably explains in part the absence of dramatic improvement in ARDS survival with drugs theoretically capable of such improvement (steroids, prostaglandin inhibitors, endotoxin antibodies) [11,74]. Solutions to the difficult general problem of defining effective therapy for ARDS require an increase in the signal-to-

noise ratio for clinical outcome results. This could come from a large increase in the signal, due for example to the introduction of a drug or support technique that had a striking effect on ARDS (such as the effect of penicillin therapy in pneumococcal pneumonia in the 1940s). Such a happening in a complicated multifactorial setting is unlikely. The low signal-to-noise ratio probably also explains why experts have difficulty predicting survival. When attempting to select a subset of ARDS patients with a 30% survival with the ECMO blood gas criteria [75], experts missed the mark (9% survival was actually observed) [46,53].

LACK OF STANDARDIZATION

Uncontrolled and frequently retrospective studies in humans have suggested improved outcomes in ARDS following mechanical ventilation support strategies that lower airway pressures [69,76,77]. However, caution must be exercised. Conclusions based upon physician judgment in the absence of scientifically valid data are frequently unreliable [3]. Retrospective studies, like other forms of observational studies, are not experiments. They do not possess the strength of inference of experiments, such as randomized clinical trials [50]. Uncontrolled studies uniformly overestimate the effectiveness of the treatment of interest [78].

The uncertainty surrounding the results of retrospective comparisons is illustrated by PCIRV. The PCIRV studies have design flaws, none being a carefully controlled prospective randomized trial [42,79]. There is no standard approach to the management of PCIRV. Many articles lack description or quantification of parameters such as end expiratory alveolar pressure and ventilatory rate (VR) without which it is difficult to define the conditions of the study [79]. Information gained from domestic and international visits to medical centers has confirmed our local experience that PCIRV is usually applied by trial and error, with changes in ventilator settings based on pathophysiologic principles. The application of PCIRV is not systematic and is therefore not reproducible in the clinical setting. Other support modes suffer from similar limitations due to nonuniformity of care [80].

Information input overload

The result of application of a computerized PCIRV protocol is particularly instructive because of its implication regarding the limited number of variables physicians are capable of managing [81,82]. The PCIRV protocol operates in a dedicated personal computer linked to a mechanical ventilator. Four variables – ratio of inspiratory time to expiratory time (I/E), VR, Ppeak and positive end expiratory pressure setting (setPEEP) – are adjusted according to protocol instructions displayed on bedside terminals. These four variables determine the end expiratory alveolar pressure [82,83] (Figure 27.4). 'Controlled air trapping' (end expiratory alveolar pressure > 0) is achieved as the clinical staff follows the protocol instructions displayed on the PCIRV computer terminal screen.

Since the initial application of the computerized protocol in our ICU, PCIRV has become simplified and more predictable. This change in our perception of PCIRV performance was noted by physicians, nurses and respiratory therapists. This suggests that the four determining variables (I/E, VR, Ppeak, setPEEP) could not have been managed systematically prior to computerized protocol control, even though PCIRV had been used by experienced pulmonary and critical care physicians within an academic training program. It indicates that, faced with the challenge of adjusting four variables (Figure 27.4), experienced physicians were not able to develop a systematic response to ventilatory support problems. This is an example of

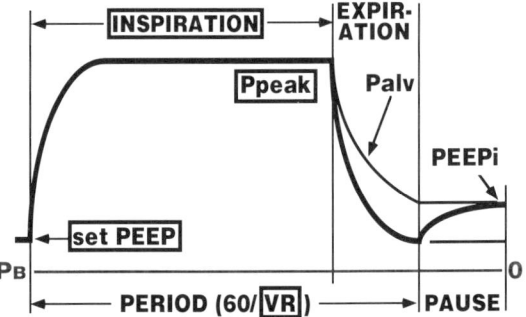

Figure 27.4 Airway pressure waveform during inverse ratio ventilation with air trapping. Ppeak = peak airway pressure; set PEEP = positive end expiratory pressure setting; Palv = alveolar pressure; P_B = barometric pressure (the reference 0); PEEPi = intrinsic PEEP (end expiratory alveolar pressure); VR = ventilatory rate; INSPIRATION = inspiration time; EXPIRATION = expiration time; PAUSE = end expiratory pause (breath hold) to allow equilibration of the airway pressure (thick waveform) with alveolar pressure (thin waveform). Boxes indicate the four controlled ventilator variables used to adjust end expiratory alveolar pressure (PEEPi).

information input overload [41,83–86], and is part of a general limitation of our ability to manage clinical problems that have at least four variable determinants. Within the more than 236 different variable categories noted in one of our patients with ARDS one morning on rounds [83] there are a number of clinically important problems involving consideration of many more than four variables, Human decision making is limited by our ability to assimilate information. In the ICU we commonly attempt to relate many more than two variables in the management of mechanical ventilation alone. Humans are, however, limited in their ability to estimate the degree of relatedness (covariation) between only two variables [87]. It is appropriate to ask how well we can expect clinicians to relate multiple clinical variables to each other and systematically generate therapeutic decisions that are coherent and that include all appropriate options.

Rescue therapy for 'life threatening problems'

Rescue therapy has been a common element in the design of trials of therapy in life threatening problems. It was included in the ECMO clinical trial of 1974–77 [53,75,88]. The decision to employ rescue therapy is based on the assumption that the physician knows the expected patient outcome with adequate certainty. In the ECMO trial, conditions that defined 'control failures' and allowed the use of ECMO as rescue therapy for control patients were: arterial oxygen partial pressure (Pa_{O_2}) $\leqslant$ 45 mmHg for $\geqslant$ 12 hours with fraction of inspired oxygen (F_{IO_2}) = 1.0 and with maximum tolerated PEEP, or Pa_{O_2} $\leqslant$ 35 mmHg for $\geqslant$ 6 hours [75, p.7; 89, p.6]. Since then, it has become clear to me that such predictions are quite uncertain. My colleagues and I have encountered patients who met these criteria but who survived in the control treatment arm of a recent randomized controlled clinical trial [59]. Rescue therapy is also an intuitive clinical response to the almost universally sensed imperative to 'do something' when the patient fails to respond to 'life saving' treatments. This is an activist position that ascribes more value to active treatment than to waiting, even though there is frequently no clinical outcome information on which to build an argument that the active treatment will lead to a favorable impact on patient outcome. This activist position is bolstered with ethical arguments that depend on the same unproved assumptions.

Ethical concerns

Many design flaws in ARDS clinical trials, and many clinical objections to performing clinical trials for patients with ARDS or other life threatening problems, are based on 'ethical concerns'. A discussion of ethical issues, and of the closely related issues of the authoritarian (expert) paradigm and of physician belief, is therefore necessary. The process of medical care is based upon the principle of beneficence [90]. All clinical practitioners intend to benefit their patients (I ignore uncommon malicious behavior, at times dramatically exposed in the press). Benefit appears to be the over-riding factor now [90,pp. 14,161] as it was for Hippocrates ('Be of benefit and do no harm') [90,p. 11]. Clinical decision making guided by the principle of beneficence is, unfortunately, confounded by both the uncertainty of medical scientific information, and by the probabilistic nature of medical decision making. The conundrum is clear: the principle of beneficence implies patient benefit, but the outcome information necessary for the physician to be confident that patient benefit would follow the intervention is frequently missing! The intention to benefit, while often necessary, is not sufficient.

The intention to do good is sometimes persuasive in itself. It is of crucial importance as a defense in litigation when someone's life has been lost. The perpetrator's intention may lead jurors to a judgment of manslaughter, rather than murder, with significant consequences in the assigned punishment. Whereas intention (motive) is important in many legal situations, the law downplays intent (motive) in medical matters. The standard of medical practice is of greater importance. However, even violation of the standard of practice with obvious malicious intent is of little consequence in the absence of harm to the patient. Patient harm becomes the focal effect that precipitates concern about the process of care. When harm has occurred, compliance with the standard of practice then becomes the cornerstone of defense. Even then, the physician's intention is of minor importance.

The intention to be beneficent can be effected at several levels, each level associated with different probabilities of actually conferring benefit on the patient. One can intend to be benevolent, seeking only 'the quality of charity or kindness' [91]. Such intentions are not directly linked to patient benefit. In contrast, the intention to be beneficent can be directed at 'the doing of good' [92,93]. This is directly linked to patient benefit but, interestingly, is not necessarily associated with benevolence. This intention to do good, widely accepted in principle by practitioners, may be the result of decisions without rational argument. Such decisions can frequently mislead clinicians, even when based on extensive personal experience (see below). When such decisions are based on rational argument, but the rational argument is not based on credible outcome data, the likelihood of actually doing good for the patient will depend on the signal-to-noise ratio for the clinical problem of interest (see below). If the signal-to-noise ratio is high enough, the decision will be sound and patient benefit likely follow. If the signal-to-noise ratio is low, as is commonly the case with difficult clinical decisions like those encountered in ARDS care, then personal experience and the best intentions will not suffice. Credible group data from well controlled clinical trials (preferably double blinded randomized clinical trials with sufficient power) will be necessary for clinical decisions that can be expected to confer benefit on the patient. With the low signal-to-noise ratio characteristic of many complex clinical problems, the problem reduces to the need to quantify the probability of benefit. When this probability cannot be quantified, clinicians are in danger of being misled by data and experience. The quantifiable probabilities established by credible group studies such as randomized clinical trials provide the foundation for decisions likely to confer benefit on the patient. Many critical care problems depend on such quantifiable probabilities. Unfortunately, the studies that could provide such data are rarely performed. The needed data base for complex decisions is sorely deficient. Physicians are thus deprived of the assistance they need in making difficult decisions in the complex clinical circumstances of ARDS.

The ICU decision making paradigm based

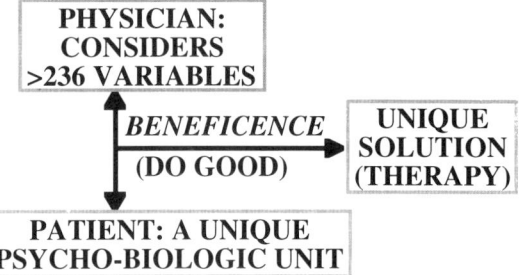

(a)

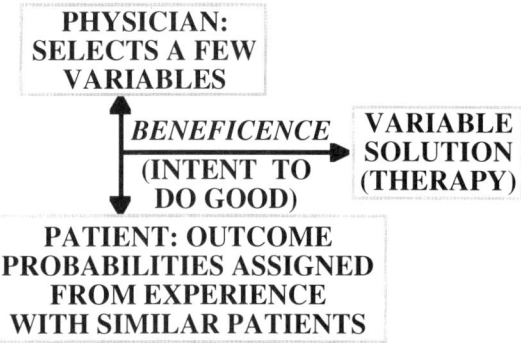

(b)

Figure 27.5 (a) Ideal ICU decision making paradigm based on the doing of good. (b) Actual ICU decision making paradigm based on the intent to do good. See text for discussion.

upon the principle of beneficence requires the physician to evaluate all of the pertinent information, to consider the patient as a unique individual (a unique psychobiologic unit) and to come to a unique solution (therapy) that will do good (favorably influence the patient outcome) (Figure 27.5a). This paradigm of 'individualized patient care' appears to be commonly taught.

In truth, the ICU decision making paradigm based on the principle of beneficence and used in critical care medicine decision making is usually not that directed at patient outcome but rather one directed at physician intent (Figure 27.5b). The physician usually chooses a few familiar and understood variables (intuitively responding to the human limitations in managing information). The patient, while always viewed as an individual, is categorized and an attempt to assign general outcome probabilities for different therapy options is made by drawing upon past experience (personal or published) with similar patients. Because of the common complexity of the decisions, the physician makes the therapeutic decision with the intent to do good, but usually without the outcome knowledge that would enable the physician to draw a conclusion about benefit. This results in therapeutic decisions that are frequently inconsistent and difficult to reproduce.

Authoritarian (expert) paradigm and physician belief

The expert or authoritarian paradigm has been the foundation of the traditional patient–physician relationship. The physician is the expert and possesses the requisite training, knowledge and experience to provide the advice necessary to guide the patient towards a favorable outcome. In this process, the patient's 'best interest' is served by provision of the 'best available' therapy [94]. The physician's 'belief' in the superiority of a therapeutic choice is cited as a foundation of ethical decision making [94] and the fiduciary nature of the physician–patient encounter [94,95]. The absence of such a belief in the face of therapeutic options constitutes the state of 'equipoise' within an individual physician (individual equipoise) or within the medical community (clinical equipoise) [94,96]. When equipoise is present, randomized clinical trials comparing therapeutic possibilities seem justified. A number of concerns can be raised in response to this traditional view. They are not responsive to general human limitations with information processing [41,82–85]. Ignoring these limitations raises physician 'belief' to a level of undeserved importance. Physician 'belief' in the

superiority of complex therapies may, in fact, undermine the fiduciary relationship that should exist between physician and patient [94,95] by exposing the patient to undesirable therapy.

The 'belief' of the adherents of a particular policy, in itself, provides no justification for the policy. The belief is no more than an opinion. The policy can only rationally be justified by data or arguments. Belief can be based on credible outcome data. It may also be based on unfounded conjecture. Belief is commonly based on considerations that fall on a continuum between credible outcome data and unfounded conjecture. Belief insufficiently grounded in credible outcome data, even when based on extensive personal and medical community experience, can mislead well intentioned clinicians to make decisions that fail to benefit and even bring harm to their patients. The results of the Vineberg procedure for angina pectoris, with its 75% positive placebo effect [50], and of the cardiac arrhythmia suppression trial (CAST), with its unexpectedly high mortality associated with effective suppression of premature ventricular beats following myocardial infarction [97–102], are graphic examples of this ever present danger. Other important examples are easily found and include oxygen therapy for neonatal respiratory distress [103], gastric freezing for upper gastrointestinal hemorrhage, internal mammary artery ligation, laetrile for cancer, rapid intravenous infusion of 5-fluorouracil for colorectal cancer, intra-arterial infusion of chemotherapeutic agents for colorectal liver metastases, hydrocortisone after myocardial infarction [49], splenectomy for Gaucher's disease and frontal lobotomy. It is therefore of interest to find belief, in itself and without supporting data, used as a justification for some of the most consequential and onerous decisions in critical care medicine [94,104,105]. To be fair, it must be acknowledged that some workers demand that physician opinion be based on reliable actuarial data [105–107], but this does not appear to be a universal expectation. It is rapidly appreciated that belief itself is neither sufficient nor even always necessary for the effectuation of correct therapy. The steadfast belief of the medical adherents of laetrile therapy did not make the therapy correct, nor could it justify the conduct of a clinical trial [105]. Just as the individual practitioner cannot invoke idiosyncratic good intentions as a defense, so also should this avenue of defense be forbidden to the expert committee that may be charged with defining a standard of care for the medical community. Poorly supported opinion, no matter how well intended, does not gain credibility by being offered by a dozen experts rather than by one practitioner.

Belief is influenced by personal experience and observation. Since memory is such a poor source of unbiased information [108,109], one can expect the opinions or beliefs of physicians, in the area of controversial and complicated ICU problems such as ARDS, to be variable and to reflect poorly the conclusions that would be drawn from well controlled systematic clinical trials. The administration of what the physician believes to be the best therapy can only discharge obligations under the Hippocratic oath when such belief is based on credible data. When reliable outcome data exist, they should take precedence over personal opinion [107]. When unfounded or conjectural physician belief is allowed to disrupt the experimental design of a randomized clinical trial, not only may the individual patient suffer, but the clinical trial may be rendered uninterpretable and the information anticipated from the trial results thereby lost. For example, rescue therapy application or other changes in the conduct of the clinical trial protocol, while based on good intentions, may destroy the credibility of the trial and thus perpetuate the therapeutic uncertainty that the trial was designed to ameliorate.

The traditional physician – patient relationship, Truog argues, is contractual for routine matters but fiduciary for critical illness [94]; I prefer to consider it fiduciary for all medical matters, as does Moline [95]. The patient expects the physician to pursue the patient's best interest, without conflict or distraction. The definition of 'best interest' for the patient is critical. If achievement of a favorable patient outcome is the goal, then reliable outcome data are necessary for clinical decision making. If good physician intention is the goal, then individual physician opinion will suffice. The expert paradigm fosters the notion that good intentions on the part of the physician will produce the desired clinical outcome. This is unlikely to be the case in the complex critical care environment in which information overload and low signal-to-noise ratio for outcome results are so common [41,110]. Although we are advised that 'physicians must recommend only therapies in which they personally believe' [94], reflection leads to the recognition that the proper object of medical therapy is the achievement of a good patient outcome, no matter what the physician's belief, not the application of the physician's good intention.

The ability of experts to come to the 'right therapeutic decision' when dealing with multivariate problems like ARDS should be questioned. This conclusion challenges the expert (authoritarian) paradigm that forms the foundation for much clinical decision making. This challenge leads to consideration of a complementary therapeutic decision making paradigm, one based on well defined rules constructed from the most scientifically credible information available, with a preference for group data obtained under well controlled circumstances [41]. Computerized protocols incorporating such rules might be used as a decision support tool in the ICU (see below).

LACK OF CONCURRENT CONTROLS

Historical control limitations

When uncontrolled studies are carried out, investigators are limited to comparisons with historical controls. Historical control comparisons should always be approached with caution. Survival of the control patients in the recent LFPPV-ECCO$_2$R randomized clinical trial at the LDS Hospital [59,71] and of non-randomized patients with ARDS meeting ECMO criteria at the LDS Hospital during the same period [68] was, quite unexpectedly, higher than that of historical controls and was similar to that reported after LFPPV-ECCO$_2$R (Chapter 25).

CONFUSION AND MIXING OF RESULTS AND QUESTIONS FROM DIFFERENT LEVELS OF INQUIRY

Mandelbrot has outlined compellingly the importance of defining the level of inquiry in investigation [111]. There may be no universally correct answer. Rather, appropriate answers may differ for different levels of inquiry. The fascinating set of responses to Mandelbrot's disarmingly simple question 'What is the shape and dimension of a 10 cm ball of twine composed of 1 mm threads' provides a dramatic illustration of this important relativistic principle (Figure 27.6). The answer to the question 'What is the length of the coastline of England?' is equally illuminating [111].

Reductionist versus holistic research

The importance of clearly defining the level or conditions of inquiry is closely related to the tension between reductionist and holistic research [41,112,113]. Feinstein has discussed the limitations of a number of common approaches to clinical research and emphasized the need for an enhanced focus on holistic investigation of the intact patient [114]. Results from reductionist research dealing with biochemical, cell biological, or physiological mechanisms are commonly extrapolated to the intact patient in the clinical decision making context. The implicit assumption that one can extrapolate such

10 cm BALL of 1 mm THREADS		
RESOLUTION	DIMENSION	SHAPE
10 cm	0	Point
1 cm	3	Sphere
1 mm	1	Line
0.1 mm	3	Column
0.01 mm	1	Line
0.001 mm	0	Point

BB Mandelbrot. The Fractal Geometry of Nature. WH Freeman. NY. 1983, 17-18

Figure 27.6 The dependence of dimension and shape on the resolution (level of inquiry). A 10 cm diameter ball is constructed of 1 mm threads of many fibered twine. The dimension and shape of the object vary as the item receiving attention progresses from the ball at a distance, the ball close at hand, the threads at a distance, the threads close at hand, the fibers at a distance and the fibers close at hand (111).

results to the clinical arena, thus mixing questions and results from different levels of inquiry, is frequently incorrect. The unsuccessful search for the 'magic bullet' for ARDS (and for sepsis, a closely related clinical problem) incorporates this assumption [11,74]. Since both questions and answers depend on level of inquiry, a focus on investigation of the intact patient in the clinical environment seems imperative.

Matching the investigative laboratory to the level of inquiry

It is not only the questions and the results that are determined by the level of inquiry. So also are the techniques, methods and laboratories required for investigations at different levels of inquiry. The different levels of inquiry represented by different levels of spatial resolution (Figure 27.6) or by different levels in the vertically integrated medical research structure (Figure 27.7) imply the existence of these different techniques, methods and laboratories. It would be as inappropriate to use the techniques of biochemistry to evaluate ultimate outcome issues of medical interest as it would be to use a wind tunnel laboratory for airfoil development to study questions of nuclear physics. Laboratories are tailored not only to the subject matter, but inextricably to the level of inquiry. This leads to a natural, but commonly only indirectly addressed question: 'What kind of **laboratory** is necessary for clinical outcomes research?'

Clinical outcomes research laboratory

Three elements form the essential building blocks of clinical research: **control**, **measurement** and **analysis** [115]. They must figure as established facets of the operation of a clinical outcomes research laboratory. Of these three central elements, **control** is the key missing ingredient. The misperception that laboratory level control is impossible to achieve in the clinical ICU environment is widespread. This misperception itself is an important determinant of the clinical research programs mounted in the medical community. It consitutes a paradigmatic view that limits the

LEVEL OF INQUIRY

Holistic

INTEREST	MEASUREMENT
Medical	Ultimate Outcome
Pathophysiol	Intermed Outcome
Organ Physiol	Isolated / *In Situ*
Cell Physiol	Isolated / Group
Chemistry	Biochemistry

Reductionist

Figure 27.7 Levels of biomedical inquiry. As one moves from the biochemical measurements of the chemist to the ultimate outcome measurements of medical outcomes research, one moves from a reductionist to a holistic approach to medical problems. The answers provided at one level of inquiry may be totally irrelevant to questions posed at another level of inquiry.

possibilities for clinical research in general and in ARDS in particular.

Kuhn has proposed that a paradigm is prerequisite for itself [116,117]. While nature or the world is the object of science (including medical science at the clinical outcome level), this world is a perceived world determined jointly by nature and by the paradigms that constitute the tools with and through which we view nature [117]. Kuhn points to the 'apparently arbitrary elements, compounded of personal and historical accident' that are 'always a formative ingredient of the beliefs espoused by a given scientific community at a given time' [116].

'The theories we hold apparently lead us to expect and predict stronger empirical relationships than actually exist' [87]. We appear to underestimate the relatedness of two variables when faced with data in the absence of theory, but overestimate the relatedness, in the absence of data, when preconceptions or theories can be applied. The preconceived notions or hypotheses we hold not only influence our estimates of relatedness of variables, but they influence what we remember and how we recall items in memory [108,118]. Items are not stored uniformly in memory and sampling from memory (recall) is not random. Items having the highest chance of being available for recall are those that are well known, familiar and important. Items that confirm our prejudices or pre-existing beliefs are more readily available from memory than items that contradict these beliefs. Recently stored items are most easily recalled, as are vivid or dramatic events. Sampling from memory is likely to be biased [108,118]. Our traditional clinical therapeutic decision making paradigm is based on the incorporation of a large number of current variable values with past information and experience by the individual physician interacting with an individual patient at the bedside [41]. Since many clinical therapeutic decisions made in the complex ICU environment are strongly influenced by items we recall from memory, it is appropriate to question the suitability of this traditional decision making process.

Revolutions in science are the result of shifts in the paradigms (the models) through which we view the world in the empiric effort called science [116]. We need a serious reassessment of the widespread clinical belief in the impossibility of **control** in the ICU for both clinical outcomes research and for clinical care.

CLINICAL TRIAL DESIGN

INFERENCE

The confidence with which we can draw inferences about causal reationships influences the likelihood of taking action – for example, changing clinical practice as a result of clinical trials. Inferences are strengthened by high predictability of the association between an intervention and the outcome of interest. Controlled trials are not needed under extraordinary circumstances, such as those associated with a striking reduction of mortality in what was a uniformly fatal disease [78]. In such a case the signal-to-noise ratio is so high that causal inferences can be confidently drawn from uncontrolled observations without the rigor of formal randomized trials.

MEASUREMENT AND CONTROL

Measurement, control and analysis are the pillars of clinical research [115]. To be of high quality, measurements must be accurate, precise, timely and representative. Precision (reliability, consistency) is reduced by random error. Such random error can be introduced by the observer, by the subject or by instrument (measurement) variability. Accuracy is reduced by systematic error (bias) originating, as well, in either the observer, the subject or the measurement. Minimizing associated random error and systematic error (bias) in

patient samples increases the likelihood of drawing correct inferences for the target population. Accuracy and precision of data assured, one is still left with the challenge of assuring that data used for clinical care decisions are representative. The representativeness of data is a difficult issue. For example, an accurate and precise measurement of Pao_2 during endotracheal suctioning, or during chest percussion in the lateral decubitus position, may not be representative of lung function for decision making purposes. A moving median based on an automated continual data acquisition scheme appears to be an advance [119–121].

Control is essential in experimental interventions. Experiments in any scientific discipline are expected to be well controlled so that the only significant difference between test groups will be due to the intervention being studied. While this is well-recognized and applied in reductionist medical research, it is commonly missing in the holistic research of clinical trials. Nonspecific effects (placebo effect, Hawthorne effect, regression to the mean) can be important [50,78,122]. The placebo effect was associated with a 75% positive clinical response in control patients in a clinical trial of the Vineberg procedure for angina pectoris [78]. It is now clear that adequate control of important elements of the process of medical care, through application of computerized protocols, is within reach [41,59,83,123–125]. It seems likely that many will be amenable to such control, but how many of the important clinical care process elements will be able to be standardized through computerized protocol control is unknown.

INTERVENTIONAL AND OBSERVATIONAL STUDIES

Interventional (experimental) studies are more powerful than observational studies (50). The results of an experimental study are usually superior to those of an observational study because they allow more credible inferences about cause and effect. They are commonly exercises in hypothesis testing. The hypotheses so tested are frequently based on the results of observational studies, either formally designed or part of routine medical practice. The outcomes used in these experiments can be divided into two broad classes, ultimate outcomes and intermediate outcomes. The high mortality rate of patients with ARDS makes survival with functional recovery the most compelling ultimate outcome for ARDS clinical trials. Other ultimate outcomes, such as length of stay and actual cost may also be valuable but should not be a substitute for, or be used in preference to, survival for hypothesis testing. Intermediate outcomes (endpoints), such as pain relief, symptoms, mental state, total thoracic compliance (Cth), Pa_{O_2}, pH, thermodilution cardiac output ($\dot{Q}t$), sleep stage, net fluid balance, etc., serve a different purpose. Intermediate outcome variables are important for treatment group comparative descriptive purposes when analyzing the performance of a clinical trial. When subjected to exploratory statistical analysis they also provide suggestions about possible associations and mechanisms that may lead to subsequent hypothesis testing with future experiments.

Alternate treatment strategies

Treatment–placebo–treatment, treatment–placebo (or vice versa), treatment A–treatment B or treatment crossover designs within individual patients are inadequate when ultimate endpoints are the basis for drawing conclusions and inferences. They are not suitable for the most compelling questions facing ARDS research. These questions must be answered with studies using ultimate clinical outcome. Alternate treatment strategies applied within groups can provide meaningful data. They require careful consideration of potential crossover of treatment effects, frequently through learning and

unlearning during different treatment periods, by members of the clinical staff (physicians, nurses, therapists). The confounding impact of crossover treatment effects can be reduced by including historical as well as concurrent control group data comparisons. The historical data should be obtained during a period immediately preceeding the initiation of the alternate treatment study.

Observational (descriptive) studies

Observational (descriptive) studies are not experiments. They are unlikely to lead to causal conclusions, except for the unusual case of large signal-to-noise ratio effects. These are unlikely in ARDS because of its complexity. They can provide the basis for hypothesis generation, but such hypotheses would have to be subjected subsequently to experimental testing. Current emphasis on outcomes research centered on examination of large clinical databases, such as the Medicare database, is unlikely to be fruitful [126–128]. Large clinical data base reviews seems particularly unlikely to contribute meaningfully to the definition of desirable care for critically ill patients, including those with ARDS.

Hypothesis testing errors

False-positive and false-negative, as well as true-positive and true-negative results are to be expected from the application of any diagnostic test. The predictive value of the test result is dependent on the incidence of the disease in question [129–131]. The same inherent limitations are present in the test of a hypothesis in a clinical trial [132,133]. Not only are false- and true-positive and -negative results possible, but the predictive value of the experimental result is dependent on the prior probability that the hypothesis in question is true (134).

α and β errors, power (1-β) and n

Two types of errors must be minimized in designing a clinical trial (Figure 27.8). The type I error (α error) is the probability of concluding that a difference between test groups exists when in fact they are not significantly different with respect to the outcome assessment (false-positive result). The type II error (β error) is the probability of concluding that no difference between test groups exists when in fact they are significantly different with respect to the outcome assessment (false-negative result). The investigator is required to specify, as part of the experimental design, the difference between treatment group outcomes that is deemed to be of sufficient clinical importance to be detected [135]. The investigator must also specify the desired probability of actually detecting this clinically important difference between treatment group outcomes. This probability is called the power (1-β) of the experiment. The power (1-β) is the true positive rate (Figure 27.8). Once the acceptable α and β errors, power level and the clinically important difference are specified, the sample size (n) can be determined [135]. A trial with fewer than n enrolled patients will risk reducing the probability of detecting the difference

between treatment group outcomes deemed **significant** to a level below (1-β). A trial with more than n enrolled patients may increase the probability of detecting a difference between treatment group outcomes deemed **trivial and insignificant** to a level greater than α. This important part of the initial experimental design requires an a priori estimation of differences in treatment group outcomes that are likely to be clinically significant and to lead to action on the part of the medical community. Such estimations should be based on the best data and scientific foundation available. If reliable estimations cannot be made there is little justification for proceeding with plans for a clinical trial [135].

The power to detect a real difference between control and LFPPV-ECCO$_2$R therapy group survival depends on the number of patients studied [48–51]. Assuming that the observed survival rates of 42% for the control group and 33% for the LFPPV-ECCO$_2$R group represent the true survival rates of these two treatment groups [59,71], the number of study patients, per treatment group, required to detect this difference in survival 80% of the time (power = 0.8) [51] is approximately 400. This explains the need for multicenter trials, even when differences in survival larger than this are predicted.

INTERNAL AND EXTERNAL VALIDITY

External validity

The population sample and the variables chosen are proxies for the target population and for the phenomena of interest, respectively. The population sample and variables make scientific studies feasible, since it is usually neither possible to study all members of a population nor to directly measure the phenomena of interest. External validity (generalizability of study results) [50] will be present only when the population sampled is an unbiased representation of the population of interest. Explicit definition of the population

	Therapy Effective (Ho False)	**Therapy Not Effective (Ho True)**
Trial + (Reject Ho)	**1-β** POWER	α TYPE I
Trial ▪ (Accept Ho)	β TYPE II	

Figure 27.8 Errors in clinical trial results. α (Type 1) = false-positive result; β (type II) = false-negative result; (1-β) (power) = true-positive result; (1-α, not shown, = true-negative result); Ho - null hypothesis.

of interest with specific and, when possible, quantifiable criteria for patient selection is essential. Unbiased identification, solicitation and enrollment of all potential candidates is essential. Maximizing use of quantifiable non-judgmental criteria is advantageous.

Dropouts, rescue therapy application and inability to obtain follow up data

Patients, once enrolled, must complete the therapy protocol and be included in data analysis for maximum external validity. Those problems that might lead to patient dropout from treatment groups should receive careful consideration during the planning phase of the trial. Excluding such patients from enrollment may be the most reasonable solution to maintaining credibility of clinical trial results. This may restrict the patient population to which the clinical trial results would then be applicable. Rescue therapy should be avoided. Since a clinical trial will only be mounted when neither of the treatments offered is clearly superior: there is little ethical justification for abandoning one form of therapy for another during the conduct of the trial. This proposal may be disconcerting to some workers (see 'Ethical concerns' and 'Authoritarian (expert) paradigm and physician belief' sections above). The absence of follow up data eliminates crucial outcome data from analysis. This absence of data can be a problem in retrospective (observational) studies as well. For example, Hickling's influential report of high survival of patients with ARDS using a therapy intended to minimize ventilatory support (permissive hypercapnia) [136] included 50 patients, but data were unavailable for a large fraction of the patients because the medical records could not be located [137].

Internal validity

Internal validity is synonymous with drawing correct causal inferences from the measurements in the population sample. It concerns the quality, credibility and truth of the experiment, but is limited to the experimental results that must be representative of the study sample and is independent of the issue of generalizability (external validity). Two approaches can be taken to the inferences drawn from the experimental clinical trial. If the 'intention to treat' principle is observed, the inferences are applicable to the decision to treat or not, when made by the clinician. If the impact of actual and successful implementation and completion of the treatment in question is the focus, then inferences about treatment efficacy, and perhaps about mechanisms of action, would be provided, but this might have little impact on the decision to treat or not to treat [49,50]. Implementation of control over the process of clinical care would lead these two approaches to converge. Control, now possible for some important elements of ICU care, would reduce dropout, rescue therapy and loss of follow up data to a low level.

Control is essential in experimental interventions. Experiments in any scientific discipline are expected to be well controlled so that the only significant difference between test groups will be due to the intervention being studied. While this is well recognized and applied in reductionist medical research, it is commonly missing in the holistic research of clinical trials. It is now clear that adequate control of important elements of the process of medical care, through application of computerized protocols, is within reach [41,59,83,123–125].

RANDOMIZATION AND DOUBLE BLINDING

The justification for and the superiority of randomized controlled double blinded clinical trials is established [49,50]. While measurements can increase the objectivity of our knowledge, reduce bias and enhance communication, they are associated with errors that can reduce and even destroy their value [50]. Both observational (descriptive) and experimental (interventive) studies contribute measurements. The randomized double blinded trial is the ideal design for an experimental, between group comparison for many important clinical care questions [50,138]. Except for chance maldistributions, randomization eliminates the effect of pre-randomization confounding variables (unintended cointerventions). Double blinding eliminates the effect of post-randomization confounding variables (unintended cointerventions). Double blinding is an essential feature and is as important an element as randomization in the design of experiments that lead to accurate causal inference. Double blinding reduces differential bias between the study groups, even though it has no effect on overall bias [50]. Controlled randomized double blinded trials provide the most credible means of defining what does and what does not work in the clinical setting. Randomized double blind controlled trials are the most scientifically rigorous clinical experiments. A concurrent control group is essential in clinical trials of ARDS. The limitations of historical control observations (see above) seriously compromise the credibility of inferences drawn from comparisons with results from historical control patient groups. The result of the LFPPV-ECCO$_2$R clinical trial [59], like that of the ECMO trial in the 1970s [53], is a potent reminder of the importance of controls in such evaluations. Without a control group, a US survival of LFPPV-ECCO$_2$R patients similar to those reported from Europe would have been reported, and the comparable survival of control patients would have been unknown [59]. Ethical objections to controlled trials of unproven therapies (not supported by credible data) should be viewed with caution. A stronger ethical argument may frequently be mounted in favor of a randomized controlled clinical trial. Such an argument is particularly pertinent in the high technology ICU environment in which information overload is intense.

REDUCING COINTERVENTIONS IN STUDIES THAT CANNOT BE DOUBLE BLINDED

The evaluation of new therapies poses a formidable challenge in ICU medicine. When therapy evaluation cannot be blinded, as in the evaluation of extracorporeal support, the problem becomes more difficult. If a study is only single blinded or is nonblinded, cointerventions due to observer bias cannot be prevented. The computerized protocol control technique of ventilator management, developed for the recent LFPPV-ECCO$_2$R clinical trial, has potential applicability here [59,123,124]. Computerized protocols may play an important role in reducing differential observer bias in single blinded studies or in studies that cannot be blinded [50,78]. Experiments that cannot be double blinded produce less credible results because of the ever present threat of differential bias between study groups. Protocols can standardize care and make clinical decision making more independent of observer or subject judgement. The use of detailed protocols in single blinded or nonblinded experiments may play an important role in reducing differential bias. They will also likely reduce the noise introduced by the clinical caregivers. The signal-to-noise ratio for outcome events will therefore increase (Figure 27.9).

Protocols

Virtually all clinical trials employ protocols. These protocols include definitions, patient selection criteria, procedural rules and guidelines for conduct of the trial. They generally provide some specific instructions, but not enough to adequately control the moment-to-moment process of care. Algorithms usually contain nonspecific, judgment-requiring suggestions like 'optimize PEEP' or 'maximize antibiotic therapy'. While these are useful general statements and concepts, they are not executable instructions. Clinical algorithm texts and other published guidelines contain many such general instructions [139–143].

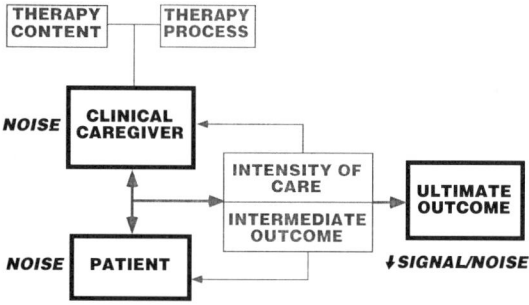

Figure 27.9 The reduction in noise from the clinical caregiver resulting from computerized protocol control of care (medical decision support). Computerized protocols standardize elements of both the content and the process of care given by the clinical caregiver. This reduces the noise introduced by the clinical caregiver and leads to an increase in the signal-to-noise ratio for the ultimate outcome observed in the clinical trial (the experiment). See Figure 27.3 and text.

While general instructions provide guidelines and are of value for their conceptual content, they fail to standardize therapy. The application of general guidelines is associated with great variation of practice by different clinicians.

Computerized protocols

While it is possible to conceive of paper based, protocol flow diagrams with the requisite detail to produce fully executable protocols that would lead to identical treatment responses in different clinical centers, this is almost impossible to achieve in practise. Unaided, humans are not capable of providing the persistent commitment to detail and to decision making logic (rules) necessary to effect standardization of care comparable with that achieved by an executable computerized protocol. Computerized protocols eliminate unnecessary variation in clinical care. This standardizes clinical care and imposes control on the clinical care process. This can be expected to reduce noise intro-

duced by the clinical caregiver and thereby increase the signal-to-noise ratio for ultimate clinical outcomes (Figure 27.9). The hectic ICU environment makes it even more difficult. Before one can evaluate the outcome of a particular medical intervention, the intervention must be applied in a uniform manner to comparable patients [49]. Computerized protocols that control medical decision making reduce the noise introduced in the clinical care team response by standardizing care at a level unachievable without computerization [41,83,123,124].

Those who question if a protocol has incorporated the 'right way' to manage a problem, imply that the right way is knowable. In fact, it is probably not possible to choose the right way when developing a specific protocol for a complicated clinical problem with a multi-factorially determined clinical outcome. The right way is generally unknown, and frequently unknowable. It is more likely that there are several defensible and reasonable approaches, no one of which is clearly superior. What is necessary is the choice of one of these reasonable approaches and its consistent clinical use [33,125]. Such an approach standardizes care and provides a basis for comparison with alternative approaches in future randomized trials. This seems to be a reasonable means of iteratively improving therapy and of advancing towards the right way of clinical care. Pursuit of protocol control of clinical care appears to be a desirable and productive medical research and clinical care aim.

Control of the process of medical care appears to be beneficial [144,145]. Computer based clinical decision support systems appear to have a favorable impact on patient outcome [146]. Standardization can avoid vexing problems in very different areas of clinical medicine [147,148]. Computerized protocols have favorable impacts on hospital pharmacy and infectious disease departments [149–154]. Computerized protocol application in both outpatient and inpatient hospital practice has been associated with favorable consequences [150–152,154–165]. They have controlled the intensity of care of patients with ARDS in both treatment groups of a randomized trial [59]. Three benefits follow the use of such specific control of care: precise description of the care of patients; assurance of equal intensity of care; and common intermediate endpoints (e.g. therapy regulated to produce the same Pa_{O_2} and arterial pH). These protocols have, to date, only controlled a small part of the unnecessary variation in critical care. Many unaddressed facets of care are likely to be as effectively controlled as has been mechanical ventilation in ARDS. Since management of mechanical ventilation in severe ARDS is perceived as a complicated and intellectually demanding process, it is likely that many other facets of critical care can be successfully addressed by computerized protocol control.

Patients with ARDS supported with computerized protocols have experienced a higher survival than expected from historical control data [59,71], but there are as yet no data supporting a causal association between computerized protocol use and patient outcome. In fact, from 1987 to 1991 at the LDS Hospital the same unexpectedly high survival was observed in ARDS patients supported with or without protocol control of mechanical ventilation [68]. Computerized protocol control of mechanical ventilation appears feasible, safe and practical (given an appropriate clinical computer infrastructure), but its impact on patient outcome remains to be explored. Other randomized clinical trials, using less detailed and manually applied protocols, have demonstrated clearly that protocol controlled care favorably affects the outcome of patients with thromboembolic disease [166–168].

This elimination of variation in medical care can be viewed as part of a widespread movement in human behavior. The elimination of unnecessary variation in industry has been the foundation of the widely acclaimed

process of continuous quality improvement [169] based largely on statistical considerations developed at the Bell Telephone Laboratories in the 1930s [93]. While this has not been subjected to experimental verification in an interventional study, these principles are generally accepted throughout industry. They have been credited with the remarkable economic recovery of Japan after the second world war [170,171].

OUTCOME

Intermediate versus untimate outcome variables

The clinical question addressed will require the choice of appropriate outcome variables. The hypothesis should be tested with the most simple ultimate outcome variable, survival being the common choice for many ARDS studies. Other variables, including intermediate outcome variables, such as Cth, Pa_{O_2}, heart rate etc., should be recorded for three purposes. Firstly, to test the randomization by exploring for nonuniformity of pertinent descriptors such as age, gender, severity of illness and study entry criteria variables. Secondly, to describe the course of the different patient groups during the clinical trial. Thirdly, to examine with exploratory descriptive statistical analysis the relationship of variables to the ultimate outcome and identify possible hypotheses for future testing.

Intermediate variables are not definitive indicators of ultimate patient outcome (Figure 27.3). Ultimate oucomes such as long term survival and functional state should be the most important determinants in most clinical situations [50]. Nevertheless, intermediate outcomes, frequently therapeutic endpoints, such as Pa_{O_2}, Cth, frequency of premature ventricular contractions, etc., are commonly used to assess interventions because they are more easily assessed than are ultimate outcomes. Such intermediate outcome variables are, however, frequently poorly reflective of the ultimate outcome. The recent cardiac arryhthmia suppression trial results on post-myocardial infarction are a striking example of how misleading intermediate outcome variables can be. Patients with effective pharmacologic suppression of premature ventricular contractions had a higher death rate than that experienced by the placebo group [97,98,100].

SUMMARY

This field is in dire need of well controlled, randomized clinical trials [172,173]. A specific definition of ARDS and the application of specific and well articulated rules for enrolling patients in clinical trials will enhance the external validity (generalizability) of study results [50]. While randomization of carefully identified and selected patients will probably resolve the problem of uneven representation of important variables in the treatment arms of the clinical trial up to the point of randomization, control of such unevenness after randomization depends upon double blinding [50]. Unfortunately, double blinding the therapies being evaluated is not possible for many of the treatments of interest (e.g. PCIRV, LFPPV-ECCO$_2$R) and this threatens the internal validity of the clinical trial [50]. The use of computerized protocols has enabled workers at the LDS Hospital to reduce variability in the mechanical ventilation therapy of patients with ARDS in a clinical trial that could not be blinded [59,123,124]. While this approach seems promising, data concerning the transferability of such protocols to other medical centers, and data concerning the impact of protocol control of care on patient outcome, are not yet available. My colleagues and I are conducting a clinical trial in independent hospitals to address these two important issues. There are, however, many improvements that can be made at present. The recognition that progress in our understanding of the management of ARDS will probably depend on the

performance of well controlled randomized clinical trials is a necessary first step.

ACKNOWLEDGEMENTS

Supported by the NIH (HL36787), the Deseret Foundation, the Respiratory Distress Syndrome Foundation, the LDS Hospital and IHC, Inc.

REFERENCES

1. Moser, M., Herebert, P. and Hennekens, C. (1991) An overview of the meta-analysis of the hypertension treatment trials. *Arch. Intern. Med.*, **151**, 1277–9.
2. Groeger, J., Strosberg, M., Halpern, N. *et al.* (1992) Descriptive analysis of critical care units in the United States. *Crit. Care Med.*, **20**, 846–63.
3. Ontario Intensive Care Study Group (1992) Evaluation of right heart catheterization in critically ill patients. *Crit. Care Med.*, **20**, 928–33.
4. Bachofen, M. and Weibel, E.R. (1977) Alterations of the gas exchange apparatus in adult respiratory insufficiency associated with septicemia. *Am. Rev. Respir. Dis.*, **116**, 589–615.
5. Tomashefski, J.F.J., Davies, P., Boggis, C., *et al.* (1983) The pulmonary vascular lesions of the adult respiratory distress syndrome. *Am. J. Pathol.*, **112**, 112–26.
6. Rinaldo, J. and Rogers, R. (1982) Adult respiratory distress syndrome – changing concepts of lung injury and repair. *N. Engl. J. Med.*, **306**, 900–9.
7. Mason, R. (1985) Pulmonary alveolar type II epithelial cells and adult respiratory distress syndrome. *West. J. Med.*, **143**, 611–5.
8. Pepe, P.E. (1986) The clinical entity of adult respiratory distress syndrome. *Crit. Care Clin.*, **2**, 377–403.
9. Maunder, R.J. and Hudson, L.D. (1991) Clinical risks associated with the adult respiratory distress syndrome, in *Adult Respiratory Distress Syndrome*, (eds W.M. Zapol and F. LeMaire), Marcel Dekker, New York, pp. 1–21.
10. Suter, P.M., Suter, S., Girardin, E. *et al.* (1992) High bronchoalveolar levels of tumor necrosis factor and its inhibitors, interleukin-1, interferon, and elastase, in patients with adult

respiratory distress syndrome after trauma, shock, or sepsis. *Am. Rev. Respir. Dis.* **145**, 1016–22.

11. Lamy, M., Deby-Dupont, G., Deby, D. *et al.* (1992) Why is our present therapy for adult respiratory distress syndrome so ineffective? *Intensive Crit. Care Dig.* **11**, 6–12.

12. Kawano, T., Mori, S., Cybulsky, M. *et al.* (1987) Effect of granulocyte depletion in a ventilated surfactant-depleted lung. *J. Appl. Physiol.*, **62**, 27–33.

13. Martin, R.R., Pistorese, B.P., Hudson, L.D. and Maunder, R.J. (1991) The function of lung and blood neutrophils in patients with the adult respiratory distress syndrome. *Am. Rev. Respir. Dis.*, **144**, 254–62.

14. Roten, R., Markert, M., Feihl, F. *et al.* (1991) Plasma levels of tumor necrosis factor in the adult respiratory distress syndrome. *Am. Rev. Respir. Dis.*, **143**, 590–2.

15. Fahey, T.J., Tracey, K.J. and Cerami, A. (1992) Tumor necrosis factor (cachectin) and the adult respiratory distress syndrome, in *Update: Pulmonary Diseases and Disorders*, (ed. A. Fishman), McGraw-Hill, New York, 175–83.

16. Romaschin, A.D., DeMajo, W.C., Winton, T. *et al.* (1992) Systemic phospholipase A_2 and cachectin levels in adult respiratory distress syndrome and multiple-organ failure. *Clin. Biochem.*, **25**, 55–60.

17. Stephenson, A.H., Lonigro, A.J., Hyers, T.M. *et al.* (1988) Increased concentrations of leukotrienes in bronchoalveolar lavage fluid of patients with ARDS or at risk for ARDS. *Am. Rev. Respir. Dis.*, **138**, 714–9.

18. Antonelli, M., Lenti, L., Bufi, M. *et al.* (1989) Differential evaluation of bronchoalveolar lavage cells and leukotrienes in unilateral acute lung injury and ARDS patients. *Intensive Care Med.*, **15**, 439–45.

19. Ratnoff, W.D., Matthay, M.A., Wong, M.Y.S. *et al.* (1988) Sulfidopeptide-leukotriene peptidases in pulmonary edema fluid from patients with the adult respiratory distress syndrome. *J. Clin. Immunol.*, **8**, 250–8.

20. Bernard, G.R., Korley, M.V., Chee, P. *et al.* (1991) Persistent generation of peptido leukotrienes in patients with the adult respiratory distress syndrome. *Am. Rev. Respir. Dis.*, **144**, 262–7.

21. Light, R.B. (1988) Intrapulmonary oxygen consumption in experimental pneumococcal pneumonia. *J. Appl. Physiol.*, **64**, 2490–5.

22. Hoffmann, B., Böhm, S., Morris, A. *et al.* (1991) *In vivo* demonstration of the Haldane effect during extracorporeal gas exchange. *Int. J. Artif. Organs*, **14**, 703–6.

23. Simms, H.H. and D'Amico, R. (1991) Increased PMN CD11b/CD18 expression following post-traumatic ARDS. *J. Surg. Res.*, **50**, 362–7.

24. Rubin, D.B., Wiener-Kronish, J.P., Murray, J.F. *et al.* (1990) Elevated von Willebrand factor antigen is an early plasma predictor of acute lung injury in nonpulmonary sepsis syndrome. *J. Clin. Invest.*, **86**, 474–80.

25. Matthay, M.A., Newman, W., Beall, D. *et al.* (1992) Elevated levels of circulating ELAM–1 in the plasma of patients with sepsis syndrome. *Am. Rev. Respir Dis.*, **145**, A452.

26. Murray, J., Matthay, M., Luce, J. and Flick, M. (1988) An expanded definition of the adult respiratory distress syndrome. *Am. Rev. Respir. Dis.*, **138**, 720–3.

27. Kraus, P., Lipman, J., Lee, C. *et al.* (1993) Acute lung injury at Baragwanath ICU. *Chest*, **103** 1832–6.

28. Petty, T., Bone, R., Gee, M. *et al.* (1992) Contemporary clinical trials in acute respiratory distress syndrome. *Chest*, **101**, 550–2.

29. Bernard, G., Artigas, A., Brigham, K. *et al.* (1994) The American–European consensus conference on ARDS: definitions, mechanisms, relevant outcomes and clinical trial coordination. *Am. J. Respir. Crit. Care Med.*, **149**, 818–24.

30. Bernard, G., Artigas, A., Brigham, K. *et al.* (1994) Report of the American–European consensus conference on acute respiratory distress syndrome: definitions, mechanisms, relevant outcomes and clinical trial coordination. *J. Crit. Care*, **9**, 72–81.

31. Glauser, F., Polatty, R. and Sessler, C. (1988) Worsening oxygenation in the mechanically ventilated patient. *Am. Rev. Respir. Dis.*, **138**, 458–65.

32. Marini, J.J. (1993) Mechanical ventilation and newer ventilatory techniques, in *Pulmonary and Critical Care Medicine* (ed. R.C. Bone), Mosby Year Book, St Louis, R:5:1–23. vol. 2.

33. Morris, A. (1994). ARDS and new modes of mechanical ventilation: reducing the complications of high volume and high pressure. *New Horizons*, **2**, 19–33.

34. Welch, B.E., Morgan, T.E.J. and Clamann, H.G. (1963) Time concentration effects in relation to oxygen toxicity in man. *Fed. Proc.*, **22**, 1053–6.

35. Hyde, R.W. and Rawson, A.J. (1969) Unintentional iatrogenic oxygen pneumonitis – response to therapy. *Ann. Intern. Med.*, **71**, 517–31.

36. Philip, A.G. (1975) Oxygen plus pressure plus time: the etiology of bronchopulmonary dysplasia. *Pediatrics*, **55**, 44–50.

37. Pratt, P.C. (1974) Pathology of pulmonary oxygen toxicity. *Am. Rev. Respir. Dis.*, **110**, 51–7.

38. Witschi, H.P., Haschek, W.M., Klein-Szanto, A.J.P. and Hakkinen P.J. (1981) Potentiation of diffuse lung damage by oxygen: determining variables. *Am. Rev. Respir. Dis.*, **123**, 98–103.

39. Register, S.D., Downs, J.B., Stock, M.C. and Kirby, R.R. (1987) Is 50% oxygen harmful? *Crit. Care Med.*, **15**, 598–601.

40. Morris, A.H. (1991) Use of monitoring information in decision making, in *Respiratory Monitoring* (ed. M.J. Tobin), Churchill Livingstone, New York, pp. 213–29.

41. Morris, A. (1993) Paradigms in management, in *Pathophysiologic Foundations of Critical Care Medicine* (eds M. Pinsky and J. Dhainaut), Williams & Wilkins, Baltimore, pp. 193–206.

42. Perel, A. (1987) Newer ventilation modes – temptations and pitfalls. [Editorial]. *Crit. Care Med.*, **15**, 707–9.

43. Petty, T.L. (1988) ARDS, refinement of a concept and redefinition. *Am. Rev. Respir. Dis.*, **138**, 724.

44. Ayres, S. and Combs, A. (1992) A tale of two intensive care units? All intensive care units are not the same! *Crit. Care Med.*, **20**, 727–8.

45. Rinaldo, J. (1986) The prognosis of the adult respiratory distress syndrome – inappropriate pessimism? [Editorial]. *Chest*, **90**, 470–1.

46. Pontoppidan, H., Wilson, R., Rie, M. and Schnieder, R. (1977) Respiratory intensive care. *Anesthesiology*, **47**, 96–116.

47. Murray, J. (1977) Mechanisms of acute respiratory failure. *Am. Rev. Respir. Dis.*, **115**, 1071–8.

48. Lachin, J.M. (1981) Introduction to sample size determinations and power analysis for clinical trials. *Controlled Clin. Trials*, **2**, 93–113.

49. Pocock, S.J. (1983) *Clinical Trials: A Practical Approach*, Wiley, New York, p. 266.

50. Hulley, S. and Cummings, S. (1988) *Designing Clinical Research*, Williams & Wilkins, Baltimore.

51. Cohen, J. (1988) *Statistical Power Analysis for the Behavioral Sciences*, 2nd edn, Lawrence Erlbaum, Hillsdale, NJ.

52. Lewandowski, K., Slama, K. and Falke, K. (1992) Approaches to improved survival in ARDS, in *Yearbook of Intensive Care and Emergency Medicine* (ed. J-L. Vincent), Springer, Berlin, pp. 372–83.

53. Zapol, W.M., Snider, M.T., Hill, J.D. *et al.* (1979) Extracorporeal membrane oxygenation in severe acute respiratory failure. *JAMA*, **242**, 2193–6.

54. Andersen, J.B. (1987) Inverse I:E ratio ventilation with pressure control in catastrophic lung disease in adults. *Intensive Care Med.*, **4**, 21–2.

55. Andersen, J.B. (1989) Ventilatory strategy in catastrophic lung disease. Inversed ratio ventilation (IRV) and combined high frequency ventilation (CHFV). *Acta Anaesthesiol. Scand.*, **90**, 145–8.

56. Morris, A. (1992) Protocols, ECCO$_2$R, and the evaluation of new therapy. *Jpn. J. Intensive Care Med.*, **16**, 61–3.

57. Zapol, W.M., Frikker, M.J., Pontoppidan, H. *et al.* (1991) The adult respiratory distress syndrome at Massachusetts General Hospital, etiology progession and survival rates, 1978–1988, in *Adult Respiratory Distress Syndrome* (eds W. Zapol and F. Lemaire), Marcel Dekker, New York, pp. 367–80.

58. Rollins, R., Morris, A., Mortensen, C. and Cipriano, P. (1986) Arterial hypoxemia in 1985 predicts a mortality identical to that in 1975. *Clin. Res.*, **34**, 79A.

59. Morris, A., Wallace, C., Menlove, R. *et al.* (1994) A randomized clinical trial of pressure-controlled inverse ratio ventilation and extracorporeal CO$_2$ removal for ARDS. *Am. J. Respir. Crit. Care Med.*, **149**, 295–305.

60. Bartlett, R.H., Morris, A.H., Fairley, H.B. *et al.* (1986) A prospective study of acute hypoxic respiratory failure. *Chest*, **89**, 684–9.

61. Artigas, A., Carlet, J., Le Gall, J. *et al.* (1991) Clinical presentation, prognostic factors, and outcome of ARDS in the European collaborative study (1985–1987): a preliminary report, in *Adult Respiratory Distress Syndrome* (eds W. Zapol and F. Lemaire), Marcel Dekker, New York, pp. 37–63.

62. Rinaldo, J. (1986) Indicators of risk, course, and prognosis in adult respiratory distress syndrome. *Am. Rev. Respir. Dis.*, **133**, 343 (letter).

63. Bell, R.C., Coalson, J., Smith, J. and Johanson, W. (1983) Multiple organ system failure and infection in adult respiratory distress syndrome. *Ann. Intern. Med.*, **99**, 293–8.

64. Montgomery, A.B., Stager, M., Carrico, C., and Hudson, L. (1985) Causes of mortality in patients with adult respiratory distress syndrome. *Am. Rev. Respir. Dis.*, **132**, 485–9.

65. Fowler, A., Hamman, R., Zerbe, G. *et al.* (1985) Adult respiratory distress syndrome: prognosis after onset. *Am. Rev. Respir. Dis.*, **132**, 472–8.

66. Artigas, A. (1988) Adult respiratory distress syndrome: changing concepts of clinical evolution and recover, in *Update in Intensive Care and Emergency Medicine 5* (ed. J. Vincent), Springer, Berlin, pp. 97–114.

67. Kolobow, T. (1988) An update on adult extracorporeal membrane oxygenation – extracorporeal CO_2 removal. *Trans. Am. Soc. Artif. Intern. Organs*, **34**, 1004–5.

68. Suchyta, M.R., Clemmer, T.P., Orme, J.F. *et al.* (1991) Increased survival of ARDS patients with severe hypoxemia (ECMO criteria). *Chest*, **99**, 951–5.

69. Hickling, K. (1992) Low volume ventilation with permissive hypercapnia in the adult respiratory distress syndrome. *Clin. Intensive Care 3*, 67–78.

70. Rossaint, R., Falke, K., Lopez, F. *et al.* (1993) Inhaled nitric oxide for the adult respiratory distress syndrome. *N. Engl. J. Med.*, **328**, 399–405.

71. Morris, A.H., Wallace, C.J., Clemmer, T.P. *et al.* (1992) Final report: computerized protocol-controlled clinical trial of new therapy which includes $ECCO_2R$ for ARDS. *Am. Rev. Respir. Dis.*, **145**, A184.

72. Shapiro, B. (1992) New ventilator technology: impact on patient care, in *Critical Care – State of the Art*, vol. 3, (eds R. Carlson and H. Reines), Society of Critical Care Medicine, Anaheim, CA, pp. 17–45.

73. East, T. (1993) The magic bullets in the war on ARDS: aggressive therapy for oxygenation failure. *Respir. Care*, **38**, 690–702.

74. Natanson, C., Hofman, W., Suffredini, A. *et al.* (1994) Selected treatment strategies for septic shock based on proposed mechanisms of pathogenesis. *Ann. Intern. Med.*, **120**, 771–83.

75. National Heart and Lung Institute (1974) *Protocol for Extracorporeal Support for Respiratory Insufficiency Collaborative Program*, NHLI, Division of Lung Diseases, Bethesda, MD.

76. Marini, J.J. and Kelsen, S.G. (1992) Re-targeting ventilatory objectives in adult respiratory distress syndrome [Editorial.] *Am. Rev. Respir. Dis.*, **146**, 2–3.

77. Marcy, T.W. and Marini, J.J. (1992) Modes of mechanical ventilation, in *Current Pulmonology*, vol. 13, (eds D.H. Simmons and D.F. Tierney), Mosby Year Book, St Louis, pp. 43–90.

78. Guyatt, G., Drummond, M., Feeny, D. *et al.* (1986) Guidelines for the clinical and economic evaluation of health care technologies. *Soc. Sci. Med.*, **22**, 393–408.

79. Kaczmarek, R.M. and Hess, D. (1990) Pressure-controlled inverse-ratio ventilation, panacea or auto-PEEP? *Respir. Care*, **35**, 945–8.

80. Garner, W., Downs, J.B., Stock, M.C. and Räsänen, J. (1988) Airway pressure release ventilation (APRV): a human trial. *Chest*, **94**, 779–81.

81. Boehm, S., Peng, L., East, T. *et al.* (1990) Computerized protocol management of pressure control inverse ratio ventilation. *Chest*, **98**, 77S (abstract).

82. East, T.D., Böhm, S.H., Wallace, C.J. *et al.* (1992) A successful computerized protocol for clinical management of pressure control inverse ratio ventilation in ARDS patients. *Chest*, **101**, 697–710.

83. Morris, A. and Gardner, R. (1992) Computer applications, in *Principles of Critical Care* (eds J. Hall, G. Schmidt and L. Wood, McGraw-Hill, New York, pp. 500–14.

84. Miller, G. (1956) The magical number seven, plus or minus two: some limits on our capacity for processing information. *Psychol. Rev.*, **63**, 81–97.

85. Miller, J. (1978) *Living Systems*, McGraw-Hill, New York.

86. Miller, J. and Miller, J. (1990) Introduction: the nature of living systems. *Behav. Sci.*, **35**, 157–63.

87. Jennings, D., Amabile, T. and Ross, L. (1982) Informal covariation assessment: data-based versus theory-based judgments, in *Judgment under Uncertainty: Heuristics and Biases* (eds D. Kahnenan, P. Slovic and A. Tversby), Cam-

bridge University Press, Cambridge, pp. 211–230.

88. National Heart, Lung, and Blood Institute. (1979) *Extracorporeal Support for Respiratory Insufficiency: A Collaborative Study in Response to RFP-NHLI-73–20, Appendices 9 and 10*, US Department of Health, Education and Welfare, National Institutes of Health, Bethesda, pp. 305–370.

89. National Heart, Lung, and Blood Institute. (1979) *Extracorporeal Support for Respiratory Insufficiency: A Collaborative Study in Response to RFP-NHLI-73–20*, US Department of Health, Education and Welfare, National Institutes of Health, Bethesda, p. 390.

90. Jonsen, A., Siegler, M. and Winslade, W. (1986) *Clinical Ethics*, 2nd edn, Macmillan, New York.

91. Morris, W. (ed.) (1979) *The American Heritage Dictionary of the English Language*, Houghton Mifflin, Boston, p. 123.

92. Flexner, S. (ed.) (1987) *The Random House Dictionary of the English Language*, 2nd edn, Random House, New York, pp. 193–4.

93. Shewart, W. (1931) *Economic Control of Quality of Manufactured Product*, Van Nostrand, New York. (Republished (1980) by American Society for Quality Control, 230 W. Wells St, Milwaukee, WI 53203.)

94. Truog, R. (1992) Randomized clinical trials: lessons from ECMO. *Clin. Res.*, **40**, 519–27.

95. Moline, J. (1986) Professionals and professions: a philosophical examination of an ideal. *Soc. Sci. Med.*, **22**, 501–8.

96. Meinert, C. (1990) Extracorporeal membrane oxygenation trials. *Pediatrics*, **85**, 365–366.

97. Cardiac Arrhythmia Suppression Trial (CAST) Investigators. (1989) Preliminary report: effect of encainide and flecainide on mortality in a randomized trial of arrhythmia suppression after myocardial infarction. *N. Engl. J. Med.*, **321**, 406–12.

98. Pratt, C., Brater, D., Harrell, F. Jr *et al.* (1990) Clinical and regulatory implications of the Cardiac Arrhythmia Suppression Trial [Editorial.] *Am. J. Cardiol.*, **65**, 103–5.

99. Passamani, E. (1991) Clinical trials – are they ethical? *N. Engl. J. Med.*, **324**, 1589–91.

100. Cardiac Arrhythmia Suppression Trial II Investigators. (1992) Effect of the antiarrhythmic agent moricizine on survival after myocardial infarction. *N. Engl. J. Med.*, **327**, 227–33.

101. Greene, H., Roden, D., Katz, R. *et al.* (1992) The Cardiac Arrythmia Suppression Trial: first CAST . . . then CAST-II. *J. Am. Coll. Cardiol.*, **19**, 894–8.

102. Clyne, C., Estes, N.I. and Wang, P. (1992) Moricizine. *N. Engl. J. Med.*, **327**, 255–60.

103. Silverman, W. (1985) *Human Experimentation: A Guided Step into the Unknown*, Oxford University Press, Oxford.

104. O'Rourke, P. and Crone, R. (1990) Pediatric applications of extracorporeal membrane oxygenation Editorial *J. Pediatr.*, **116**, 393–4.

105. Levine, R. (1988) *Ethics and Regulation of Clinical Research*, 2nd edn, Yale University Press, New Haven.

106. Chalmers, I. (1986) Minimizing harm and maximizing benefit during innovation in health care: controlled or uncontrolled experimentation? *Birth*, **13**, 155–64.

107. Chalmers, T. (1990) A belated randomized controlled trial. *Pediatrics*, **85**, 366–9.

108. Beyth-Marom, R. and Dekel, S. (1985) *An Elementary Approach to Thinking Under Uncertainty*, Lawrence Erlbaum, Hillsdale, NJ, p. 154.

109. Hirsch, E. (1987) *Cultural Literacy*, Houghton Mifflin, Boston, p. 251.

110. Morris, A. (1994) Uncertainty in the management of ARDS: lessons for the evaluation of a new therapy. [Editorial.] *Intensive Care Med.*, **20**, 87–9.

111. Mandelbrot, B. (1983) *The Fractal Geometry of Nature*, W.H. Freeman, New York, p. 468.

112. Engel, G. (1977) The need for a new medical model: a challenge for biomedicine. *Science*, **196**, 129–36.

113. Foss, L. and Rothenberg, K. (1988) *The Second Medical Revolution*, New Science Library, Shambhala, Boston.

114. Feinstein, A. (1994) *Clinical Judgment* revisited: the distraction of quantitative models. *Ann. Intern. Med.*, **120**, 799–805.

115. Atkins, H. (1958) The three pillars of clinical research. *BMJ*, **27 Dec.**, 1547–53.

116. Kuhn, T. (1970) The structure of scientific revolutions, in *International Encyclopedia of Unified Science*, 2nd edn, vol. 2, no. 2, University of Chicago Press, Chicago.

117. Hoyningen-Huene, P. (1993) *Reconstructing Scientific Revolutions: Thomas S. Kuhn's Philosophy of Science*, University of Chicago Press, Chicago.

118. Tversky, A. and Kahneman, D. Availability: a heuristic for judging frequency and probability, in *Judgment Under Uncertainty: Heuristics and Biases* (eds D. Kahneman, P. Slovic and A. Tversky), Cambridge University Press, Cambridge, pp. 163–78.

119. Morris, A., Gardner, R. and East, T. (1995) Clinical applications of computers in monitoring, in *Acute Care Monitoring* (eds R. Levine, R. Fromm and A. Davies), Mosby Year Book, St Louis, pp. 413–41.

120. Gardner, R., Hawley, W., East, T. *et al.* (1992) Real time data acquisition: recommendations for the Medical Information Bus (MIB). *Int. J. Clin. Monit. Comput.*, **8**, 251–8.

121. Oniki, T. and Gardner, R. (1993) Computerized detection of arterial oxygen desaturation in an intensive care unit, in *Proceedings of the 17th Annual Symposium on Computer Applications in Medical Care (SCAMC)*, October 30–November 3, 1993, McGraw-Hill, Washington, pp. 356–360.

122. Whitney, C. and Von Korff, M. (1992) Regression to the mean in treated versus untreated chronic pain. *Pain*, **50**, 281–5.

123. Henderson, S., Crapo, R., Wallace, C. *et al.* (1992) Performance of computerized protocols for the management of arterial oxygenation in an intensive care unit. *Int. J. Clin. Monit. Comput.*, **8**, 271–80.

124. East, T., Morris, A., Wallace, C. *et al.* (1992) A strategy for development of computerized critical care decision support systems. *Int. J. Clin. Monit. Comput.*, **8**, 263–9.

125. Morris, A. (1993) Protocol management of ARDS. *New Horizons*, **1**, 593–602.

126. Anderson, C. (1994) Measuring what works in health care. *Science*, **263**, 1080–3.

127. Kasssirer, J. (1993) The quality of care and the quality of measuring it. *N. Engl. J. Med.*, **329**, 1263–5.

128. Tanenbaum, S. (1993) What physicians know. *N. Engl. J. Med.*, **329**, 1268–71.

129. Vecchio, T. (1966) Predictive value of a single diagnostic test in unselected populations. *N. Engl. J. Med.*, **274**, 1171–3.

130. Komaroff, A. and Berwick, D. (1980) Decision theory and medical practice, *Harrison's Principles of Internal Medicine*, vol. Update IV (eds K. Isselbacher, R. Adams, E. Braunwald *et al.*), McGraw-Hill, New York, pp. 243–4.

131. Griner, P., Mayewski, R., Mushlin, A. and Greenland, P. (1981) Selection and interpretation of diagnostic tests and procedures. *Ann. Intern. Med.*, **94**, 553–600.

132. Feinstein, A. (1977) *Clinical Biostatistics*, C.V. Mosby, St Louis.

133. Browner, W. and Newman, T. (1987) The analogy between diagnostic tests and clinical research. *JAMA*, **257** 2459–63.

134. Diamond, G. and Forrester, J. (1983) Clinical trials and statistical verdicts: probable grounds for appeal. *Ann. Intern. Med.*, **98**, 385–94.

135. Fleiss, J. (1981) *Statistical Methods for Rates and Proportions*, Wiley, New York.

136. Kaczmarek, R.M. and Hickling, K. (1993) Permissive hypercapnea. *Respir. Care*, **38**, 373–87.

137. Hickling, K.G. (1990) Ventilatory management of ARDS: can it affect the outcome? *Intensive Care Med.*, **16**, 219–26.

138. Levine, M. (1992) Reader's guide for causation: Was a comparison group for those at risk clearly identified? *ACP J. Club*, **January/February**, A12–3.

139. Don, H. (ed.) (1985) *Decision Making in Critical Care*, B.C. Decker, Philadelphia.

140. Karlinsky, J., Lau, J. and Goldstein, R. (1991) *Decision Making in Pulmonary Medicine*, B.C. Decker, Philadelphia.

141. Armstrong, R., Bullen, C., Cohen, S. *et al.* (1991) *Critical Care Algorithms*, Oxford University Press, New York, p. 100.

142. Boutros, A.R., Hoyt, J.L., Boyd, W.C. and Harford, C.E. (1977) Algorithm for management of pulmonary complications in burn patients. *Crit. Care Med.*, **5**, 89.

143. Guidelines Committee Society of Critical Care Medicine. (1992) Guidelines for the care of patients with hemodynamic instability associated with sepsis. *Crit. Care Med.*, **20**, 1057–9.

144. Wirtschafter, D.D., Scalise, M., Henke, C. and Gams, R.A. (1981) Do information systems improve the quality of clinical research? Results of a randomized trial in a cooperative multi-institutional cancer group. *Comput. Biomed. Res.*, **14**, 78–90.

145. Dawes, R., Faust, D. and Meehl, P. (1989) Clinical versus actuarial judgement. *Science*, **243**, 1668–74.

146. Johnston, M., Langton, K., Haynes, B. and Mathieu, A. (1994) Effects of computer-based

clinical decision support systems on clinician performance and patient outcome. *Ann. Intern. Med.*, **120**, 135–42.

147. Leiner, G., Abramowitz, S. and Small, M. (1969) Pulmonary function testing in laboratories associated with residency training programs in pulmonary diseases. *Am. Rev. Respir. Dis.*, **100**, 240–4.

148. Hirsh, J. (1991) Oral anticoagulant drugs. *N. Engl. J. Med.*, **324**, 1865–75.

149. Gardner, R.M., Hulse, R.K. and Larsen, K.G. (1990) Assessing the effectiveness of a computerized pharmacy system, in *Proceedings of the 14th Annual Symposium on Computer Applications in Medical Care*, Baltimore, IEEE Computer Society Press, Los Alamitos, CA, pp. 668–72.

150. Evans, R.S., Burke, J.P., Pestotnik, S.L. *et al.* (1990) Prediction of hospital infections and selection of antibiotics using an automated hospital database, in *Proceedings of the 14th Annual Symposium on Computer Applications in Medical Care*, Baltimore, IEEE Computer Society Press, Los Alamitos, CA, pp. 663–67.

151. Evans, R.S., Pestotnik, S.L., Burke, J.P. *et al.* (1990) Reducing the duration of prophylactic antibiotics use through computer monitoring of surgical patients. *Ann. Pharmacother.*, **24**, 351–4.

152. Classen, D.C., Pestotnik, S.L., Evans, R.S. and Burke, J.P. (1991) Computerized surveillance of adverse drug events in hospital patients. *JAMA*, **266**, 2847–51.

153. Classen, D.C., Evans, R.S., Pestotnik, S.L. *et al.* (1992) The timing of prophylactic administration of antibiotics and the risk of surgical-wound infection. *N. Engl. J. Med.*, **326**, 281–6.

154. Evans, R., Pestotnik, S., Classen, D. *et al.* (1992) Prevention of adverse drug events through computerized surveillance, in *Proceedings of the 16th Annual Symposium on Computer Applications in Medical Care*, Baltimore, IEEE Computer Soc Press, Los Alamitos, CA, pp. 437–41.

155. McDonald, C.J. (1976) Protocol-based computer reminders, the quality of care and the non-perfectability of man. *N. Engl. J. Med.*, **295**, 1351–5.

156. McDonald, C.J. (1976) Use of a computer to detect and respond to clinical events: its effect on clinician behavior. *Ann. Intern. Med.*, **84**, 162–7.

157. McDonald, C., Wilson, G. and McCabe, G. Jr (1980) Physician response to computer reminders. *JAMA*, **244**, 1579–81.

158. Tierney, W., McDonald, C., Martin, D. *et al.* (1987) Computerized display of past test results. *Ann. Intern. Med.*, **107**, 569–74.

159. McDonald, C. and Tierney, W. (1988) Computer-stored medical records: their future role in medical practice. *JAMA*, **259**, 3433–40.

160. Tierney, W., McDonald, C., Hui, S. and Martin, D. (1988) Computer predictions of abnormal test results: effects on outpatient testing. *JAMA*, **259**, 1194–8.

161. Tierney, W., Miller, M. and McDonald, C. (1990) The effect on test ordering of informing physicians of the charges for outpatient diagnostic tests. *N. Engl. J. Med.*, **322**, 1499–504.

162. Tierney, W., Miller, M., Overhage, J. and McDonald, C. (1993) Physician inpatient order writing on microcomputer work stations. *JAMA*, **269**, 379–83.

163. Pestotnik, S.L., Evans, R.S., Burke, J.P. *et al.* (1990) Development of a computerized infectious disease monitor (CIDM). *Comput. Biomed. Res.*, **18**, 103–13.

164. Evans, R.S., Burke, J.P., Classen, D.C. *et al.* (1992) Computerized identification of patients at high risk of hospital-acquired infection. *Am. J. Infect. Control*, **20**, 4–10.

165. Classen, D.C., Pestotnik, S.L., Evans, R.S. and Burke, J.P. (1992) Intensive surveillance of midazolam use in hospitalized patients and the occurrence of cardiorespiratory arrest. *Pharmacotherapy*, **12**, 213–6.

166. Hull, R.D., Raskob, G.E. and Rosenbloom, D. (1990) Heparin for 5 days as compared with 10 days in the initial treatment of proximal venous thrombosis. *N. Engl. J. Med.*, **322**, 1260–4.

167. Cruikshank, M.K., Levine, M.H., Hirsh, J. *et al.* (1991) A standard heparin nomogram for the management of heparin therapy. *Arch. Intern. Med.*, **151**, 333–8.

168. Hull, R.D., Raskob, G.E., Rosenbloom, D. *et al.* (1992) Optimal therapeutic level of heparin therapy in patients with venous thrombosis. *Arch. Intern. Med.*, **152**, 1589–95.

169. Deming, W. (1986) *Out of the Crisis*, Massachusetts Institute of Technology, Center for Advanced Engineering Study, Cambridge, MA.

170. Imai, M. (1986) *Kaizen – The key to Japan's*

Competitive Success, McGraw-Hill, New York, p. 259.

171. Walton, M. (1986) *The Deming Management Method*, Putnam, New York.

172. Morris, A. (1989) Randomized clinical trials urged in critical care medicine. [Editorial.] *Contemp. Intern. Med.*, **9**, 9–10.

173. Morris, A. (1991) Randomized clinical trials. [Editorial.] *Trans. Am. Soc. Artif. Intern. Organs*, **37**, 41–2.

PART FIVE

THERAPEUTIC INTERVENTIONS

FLUID BALANCE AND RENAL FUNCTION

Phillip Factor, David Ciccolella and Jacob I. Sznajder

Acute hypoxemic respiratory failure can be a consequence of alveolar edema accumulation due either to increased pulmonary capillary hydrostatic pressure, as in congestive heart failure, or through increased alveolar capillary permeability, as in the syndrome of acute respiratory distress in adults (ARDS) [1,2]. Increased capillary permeability allows extravasation of plasma constituents into the interstitial space. The interstitium is a compliant compartment normally able to accommodate large amounts of fluid. However, when it is overwhelmed, fluid spills into the alveolar air spaces [3]. Extravascular lung water must increase by at least 20% before alveolar flooding occurs [4]. The etiology of ARDS remains unknown, but in several large studies sepsis, gastric acid aspiration, trauma and blood product transfusion following trauma accounted for most cases of [5].

Katzenstein and coworkers have proposed a pathologic model of acute lung injury termed diffuse alveolar damage, composed of two sequential phases (Figure 28.1), which is applicable to the many conditions associated with acute lung injury [6]. During the initial exudative phase (usually lasting for 1–3 days), proteinaceous fluid accumulates in the interstitial and alveolar air spaces. This is characterized by inhomogeneous ultrastructural changes that include denudation of the alveolar basement membrane, formation of hyaline membranes, widening of intercellular junctions and increased alveolar-capillary permeability (Chapter 4). During the late exudative phase there is progressive thickening of the alveolar interstitium, heralding the onset of a subsequent proliferative phase [7]. Clinically the exudative phase is characterized by 'leaky' capillaries and progressive edema accumulation. Thus we postulate that therapeutic strategies designed to reduce edema formation (see below) should have the greatest impact during the early exudative phase when the alveolus is 'leaky'.

The exudative phase may be followed by proliferation of interstitial components (i.e. myoblasts and fibroblasts) and alveolar type II cells. This proliferative phase results in thickening of the alveolar wall with deposition of collagenous/fibrous material in the interstitial space. The factors contributing to the development of fibrosis are not completely understood, although growth factors produced by platelets, macrophages and fibroblasts (e.g. platelet derived growth factor, keratinocyte growth factor, fibroblast growth factor, epidermal growth factor, transforming growth factor and hepatocyte growth factor) have been implicated [7]. For normal lung repair, the restoration of extracellular matrix and connective tissues and the controlled replication of fibroblasts are critical. If these steps do not occur, hyperplasia of type II pneumo-

ARDS Acute Respiratory Distress in Adults. Edited by Timothy W. Evans and Christopher Haslett. Published in 1996 by Chapman & Hall, London. ISBN 0 412 56910 8

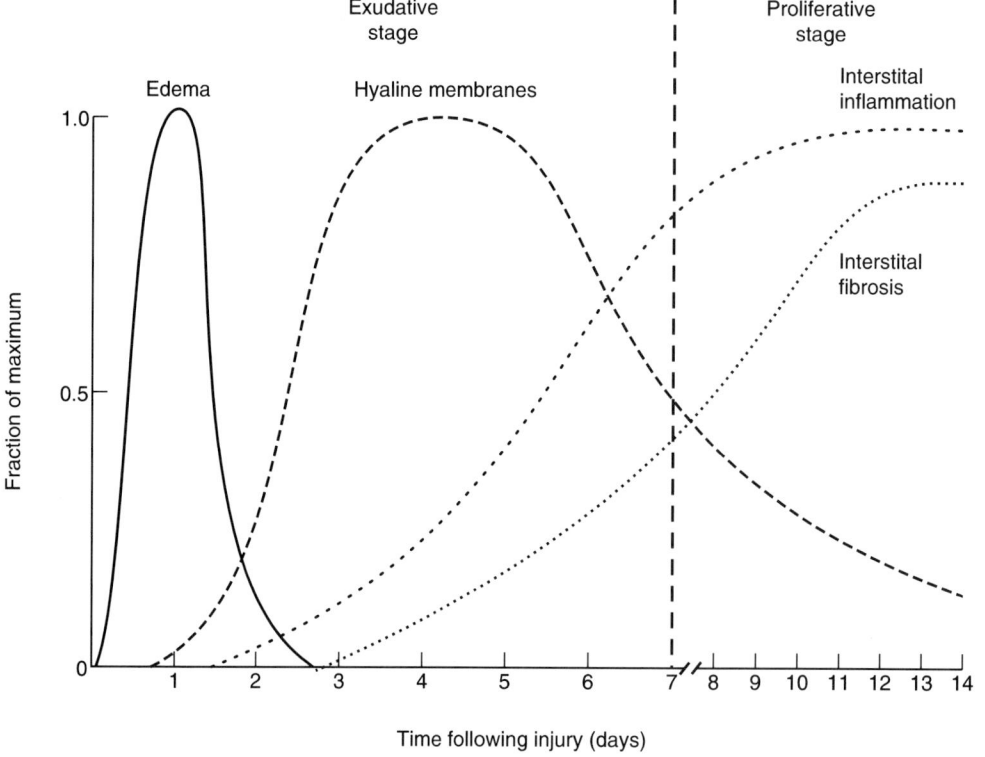

Figure 28.1 Time course of diffuse alveolar damage. The initial, exudative, phase is characterized by alveolar edema accumulation and formation of hyaline membranes. The subsequent exudative phase is typified by interstitial inflammation and collagen deposition. (Reproduced from Katzenstein, A. and Askin, F.B. (1982) *Surgical Pathology of Non-Neoplastic Lung Disease*, W.B. Saunders, Philadelphia.)

cytes and an abnormal proliferation of interstitial cells, including fibroblasts, occurs. If healing is disordered, intravascular coagulation, chemotaxins and proinflammatory agents may amplify this anomalous repair, with deposition of abnormal interstitial collagen and distortion of alveolar architecture [7]. While resolution of the lung injury may still occur, there is a risk of progression to severe fibrosis. In such cases pulmonary hypertension and a large dead space fraction develop, minute ventilation requirements are high, and there is intrapulmonary shunt which is poorly responsive to therapeutic interventions [2]. As the alveolar septae during the proliferative phase of ARDS are no longer leaky, these patients typically do not respond

to positive end expiratory presure (PEEP) or reductions in pulmonary hydrostatic pressure.

MECHANISMS OF PULMONARY EDEMA ACCUMULATION AND CLEARANCE

LUNG EDEMA ACCUMULATION

When alveolar-capillary permeability is normal, the lung is relatively resistant to the accumulation of alveolar edema, even at elevated hydrostatic pressures [4]. In the presence of pulmonary capillary leak, lung edema can develop at low pulmonary microvascular pressures. The forces governing alveolar fluid movement across semipermeable membranes are summarized in the Starling equation (Chapter 20):

$$\text{edema flux} = K_f[(P_{mv} - P_{is}) - \sigma(\pi_{mv} - \pi_{is})],$$

where K_f is the capillary filtration coefficient for fluid across the capillary; P_{mv} and P_{is} are the hydrostatic pressures in the microvessels and interstitium, respectively; σ is the protein reflection coefficient of the membrane, and π_{mv} and π_{is} are the oncotic pressures in the pulmonary vessels and the interstitium. Normally, a positive hydrostatic pressure gradient ($P_{mv} - P_{is}$) tends to move liquid from the circulation to the interstitial space. This is opposed by an oncotic pressure gradient ($\pi_{mv} - \pi_{is}$) that promotes movement of liquid back into the vascular compartment [8]. The net Starling forces favor movement of fluid into the lung interstitium, resulting in net edema accumulation. Lung lymphatics serve a protective role by draining this 'excess' fluid from the interstitium. When this mechanism fails, or is overwhelmed, alveolar edema develops [4,8].

In contrast to high pressure 'cardiogenic' pulmonary edema where P_{mv} is increased and π_{is} reduced (due to interstitial protein washout), the pulmonary hydrostatic pressures in ARDS are low and edema accumulates as a result of increased alveolar capillary permeability. Thus pulmonary edema does not accumulate in normal dogs until left atrial pressure exceeds ~25 Torr (3.3 kPa) [9]. However, when the oncotic pressure is reduced by 50% in normal lungs, edema accumulates at lower left atrial pressures. Normal lungs perfused at a low atrial pressure (5 Torr) (0.7 kPa) gain only small amounts of extravascular lung water over time. During lung injury, in the presence of capillary leak, edema increases moderately with a similarly low left atrial pressure. However, increasing the microvascular pressure moderately (to 10 Torr (1.3 kPa)) results in a significant increase in lung edema accumulation over time (Figure 28.2). During ARDS, damage to pulmonary epithelial and endothelial structures

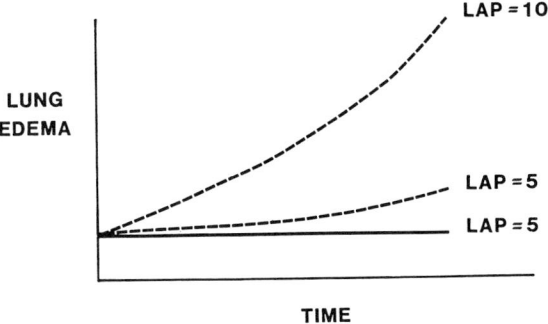

Figure 28.2 At low left atrial pressures (LAP) and normal alveolar permeability no significant increases in extravascular water are observed in isolated dog lungs over time. In the presence of injury, lung edema accumulates, even at a normal LAP of 5 mmHg. If LAP is increased moderately to 10 mmHg edema accumulation increases severalfold over the same period of time.

causes σ to fall towards zero (permeability to proteins increases) and K_f to increase, decreasing the opposing, protective interstitial oncotic gradient that promotes movement of fluid back into the pulmonary vasculature [8]. In this setting, protective mechanisms (lymphatic drainage and active transport mechanisms) are overwhelmed and the air spaces fill with proteinaceous fluid, leading to excessive intrapulmonary shunt and refractory hypoxemia [10].

Recently it has been reported that ultrastructural changes in the pulmonary microvasculature of animals with high pressure pulmonary edema resemble those found in low pressure pulmonary edema [11,12]. These observations suggest that these two models of pulmonary edema accumulation have more in common than previously thought. Thus, their treatment will also have much in common.

LUNG EDEMA CLEARANCE

Pulmonary edema accumulation occurs as a result of hydrostatic and oncotic pressure gradients across the semipermeable alveolar septae [13]. By contrast, removal of alveolar edema is predominantly dependent on osmotic gradients generated by active ion transport [14–16] (Chapter 20). The importance of active Na^+ transport in edema clearance has been demonstrated in live sheep, rabbits, dogs and in normal isolated rat and rabbit lungs [14–17]. Osmotic gradients are generated by the active transport of Na^+ out of cells by Na^+,K^+-ATPases located in the basolateral portion of the cell membrane of alveolar type II epithelial cells [18]. Na^+ enters the cell through amiloride sensitive Na^+ channels that are located on the apical (e.g. air space) surface of alveolar type II cells [19]. Other cell membrane components, such as Na^+,H^+ exchanger, Na^+,Cl^- co-transporter, Na^+,K^+-$2Cl^-$ co-transporter, Na^+, glucose co-transporter and Na^+, bicarbonate co-transporter, also play roles in effecting Na^+ transport [20,21]. Current data support the hypothesis that Na^+ transport across the alveolar epithelium, and hence edema clearance, is primarily dependent on the function of the alveolar apical Na^+ channels and the basolaterally located Na^+,K^+-ATPase [18,19,22,23]. Water moves along these osmotic gradients, out of the alveolus, via transmembrane water channels [24]. Supporting the importance of active Na^+ transport in effecting lung edema clearance are studies in isolated rat lungs which demonstrated that lung liquid clearance was completely stopped by hypothermia (possibly by inhibiting active solute transport) [25,26] and decreased by both the Na^+ channel antagonist amiloride, and by ouabain, a Na^+,K^+-ATPase antagonist [14,27,28].

Investigations are being conducted to develop methods to accelerate pulmonary edema clearance during lung injury. Increasing active Na^+ transport in sheep and dogs with terbutaline increases lung edema clearance [29]. In a model of proliferative lung injury induced by chronic exposure of rats to 85% hyperoxia, we have observed that active

alveolar Na^+ transport is increased when compared with controls. The augmented transport was associated with increased Na^+,K^+-ATPase expression in the alveolar type II cells isolated from these same rats [30] and increased numbers of perialveolar lymphatic vessels [31]. These studies suggest that upregulation of alveolar Na^+,K^+-ATPase can increase lung edema clearance in injured lungs once edema has accumulated. The importance of active transport in patients with hypoxemic respiratory failure has been recently demonstrated [32]. Patients with respiratory failure who were able to increase the concentration of air space sampled protein 24 hours after intubation had better outcomes than patients who were not. This observation has been interpreted to mean that the processes responsible for edema clearance (i.e. active ion transport) are functional and contribute to recovery from pulmonary edema. Hence, investigations focusing on strategies to accelerate lung edema clearance by modulating the expression and function of lung apical Na^+ channels and Na^+,K^+-ATPase are warranted. Also, hormones such as aldosterone can increase Na^+,K^+-ATPase expression in the lungs and increase active Na^+ transport [33,34].

STRATEGIES FOR TREATMENT

Despite extensive research no specific therapy for the treatment of ARDS has come to light. This is not surprising given the many underlying conditions that can precipitate the clinical syndrome. Improved intensive care and supportive therapies have produced modest improvements in survival of these critically ill patients [35]. As our ability to support these patients improves, we are faced with a host of new problems and complications that further threaten their survival. Athough very important in the supportive therapy of these patients, PEEP, mechanical ventilation and high concentrations of inspired oxygen also have adverse effects that may impact on patient outcome [36,37]. Ideally, edema formation would be reduced and clearance accelerated during the early phase of ARDS, such that the complications attendant upon prolonged mechanical ventilation and intensive care unit (ICU) stays would be avoided, thereby preventing progression to the abnormal proliferative phase of ARDS. Specifically, if pulmonary edema accumulation can be limited [38], or its clearance accelerated [34,39], then improved survival or reduced ICU stays might be achievable, as has been suggested in a recent clinical study [32].

PEEP

The institution of PEEP has been shown to improve lung compliance and gas exchange in ARDS by redistributing edema to the peribronchial and perivascular interstitial spaces [40]. Although PEEP may improve gas exchange and lung compliance, total lung water may actually increase [41,42]. This probably occurs due to a PEEP induced reduction in interstitial hydrostatic pressure (P_{is}), resulting in an increased hydrostatic gradient (P_{mv} − P_{is}) favoring movement of liquid from the vessels into the interstitium. This lowering of interstitial pressures increases the pressure gradient that moves water to the peribronchovascular spaces where no lymphatics are available to drain the fluid [13]. Secondly, the beneficial effects of PEEP may be outweighed if hemodynamic impairment reduces oxygen delivery (D_{O_2}) by reducing venous return [43]. The PEEP induced increment in intrathoracic pressure may increase right ventricular afterload and shift the intraventricular septum leftward, reducing effective left ventricular compliance and cardiac output [43–45]. Since PEEP does not reduce total lung water, but rather redistributes it from the air spaces to the interstitium, the discontinuation of PEEP can be associated with reflooding of alveoli. Thus, even during brief endotracheal tube suctioning, patients with ARDS in the exudative

phase of the condition may develop arterial desaturation.

PRELOAD REDUCTION

The observation that most patients with ARDS do not die of respiratory failure but rather as a consequence of subsequent nosocomial infection and associated multiple system organ failure (MSOF) [7,32] would seem to justify therapeutic strategies to limit early edema formation [46]. These could potentially reduce the magnitude and duration of potentially harmful interventions. Inspection of the Starling equation has led researchers to study various approaches towards this end. After acute lung injury, K_f increases and σ falls. In the clinical setting neither variable can be intentionally altered. Animal studies have shown that, during lung injury, increasing π_{mv} with colloid infusions does not protect against alveolar flooding because permeability to protein is high [2,8]. The prevention of edema accumulation by reductions in pulmonary artery occlusion pressure (PAOP) is an adjunctive therapy designed to support ARDS patients until the primary etiology can be treated and normal capillary permeability restored. Reducing the hydrostatic gradient (P_{mv} − P_{is}) by decreasing P_{mv}, as shown in Figure 28.3, has proved to be successful in limiting edema formation in canine models of acute lung injury caused by intravenous oleic acid, intratracheal administration of hydrochloric acid or kerosene [38,43,44,47]. These concepts have subsequently been confirmed in patients with hypoxemic respiratory failure [48–50].

In a retrospective study of patients with ARDS it was observed that when preload (PAOP) was reduced and maintained at 75% or less of initial values, survival rate was ~75%, compared with ~29% in patients with ARDS where preload reduction was not attempted. This reduction in mortality was also associated with shorter ICU stays [48]. A second study used diuretics to reduce PAOP

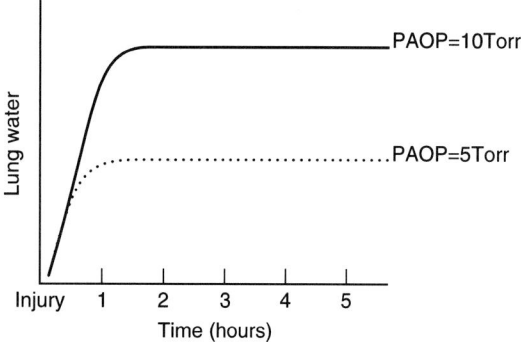

Figure 28.3 Following acute lung injury in dogs, pulmonary edema rapidly accumulates when PAOP = 10 Torr (1.3 kPa) and plateaus after 2 hours. If preload is reduced to a PAOP of 5 Torr (0.7 kPa) 1 hour after inducing lung injury, pulmonary edema accumulation stops.

from 16 to 12 Torr (2.1 to 1.6 kPa) in ARDS patients, which resulted in lower PEEP requirements and increased survival rates (80% versus 40%) in the group of patients in whom the PAOP could be reduced [49]. Finally, investigators recently found a decrease in the duration of mechanical ventilation and ICU stay in patients who had negative fluid balance in the first 72 hours of ICU care, as compared with patients having a moderate fluid gain of 2–3 liters [50]. Although further controlled prospective studies are warranted, these observations suggest that therapies designed to reduce pulmonary edema are beneficial in patients with ARDS. It should be noted that this form of therapy is most likely to impact on patients during the early exudative phase of ARDS while the alveoli are 'leaky' (Chapter 4).

While preload reduction may decrease edema formation, excessive reduction can produce an inadequate cardiac output and a hypotensive, hypoperfused state. Our approach is to strive for the lowest PAOP that allows an adequate cardiac output and Do_2 (Chapter 19). This can be best achieved with judicious limitation of fluid administration and careful diuresis [48–50]. In patients with systolic dysfunction, inotropic support may be used to maintain peripheral perfusion at low preload pressures. If preload is low, consideration should be given to the utilization of intravascular volume expanders such as red blood cells. This allows iso-osmotic expansion of the intravascular space, increasing preload and Do_2. The choice of fluids to be used in these circumstances has long been a topic of controversy. As capillaries become leaky and the reflection coefficient for protein (σ) falls towards zero, large molecules are no longer retained within the intravascular space. Unlike crystalloid solutions, which can be cleared from the interstitium by active transport mechanisms, larger molecules (i.e. albumin, dextrans, hespan) can only be cleared by metabolism or through the already overwhelmed lymphatics. Data exist suggesting that colloids may impair pulmonary edema clearance by increasing alveolar interstitial oncotic pressures and reducing glomerular filtration rates by increasing renal interstitial oncotic pressures [51,52]. Although we recommend the administration of crystalloid solutions, which are more readily cleared from the lung than are colloid solutions [53], no prospective data exist to show that any particular type of fluid therapy alters the prognosis of ARDS.

The utilization of an aggressive approach such as preload reduction in these patients requires invasive hemodynamic monitoring in most cases. Thus, right heart catheterization is often performed in patients with ARDS to guide cardiovascular management. This procedure should be performed by experienced clinicians such that the data generated can be interpreted correctly [54,55], and then only to obtain objective data that are essential for patient management (calculation of intra-pulmonary shunt fraction, oxygen delivery, cardiac output, pulmonary capillary occlusion pressure), and cannot otherwise be obtained by more subjective means (e.g. mental status, urine output, cardiovascular examination, capillary refill, etc.). Echocardiography can also be used in these patients to help rule out cardiogenic etiologies of pulmonary edema and guide hemodynamic management.

EFFECTS OF PRELOAD REDUCTION ON OXYGEN DELIVERY AND UPTAKE

Defining the adequacy of cardiac output and D_{O_2} is difficult in patients with ARDS. Lactic acidosis is frequently noted and it has been postulated that D_{O_2} may be inadequate in these patients [56–58]. In normal animals and humans, a D_{O_2} of 8–10 ml/kg/min is considered to be adequate to ensure aerobic metabolism. In adult patients with ARDS it has been suggested that this critical threshold is increased to approximately 20 ml/kg/min and that a D_{O_2} below this level is associated with cellular hypoxia [58,59]. The fact that mixed venous oxygen saturation is typically normal or elevated in these patients despite increased total body oxygen consumption has been interpreted to mean that there is a peripheral defect in D_{O_2} or oxygen extraction. This has been attributed to the shunting of blood past peripheral capillary beds. These hypotheses were generated from early studies of oxygen consumption and utilization in critically ill patients [56–58]. Subsequent review of this data has revealed methodological problems that confound the results of these studies [60–62] (Chapter 19). More recent studies utilizing independent measures of V_{O_2} and D_{O_2} have been unable to demonstrate whole body oxygen supply dependency in patients [63–65]. Furthermore, careful review of prospective studies in which D_{O_2} was intentionally augmented demonstrates no overall increased survival [66]. Other studies have suggested that rather than cellular oxygen supply limitation there is a defect in cellular oxygen utilization [63]. It has been shown in models of sepsis that cells have disordered redox states and abnormal pyruvate metabolism, both of which lead to excess lactate production [59,67–69]. Thus, while it is extremely important to maintain adequate cardiac output in critically ill patients, we

believe that modest reductions in cardiac output to reduce edemagenesis are well tolerated [48,50].

FLUID MANAGEMENT STRATEGIES AND RENAL FUNCTION

We recommend reducing PAOP in patients with ARDS whenever possible. Likewise, we avoid large volume fluid administration in patients felt to be at risk for the development of pulmonary capillary leak. Typically we use a combination of Na^+ and water restriction with diuretics. Another, albeit more cumbersome, option is phlebotomy with plasmapheresis and return of red blood cells to the patient. In patients with impaired renal function continuous arteriovenous hemofiltration (CAVH) with or without dialysis can be effective in reducing intravascular volume. However, some patients demonstrate continuing volume requirements, making it difficult to reduce PAOP without significantly compromising cardiac output, probably reflecting persistent capillary leak and possibly conferring a poor prognosis [70].

As stated above, the development of MSOF is associated with a high mortality in patients with ARDS [71,72]. Among the major contributors to MSOF is renal impairment [73]. Renal failure developing during the course of ARDS has not been well characterized. During respiratory failure from multiple etiologies the development of renal failure increases mortality up to 80% [57,74,75]. Frequent predisposing factors for renal failure include hypotension due to gastrointestinal bleeding, sepsis and cardiac dysfunction and nephrotoxicity from drugs such as aminoglycoside antibiotics [75]. Septic shock and nonhypotensive sepsis as causes of ARDS are frequently associated with acute renal failure [76,77]. This is typically oliguric, although nonoliguric renal failure may also occur. Proteinuria may be manifested in diverse causes of ARDS such as sepsis [78] or trauma [79]. A temporal relationship between the development of pulmonary edema and increased urinary protein concentrations in ARDS suggests a common underlying mechanism of increased capillary permeability [79].

The use of preload reduction therapy to lower pulmonary microvascular pressures to minimize pulmonary edema may decrease cardiac output and increase the risk for renal failure. Low dose dopamine to increase renal blood flow is frequently used in this setting, but there are no prospective data in humans to support this therapeutic approach.

The utilization of CAVH and CAVH with countercurrent dialysis (CAVH-D) has been studied in patients with ARDS. In addition to hemofiltration it has been postulated that CAVH can be of therapeutic benefit in these patients. Uncontrolled studies have reported reductions in F_{IO_2}, PEEP, intrapulmonary shunt and PAOP in children and adults treated with CAVH [70,80,81]. The exact mechanisms responsible for these changes are unclear. Clearance of intravascular water with subsequent increases in colloid oncotic pressure, filtration of low molecular weight substances such as bradykinin and 'myocardial depressant factors', histamine and complement activating factor have been proposed as possible mechanisms. Studies from animal models of sepsis have demonstrated increased clearance of thromboxane B_2 and 6-keto-prostaglandin F_2 in response to hemofiltration [82]. However, to date no randomized, prospective clinical trials are available to recommend utilization of CAVH or CAVH-D as specific therapeutic modalities for the treatment of capillary leak *per se*. These methods continue to be useful in reducing total body salt and water burdens in critically ill patients.

Supportive therapeutic measures for ARDS, such as mechanical ventilation and PEEP, may also cause alterations in renal function. Respiratory failure [83] and mechanical ventilation [84] have been associated with increased antidiuretic hormone release and increased plasma aldosterone and renin activ-

ity [85]. These changes lead to increased tubular reabsorption of Na^+ and water, contributing to positive fluid balance and, potentially, worsened pulmonary edema. They can be reversed by the discontinuation of PEEP and/or improving cardiac output [85,86]. A decrease in plasma atrial natriuretic factor may also contribute to fluid retention and renal dysfunction in mechanically ventilated patients [87,88].

A prospective study of ARDS in which a negative fluid balance was maintained

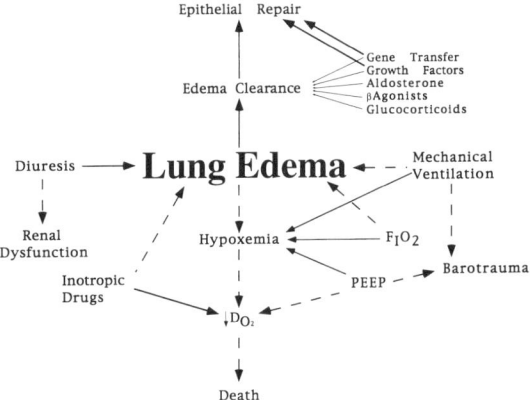

Figure 28.4 Although therapeutic strategies are utilized for their beneficial effects (solid arrows) on lung edema and oxygen delivery, they may also have deleterious effects (dashed arrows) that contribute to lung injury. For example, mechanical ventilation is used to improve oxygenation; however, it may increase lung edema and produce barotrauma. PEEP is utilized to maintain alveolar volume and improve oxygenation but it may increase lung edema, cause baratrauma and decrease cardiac output. Diuresis decreases preload and reduces edema formation, but when utilized excessively it can reduce cardiac output and cause renal dysfunction. High F_{IO_2} is utilized initially for treatment of hypoxemia but when used for prolonged periods of time it can cause oxidative lung injury. Inotropic drugs are utilized to increase cardiac output and D_{O_2} but they can also produce a flow dependent increase in lung edema. The agents listed in the upper right portion of the figure represent experimental concepts that may become part of the therapeutic armamentarium for the treatment of ARDS in the future.

showed that most survivors had a negative cumulative fluid balance [50]. In this and other studies no renal failure was observed nor did negative fluid balance influence weight loss or fluid balance. Although we know of no specific approach to prevent renal failure, careful attention to cardiac output, renal perfusion and urine output, monitoring of nephrotoxic drug levels and the possible use of dopamine, especially when using potent vasoconstrictors, may aid in attenuation or prevention of renal failure.

The approach to managing fluid balance and decreasing lung edema in patients with ARDS requires close and careful attention to clinical conditions. As shown in Figure 28.4, many therapeutic interventions, although necessary and life saving, can potentiate acute lung injury (i.e. high concentrations of oxygen, PEEP, mechanical ventilation, diuresis, inotropic drugs). Thus there exists, for every therapeutic endeavor, a balance between risk and benefit. We recommend an early and aggressive approach for edema reduction that includes preload reduction whenever possible. We anticipate that future therapeutic directions will include new strategies to increase edema clearance by intentional, lung specific processes that enhance active transport and repair mechanisms.

SUMMARY

- The early, exudative phase of ARDS is characterized by increased pulmonary capillary permeability, the accumulation of proteinaceous alveolar edema and the formation of hyaline membranes. Despite ongoing investigations, no specific pharmacological interventions been developed. As such, supportive therapies must be employed until the primary etiology responsible for ARDS can be identified and treated.
- To prevent further edema accumulation during the early exudative phase, pulmonary microvascular pressures (PAOP) should

be reduced (by diuresis and fluid restriction) to the lowest level that is compatible with an adequate cardiac output.
- In contrast to accumulation, the clearance of alveolar edema is dependent on the active transport of Na^+ out from the alveolus. Therapeutic strategies are being designed to enhance active Na^+ transport mechanisms and accelerate lung edema clearance.

ACKNOWLEDGEMENTS

This work was supported in part by a Grant in-Aid from the American Heart Association of Metropolitan Chicago, by a Career Investigator Award from the American Lung Association (J.I. Sznajder) and Michael Reese Hospital and Medical Center.

REFERENCES

1. Montaner, J.S.G., Tsang, J. and Evans, K.G. (1986) Alveolar epithelial damage: a critical difference between high pressure and oleic acid induced low pressure edema. *Journal of Clinical Investigation*, **77**, 1786–96.
2. Hall, J.B. and Wood, L.D.H. (1986) Pulmonary edema, in *Current Therapy in Respiratory Medicine* (ed. R. Cherniack), B.C. Dekker, Toronto, pp. 222–7.
3. Sznajder, J.I., Evanders, A., Pollak, E.R. *et al.* (1987) Pericardial effusion causes interstitial pulmonary edema in dogs. *Circulation*, **76**, 843–9.
4. Staub, N.C., Nagano, H. and Pearce, M.L. (1967) Pulmonary edema in dogs, especially the sequence of fluid accumulation in lung. *Journal of Applied Physiology*, **22**, 227–43.
5. Hyers, T.M. and Fowler, A.A. (1986) Adult respiratory distress syndrome: causes, morbidity and mortality, *Federation Proceedings*, **45**, 25–9.
6. Katzenstein, A.L., Bloor, C.M. and Liebow A. (1976) Diffuse alveolar damage: the role of oxygen, shock and related factors. *American Journal of Pathology*, **85**, 210–28.
7. Bitterman, P.B. (1992) Pathogenesis of fibrosis in acute lung injury. *American Journal of Medicine*, **92**(6A), 39S–43S.
8. Taylor, A.E. (1981) Capillary fluid filtration,

Starling forces and lymph flow. *Circulation Research*, **49**, 557–75.

9. Guyton, A.C. and Lindsey, A.W. (1959) Effect of elevated left atrial pressure and decreased plasma protein concentration on the development of pulmonary edema. *Circulation Research*, **7**, 649–57.

10. Dantzker, D. (1982) Gas exchange in the adult respiratory distress syndrome. *Clinics in Chest Medicine*, **3**, 57–67.

11. Bahofen, H., Schurch, S., Michel, P.P. and Weibel E.R. (1993) Experimental hydrostatic pulmonary edema in rabbit lungs: morphology. *American Review of Respiratory Disease*, **147**, 989–96.

12. Bahofen, H., Schurch, S. and Weibel, E.R. (1993) Experimental hydrostatic pulmonary edema in rabbit lungs: barrier lesions. *American Review of Respiratory Disease*, **147**, 997–1004.

13. Staub, N.C. (1983) Alveolar flooding and clearance. *American Review of Respiratory Disease*, **127**, S44–51.

14. Crandall, E.D., Heming, T.A., Palombo, R.L. and Goodman, B.E. (1986) Effects of terbutaline on sodium transport in isolated perfused rat lung. *Journal of Applied Physiology*, **60**, 289–94.

15. Berthiaume, Y., Staub, N.C. and Matthay, M.A. (1987) Beta-adrenergic agonists increase lung liquid clearance in anesthetized sheep. *Journal of Clinical Investigation*, **79**, 335–43.

16. Effros, R.M., Mason, G.R., Hukkanen, J. and Silverman, P. (1989) New evidence for active sodium transport from fluid filled rat lungs. *Journal of Applied Physiology*, **66**, 909–19.

17. Olver, R.E. (1983) Fluid balance across the fetal alveolar epithelium. *American Review of Respiratory Disease*, **127**, S33–36.

18. Schneeberger, E.E. and McCarthy, K.M. (1986) Cytochemical localization of Na, K-ATPase in rat type II pneumocytes. *Journal of Applied Physiology*, **20**, 1584–9.

19. O'Brodovich, H., Ueda, J., Canessa, C. *et al.* (1993) Expression of the Na^+ channel in the developing rat lung. *American Journal of Physiology*, **265**, C491–6.

20. Nord, E.P., Brown, S.E.S. and Crandall, E.D. (1987) Characterization of Na^+-H^+ antiport in type II alveolar epithelial cells. *American Journal of Physiology*, **252**, C490–8.

21. Stormo, M.L. and Goodman, B.E. (1991) Investigation of Na^+-coupled glucose cotransport in isolated hamster lungs. *FASEB Journal*, **5**, A1339.

22. Russo, R.M., Lubman, R.L. and Crandall, E.D. (1992) Evidence for amiloride sensitive sodium channels in alveolar epithelial cells. *American Journal of Physiology*, **262**, L405–11.

23. Voilley, N., Lingueglia, E., Champigny, G. *et al.* (1994) The lung amiloride-sensitive Na^+ channel: biophysical properties, pharmacology, ontogenesis, and molecular cloning. *Proceedings of the National Academy of Sciences of the USA*, **91**, 247–51.

24. Folkesson, H.G., Matthay, M.A., Hasegawa, H. *et al.* (1994) Transcellular water transport in lung alveolar epithelium through mercurial sensitive water channels. *Proceedings of the National Academy of Sciences of the USA*, **91**, 4970–4.

25. Serikov, V.B., Grady, M. and Matthay, M.A. (1993) Effect of temperature on alveolar liquid and protein clearance in an *in situ* goat lung. *Journal of Applied Physiology*, **75**, 940–7.

26. Rutschman, D.H., Olivera, W. and Sznajder, J.I. (1993) Active and passive fluid movement in isolated perfused rat lungs. *Journal of Applied Physiology*, **75**, 1574–80.

27. Saumon, G. and Basset, G. (1993) Electrolyte and fluid transport across the mature alveolar epithelium. *Journal of Applied Physiology*, **74**, 1–15.

28. Olivera, W., Ridge, K., Wood, L.D.H. and Sznajder, J.I. (1993) Atrial naturetic factor decreases active sodium transport and increases alveolar epithelial permeability. *Journal of Applied Physiology*, **75**, 1581–6.

29. Matthay, M.A. (ed.) (1985) Symposium on pulmonary edema. *Clinics in Chest Medicine*, **11**, 575–80.

30. Olivera, W., Ridge, K., Wood, L.D.H. and Sznajder, J.I. (1994) Active sodium transport and alveolar epithelial Na, K-ATPase increase during subacute hyperoxia in rats. *American Journal of Physiology*, **266**, L577–84.

31. Schraufnagel, D.E., Basterra, J.L., Haines, K.D. and Sznajder, J.I. (1994) Lung lymphatics increase after hyperoxic injury: an ultrastructural study of casts. *American Journal of Pathology*, **144**, 1393–1402.

32. Matthay, M.A. and Wiener-Kronish, J.P. (1990) Intact epithelial barrier function is critical for the resolution of alveolar edema in humans. *American Review of Respiratory Disease*, **142**, 1250–7.

33. Ciccolella, D.E., Ridge, K., Surani, S. and Sznajder, J.I. (1992) Aldosterone upregulates

the Na, K-ATPase β-1 subunit mRNA in cultured alveolar rat type 2 cells. *FASEB Journal*, **6**, A1190.

34. Olivera, W., Ridge, K., Yeates, D. and Sznajder, J.I. (1992) Aerosolized aldosterone increases lung liquid clearance in isolated rat lungs. *American Review of Respiratory Disease*, **145**, A366.

35. Morris, A.H., Wallace, C.J., Menlove, R. *et al.* (1994) Randomized clinical trial of pressure-controlled inverse ratio ventilation and extracorporeal CO_2 removal for adult respiratory distress syndrome. *American Journal of Respiratory and Critical Care Medicine*, **149**, 295–305.

36. Pingleton, S.K. and Hall, J.B. (1992) Complications of critical care: prevention and early detection, in *Principles of Critical Care* (eds J.B. Hall, G. Schmidt and L.D.H. Wood), McGraw-Hill, New York, pp. 587–611.

37. Peterson, G.W. and Horst, B. (1983) Incidence of pulmonary barotrauma in a medical ICU. *Critical Care Medicine*, **11**, 67–74.

38. Sznajder, J.I., Zucker, A.R., Wood, L.D.H. and Long, G.R. (1986) Effects of plasmapheresis and hemofiltration on acid aspiration pulmonary edema. *American Review of Respiratory Disease*, **134**, 222–8.

39. Olivera, W., Yeates, D., Ilekis, J. and Sznajder, J.I. (1992) Epidermal growth factor (EGF) increases lung liquid clearance and active Na^+ transport in isolated rat lungs. *American Review of Respiratory Disease*, **145**, A366.

40. Malo, J., Ali, J. and Wood, L.D.H. (1984) How does positive end-expiratory pressure reduce intrapulmonary shunt in canine pulmonary edema? *Journal of Applied Physiology*, **57**, 1002.

41. Pare, P.D., Warriner, E., Baile, M. and Hogg, J.C. (1983) Redistribution of pulmonary extravascular water with positive end-expiratory pressure in canine pulmonary edema. *American Review of Respiratory Disease*, **127**, 590–3.

42. Crandall, E.D., Staub, N.C., Goldberg, H.S. and Effros, R.M. (1983) Recent developments in pulmonary edema. *Annals of Internal Medicine*, **99**, 808–22.

43. Wood, L.D.H. and Prewitt, R.M. (1981) Cardiovascular management in acute hypoxemic respiratory failure. *American Journal of Cardiology*, **47**, 963–72.

44. Permutt, S., Wise, R.A. and Sylvester, J.T. (1985) Interaction between the circulatory and ventilatory pumps, in *The Thorax* (part b) (eds C. Roussos and P.T. Macklem), Marcel Dekker, New York, p. 701.

45. Fessler, H.E., Brower, R.G., Wise, R.A. and Permutt, S. (1991) Effects of positive end-expiratory pressure on the gradient for venous return. *American Review of Respiratory Disease*, **143**, 19–24.

46. Sznajder, J.I. and Wood, L.D.H. (1991) Beneficial effects of reducing pulmonary edema in patients with hypoxemic respiratory failure. *Chest*, **100**, 890–2.

47. Zucker, A., Holm, B., Wood, L.D.H. *et al.* (1992) Positive end expiratory pressure allows exogenous surfactant to reduce canine acid aspiration pneumonitis. *Journal of Applied Physiology*, **73**, 679–86.

48. Humphrey, H., Hall, J.B. and Sznajder, J.I. (1990) Improved survival in ARDS patients associated with a reduction in pulmonary capillary wedge pressure. *Chest*, **97**, 1176–80.

49. Eisenberg, P.R., Hansrough, J.R., Anderson, D. and Schuster, D.P. (1987) A prospective study of lung water measurements during patient management in an intensive care unit. *American Review of Respiratory Disease*, **136**, 662.

50. Schuller, D., Mitchell, J.P., Calandrino, F.S. and Schuster, D.P. (1991) Fluid balance during pulmonary edema: is fluid gain a marker of poor outcome? *Chest*, **100**, 1068–75.

51. Lucas, C.E., Ledgerwood, A.M. and Higgins, R.F. (1979) Impaired salt and water excretion after albumin resuscitation for hypovolemic shock. *Surgery*, **86**, 544–9.

52. Lucas, C.E., Ledgerwood, A.M., Higgins, R.F. and Weaver, D.W. (1980) Impaired pulmonary function after albumin resuscitation from hemorrhagic shock. *Journal of Trauma*, **20**, 446–51.

53. Matthay, M.A., Landolt, C.C. and Staub, N.C. (1982) Differential liquid and protein clearance from the alveoli of anesthetized sheep. *Journal of Applied Physiology*, **53**, 96–104.

54. Iberti, T.J., Fischer, E.P. and Leibowitz, A.B. (1990) A multicenter study of physicians' knowledge of the pulmonary artery catheter. *JAMA*, **264**, 2928–32.

55. Chatterjee, K., Parmley, W.W. and Ganz, W. (1989) Hemodynamic studies: their uses and limitations. *American Journal of Cardiology*, **64**, 30.

56. Powers, S.R., Mannal, R. and Neclerio, M. (1973) Physiologic consequences of positive

end-expiratory pressure (PEEP) ventilation. *Annals of Surgery,* **178**, 265–72.

57. Rhodes, G.R., Newell, J.C. and Shah, D. (1978) Increased oxygen consumption accompanying increased oxygen delivery with hypertonic mannitol in adult respiratory distress syndrome. *Surgery,* **84**, 490–7.

58. Schumaker, W., Appel, P. and Kram, H. (1988) Prospective trial of supranormal values of survivors as therapeutic goals in high risk surgical patients. *Chest,* **94**, 1176–86.

59. Hall, J.B., Schmidt, G.A. and Wood, L.D.H. (1992) *Principles of Critical Care,* McGraw-Hill, New York.

60. Stfatton, H.H., Feustel, P.J. and Newell, J.C. (1987) Regression of calculated variables in the presence of shared measurement error. *Journal of Applied Physiology,* **62**, 2083–93.

61. Archie, J.P. (1981) Mathematic coupling of data: a common source of error. *Annals of Surgery,* **193**, 296–303.

62. Russell, J.A. and Phang, P.T. (1994) The oxygen delivery/consumption controversy. *American Journal of Respiratory and Critical Care Medicine,* **149**, 533–7.

63. Manthous, C.A., Schumacker, P.T., Pohlman, A. *et al.* (1993) Absence of supply dependence of oxygen consumption in patients with septic shock. *Journal of Critical Care,* **8**, 203–11.

64. Ronco, J.J., Fenwick, J.C., Wiggs, B.R. *et al.* (1993) Oxygen consumption is independent of increases in oxygen delivery by dobutamine in septic patients who have normal or increased plasma lactate. *American Review of Respiratory Disease,* **147**, 25–31.

65. Ronco, J.J., Phang, P.T., Walley, K.R. *et al.* (1991) Oxygen consumption is independent of changes in oxygen delivery in severe adult respiratory distress syndrome. *American Review of Respiratory Disease,* **143**, 1267–73.

66. Tuchschmidt, J., Fried, I. and Astiz, M. (1992) Elevation of cardiac output and oxygen delivery improves outcome in septic shock. *Chest,* **102**, 216–20.

67. Siegal, J.H., Cerra, F.B. and Coleman B. (1979) Physiological and metabolic correlations in human sepsis. *American Journal of Physiology,* **186**, 163–93.

68. Vary, T.C. (1991) Increased pyruvate dehtdrogenase kinase activity in response to sepsis. *American Journal of Physiology,* **260**, E669–774.

69. Curtis, S.E. and Cain, S.M. (1992) Regional and systemic oxygen delivery/uptake relations and lactate flux in hyperdynamic endotoxin treated dogs. *American Review of Respiratory Disease,* **145**, 348–54.

70. Garzia, F. Todor, R. and Scalea, T. (1991) Continuous arteiovenous hemofiltration countercurrent dialysis (CAVH-D) in acute respiratory failure. *Journal of Trauma,* **31**, 1277–85.

71. Knaus, W.A., Draper, E.A., Wagner, D.P. and Zimmerman, J.E. (1985) APACHE II a severity of disease classification system. *Critical Care Medicine,* **13**, 818–29.

72. Montgomery, A.B., Stager, M.A. and Carrico, C.J. (1985) Causes of mortality in patients with the adult respiratory distress syndrome. *American Review of Respiratory Disease,* **132**, 485–9.

73. Dorinsky, P.M. and Gadek, J.E. (1989) Mechanisms of multiple non-pulmonary organ failure in ARDS. *Chest,* **96**, 885–92.

74. Simmons, R.S., Berdine, G.G. and Seidenfeld, J.J. *et al.* (1987) Fluid balance and the adult respiratory distress syndrome. *American Review of Respiratory Disease,* **135**, 924–9.

75. Kraman, S., Kahn, F. Patel, S. and Seriff N. (1979) Renal failure in the respiratory intensive care unit. *Critical Care Medicine,* **7**, 263–6.

76. Cumming, A.D., Kline, R. and Linton, A.L. (1988) Association between renal and sympathetic responses to nonhypotensive systemic sepsis. *Critical Care Medicine,* **16**, 1132–7.

77. Zager, R.A. (1986) *Escherichia coli* endotoxin injections potentiate experimental ischemic renal injury. *American Journal of Physiology,* **251**, F988–94.

78. Richmond, J.M., Sibbald, W.J., Linton, A.M. and Linton, A.L. (1982) Patterns of urinary protein excretion in patients with sepsis. *Nephron,* **31**, 219–23.

79. Kreuzfelder, E., Joka, T. and Keinecke, H. *et al.* (1988) Adult respiratory distress syndrome as a specific manifestation of a general permeability defect in trauma patients. *American Review of Respiratory Disease,* **137**, 95–9.

80. Gotloib, L., Barzilay, E., Shustak, A. and Lev A. (1984) Sequential hemofiltration in non-oliguric high capillary permeability pulmonary edema of severe sepsis. *Critical Care Medicine,* **12**, 997–1000.

81. DiCarlo, J.V., Dudley, T.E. and Sherbotie, J.R. (1990) Continuous arteriovenous hemofiltration improves pulmonary gas exchange in children with multiple organ failure. *Critical Care Medicine,* **18**, 882–6.

82. Staubach, K.H., Rau, H.G. and Koolstra, A. *et*

al. (1989) Can hemofiltration increase survival time in acute endotoxemia – a porcine shock model. *Progress in Clinical and Biological Research*, **308**, 821–6.

83. Szatalowicz, V.L., Goldberg, J.P. and Anderson, R.J. (1982) Plasma antidiuretic hormone in acute respiratory failure. *American Journal of Medicine*, **72**, 583–7.

84. Sladen, A., Laver, M.B. and Pontoppidan H. (1968) Pulmonary complications and water retention in prolonged mechanical ventilation. *New England Journal of Medicine*, **279**, 448–53.

85. Annat, G., Viale, J.P. and Xuan, B.B. *et al.* (1983) Effect of PEEP ventilation on renal function, plasma renin, aldosterone, neurophysins and urinary ADH, and prostaglandins. *Anesthesiology*, **58**, 136–41.

86. Gammanpila, S., Bevan, D.R. and Bhudu R. (1977) Effect of positive and negative expiratory pressure on renal function. *British Journal of Anaesthesia*, **49**, 199–205.

87. Andrivet, P., Adnot, S., and Brun-Buisson, C. *et al.* Involvement of ANF in the acute antidiuresis during PEEP. *Journal of Applied Physiology*, **65**, 1967–74.

88. Leithner, C., Frass, M. and Pacher, R. *et al.* (1987) Mechanical ventilation with positive end-expiratory pressure decreases release of alpha-atrial naturetic peptide. *Critical Care Medicine*, **15**, 484–8.

E. Robert Grover and David Bihari

Since the first description of the syndrome of acute respiratory distress in adults (ARDS) in 1967 [1], there has been considerable debate concerning its exact definition. Specifically, distinguishing the syndrome from acute lung injury (ALI) has only recently been addressed. The relevance of the pulmonary hypertension that complicates ARDS and its role in the pathophysiology of the accompanying acute respiratory failure has also been the subject of investigation. ARDS has been defined recently as noncardiogenic pulmonary edema with refractory hypoxemia (Pa_{O_2} / F_{IO_2} ratio < 27 kPa), associated with bilateral infiltrates on chest radiography [2]. It represents the most extreme form of ALI, the latter term being used to describe a broad spectrum of pulmonary disease ranging from subclinical respiratory compromise to a total dependence upon extracorporeal lung support.

ALI may complicate a wide variety of insults such as systemic infection, trauma and pulmonary infection or aspiration. The underlying pathophysiological mechanisms are assumed to be essentially the same and include increased pulmonary capillary permeability; mismatching of alveolar perfusion ($\dot{Q}$) with ventilation ($\dot{V}$); hypoxic pulmonary vasoconstriction and pulmonary capillary microthrombosis. This assumption is of some importance since by implication it suggests that a single therapeutic regimen should be appropriate for all patients with ARDS, whatever the precipitating cause. In those cases in whom the disease process is particularly severe, the pulmonary edema is associated with the clinical abnormalities typical of ARDS – severe refractory hypoxemia, hypercarbia and pulmonary hypertension.

The presence of acute pulmonary hypertension (defined as a mean pulmonary artery pressure $>$ 20 mmHg) in ALI/ARDS is known to be a poor prognostic indicator, although it has not yet been causally related to increased mortality [3,4] (Chapter 17). Nevertheless, as a result there have been repeated attempts to identify a suitable and specific pulmonary vasodilator therapy. Numerous agents have been studied (including isoprenaline, sodium nitroprusside, prostaglandin (PG) E_1 and prostacyclin (PGI_2), infused both intravenously and via the pulmonary artery [5–8]. Although all these compounds can lower pulmonary artery pressure, none has proved to be ideal, mainly due to their nonspecific vasodilator action leading to systemic hypotension, increased intrapulmonary shunt and worsening hypoxemia. For this reason, the discovery that the very short acting endogenous vasodilator, endothelium derived relaxing factor (EDRF) is synonymous with nitric oxide (NO) [9], which can be administered to the critically ill via the respiratory tract, has particular therapeutic significance for patients with ARDS.

ARDS Acute Respiratory Distress in Adults. Edited by Timothy W. Evans and Christopher Haslett. Published in 1996 by Chapman & Hall, London. ISBN 0 412 56910 8

HISTORY

The properties of NO were first investigated and reported by Humphrey Davy at the end of the seventeenth century [10]. At that time his principal interest was **nitrous oxide** (N_2O), while the higher oxides of nitrogen were byproducts of N_2O synthesized by the combustion of ammonium nitrate. Davy described an attempt to inhale purified NO as follows: 'I made three inspirations and expirations of nitrous oxide to free my lungs ... from oxygen, then attempted to inspire the nitrous gas (NO) ... It tasted astringent and highly disagreeable ... aeriform nitrous acid was instantly formed in my mouth, which burnt the tongue and palate ... I never design again to attempt so rash an experiment.' As a result of these and other experiments, NO and **nitrogen dioxide** (NO_2) were identified as poisonous gases. The higher oxides of nitrogen are now also recognized to be important environmental pollutants as a result of their production from many combustion processes. The poisonous nature of these gases was tragically reconfirmed in 1966 when at least three patients were inadvertently exposed to N_2O, contaminated with NO and NO_2 during induction of anesthesia [11]. They rapidly developed profound cyanosis unresponsive to oxygen therapy, which was due to the avid reaction of NO with the heme moiety of hemoglobin resulting in methemoglobinemia. Despite prompt treatment with methylene blue, two of these victims subsequently died of acute respiratory failure, associated with fulminant pulmonary edema.

In view of their demonstrable toxicity, the Health and Safety Executive, via the Control of Substances Hazardous to Health (COSHH) document, specify employee environmental exposure limits for NO and NO_2 of 25 and 3 parts per million (p.p.m.) respectively over an 8 hour time-weighted average period [12]. Indeed, it is now appreciated that inhalation of NO_2 is responsible for silo fillers' disease,

which is characterized by a potentially fatal acute pneumonitis [13]. The toxicity of pure inhaled NO is unclear, other than that it reacts with hemoglobin to form methemoglobin. Elevated levels of this substance can be detected readily in the blood of smokers after inhaling cigarettes, the smoke of which may contain NO at concentrations of 600–1000 p.p.m. [14,15].

ARGININE–NO PATHWAY (Chapter 17)

In 1980 Furchgott and Zawadzki found that rabbit aortic rings, preconstricted with phenylephrine, would relax in response to acetylcholine but only if the endothelial intima was intact [16]. As a result, they postulated that the endothelium released a previously unknown mediator stimulated by acetylcholine which they named 'endothelium derived relaxing factor' (EDRF). The search for the chemical identity of this substance appeared to be resolved in 1987 when a biological and chemical assay system was employed to demonstrate that the properties of EDRF were essentially identical to those of NO [9]. Nowadays, it is generally accepted that EDRF may exist in several forms with varying half lives, although NO is probably the active moiety in each instance [17].

It has become apparent that NO is a fundamental mediator released by a large variety of cell types under different physiological circumstances within many, if not all, organisms for diverse purposes [18]. It is synthesized from the substrates L-arginine (a semiessential basic amino acid in man) and molecular oxygen by a group of enzymes known as nitric oxide synthases (NOS), with the byproduct L-citrulline [19] (Figure 29.1). These are closely related to, if not part of, the P_{450} reductase enzyme series [20]. The NOS enzyme family can be divided functionally into two main subtypes, the constitutive (cNOS) and inducible (iNOS) forms [18,21]. The former exists in at least two isoforms, endothelial and neuronal, which constantly

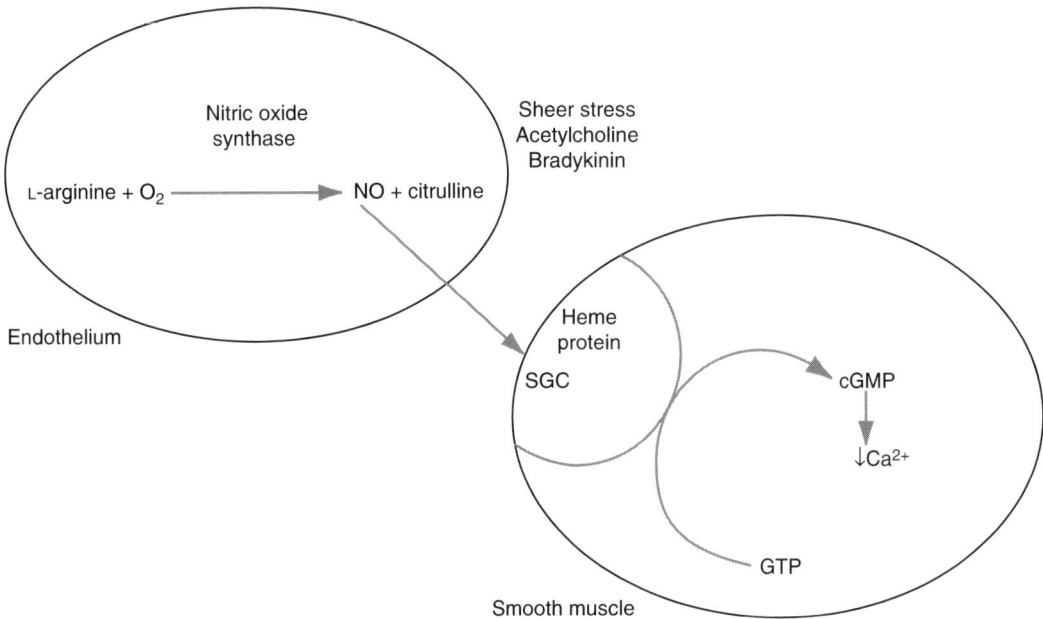

Figure 29.1 L-arginine – nitric oxide pathway within the vasculature. SGC = soluble guanylate cyclase; cGMP = cyclic guanosine monophosphate; GTP = guanosine triphosphate.

produce NO under tight physiological control (Table 29.1).

Endothelium derived NO stimulates the soluble guanylate cyclase of adjacent smooth muscle cells, leading to a rise in cyclic guanosine monophosphate, a fall in free intracellular calcium and ultimately vascular smooth muscle relaxation. A rise in luminal shear stress stimulates endothelial cells to release NO, thereby accounting for the reflex vasodilatation observed in response to increased blood flow [22]. Thus, the tone of the circulation at any time is determined by a balance of counteracting vasodilator and vasoconstrictor substances, of which NO is only one. Many neurons also generate NO, which may act as a

Table 29.1 Comparative features of the nitric oxide synthase (NOS) enzyme family

Constitutive *(Endothelial/neuronal)*	*Inducible* *(Macrophage)*
Active in limited range of cell types (e.g. endothelial, neuronal, platelets)	Potentially active in wide range of cell types (e.g. reticuloendothelial, smooth muscle, stromal)
Activity does not require enzyme induction	Activity requires trigger for enzyme induction/ synthesis
Physiological mediator	Pathophysiological mediator
Associated with low levels of NO	Associated with high levels of NO
Continuous modulator activity (vascular tone)	Intermittent effector activity (cytotoxicity)
Calcium/calmodulin dependent	Calcium/calmodulin independent
Activity unaffected by steroids	Induction but not activity inhibited by steroids

Tetrahydrobiopterin/flavin adenine dinucleotide dependent
Activity inhibited by various arginine analogs

neurotransmitter within both the central and peripheral nervous systems. Nitroxergic neurons are now known to constitute a major part of the nonadrenergic, noncholinergic autonomic nervous system [23,24]. They have a potent influence on splanchnic and bronchial smooth muscle tone [25,26]. Further discussion of the emerging roles of NO within the nervous system is beyond the scope of this chapter, but these are well reviewed elsewhere [27,28].

The iNOS system is thought to be absent under normal physiological conditions within the vasculature. The potential for iNOS gene expression, however, is present in many cell types, including endothelial, vascular smooth muscle, reticuloendothelial and immunocompetent cells [18,29]. Gene expression and the subsequent synthesis of the enzyme may be induced by a number of stimuli, including endotoxin and various mediators of the acute inflammatory response. Its principal function appears to be as a part of the host immune response whereby phagocytes use NO derivatives to assist with intracellular microbial killing [30,31]. Vascular iNOS activity may also be responsible in part for the hyperemia characteristic of acute inflammation. However, excess NO production by iNOS in endothelial and vascular smooth muscle cells may lead to profound loss of vasomotor tone and contribute to the hypotension typical of septic shock [32,33]. A pathological role for iNOS has also been postulated in several chronic inflammatory and autoimmune disorders, including rheumatoid arthritis, diabetes mellitus and inflammatory bowel disease [34,37].

INHALED NO AND PULMONARY HYPERTENSION

Until 1987, NO was of little clinical or scientific interest, other than to toxicologists and environmentalists. The discovery that it has all the chemical and biological properties of EDRF, making it the first true gas to be identified as an endogenous mediator, has stimulated an enormous amount of published and ongoing research. One of the first clinical applications of NO described was its use to measure pulmonary diffusing capacity [38]. Subsequently, the effects of inhaled NO (40 p.p.m. in air) were investigated in normal volunteers and in patients with either primary pulmonary hypertension (PPH), mitral valve disease or ischemic heart disease [39,40]. In every patient, pulmonary vascular resistance (PVR) was noted to fall whilst systemic vascular resistance (SVR) was unchanged. This effect was compared with a PGI_2 infusion in the same patients with PPH; PGI_2 induced a significant reduction in both PVR and SVR [39]. It was concluded that NO was both an effective and selective pulmonary vasodilator. A more detailed study of inhaled NO (5–80 p.p.m.) in awake lambs with induced pulmonary hypertension (either by the infusion of a thromboxane analogue U46619, or by exposure to an hypoxic gas mixture), confirmed its potency as a pulmonary vasodilator with a rapid onset and offset, and its lack of systemic hemodynamic effects [41].

These results encouraged further clinical studies of inhaled NO for pulmonary hypertension secondary to a variety of diseases. In particular, two independent research groups published short reports, each describing the successful application of short term NO inhalation to neonates with severe persistent pulmonary hypertension of the newborn (PPHN) [42,43]. This syndrome can be idiopathic or associated with various neonatal cardiorespiratory diseases, including meconium aspiration and group B streptococcal infection. In severe cases it is associated with profound hypoxemia due to right to left shunting of blood away from the pulmonary artery via a patent ductus arteriosus and foramen ovale. The treatment of last resort is extracorporeal membrane oxygenation (ECMO), an expensive and complex technique with significant morbidity administered in combination with conventional vasodilators (e.g. PGI_2, tolazoline), in an attempt to reduce the pulmonary vasospasm. As in adults, these agents are often dose limited by their systemic hypotensive effects. The observation that inhaled NO therapy (6–80 p.p.m.) could dramatically improve oxygenation in neonates with PPHN was suggested by some to herald the discovery of a major advance in the treatment of this life threatening condition.

Pulmonary hypertension can also become a critical problem in patients with cardiac valvular lesions (especially mitral valve disease) and during the perioperative phase of cardiac surgery. Several early reports suggested that inhaled NO might be beneficial, although many such patients have undoubtedly developed an irreversible increase in PVR, due to vascular remodeling [40,44]. NO therapy seems to be particularly promising for the management of perioperative acute pulmonary hypertensive crises in both adults and children (unpublished observations).

INHALED NO AND ARDS

The pulmonary hypertension accompanying severe ARDS is an obvious potential target for NO therapy. Several groups worldwide have now published results confirming that inhaled NO at concentrations of 5–40 p.p.m. significantly reduces pulmonary artery pressure (PAP) in these patients [45–47]. A more surprising observation is the associated improvement in arterial oxygenation, which shows wide and generally unpredictable variation between individuals. A careful analysis of this phenomenon was reported using the multiple inert gas elimination technique in nine patients with severe ARDS (six receiving concurrent venovenous ECMO) [45]. This revealed that NO improved oxygenation by reducing venous admixture, while increasing the fraction of pulmonary blood flowing to lung regions with normal $\dot{V}/\dot{Q}$ ratios. There was also a small increase in cardiac output

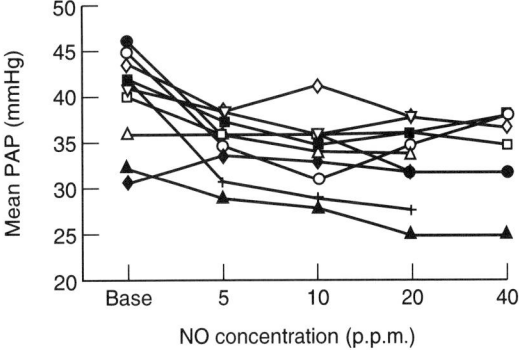

Figure 29.2 Dose profile of inhaled nitric oxide and mean pulmonary artery pressure in 10 patients with ARDS. $P < 0.003$ by Friedman's nonparametric analysis of variance.

within the group, but no significant change in blood pressure or SVR. By contrast, an infusion of PGI_2 (4 ng/kg/min) in the same patients demonstrated an increase in venous admixture, a worsening of arterial oxygenation and a fall in systemic blood pressure, although cardiac output (and hence arterial oxygen delivery) was increased significantly. Prolonged NO therapy (3–53 days) was given subsequently to seven of these patients, of whom six ultimately survived; a remarkable achievement.

A dose profile study of inhaled NO (5–40 p.p.m.) in 10 patients with ARDS, performed within our own institution, confirmed its unique physiological properties (Figures 29.2 and 29.3). It was also noted that the optimal dose for reversal of pulmonary hypertension clearly exceeded that required for maximal arterial oxygenation. Indeed, PAP continued to fall as the dose of NO was increased, whereas gas exchange improved with increasing NO concentration up to approximately 10 p.p.m. and subsequently declined. This interesting observation is not fully understood. It has been suggested that relatively low concentrations of inhaled NO (i.e. less than 10 p.p.m.) may act locally on well ventilated lung units, inducing vasodilatation of adjacent blood vessels, thereby

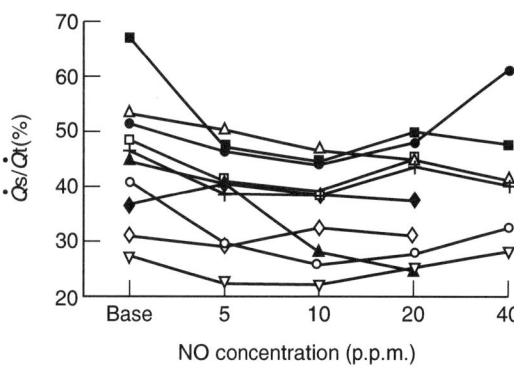

Figure 29.3 Dose profile of inhaled nitric oxide and intrapulmonary shunt in 10 patients with ARDS. $P < 0.02$ by Friedman's nonparametric analysis of variance.

improving the matching of perfusion with ventilation. As the concentration of inhaled NO increases, it may generate a more global effect throughout the pulmonary vasculature, thereby increasing intrapulmonary shunt. Therefore, NO can be considered to show selectivity at two levels: well ventilated versus poorly ventilated lung vasculature (dose dependent) and the pulmonary versus systemic circulations (dose independent). The optimal dose for any individual requires careful titration against the desired effect, with continuous monitoring of the concentrations of NO and NO_2 delivered via the inspiratory limb of the ventilator. It is of some concern to note that in all the patients subsequently treated with prolonged and continuous NO inhalation (2–44 days) a profound 'dependence' on the therapy seemed to develop, such that interruption of the gas supply even for a brief period (e.g. to change an empty cylinder) could provoke a life threatening cardiovascular collapse associated with fulminant pulmonary hypertension and extreme hypoxemia. In one case this proved to be an irreversible decline. The mechanism to explain this phenomenon is not understood, although it has been observed by other investigators (personal communications). It is tempting to speculate that exogenous NO

leads to downregulation of endogenous NO production by cNOS within the pulmonary vasculature. This obviously makes it extremely important that the integrity of the NO supply and delivery system is monitored constantly at the bedside with the same vigilance that is applied to inspired oxygen therapy.

POTENTIAL RISKS AND BENEFITS OF NO THERAPY

The attraction of inhaled NO therapy in ARDS lies in its ability to reduce PAP and, more importantly, improve arterial oxygenation. A raised PAP leads to an increase in pulmonary capillary pressure, thereby worsening the increased pulmonary capillary permeability associated with ARDS (Chapter 28). Any improvement in arterial oxygenation enables the clinician to reduce the mean airway pressure and/or the inspired oxygen concentration required, both of which predispose to further lung injury. NO, however, is a toxic, highly reactive free radical and there are a variety of potential hazards associated with its medical use (Chapter 11).

Short term exposure of healthy adults to modest concentrations of NO does not appear to cause any serious adverse effects. Indeed, NO can be detected in the expirate of animals and man due to endogenous production, although the site(s) and mechanism of synthesis within the respiratory tract have not been clearly defined. While the NO has been assumed to originate from the host's lower airway, it may be derived from the nasopharynx of the upper airway. Furthermore, the source may be exogenous and due to bacterial colonization of the nasopharynx [48]. This has considerable implications for the intubated patient, who may be denied an important natural source of inspired NO.

It is well known that inhaling NO at high concentrations causes methemoglobinemia, a not infrequent phenomenon in heavy smokers. An increase in the concentration of methemoglobin reduces the oxygen carrying capacity of red blood cells, but is usually self-limiting due to the enzyme methemoglobin reductase. Levels of high exposure can overwhelm this mechanism, causing profound central cyanosis unresponsive to oxygen therapy, which can be reversed with intravenous methylene blue (1 mg/kg).

NO reacts readily with oxygen to form NO_2 at a rate that is proportional to the concentration of oxygen and the square of the NO concentration [49]. Patients with ARDS given NO are usually undergoing mechanical ventilation with high inspired levels of oxygen. There is little doubt that NO_2 is a very toxic gas that can cause significant lung damage even at low concentrations. Consequently, every effort should be made to limit patient exposure, and the inspired gas should ideally be monitored constantly for NO and NO_2 content during inhaled NO therapy [50,51].

To exert a pharmacological effect within the lungs, inhaled NO must first enter the aqueous phase. It can then diffuse freely into the tissues of the respiratory tract. It also reacts avidly with superoxide anion radical (O_2^-) to form peroxynitrite ($ONOO^-$) [52]. This is a relatively stable anion with a half life of 1.9 s at pH 7.4, permitting its diffusion over several cell diameters. Peroxynitrite decomposes to generate a highly reactive and cytotoxic oxidant, similar to the hydroxyl radical, that mediates lipid peroxidation and sulfhydryl oxidation. In patients with an acute lung injury, inflammatory cells accumulate within the lung parenchyma and provide a potent source of reactive oxygen species. This high level of oxidant stress can overwhelm the host's normal antioxidant mechanisms (e.g. superoxide dismutase, catalase, glutathione peroxidase), which may be compounded further by the introduction of exogenous NO.

Inhaled NO undoubtedly improves $\dot{V}/\dot{Q}$ matching and hence arterial oxygenation in most, if not all, patients with ARDS. There is usually, however, no significant change in cardiac output, other than in patients with severe pulmonary hypertension [47]. Hence, for the intrapulmonary shunt to be reduced there must be a general redistribution of pulmonary blood flow away from the damaged, hypoxic regions of the lung toward healthy lung segments with relatively normal gas exchange. This may deprive the damaged lung parenchyma of an adequate blood supply necessary for tissue repair and functional recovery. It is of some concern therefore that, while inhaled NO therapy can improve the arterial oxygen tension of patients with ARDS, it may at the same time act to worsen underlying lung injury and impede the healing process.

SYSTEMIC EFFECTS OF INHALED NO

It is stated generally that the pharmacological effects of inhaled NO are restricted to the lungs. This can be explained by the high affinity of hemoglobin for NO, which acts as an efficient scavenger of any NO that enters the pulmonary circulation. NO is a potent inhibitor of platelet adhesion and aggregation. It has been reported that patients treated with inhaled NO can develop a prolonged bleeding time, which usually reflects platelet dysfunction [53]. This is the only extrapulmonary physiological effect that has been reported to date. There remains some debate, however, about whether NO can enter the systemic circulation in a potentially active form, bound to a carrier molecule, to generate other effects that remain unknown [17].

DELIVERY AND ANALYSIS OF NO IN THE INTENSIVE CARE UNIT

Due to the experimental nature of inhaled NO therapy, commercial delivery systems are only now becoming available. Several methods have been described in the literature by researchers in the field, each with their merits and problems [46,54]. Some of the features required of an ideal system are listed in Table 29.2. The technique chosen must obviously be

Table 29.2 Some optimal features of an inhaled NO delivery system

---

Minimum nitric oxide and oxygen mixing time
Prevention of environmental contamination with nitrogen oxides
Constant monitoring of the inspired nitric oxide and nitrogen dioxide gas concentrations
Maintenance of a constant, known concentration of inspired nitric oxide and oxygen
Provision for a range of inspired oxygen concentrations up to a nominal 100%
Prevention of clinical staff exposure to nitrogen oxides
Minimum exposure of the breathing system/ventilator to nitrogen oxides
Provision for precise adjustment of the inspired nitric oxide concentration over a wide
range (i.e. typically 50 ppb–50 ppm)

---

appropriate for the type of ventilator to be used. In particular, variations in the design of modern ventilators have demanded different methods of NO administration. Critical factors include the presence or absence of a facility to introduce and regulate an additional gas source (high or low pressure), and whether an intermittent or continuous flow of fresh gas is generated in the inspired limb of the breathing system. Depending upon the design of the ventilator, the NO gas (in nitrogen) may be entrained into the fresh gas supply either upstream, within or downstream of the ventilator. The system used currently at Guy's Hospital, London, UK, is illustrated in Figure 29.4. It has been designed specifically for use with the Siemens Servo ventilator series.

It is a generally accepted principle of good medical practice that the composition of any fresh gas mixture used to ventilate a patient should be monitored constantly. This is particularly important during NO therapy in view of its potent and potentially toxic effects. Chemiluminescence is the 'gold standard' and is used routinely for the monitoring of environmental NO pollution [55]. The typical apparatus samples ambient air continuously and mixes it with ozone, which oxidizes any NO present to 'high energy' NO_2. Each NO_2 molecule liberates a photon as it decays to its ground state. The radiation is quantified by a photomultiplier, which enables the concentration of NO to be derived. This method is relatively specific and extremely sensitive, such that NO can be detected reliably at concentrations less than 1 part per billion. NO_2 can also be measured indirectly by reducing it to NO prior to entry into the reaction chamber.

However, most commercially available chemiluminescence analyzers have a number of practical disadvantages when used in a clinical setting for which they were not designed. They tend to be bulky, noisy, expensive and generate excessive heat, as well as requiring considerable expertise for correct calibration and maintenance. Furthermore, they generally have a sample gas flow rate set at up to 1 l/min which cannot be returned easily to the breathing system due to the presence of ozone in the discharged gases. This ozone must be scrubbed from the exhaust gases with activated charcoal to prevent environmental contamination. The accuracy of the device also requires that the source gas is sampled at ambient pressure, which is clearly not the case during positive pressure ventilation.

The principal alternative method for NO and NO_2 analysis uses an electrochemical (fuel cell) sensor. Several devices have been developed recently for medical application [56]. Although not as accurate as chemiluminescence (with a sensitivity typically of + 0.5 p.p.m.), they have a number of significant advantages. These include mainstream (as apposed to sidestream) gas sampling; a rapid response time to changes in NO concentration; insensitivity to sample gas pressure fluctuation; ease of use and low cost. Fuel cell sensors are probably the best choice for mon-

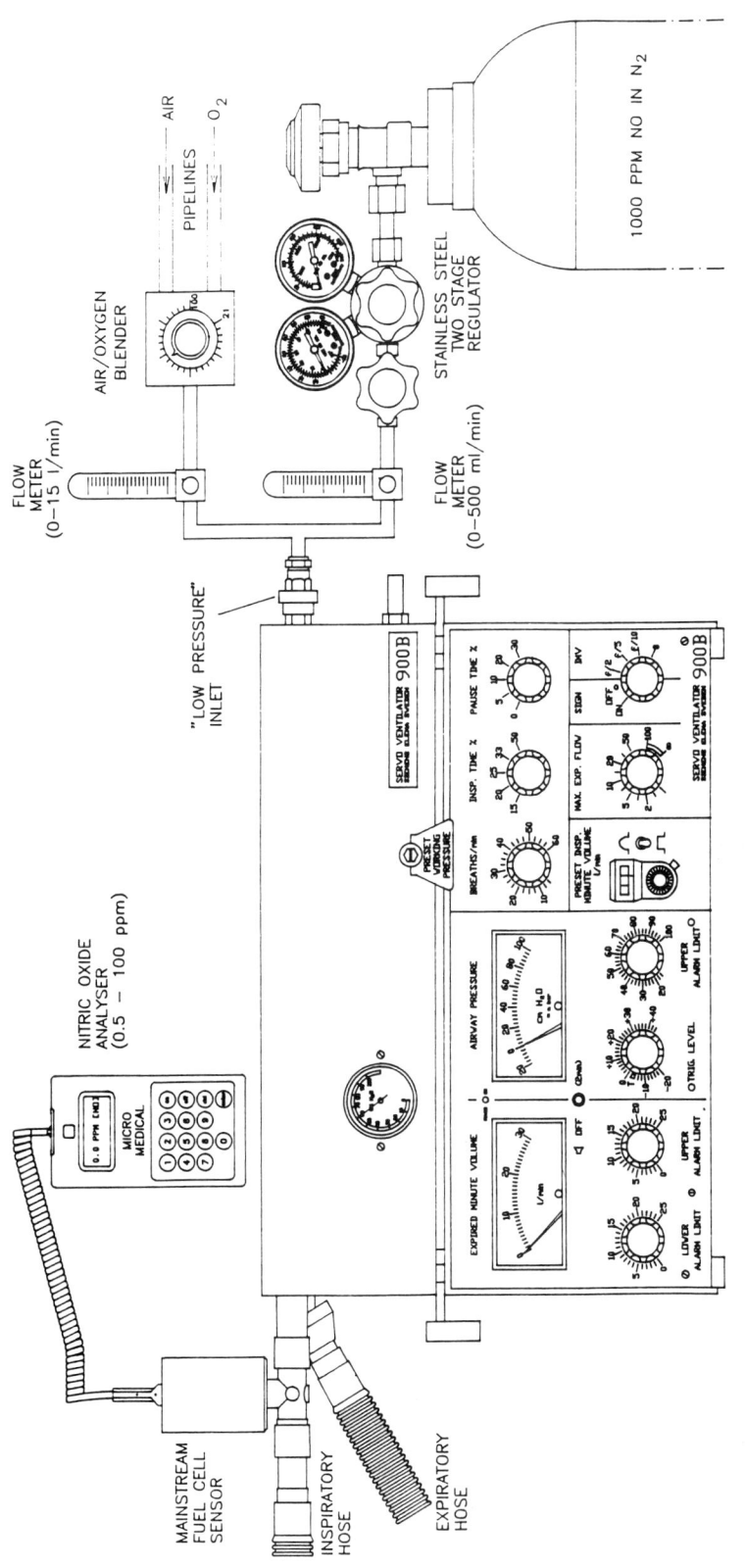

Figure 29.4 An inhaled nitric oxide delivery and monitoring system.

itoring inhaled NO therapy in the ICU, although they would probably be unsuitable if NO concentrations below 1 p.p.m. were used routinely.

CONCLUSION

The use of NO inhalation for the treatment of critically ill patients with severe ARDS, whilst undoubtedly an exciting and innovative area for investigation, remains experimental and of unproven efficacy. The physiological effects of inhaled NO – a reduction in PAP with an improvement in $\dot{V}/\dot{Q}$ matching – have been well documented, but the incidence of side effects and toxicity remains to be elucidated. The concern that NO therapy is only 'cosmetic', improving a set of physiological variables while having no effect on, or even exaggerating, the underlying disease process remains to be addressed. Whether or not the introduction of inhaled NO improves survival in ARDS remains to be seen but, given that the majority of patients die from sepsis and multiple organ failure, it is important to re-emphasize a point made some time ago: *'the obsession with arterial oxygen tension is unhealthy'* [57].

REFERENCES

1. Ashbaugh, D.G., Bigelow, D.B., Petty, T.L. and Levine, B.E. (1967) Acute respiratory distress in adults. *Lancet*, **ii**, 319–23.
2. Bernard, G.R., Artigas, A., Brigham, K.L. *et al.* (1994) Report of the American–European consensus conference on ARDS: definitions, mechanisms, relevant outcomes and clinical trial coordination. *Intensive Care Med.*, **20**, 225–32.
3. Zapol, W.M. and Snider, M.T. (1977) Pulmonary hypertension in severe acute respiratory failure. *N. Engl. J. Med.*, **296**, 476–80.
4. Villar, J., Blazquez, M.A., Lubillo, S. *et al.* (1989) Pulmonary hypertension in acute respiratory failure. *Crit. Care Med.*, **17**, 523–6.
5. Radermacher, P., Huet, Y., Pluskwa, F. *et al.* (1988) Comparison of ketanserin and sodium nitroprusside in patients with severe ARDS. *Anesthesiology*, **68**, 152–7.
6. Bone, R.C., Slotman, G., Maunder, R.J. *et al.* (1989) Randomized double-blind, multicenter study of prostaglandin E1 in patients with the adult respiratory distress syndrome. *Chest*, **96**, 114–9.
7. Morgan, J.M., McCormack, D.G., Griffiths, M.J.D. *et al.* (1991) Adenosine as a vasodilator in primary pulmonary hypertension. *Circulation*, **84**, 1145–9.
8. Radermacher, P., Santak, B., Wust, H.J. *et al.* (1990) Prostacyclin for the treatment of pulmonary hypertension in the adult respiratory distress syndrome: effects on pulmonary capillary pressure and ventilation–perfusion distributions. *Anesthesiology*, **72**, 238–44.
9. Palmer, R.M.J., Ferrige, A.G., and Moncada, S. (1987) Nitric oxide release accounts for the biological activity of endothelium-derived relaxing factor. *Nature*, **327**, 524–6.
10. Davy, H. (1800) *Researches, Chemical and Philosophical; Chiefly Concerning Nitrous Oxide, or Dephllogisticated Nitrous Air, and its Respiration*, J. Johnson, London.
11. Clutton-Brock, J. (1967) Two cases of poisoning by contamination of nitrous oxide with higher oxides of nitrogen during anaesthesia. *Br. J. Anaesth.*, **39**, 388–92.
12. Health and Safety Executive (1991) EH40/91 *Occupational Exposure Limits for use with the Control of Substances Hazardous to Health Regulations 1988*, HMSO, London, pp 21.
13. Scott, E.G. and Hunt, W.B. Jr (1973) Silo filler's disease. *Chest*, **63**, 701–6.
14. Norman, V., and Keith, C.H. (1965) Nitrogen oxides in tobacco smoke. *Nature*, **205**, 915–6.
15. Higenbottam, T.W., and Borland, C. (1987) NO yields of contemporary UK, US and French cigarettes. *Int. J. Epidemiol.*, **16**, 31–4.
16. Furchgott, R.F. and Zawadzki, J.V. (1980) The obligatory role of endothelial cells in the relaxation of arterial smooth muscle by acetylcholine. *Nature*, **288**, 373–6.
17. Stamler, J.S., Jaraki, O., Osborne, J. *et al.* (1992) Nitric oxide circulates in mammalian plasma primarily as an *S*-nitroso adduct of serum albumin. *Proc. Natl Acad. Sci. USA*, **89**, 7674–7.
18. Moncada, S., Palmer, R.M.J. and Higgs, E.A. (1991) Nitric oxide: physiology, pathophysiology, and pharmacology. *Pharmacol. Rev.*, **43**, 109–42.
19. Palmer, R.M.J., Ashton, D.S. and Moncada, S. (1988) Vascular endothelial cells synthesize

nitric oxide from L-arginine. *Nature*, **333**, 664–6.

20. Bredt, D.S., Hwang, P.M., Glatt, C.E. *et al.* (1991) Cloned and expressed nitric oxide synthase structurally resembles cytochrome P450 reductase. *Nature*, **351**, 714–8.

21. Radomski, M.W., Palmer, R.M.J. and Moncada, S. (1990) Glucocorticoids inhibit the expression of an inducible, but not the constitutive, nitric oxide synthase in vascular endothelial cells. *Proc. Natl Acad. Sci. USA*, **87**, 10043–7.

22. Rees, D.D., Palmer, R.M.J. and Moncada, S. (1989) Role of endothelium-derived nitric oxide in the regulation of blood pressure. *Proc. Natl Acad. Sci. USA*, **86**, 3375–8.

23. Rand, M.J. (1992) Nitrergic transmission: nitric oxide as a mediator of non-adrenergic, non-cholinergic neuroeffector transmission. *Clin. Exp. Pharmacol. Physiol.*, **19**, 147–69.

24. Rajfer, J., Aronson, W.J., Bush, P.A. *et al.* (1992) Nitric oxide as a mediator of relaxation of the corpus cavernosum in response to nonadrenergic, noncholinergic neurotransmission. *N. Engl. J. Med.*, **326**, 90–4.

25. Desai, K.M., Zembowicz, A., Sessa, W.C. and Vane, J.R. (1991) Nitroxergic nerves mediate vagally induced relaxation in the isolated stomach of the guinea pig. *Proc. Natl Acad. Sci. USA*, **88**, 11490–4.

26. Belvisi, M.G., Stretton, C.D. and Barnes, P.J. (1992) Nitric oxide is the endogenous neurotransmitter of bronchodilator nerves in human airways. *Eur. J. Pharmacol.*, **210**, 221–2.

27. Sanders, K. (1992) Nitric oxide and the nervous system. *Lancet*, **339**, 50–1.

28. Garthwaite, J. (1993) Nitric oxide signalling in the nervous system. *Neuroscience*, **5**, 171–80.

29. Knowles, R.G., Merrett, M., Salter, M. and Moncada, S. (1990) Differential induction of brain, lung and liver nitric oxide synthase by endotoxin in the rat. *Biochem. J.*, **270**, 833–6.

30. Nathan, C. and Hibbs, J.B. Jr (1991) Role of nitric oxide synthesis in macrophage antimicrobial activity. *Curr. Opin. Immunol.*, **3**, 65–70.

31. Hibbs, J.B. Jr (1992) Overview of cytotoxic mechanisms and defence of the intracellular environment against microbes, in *The Biology of Nitric Oxide*, Part 2 (eds S. Moncada, M.A. Marletta, J.B. Bibbs Jr and E.A. Higgs), Portland Press, London, pp. 201–6.

32. Rees, D.D., Cellek, S., Palmer, R.M.J. and Moncada, S. (1990) Dexamethasone prevents the induction by endotoxin of a nitric oxide syn-

thase and the associated effects on vascular tone: an insight into endotoxin shock. *Biomed. Biophys. Res. Commun.*, **173**, 541–7.

33. Kilbourn, R.G., Jubran, A., Gross, S.S. *et al.* (1990) Reversal of endotoxin-mediated shock by N-methyl-L-arginine, an inhibitor of nitric oxide synthesis. *Biomed. Biophys. Res. Commun.*, **172**, 1132–8.

34. Kolb, H. and Kolb-Bachofen, V. (1992) Nitric oxide, a pathogenetic factor in autoimmunity. *Immunol. Today*, **13**, 157–60.

35. McCartney, F.N., Allen, J.B., Mizel, D.E. *et al.* (1993) Suppression of arthritis by an inhibitor of nitric oxide synthase. *J. Exp. Med.*, **178**, 749–54.

36. McVeigh, G.E., Brennan, G.M. and Johnston, G.D. (1992) Impaired endothelium-dependent and independent vasodilation in patients with type 2 (non-insulin dependent) diabetes mellitus. *Diabetologia*, **35**, 771–6.

37. Middleton, S.J., Shorthouse, M. and Hunter, J.O. (1993) Increased nitric oxide synthesis in ulcerative colitis. *Lancet*, **341**, 465–6.

38. Borland, C.D.R. and Higenbottam, T.W. (1989) A simultaneous single breath measurement of pulmonary diffusing capacity with nitric oxide and carbon monoxide. *Eur. Respir. J.*, **2**, 56–63.

39. Pepke-Zaba, J., Higenbottam, T.W., Dinh-Xuan, A.T. *et al.* (1991) Inhaled nitric oxide as a cause of selective pulmonary vasodilatation in pulmonary hypertension. *Lancet*, **338**, 1173–4.

40. Snow, D.J., Gray, S.J., Foubert, L. *et al.* (1994) Inhaled nitric oxide in patients with normal and increased pulmonary vascular resistance after cardiac surgery. *Br. J. Anaesth.*, **72**, 185–9.

41. Frostell, C., Fratacci, M.D., Wain, J.C. *et al.* (1991) Inhaled nitric oxide – a selective vasodilator reversing hypoxic pulmonary vasoconstriction. *Circulation*, **83**, 2038–47.

42. Roberts, J.D., Polaner, D.M., Lang, P. and Zapol, W.M. (1992) Inhaled nitric oxide in persistent pulmonary hypertension of the newborn. *Lancet*, **340**, 818–9.

43. Kinsella, J.P., Neish, S.R., Shaffer, E. and Abman, S.H. (1992) Low-dose inhalational nitric oxide in persistent pulmonary hypertension of the newborn. *Lancet*, **340**, 819–20.

44. Girard, C., Lehot, J.J., Pannetier, J.C. *et al.* (1992) Inhaled nitric oxide after mitral valve replacement in patients with chronic pulmonary artery hypertension. *Anesthesiology*, **77**, 880–3.

45. Rossaint, R., Falke, K.J., Lopez, F. *et al.* (1993)

Inhaled nitric oxide for the adult respiratory distress syndrome. *N. Engl. J. Med.*, **328**, 399–405.

46. Wessel, D.L., Adatia, I., Thompson, J.E. and Hickey, P.R. (1994) Delivery and monitoring of inhaled nitric oxide in patients with pulmonary hypertension. *Crit. Care. Med.*, **22**, 930–8.

47. Grover, E.R., Smithies, M. and Bihari, D.J. (1993) A dose profile of the physiological effects of inhaled nitric oxide in acute lung injury. *Am. Rev. Respir. Dis.*, **147** A350.

48. Gerlach, H., Rossaint, R., Pappert, D. *et al.* (1994) Autoinhalation of nitric oxide after endogenous synthesis in nasopharynx. *Lancet*, **343**, 518–9.

49. Baulch, D.L. and Drysdale, D.D. (1973) *Evaluated Kinetic Data for High Temperature Reactions*, Butterworth, London.

50. Hurford, W.E. and Zapol, W.M. (1994) Nitric oxide inhalation in the intensive care unit. *Curr. Opin. Anaesth.*, **7**, 153–60.

51. Foubert, L. Fleming, B. Latimer, R. *et al.* (1992) Safety guidelines for use of nitric oxide. *Lancet*, **339**, 1615–6.

52. Beckman, J.S., Beckman, T.W., Chen, J. *et al.* (1990) Apparent hydroxyl radical production by peroxynitrite: implications for endothelial injury from nitric oxide and superoxide. *Proc. Natl Acad. Sci. USA*, **87**, 1620–4.

53. Hogman, M., Frostell, C., Arnberg, H. and Hedenstierna, G. (1993) Bleeding time prolongation and NO inhalation. *Lancet*, **341**, 1664–5.

54. Watkins, D.N., Jenkins, I.R., Rankin, J.M. and Clarke, G.M. (1993) Inhaled nitric oxide in severe acute respiratory failure – its use in intensive care and description of a delivery system. *Anaesth. Intensive Care*, **21**, 861–75.

55. Fontijin, A., Sabadell, A.J. and Ronco, R.J. (1970) Homogeneous chemiluminescent measurement of nitric oxide with ozone. *Anal. Chem.*, **42**, 575–9.

56. Petros, A. Cox, P. and Bohn, D. (1994) A simple method for monitoring the concentration of inhaled nitric oxide. *Anaesthesia*, **49**, 317–9.

57. Bihari, D.J. (1987) Indomethacin and arterial oxygenation in critically ill patients with severe bacterial pneumonia. *Lancet*, **1**, 755.

Mark J.D. Griffiths and Timothy W. Evans

The clinical conditions most commonly associated with the syndrome of acute respiratory distress in adult (ARDS) can be divided into those that directly damage the lung, for example aspiration of gastric contents, and those that cause ARDS as part of a systemic inflammatory response typified by sepsis (*Chapter 3*). The spread of inflammation outside areas directly involved by the former [1] and the perpetuation of pulmonary damage after the initial insult suggest that mediators of inflammation play a major role in acute lung injury regardless of the cause. Experimental [2] and clinical [3] studies have shown that ARDS is a multisystem vascular disorder, characterized not only by impaired pulmonary gas exchange, but also by failure of oxygen uptake in the periphery leading ultimately to multiple organ failure. Indeed, in one study respiratory failure accounted for only 16% of deaths in patients with ARDS, the majority being attributable to multisystem organ failure [4]. Sepsis is the archetypal systemic insult resulting in panendothelial damage [5], cardiovascular dysfunction [6] and ultimately multiple organ failure, which includes ARDS in approximately 25% of cases [7]. Recent reports have described patients fulfilling the criteria for sepsis syndrome [8], but who have no demonstrable focus of infection, suggesting that uncontrolled inflammation regardless of cause can reproduce clinical sepsis [9]. This phenomenon has also been described in patients with ARDS in whom

rigorous efforts were made to exclude infection [10].

A model of interactions between some of the inflammatory cells and mediators thought to contribute to acute lung injury associated with the systemic inflammatory response syndrome (SIRS) is shown in Figure 30.1. It is likely that ARDS results from the combination of factors that include initiating stimuli, recruitment and activation of inflammatory cells, amplification via cascades of inflammation and coagulation and ultimately elaboration of cytotoxic enzymes, reactive oxygen species and vasoactive mediators. Blocking the effects of individual mediators has been used to elucidate their role in acute lung injury in animal models and forms the basis of much of our discussion of proposed therapies.

STRATEGIES FOR PHARMACOLOGICAL INTERVENTION

Figure 30.2 illustrates the levels at which pharmacological intervention may be useful in a patient with ARDS. We shall not discuss the supportive therapies that aim to preserve oxygen delivery to other organs, such as inotropes and vasopressors, nor the various treatments of clinical conditions associated with ARDS. Presently there are no established pharmacological treatments for ARDS. However, the enormous amount of research investigating the pathogenesis and pathophy-

ARDS Acute Respiratory Distress in Adults. Edited by Timothy W. Evans and Christopher Haslett. Published in 1996 by Chapman & Hall, London. ISBN 0 412 56910 8

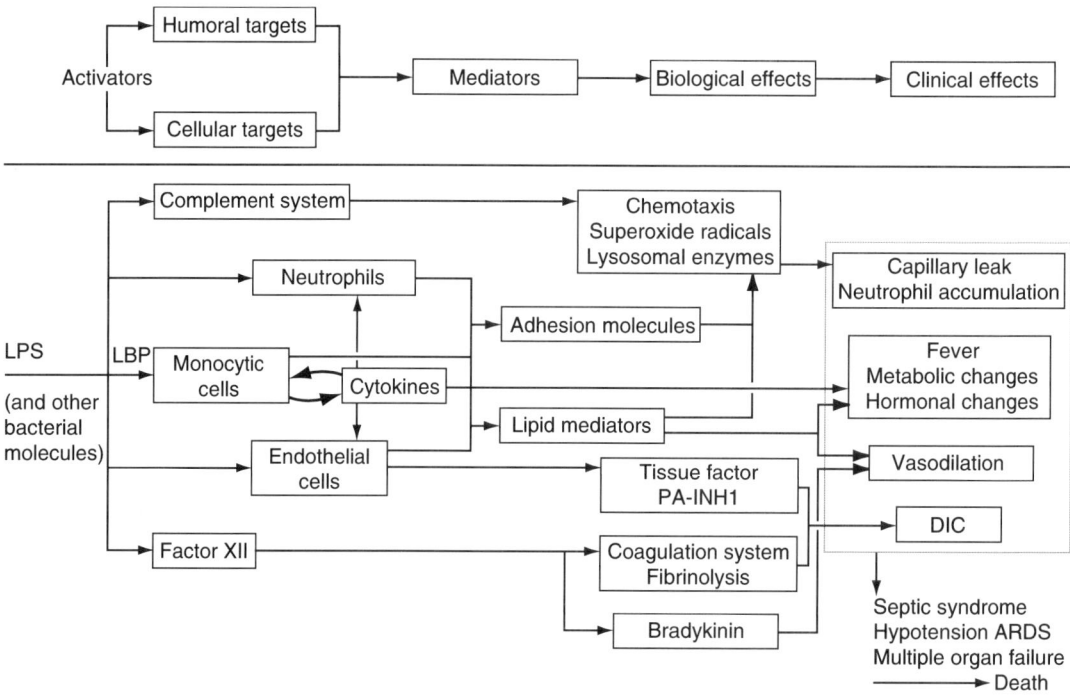

Figure 30.1 Proposed pathway for the interactions of humoral factors in the pathogenesis of sepsis. LPS = lipopolysaccharide; LBP = lipopolysaccharide binding protein; DIC = disseminated intravascular coagulation; PA-INH = plasminogen activation inhibitor. (Reproduced with permission from Glauser, M.P. *et al.* (1991) *Lancet*, **338**, 732—6.)

siology of acute lung injury has produced a plethora of potential targets and therapies, the majority of which have yet to be assessed in clinical trials. These can be divided into two groups: the first are anti-inflammatory or immunomodulatory agents that aim to interrupt or suppress the inflammatory cascade that ultimately damages the alveolar-capillary unit. The discovery of an increasing number of inflammatory mediators has provided new targets for immune therapy, but has also revealed a complex system with enormous redundancy, implying that an antagonist of a single agent is unlikely to arrest the process once initiated [11]. Thus, the inflammatory process resembles a spider's web – the loss of one or several strands (cells or mediators) may not necessarily reduce the effectiveness of the whole web, unless key strands can be identified, ideally before the web is finished.

In this respect, targeting initiators or mediators that appear early may 'nip the process in the bud' and prevent end organ damage. However, this strategy depends upon instituting therapy immediately after the insult, which is rarely feasible in the clinical setting, and which may result in many patients being treated unnecessarily. The prescribing of unnecessary treatments would be minimized by improvements in the detection of early or mild forms of acute lung injury using a sensitive severity scoring system, and in prediction of which patients at risk will develop ARDS, perhaps using biochemical markers [12,13].

Once the problem of redundancy has been overcome, it is important to recognize that any effective anti-inflammatory therapy is likely also to impair host defense. Whilst it may be possible to dissect mainly damaging mechanisms from mainly beneficial ones, it is

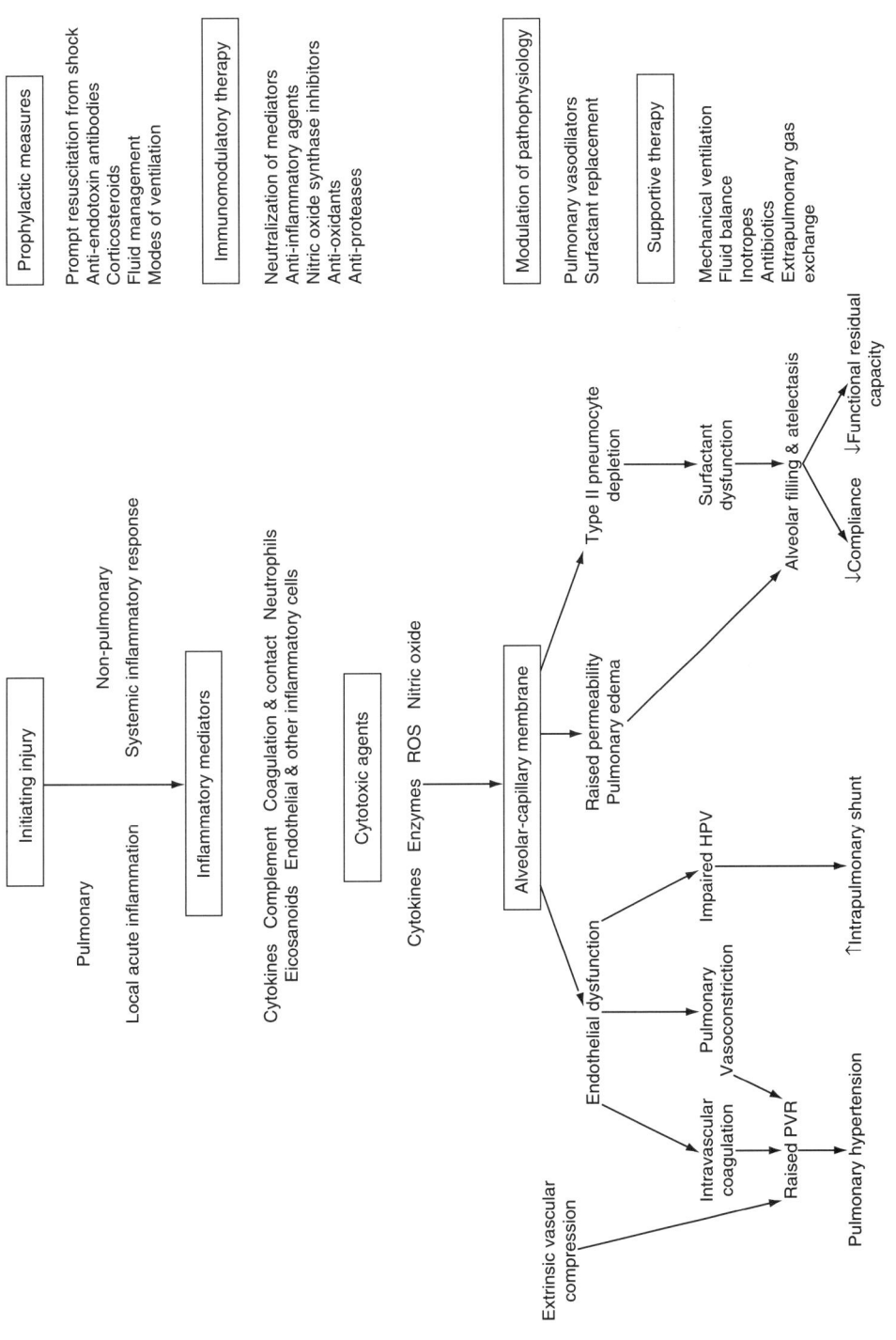

Figure 30.2 Potential targets for intervention in the development of ARDS. ROS = reactive oxygen species.

Table 30.1 Pulmonary vascular pathophysiology of ARDS

Site	Pathophysiology	Clinical correlate
Resistance vessels	Increased PVR → increased right ventricular afterload	Pulmonary hypertension → decreased cardiac index and oxygen delivery
	Loss of HPV/shunting	Decreased oxygen uptake
Microvasculature	Increased permeability	Nonhydrostatic edema
	Intravascular thrombosis/ microembolism	Microinfarction/disseminated intravascular coagulation
		Decreased oxygen uptake
Heart	Decreased contractility	Decreased cardiac index and oxygen delivery

more likely that clearer definitions of the temporal sequence of pathological events in ARDS will identify phases when particular mediators are more critical to the evolving disease than they are to host defense.

The second group of treatments aims to correct existing pathophysiology; examples include surfactant replacement and pulmonary vasodilators. Surfactant replacement therapy is covered in Chapter 16 and will not be further discussed here. Pulmonary vascular dysfunction is an important feature of ARDS (Table 30.1). Pulmonary vascular resistance (PVR) and pulmonary artery pressure are elevated in patients with respiratory failure [14–16] and in animal models of acute lung injury [17,18]. PVR is increased in early ARDS, even after correction for arterial hypoxemia, probably through a combination of increased vascular tone and structural factors such as extrinsic compression (caused by edema fluid and positive pressure ventilation) and thromboemboli [19]. Later in the clinical course vascular remodeling reduces the capillary surface area for gas exchange, which probably accounts for the exercise-induced increase in the alveolar–arterial oxygen gradient (A-aDo_2) seen in the majority of survivors [20]. Pulmonary hypertension contributes to pulmonary edema formation [21], impaired right ventricular performance [22] and may be associated with increased mortality in patients with ARDS [23]. Whether pulmonary hypertension is merely a marker of

severe vascular dysfunction or itself has an important influence on outcome is debatable. For example, loss of hypoxic pulmonary vasoconstriction (HPV) in acute lung injury [24] has an especially marked effect on gas exchange because the alveolar edema and atelectasis that occur cause enormous increases in physiological dead space. Studies using the multiple inert gas technique have demonstrated that the degree of intrapulmonary shunting is large enough to account for the observed A-aDo_2, without invoking a reduction in diffusion capacity [25]. Hence, potentially beneficial effects of vasodilators have to be weighed against adverse effects on gas exchange caused by further impairment of HPV as well as effects on the systemic circulation. In patients with acute lung injury, nitrate based vasodilators [15,26] and calcium antagonists [27] decrease PVR and pulmonary artery pressure. Whilst some studies have demonstrated improvements in cardiac index using vasodilators, none have demonstrated improved oxygen delivery and consumption [15,26]

Intravenously administered vasodilators have two drawbacks that limit their usefulness in ARDS. Most show no selectivity for the pulmonary circulation and so may destabilize a patient by causing systemic hypotension. Secondly, they act on all pulmonary vessels so that dilation of vessels supplying nonventilated areas occurs equally in ventilated and nonventilated areas. The net effect is to increase shunt fraction, which leads to a deterioration in oxygenation. Drug delivery by inhalation is theoretically attractive as it leads to selective dilation of vessels supplying ventilated alveoli, improving ventilation–perfusion matching. In the absence of an agent with intrinsic pulmonary vascular selectivity, this attribute may be conferred by the route of administration. For example, the vasodilator action of inhaled nitric oxide (NO) is rapidly lost in the circulation following reaction with hemoglobin [28]; similarly the short half life of adenosine enables it to be used as a selective pulmonary vasodilator when it is given directly into the pulmonary artery [29].

PHARMACOLOGICAL AGENTS

There is considerable overlap between the two treatment stategies discussed above, therefore each potential therapeutic agent or group of agents is discussed separately.

Corticosteroids

Corticosteroids are potent anti-inflammatory agents whose principal action was thought to depend on inhibition of phospholipase A_2 (Figure 30.3). It has been discovered recently, using molecular techniques, that glucocorticoids influence the production of several inflammatory mediators by up- or down-regulating gene transcription, for example inhibition of nitric oxide synthase induction in endothelial cells [30] and interleukin (IL)-1 production by human macrophages [31]. Furthermore, complex subcellular interactions between corticosteroids and cytokines are emerging that may uncover new mechanisms by which each affects the inflammatory process [32].

Corticosteroids are protective when given prophylactically in animal models of acute lung injury [33,34]. However, in large, well designed studies, high dose, short duration steroid therapy given before or early in the

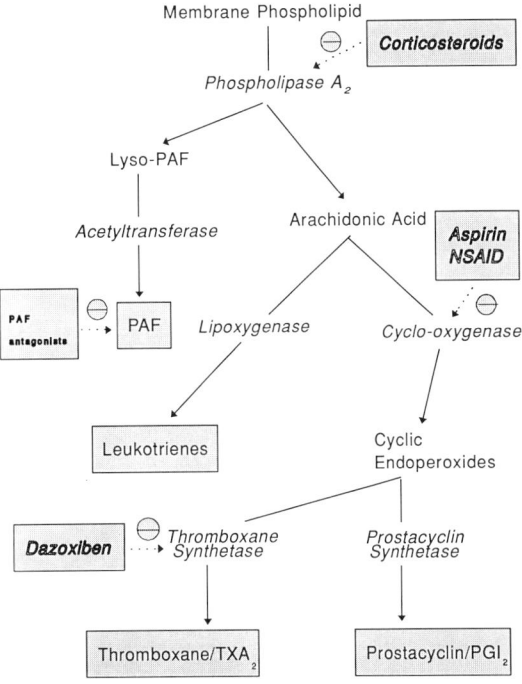

Figure 30.3 Synthetic pathway of lipid mediators in ARDS and sites of possible pharmacological manipulation. PAF = platelet activating factor.

course of ARDS was ineffective both as a treatment and a prophylactic [35,36]. Recent controlled trials suggest that steroids may confer benefit following fat embolism [37], but their use may be deleterious in postoperative patients with early respiratory failure [38]. Three small uncontrolled studies provide evidence that sustained courses of high dose steroids shorten the clinical course of uninfected patients in the fibroproliferative phase of ARDS, with few steroid related complications [10,39,40].

ANTIENDOTOXIN ANTIBODIES

Infusion of large doses of endotoxin, a Gram-negative bacterial cell wall component, can reproduce clinical sepsis, including acute lung injury in animal models [41–43]. A study on sera from patients in intensive care units demonstrated predictably high levels of endotoxin in patients with recognized sepsis [44]. However, elevated levels were also been found in patients with hemodynamic compromise secondary to variceal bleeding and major trauma. Translocation of bacteria or their cell wall constituents into the systemic circulation via an ischemic gut mucosa with impaired mucosal barrier function and diminished hepatic clearance of toxins from the portal circulation may occur [45,46]. All patients with ARDS in this study had detectable endotoxemia [44], supporting the association between circulating levels of endotoxin and the development of ARDS that has been demonstrated in some [47], but not all [48], studies of patients at risk.

Two large trials have been published recently describing the effects of monoclonal antibodies to endotoxin core glycoprotein in human sepsis syndrome [49,50]. Both demonstrated advantages, in terms of survival and resolution of system failures, but only in subgroups of patients. E5, a murine immunoglobulin (Ig)M antibody, significantly decreased mortality in patients with Gramnegative sepsis with no evidence of circulatory shock. In this group, 28% of the total, ARDS resolved in 4 of 10 patients who received E5 compared with 2 of 9 patients given placebo. By contrast, a human monoclonal IgM antibody (HA-1A: Centoxin), was found to be effective regardless of shock, but only in patients with proven Gram-negative bacteremia. Data specific to ARDS were not given. Since the publication of these encouraging data, HA-1A has received a license and subsequently been voluntarily withdrawn because further studies revealed a trend towards increased mortality in patients with Gram-positive bacteremia who had been given the drug.

CYTOKINE MANIPULATION

Technological advances since the 1980s have facilitated the identification, cloning, recombinant synthesis and functional study of many cytokines [51]. The large number of molecules, their complex interactions and overlapping effects have complicated assessment of the role of individual agents. However, there is now compelling evidence that the monokines (monocyte derived cytokines), interferon γ, interleukins IL-1, IL-6, IL-8 and especially tumor necrosis factor alpha (TNF), contribute to the uncontrolled inflammatory cascade that produces the sepsis syndrome and ARDS [13,48,52–55].

Many toxic effects of lipopolysaccharide (LPS) are mediated by the local and systemic release of these low molecular weight glycoproteins. After challenging normal humans with LPS, TNF can be detected in the serum, levels peaking about 2 hours after the dose [56]. Injecting TNF into rats produces pulmonary pathology indistinguishable from ARDS [57], and raised levels of TNF and IL-1 have been demonstrated in blood samples and bronchoalveolar lavage fluid taken from patients with the clinical syndrome [54,58]. Further evidence implicating cytokines in the pathogenesis of human ARDS has come from their therapeutic use in patients with malignant disease. In a retrospective study of 54 patients receiving high dose IL-2, 72% developed new lesions on their chest radiograph [59]. However, relative contributions of direct toxic effects of cytokines and those caused indirectly by products of activated cells and secondary mediators remain unclear. It is possible to block the damaging effects of cytokines at a number of different levels (Table 30.2), although the majority of these potential therapies are untested *in vivo* [61]. When administered prophylactically, neutralizing antibodies for TNF are protective in animal models of sepsis [71,72], although only one study has demonstrated benefit when such antibodies were given after injury [73]. Results from a study examining the safety and efficacy of a murine monoclonal anti-TNF antibody in 80 patients with severe sepsis have recently been reported [74]. Administration of the antibody was well tol-

Table 30.2 Modulation of the cytokine response in ARDS

Cytokine target	Mechanism of action	Examples
Synthesis	Gene transcription	Cyclosporin on T cell lymphokines[60]
		Glucocorticoids and PGE$_2$ on IL-2[61]
Synthesis	Translation of mRNA	Antisense oligonucleotides
Release	(unknown)	Pentamidine inhibits TNFα and IL-1 release[61-63]
Soluble cytokines	Neutralizing antibodies	IL-6 in murine bacteremia[64]
Soluble cytokines	Neutralization by soluble receptors	IL-1 downregulates alloreactivity[65] TNFα in septic shock[66]
Soluble cytokines	Enhanced clearance	High volume hemofiltration[67] Polyacrylnitrite hemofilters[68]
Receptors	Soluble antagonists	Recombinant Il-1ra in endotoxemia[69]
Effector cell	Induction of cellular protection	Induction of antioxidants and heat shock proteins by IL-1?[70]

erated despite the almost universal development of antimurine antibodies. No survival benefit was found for the total study population, but subgroup analysis suggested that the patients with increased circulating TNF levels at entry benefited from high dose anti-TNF antibody treatment. Future investigations using humanized monoclonal antibodies are awaited [75].

Pentoxifylline is a methylxanthine derivative and a phosphodiesterase inhibitor. Its actions include decreasing the production of TNF and IL-1 and the response of neutrophils and the pulmonary endothelium to these cytokines [76–78], improving red and white cell deformability and decreasing platelet aggregation. Finally, the inhibitory action of pentoxifylline on smooth muscle migration *in vitro* [79] may have have a beneficial effect on pulmonary remodeling in the fibrotic phase of ARDS. When administered before or shortly after an initiator of sepsis and ARDS, pentoxifylline attenuates acute lung injury and improves hemodynamics in animal models of shock [80–82]. This experimental work suggests a potential therapeutic role for pentoxifylline and other phosphodiesterase inhibitors in sepsis and ARDS [83], although this is yet to be defined by clinical studies.

In the fibroproliferative phase of ARDS,

locally produced cytokines are thought to regulate the growth, chemotaxis and metabolic activity of lung fibroblasts, influencing the ultimate balance between fibrosis and remodeling of normal lung tissues [84]. For example, the potent mitogenic effect of platelet derived growth factor on fibroblasts may be important in pulmonary vascular remodeling [85].

NEUTROPHIL DIRECTED THERAPIES

Overwhelming evidence points to neutrophils [86–88] and their products (such as proteolytic enzymes [53,89] and reactive oxygen species [90–93]) as mediators of the lung inflammation associated with ARDS. However, the dysfunction of lung and blood neutrophils taken from patients with ARDS [94] and the already high incidence of pneumonia complicating ARDS [95] emphasize the importance of the timing of antineutrophil therapies in these patients because of the risk of interfering with neutrophil function and thereby rendering the host defenseless against bacterial invasion.

Monoclonal antibodies have been raised against leukocyte and endothelial cell adhesion molecules: these attenuate lung injury when used prophylactically in a variety of animal models of pulmonary inflammation

[96]. The effects of an anti-CD18 monoclonal antibody on the development of multiple organ failure following trauma is currently undergoing clinical trial. However, in a canine dog model of human sepsis treatment with anti-CD18 resulted in a trend towards decreased survival [97], which may be related to the depressant effects of anti-CD18 on neutrophil function. Similarly, greater understanding of the complex interaction between proteinases, their inhibitors and inflammatory cells [98] has led to the development of elastase inhibitors with potential therapeutic applications [99]. Antioxidants, such as *N*-acetylcysteine [100] and recombinant human superoxide dismutase [101], reduce indices of acute lung injury in endotoxemic sheep, and improve hemodynamics in human fulminant hepatic failure [102]. However, in a prospective, double blind, placebo controlled trial in 66 patients with ARDS, *N*-acetylcysteine failed to improve survival or the indices of acute lung injury that were measured [103]. Assessment of the clinical use of antioxidants is complicated by the effects of high inspired oxygen concentrations and concentration dependent pro-oxidant effects of many of these compounds. For example, under certain circumstances vitamin E may promote lipid peroxidation [104]. Delivery of sufficient concentrations of antioxidants and chelators of the metal ions to sites of oxidative damage, such as the interface between bound neutrophils and endothelial cells or the intracellular milieu, represents a major theoretical problem limiting the efficacy of antioxidants *in vivo*.

MANIPULATION OF THE L-ARGININE/NITRIC OXIDE PATHWAY

Nitric oxide, which is synthesized from L-arginine, is a potent vasodilator. Two isoforms of NO synthase can be found in vascular tissues; however, in the absence of acute inflammation NO synthase is confined to the endothelium. In most vessels there is a constant production of NO that helps to maintain flow by vasodilation and inhibition of platelet adhesion [28]. Low dose infusions of NO synthase inhibitors in normal humans cause large changes in systemic vascular resistance (SVR) and PVR [105], suggesting an important role for endogenous NO in determining vascular tone in healthy human [106, 107]. Similarly, NO synthase inhibitors have been used to demonstrate the role of endogenous NO in modulating HPV [108]. Inhaled NO at concentrations of 5–80 p.p.m. produces selective and rapidly reversible pulmonary vasodilatation in animal models of pulmonary hypertension [109,110]. In healthy humans inhaling NO has no effect on pulmonary hemodynamics, but reverses the pulmonary hypertension and increase in PVR induced by breathing 12% oxygen without affecting systemic hemodynamics [111]. Concern about the toxicity of low concentrations of inhaled NO has been allayed by experiments involving long term exposure in mice [112] and more recently in patients with ARDS [113]. Concentrations of inhaled NO in the parts per billion range improved oxygenation without affecting PVR in three patients with ARDS [114]. However, given the toxicity of nitrogen oxides, monitoring of inspired gases and assessment of methemoglobin levels is advisable. The experience of Zapol and colleagues in treating 10 young patients with severe ARDS with inhaled NO has been published recently [113]. Used over short periods 18 p.p.m. NO caused small but significant decrements in mean pulmonary artery pressure, PVR and shunt fraction, without affecting cardiac output or systemic pressures. Oxygenation improved during NO inhalation, but deteriorated significantly, as did systemic pressures, during intravenous infusion of the vasodilator prostacyclin. NO was inhaled by seven patients for 3–53 days without loss of beneficial hemodynamic effect or evidence of toxicity.

The second form of NO synthase can be induced, requiring *de novo* protein synthesis, in endothelial and nonendothelial vascular tissue by endotoxin/LPS and certain 'proinflammatory' cytokines [115]. The inducible enzyme produces comparatively large amounts of NO and once synthesized activity seems not to be regulated [116]. Overproduction of NO by the inducible enzyme in vascular smooth muscle probably plays a major role in the vasodilatation and hyporesponsiveness to vasopressors that characterizes the systemic circulation of patients with SIRS [117, 118]. NO synthase inhibitors restore blood pressure in animal models of SIRS and their therapeutic potential in patients is beginning to be explored [119,120].

NO synthase can be induced in rat pulmonary vascular smooth muscle [121,122], suggesting that increased NO production in the pulmonary microvasculature is beneficial, at least in its ability to counteract pulmonary hypertension. In the common scenario of a patient with ARDS and sepsis it may be logical to combine the use of an NO synthase inhibitor with inhaled NO. These agents are exciting tools that may enable intensive care physicians to gain improved control over basic hemodynamics in this patient group. However, NO has a wide variety of physiological roles whose antagonism by complete inhibition of NO synthase would be deleterious to the host [120]. Potentially damaging effects of supplementing NO in the lung include increasing vascular permeability, as shown in the rat intestine [123], and enhanced NO mediated cytotoxicity, for example by formation of damaging reactive oxygen species [124], damage to DNA [125] and inactivation of mitochondrial enzymes [126]. Such theoretical objections will hopefully be further investigated as the therapeutic potential of NO manipulation is realized.

NONSTEROIDAL ANTI-INFLAMMATORY AGENTS

Possible beneficial effects of nonsteroidal inflammatory agents (NSAIDs) in ARDS include diminished aggregation of platelets and neutrophils, and impaired release of reactive oxygen species and neutrophil lysosomal products. As yet, no large clinical trial supports the use of NSAIDs in ARDS despite experimental data implicating eicosanoids in the pathogenesis and demonstrating the ability of their antagonists to attenuate acute lung injury [127]. Conflicting evidence has been provided by small studies in patients with established sepsis or ARDS, for example showing that indomethacin [128] and ibuprofen [129] improve gas exchange, but that dazoxiben, a specific antagonist of thromboxane A_2 synthetase, has no effect on pulmonary hemodynamics or gas exchange [130]. The recent discovery of a cyclo-oxygenase inducible by proinflammatory cytokines in human endothelial cells [131] and NSAIDs selective for this isoform [132] may provide a clinically useful inhibitor. Currently, however, the adverse effects of nonselective NSAIDs (impaired gastric cytoprotection and glomerular filtration) have limited their use in critically ill patients.

PROSTANOIDS

Prostaglandin (PG) E_1 is a vasodilator that also inhibits platelet aggregation, impairs neutrophil chemotaxis and release of toxic products and decreases macrophage activation. Continuous PGE_1 infusion into patients with ARDS influences neither survival nor the incidence of multiple organ failure [133, 134], and causes significant systemic hypotension and increased intrapulmonary shunt [133, 135]. Beneficial effects on oxygen transport have been claimed both for PGE_1 [127, 136] and prostacyclin (PGI_2) [137] in patients with sepsis and ARDS, which has encouraged further investigation into the mode of action of these vasodilating prostanoids. Preliminary experience using aerosolized PGI_2 in three patients with ARDS suggests that pulmonary vasodilatation and decreased intrapulmonary shunting can be achieved without significantly decreasing systemic blood pressure [138]. It will be interesting to compare the efficacy of aerosolized PGI_2 with that of inhaled NO, and to investigate the former's effects on inflammatory cell activity in the lung and on oxygen transport variables.

CONCLUSIONS AND FUTURE PROSPECTS

Advances in basic science have greatly increased understanding of the inflammatory systems that cause acute lung injury and the pathophysiology of the disease process that ultimately manifests as ARDS. Hence the targets for intervention have proliferated. Examples include the cytokine network and its receptors, heat shock proteins [139] and the endothelins, the most potent vasopressors known, whose role in the vascular dysfunction of sepsis and ARDS remains largely unexplored [140]. Similarly, novel agents targeting known inflammatory mediators are under development; for example, antagonists of platelet activating factor [141] and monoclonal antibodies against clotting factor VIIa [142]. Apart from the challenge of testing these agents in experimental models, it seems likely that determination of the optimum combination of agents will become an equally important preoccupation. Novel routes of administration are being explored and have already given rise to the notable success of inhaled NO and potential of aerosolized PGI_2. Drug delivery in liposomes [34] and the use of gene therapy [143] hold the promise of specific targeting of agents to inaccessable sites; for example, inducing a pulmonary endothelial cell to produce increased amounts of an intracellular antioxidant.

Efficiency of therapies may in future be improved by better methods of predicting which of the many 'at risk' patients will go on to full blown ARDS and which of the survivors will develop disabling pulmonary fibrosis, thereby targeting subgroups of patients most likely to benefit. Similarly, the adverse effects of immunosupressive therapy may be diminished by improved, perhaps molecular, techniques to detect invading organisms and permit differentiation between SIRS with and without infection.

Large prospective randomized trials will be required to determine the efficacy of new therapeutic agents. Apart from the huge cost of all such trials, studying patients with ARDS poses particular problems. There is no standard definition of ARDS, hence there is a choice as to the physiological criteria that define the study population. A multicenter trial using a more liberal definition of ARDS (Pao_2 Fio_2 ≤ 250 and bilateral infiltrates on chest radiograph within 7 days of enrollment) identified a group of patients at risk of ARDS, 98% of whom developed the full blown syndrome within 7 days [144]. Using more liberal criteria may facilitate patient enrollment and permit the use of novel therapies early in the course of the disease when interventions may be most effective. However, such a group will inevitably contain patients recovering from mild acute lung injury, which will devalue the results and which, if the end point is mortality, will decrease the power of the trial to show a significant difference between two treatments. Furthermore, there is a natural reluctance to use new and possibly dangerous agents in patients who would be expected to survive if managed conventionally. Conversely, selecting patients with severe ARDS may result in the application of management strategies after the time when the pathophysiology can be reversed. Finally, dividing patients with ARDS according to the presumed cause might allow more appropriate use of available treatments. The problems with this approach are that ARDS is commonly multifactorial and that the study will take longer to complete.

We believe there is some cause for optimism that the developments in supportive management that embody the modern intensive care unit will soon be joined by effective pharmacological therapies, which will lead to an improved outlook for patients with ARDS.

ACKNOWLEDGEMENTS

M.J.D.G. is a Wellcome Training Fellow.

REFERENCES

1. St John, R.C., Mizer, L.A. Kindt, G.C. *et al.* (1993) Acid aspiration-induced acute lung injury causes leukocyte-dependent systemic organ injury. *Journal of Applied Physiology,* **74**, 1994–2003.

2. Mizer, L.A., Weisbrode, S.E. and Dorinsky, P.M. (1989) Neutrophil accumulation and structural changes in nonpulmonary organs after acute lung injury induced by phorbol myristate acetate. *American Review of Respiratory Disease,* **139**, 1017–26.

3. Bone, R.C., Balk, R., Slotman, G. *et al.* (1992) Adult respiratory distress syndrome. Sequence and importance of development of multiple organ failure. The Prostaglandin E1 Study Group. *Chest,* **101**, 320–6.

4. Montgomery, A.B., Stager, M.A., Carrico, C.J. and Hudson, L.D. (1985) Causes of mortality in patients with the adult respiratory distress syndrome. *American Review of Respiratory Disease,* **132**, 485–9.

5. Rubin, D.B., Wiener-Kronish, J.P. and Murray, J.F. (1990) Elevated von Willebrand factor antigen is an early predictor of impending acute lung injury in nonpulmonary sepsis syndrome. *Journal of Clinical Investigation,* **86**, 474–80.

6. Thijs, L.G., Schneider, A.J., and Groeneveld, A.J.B. (1990) The haemodynamics of septic shock. *Intensive Care Medicine,* **16**(suppl. 3); S182–6.

7. Weinberg, PF, Matthay, MA, Webster, RO *et al.* (1984) Biologically active products of complement and acute lung injury in patients with the sepsis syndrome. *American Review of Respiratory Disease,* **130**; 791–6.

8. Bone, R.C., Sibbald, W.J. and Sprung, C.L. (1992) The ACCP-SCCM consensus conference on sepsis and organ failure. *Chest,* **101**, 1481–3.

9. Leatherman, J.W. and Schmitz, P.G. (1991) A pseudo-sepsis syndrome associated with chronic salicylate intoxication. *Chest,* **100**; 1391–6.

10. Meduri, G.U., Belenchia, J.M., Estes, R.J. *et al.* (1991) Fibroproliferative phase of ARDS. Clinical findings and effects of corticosteroids. *Chest,* **100**, 943–52.

11. St John, R.C. and Dorinsky, P.M. (1993) Immunologic therapy for ARDS, septic shock, and multiple-organ failure. *Chest,* **103**; 932–43.

12. Leff, J.A., Parsons, P.E., Day, C.E. *et al.* (1993) Serum antioxidants as predictors of adult respiratory distress syndrome in patients with sepsis. *Lancet,* **341**, 777–80.

13. Donnelly, S.C., Strieter, R.M., Kunkel, S.L. *et al.* (1993) Interleukin-8 and development of adult respiratory distress syndrome in at-risk patient groups. *Lancet,* **341**, 643–7.

14. Zapol, W.M. and Snider, M.T. (1977) Pulmonary hypertension in severe acute respiratory failure. *New England Journal of Medicine,* **296**; 476–80.

15. Zapol, W.M., Snider, M.T. and Rie, M (1992) Pulmonary circulation in adult respiratory distress syndrome, in *Adult respiratory Distress Syndrome,* (eds A. Artigas, F. Lemaire, P.M. Suter and W.M. Zapol) Churchill Livingstone, New York, pp. 78.

16. Leeman, M. (1991) The pulmonary circulation in acute lung injury: a review of some recent advances. *Intensive Care Medicine,* **17**, 254–60.

17. Christman, B.W., Lefferts, P.L., Blair, I.A. and Snapper, J.R. (1990) Effect of platelet-activating factor receptor antagonism on endotoxin-induced lung dysfunction in awake sheep. *American Review of Respiratory Disease,* **142**; 1272–8.

18. Jones, R. and Reid, L. (1992) Pulmonary vascular changes in adult respiratory distress syndrome, in *Adult Respiratory Distress Syndrome* (eds A. Artigas, F. Lemaire, P.M. Suter and W.M. Zapol), Churchill Livingstone, New York, 45–59.

19. Fox, G.A. and McCormack, D.G. (1992) The pulmonary physician and critical care. 4. A new look at the pulmonary circulation in acute lung injury. *Thorax* **47**, 743–7.

20. Buchser, E., Leuenberger, P., Chiolero, R. *et al.* (1985) Reduced pulmonary capillary blood volume as a long-term sequel of ARDS. *Chest,* **87**, 608–11.

21. Prewitt, R.M., McCarthy, J. and Wood L.D.H. (1981) Treatment of acute low pressure pul-

monary oedema in dogs. *Journal of Clinical Investigation.* **67**, 409–18.

22. Sibbald, W.J. and Driedger, A.A. (1983) Right ventricular function in acute disease states: pathophysiologic considerations. *Critical Care Medicine*, **11**, 339–45.

23. Bernard, G.R., Rinaldo, J., Harris, T. *et al.* (1985) Early predictors of ARDS reversal in patients with established ARDS. *American Review of Respiratory Disease*, **131**; A143.

24. Weir, E.K., Milczoch, J., Reeves, J.T. and Grover R.F. (1976) Endotoxin and prevention of hypoxic pulmonary vasoconstriction. *Journal of Laboratory and Clinical Medicine*, **68**; 975–83.

25. Dantzker, D.R., Brook, C.J., Dehart, P. *et al.* (1979) Ventilation-perfusion distributions in the adult respiratory distress syndrome. *American Review of Respiratory Disease*, **120**, 1039–52.

26. Sibbald, W.J., Driedger, A.A., McCallum, D. *et al.* (1986) Nitroprusside infusion does not improve biventricular performance in patients with acute hypoxaemic respiratory failure. *Journal of Critical Care*, **1**, 197–203.

27. Melot, C., Naeije, R., Mols, P. *et al.* (1987) Pulmonary vascular tone improves pulmonary gas exchange in the adult respiratory distress syndrome. *American Review of Respiratory Disease*, **136**, 1232–6.

28. Moncada, S., Palmer, R.M. and Higgs, E.A. (1991) Nitric oxide: physiology, pathophysiology, and pharmacology. *Pharmacological Reviews*, **43**, 109–42.

29. Morgan, J.M., McCormack, D.G., Griffiths, M.J. *et al.* (1991) Adenosine as a vasodilator in primary pulmonary hypertension. *Circulation,* **84**; 1145–9.

30. Radomski, M.W., Palmer, R.M. and Moncad S. (1990) Glucocorticoids inhibit the expression of an inducible, but not the constitutive, nitric oxide synthase in vascular endothelial cells. *Proceedings of the National Academy of Sciences of the USA*, **87**, 10043–7.

31. Kern, J.A., Lamb, R.J., Reed, J.C. *et al.* (1988) Dexamethasone inhibition of interleukin-1 beta production by human monocytes. *Journal of Clinical Investigation* **81**, 1386–92.

32. Barnes, P.J. and Adcock, I. (1993) Anti-inflammatory actions of steroids: molecular mechanisms. *Trends in Pharmacological Sciences*, **14**, 436–41.

33. Chiara, O., Giomarelli, P.P., Borrelli, E. *et al.*

(1991) Inhibition by methylprednisolone of leukocyte-induced pulmonary damage. *Critical Care Medicine*, **19**, 260–5.

34. Forsgren, P.E., Modig, J.A., Dahlback, C.M. and Axelsson B.I. (1990) Prophylactic treatment with an aerosolized corticosteroid liposome in a porcine model of early ARDS induced by endotoxaemia. *Acta Chirurgica Scandinavica*, **156**, 423–31.

35. Bernard, G.R., Luce, J.M., Sprung, C.L. *et al.* (1987) High-dose corticosteroids in patients with the adult respiratory distress syndrome. *New England Journal of Medicine*, **317**, 1565–70.

36. Bone, R.C., Fisher, C.J. Jr, Clemmer, T.P. *et al.* (1987) Early methylprednisolone treatment for septic syndrome and the adult respiratory distress syndrome. *Chest*, **92**, 1032–36.

37. Schonfeld, S.A., Ploysongsang, Y., Dilisio, R. *et al.* (1983) Fat embolism prophylaxis with corticosteroids. *Annals of Internal Medicine*, **99**, 438–43.

38. Weigelt, J.A., Norcross, J.F., Borman, K.R. and Snyder, W.H. (1985) Early steroid therapy for respiratory failure. *Archives of Surgery*, **120**, 536–40.

39. Ashbaugh, D.G. and Maier, R.V. (1985) Idiopathic pulmonary fibrosis in adult respiratory distress syndrome. *Archives of Surgery*, **120**, 530–5.

40. Hooper, R.G. and Kearl, R.A. (1990) Established ARDS treated with a sustained course of adrenocortical steroids. *Chest*, **97**, 138–43.

41. Brigham, K.L. and Meyrick, B. (1986) Endotoxin and lung injury. *American Review of Respiratory Disease*, **133**, 913–27.

42. Simons, R.K., Maier, R.V. and Chi, E.Y. (1991) Pulmonary effects of continuous endotoxin infusion in the rat. *Circulatory Shock*, **33**, 233–43.

43. Pearl, R.G., Baer, E.R., Siegel, L.C. *et al.* (1992) Longitudinal distribution of pulmonary vascular resistance after endotoxin administration in sheep. *Critical Care Medicine*, **20**, 119–25.

44. Vijaykumar, E., Raziuddin, S. and Wardle E.N. (1991) Plasma endotoxin in patients with trauma, sepsis and severe haemorrhage. *Clinical Intensive Care*, **2**, 4–9.

45. Van Goor H., Rosman C., Grand J. *et al.* (1994) Translocation of bacteria and endotoxin in organ donors. *Archives of Surgery*, **129**, 1063–6.

46. Roumen, R.M., Hendriks, T., Wevers, R.A. and Goris J.A. (1993) Intestinal permeability after severe trauma and hemorrhagic shock is increased without relation to septic complications. *Archives of Surgery*, **128**, 453–7.

47. Parsons, P.E., Worthen, G.S., Moore, E.E. *et al.* (1989) The association of circulating endotoxin with the development of the adult respiratory distress syndrome. *American Review of Respiratory Disease*, **140**, 294–301.

48. Hoch, R.C., Rodriguez, R., Manning, T. *et al.* (1993) Effects of accidental trauma on cytokine and endotoxin production. *Critical Care Medicine*, **21**, 839–45.

49. Greenman, R.L., Schein, R.M., Martin, M.A. *et al.* (1991) A controlled clinical trial of E5 murine monoclonal IgM antibody to endotoxin in the treatment of Gram-negative sepsis. The XOMA Sepsis Study Group. *JAMA*, **266**, 1097–102.

50. Ziegler, E.J., Fisher, C.J. Jr, Sprung, C.L. *et al.* (1991) Treatment of Gram-negative bacteremia and septic shock with HA-1A human monoclonal antibody against endotoxin. A randomized, double-blind, placebo-controlled trial. The HA-1A Sepsis Study Group. *New England Journal of Medicine*, **324**, 429–36.

51. Arai, K.I., Lee, F., Miyajima, A. *et al.* (1990) Cytokines: coordinators of immune and inflammatory responses. *Annual Review of Biochemistry*, **59**, 783–836.

52. Donnelly, S.C. and Haslett, C. (1992) Cellular mechanisms of acute lung injury: implications for future treatment in the adult respiratory distress syndrome. *Thorax*, **47**, 260–3.

53. Suter, P.M., Suter, S., Girardin, E. *et al.* (1992) High bronchoalveolar levels of tumor necrosis factor and its inhibitors, interleukin-1, interferon, and elastase, in patients with adult respiratory distress syndrome after trauma, shock, or sepsis. *American Review of Respiratory Disease*, **145**, 1016–22.

54. Jacobs, R.F., Tabor, D.R., Burks, A.W. and Campbell, G.D. (1989) Elevated interleukin-1 release by human alveolar macrophages during the adult respiratory distress syndrome. *American Review of Respiratory Disease*, **140**, 1686–92.

55. Tran Van Nhieu, J., Misset, B., Lebargy, F. *et al.* (1993) Expression of tumor necrosis factor-alpha gene in alveolar macrophages from patients with the adult respiratory distress syndrome. *American Review of Respiratory Disease*, **147**, 1585–9.

56. Michie, H.R., Manogue, K.R. and Spriggs, D.R. (1988) Detection of circulating tumour necrosis factor after endotoxin administration. *New England Journal of Medicine*, **318**, 1481–6.

57. Ferrari-Baliviera, E., Mealy, K., Smith, R.J. and Wilmore, D.W. (1989) Tumor necrosis factor induces adult respiratory distress syndrome in rats. *Archives of Surgery*, **124**, 1400–5.

58. Hyers, T.M., Tricomi, S.M., Dettenmeier, P.A. and Fowler A.A. (1991) Tumor necrosis factor levels in serum and bronchoalveolar lavage fluid of patients with the adult respiratory distress syndrome. *American Review of Respiratory Disease*, **144**, 268–71.

59. Vogelzang, P.J., Bloom, S.M., Mier, J.W. and Atkins M.B. (1992) Chest roentgenographic abnormalities in IL-2 recipients. Incidence and correlation with clinical parameters. *Chest*, **101**, 746–52.

60. Granelli-Piperno, A., Nolan, P., Inaba, K. and Steinman, R.M. (1990) The effect of immunosuppressive agents on the induction of nuclear factors that bind to sites on the interleukin 2 promoter. *Journal of Experimental Medicine*, **172**, 1869–72.

61. Henderson, B. and Blake, S. (1992) Therapeutic potential of cytokine manipulation. *Trends in Pharmacological Sciences*, **13**, 145–52.

62. Corsini, E., Craig, W.A. and Rosenthal, G.J. (1992) Modulation of tumor necrosis factor release from alveolar macrophages treated with pentamidine isethionate. *International Journal of Immunopharmacology*, **14**, 121–30.

63. Rosenthal, G.J., Craig, W.A., Corsini, E. *et al.* (1992) Pentamidine blocks the pathophysiologic effects of endotoxemia through inhibition of cytokine release. *Toxicology and Applied Pharmacology*, **112**, 222–8.

64. Starnes, H.F. Jr, Pearce, M.K., Tewari, A. *et al.* (1990) Anti-IL-6 monoclonal antibodies protect against lethal *Escherichia coli* infection and lethal tumor necrosis factor-alpha challenge in mice. *Journal of Immunology*, **145**, 4185–91.

65. Fanslow, W.C., Sims, J.E., Sassenfeld, H. *et al.* (1990) Regulation of alloreactivity *in vivo* by a soluble form of the interleukin-1 receptor. *Science*, **248**, 739–42.

66. Kohno, T., Brewer, M.T., Baker, S.L. *et al.* (1990) A second tumor necrosis factor receptor gene product can shed a naturally occur-

ring tumor necrosis factor inhibitor. *Proceedings of the National Academy of Sciences of the USA*, **87**, 8331–5.

67. Storck, M., Hartl, W.H., Zimmerer, E. and Inthorn, D. (1991) Comparison of pump-driven and spontaneous continuous haemofiltration in postoperative acute renal failure. *Lancet*, **337**, 452–5.

68. Bysani, G.K., Shenep, J.L., Hildner, W.K. *et al.* (1990) Detoxification of plasma containing lipopolysaccharide by adsorption. *Critical Care Medicine*, **18**, 67–71.

69. Dinarello, C.A. and Thompson, R.C. (1991) Blocking IL-1: interleukin 1 receptor antagonist *in vivo* and *in vitro*. *Immunology Today*, **12**, 404–10.

70. Kuruvilla, A.P., Shah, R., Hochwald, G.M. *et al.* (1991) Protective effect of transforming growth factor beta 1 on experimental autoimmune diseases in mice. *Proceedings of the National Academy of Sciences of the USA*, **88**, 2918–21.

71. Beutler, B., Milsark, I.W. and Cerami, A. (1985) Passive immunisation against cachectin/TNF protects mice from the lethal effects of endotoxin. *Science*, **229**, 869–71.

72. Windsor, A.C., Walsh, C.J., Mullen, P.G. *et al.* (1993) Tumor necrosis factor-alpha blockade prevents neutrophil CD18 receptor upregulation and attenuates acute lung injury in porcine sepsis without inhibition of neutrophil oxygen radical generation. *Journal of Clinical Investigation*, **91**, 1459–68.

73. Hinshaw, L., Olson, P. and Kuo, G. (1989) Efficacy of post-treatment with anti-TNF monoclonal antibody in preventing the pathophysiology and lethality of sepsis in the baboon. *Circulatory Shock*, **27**, 362–6.

74. Fisher, C.J. Jr, Opal, S.M., Dhainaut, J.F. *et al.* (1993) Influence of an anti-tumor necrosis factor monoclonal antibody on cytokine levels in patients with sepsis. The CB0006 Sepsis Syndrome Study Group. *Critical Care Medicine*, **21**, 318–27.

75. Mayforth, R.D. and Quintas J. (1990) Designer and catalytic antibodies. *New England Journal of Medicine*, **323**, 173–8.

76. Sullivan, G.W., Carper, H.T. and Novick, W.J. Jr and Mandell G.L. (1988) Inhibition of the inflammatory action of interleukin-1 and tumor necrosis factor (alpha) on neutrophil function by pentoxifylline. *Infection and Immunity*, **56**, 1722–9.

77. Bessler, H., Gilgal, R., Djaldetti, M. and Zahavi, I. (1986) Effect of pentoxifylline on the phagocytic activity, cAMP levels, and superoxide anion production by monocytes and polymorphonuclear cells. *Journal of Leukocyte Biology*, **140**, 747–54.

78. Strieter, R.M., Remick, D.G., Ward, P.A. *et al.* (1988) Cellular and molecular regulation of tumor necrosis factor-alpha production by pentoxifylline. *Biochemical and Biophysical Research Communications*, **155**, 1230–6.

79. Kullmann, A., Vaillant, P., Muller, V. *et al.*(1993) *In vitro* effects of pentoxifylline on smooth muscle cell migration and blood monocyte production of chemotactic activity for smooth muscle cells: potential therapeutic benefit in the adult respiratory distress syndrome. *American Journal of Respiratory Cell and Molecular Biology*, **8**, 83–8.

80. Seear, M.D., Hannam, V.L., Kaapa, P. *et al.* (1990) Effect of pentoxifylline on hemodynamics, alveolar fluid reabsorption, and pulmonary edema in a model of acute lung injury. *American Review of Respiratory Disease*, **142**, 1083–7.

81. Coccia, M.T., Waxman, K., Soliman, M.H. *et al.* (1989) Pentoxifylline improves survival following hemorrhagic shock. *Critical Care Medicine*, **17**, 36–8.

82. Welsh, C.H., Lien, D., Worton, G.S. *et al.* (1988) Pentoxifylline decreases endotoxin-induced pulmonary neutrophil sequestration and extravascular protein accumulation in the dog. *American Review of Respiratory Disease*, **138**, 1106–14.

83. Mandell, G.L. (1988) ARDS, neutrophils, and pentoxifylline. *American Review of Respiratory Disease*, **138**, 1103–5.

84. Knighton, D.R. and Fiegel, V.D. (1989) Growth factors and repair, in *Multiple Organ Failure* (eds D.G. Bihari and F.B. Cerra), New Horizons III, Fullerton, CA. pp. 371–89.

85. Deuel, T.F. and Huang, J.S. (1982) Platelet-derived growth factor: structure, function and roles in normal and transformed cells. *Journal of Clinical Investigation*, **69**, 1046–9.

86. Gadek, J.E. (1992) Adverse effects of neutrophils on the lung. *American Journal of Medicine*, **92**, 27S–31S.

87. Chollet-Martin, S., Montravers, P., Gibert, C. *et al.* (1992) Subpopulation of hyperresponsive polymorphonuclear neutrophils in patients with adult respiratory distress syn-

drome. Role of cytokine production. *American Review of Respiratory Disease*, **146**, 990–6.

88. Repine, J.E. and Beehler, C.J. (1991) Neutrophils and adult respiratory distress syndrome: two interlocking perspectives in 1991. *American Review of Respiratory Disease*, **144**, 251–2.

89. Birrer, P. (1993) Consequences of unbalanced protease in the lung: protease involvement in destruction and local defense mechanisms of the lung. *Agents and Actions*, **40**, 3–12.

90. Krsek-Staples, J.A., Kew, R.R. and Webster, R.O. (1992) Ceruloplasmin and transferrin levels are altered in serum and bronchoalveolar lavage fluid of patients with the adult respiratory distress syndrome. *American Review of Respiratory Disease*, **145**, 1009–15.

91. Sznajder, J.I., Fraiman, A., Hall, J.B. *et al.* (1989) Increased hydrogen peroxide in the expired breath of patients with acute hypoxemic respiratory failure. *Chest*, **96**, 606–12.

92. Richard, C., Lemonnier, F., Thibault, M. *et al.* (1990) Vitamin E deficiency and lipoperoxidation during adult respiratory distress syndrome. *Critical Care Medicine*, **18**, 4–9.

93. Brigham, K.L. (1990) Oxidant stress and adult respiratory distress syndrome. *European Respiratory Journal*, **11**, 482s–484s.

94. Martin, T.R., Pistorese, B.P., Hudson, L.D. and Maunder, R.J. (1991) The function of lung and blood neutrophils in patients with the adult respiratory distress syndrome. Implications for the pathogenesis of lung infections. *American Review of Respiratory Disease*, **144**, 254–62.

95. Niederman, M.S. and Fein, A.M. (1990) Sepsis syndrome, the adult respiratory distress syndrome, and nosocomial pneumonia. A common clinical sequence. *Clinics In Chest Medicine*, **11**, 633–56.

96. Hellewell, P.G. (1993) Cell adhesion molecules and potential for pharmacological intervention in lung inflammation. *Pulmonary Pharmacology*, **6**, 109–18.

97. Eichacker, P.Q., Hoffman, W.D., Farese, A. *et al.* (1993) Leukocyte CD18 monoclonal antibody worsens endotoxemia and cardiovascular injury in canines with septic shock. *Journal of Applied Physiology*, **74**, 1885–92.

98. Tetley, T.D. (1993) New perspectives on basic mechanisms in lung disease. 6. Proteinase imbalance: its role in lung disease. *Thorax*, **48**, 560–5.

99. Travis, J. and Fritz, H. (1991) Potential problems in designing elastase inhibitors for therapy. *American Review of Respiratory Disease*, **143**, 1412–5.

100. Bernard, G.R., Lucht, W.D., Niedermeyer, M.E. *et al.* (1984) Effect of *N*-acetylcysteine on the pulmonary response to endotoxin in the awake sheep and upon *in vitro* granulocyte function. *Journal of Clinical Investigation*, **73**, 1772–84.

101. Koyama, S., Kobayashi, T., Kubo, K. *et al.* (1992) Recombinant-human superoxide dismutase attenuates endotoxin-induced lung injury in awake sheep. *American Review of Respiratory Disease*, **145**, 1404–9.

102. Harrison, P.M., Wendon, J.A., Gimson, A.E. *et al.* (1991) Improvement by acetylcysteine of hemodynamics and oxygen transport in fulminant hepatic failure. *New England Journal of Medicine*, **324**, 1852–7.

103. Jepsen, S., Herlevsen, P., Knudsen, P. *et al.* (1992) Antioxidant treatment with *N*-acetylcysteine during adult respiratory distress syndrome: a prospective, randomized, placebo-controlled study. *Critical Care Medicine*, **20**, 918–23.

104. Halliwell, B. and Gutteridge, J.M.C. (1988) Free radicals and antioxidant protection: mechanisms and significance in toxicology and disease. *Human Toxicology*, **7**, 7–13.

105. Stamler, J.S., Loh, E., Roddy, M. *et al.* (1994) Nitric oxide regulates systemic and pulmonary vascular resistance in normal subjects. *Circulation*, **89**, 2035–40.

106. Vallance, P., Collier, J. and Moncada, S. (1989) Nitric oxide synthesised from L-arginine mediates endothelium dependent dilatation in human veins *in vivo*. *Cardiovascular Research*, **23**, 1053–7.

107. Vallance, P., Collier, J. and Moncada, S. (1989) Effects of endothelium-derived nitric oxide on peripheral arteriolar tone in man. *Lancet*, **ii**, 997–1000.

108. Liu, S.F., Crawley, D.E., Barnes, P.J. and Evans, T.W. (1991) Endothelium-derived relaxing factor inhibits hypoxic pulmonary vasoconstriction in rats. *American Review of Respiratory Disease*, **143**, 32–7.

109. Frostell, C., Fratacci, M.D., Wain, J.C. *et al.* (1991) Inhaled nitric oxide. A selective pulmonary vasodilator reversing hypoxic pulmonary vasoconstriction *Circulation*, **83**, 2038–47.

110. Fratacci, M.D., Frostell, C.G., Chen, T.Y. *et al.* (1991) Inhaled nitric oxide. A selective pulmonary vasodilator of heparin-protamine vasoconstriction in sheep. *Anesthesiology*, **75**, 990–9.

111. Frostell, C.G., Blomqvist, H., Hedenstierna, G. *et al.* (1993) Inhaled nitric oxide selectively reverses human hypoxic pulmonary vasoconstriction without causing systemic vasodilation. *Anesthesiology*, **78**, 427–35.

112. Oda, H., Nogami, H., Kusomoto, S. *et al.* (1976) Long-term exposure to nitric oxide in mice. *Journal of the Japanese Society for Air Pollution*, **11**, 150–60.

113. Rossaint, R., Falke, K.J., Lopez, F. *et al.* (1993) Inhaled nitric oxide for the adult respiratory distress syndrome. *New England Journal of Medicine*, **328**, 399–405.

114. Gerlach, H., Pappert, D., Lewandowski, K. *et al.* (1993) Long-term inhalation with evaluated low doses of nitric oxide for selective improvement in oxygenation in patients with adult respiratory distress syndrome. *Intensive Care Medicine*, **19**, 443–9.

115. MacNaul, K.L. and Hutchinson N.I. (1993) Differential expression of iNOS and cNOS mRNA in human vascular smooth muscle cells under normal and inflammatory conditions. *Biochemical and Biophysical Research Communications*, **196**, 1330–4.

116. Stoclet J.-C., Fleming I., Gray G. *et al.* (1993) Nitric oxide and endotoxaemia. *Circulation*, **87**, V77–V80.

117. Hibbs, J.B. Jr, Westenfelder, C., Taintor, R. *et al.* (1992) Evidence for cytokine-inducible nitric oxide synthesis from L-arginine in patients receiving interleukin-2 therapy. *Journal of Clinical Investigation*, **89**, 867–77.

118. MacMicking, J.D., Nathan, C., Hom, G. *et al.* (1995) Altered response to bacterial infection and endotoxic shock in mice lacking inducible nitric oxide synthase. *Cell*, **81**, 641–50.

119. Lorente, J.A., Landin, L., de Pablo, R. *et al.* (1993) L-arginine pathway in the sepsis syndrome. *Critical Care Medicine*, **21**, 1287–95.

120. Griffiths, M.J.D. and Evans T.W. (1994): Nitric oxide synthase inhibitors in septic shock: theoretical considerations. *Clinical Intensive Care*, **5**, 29–36.

121. Nakayama, D.K., Geller, D.A., Lowenstein, C.J. *et al.* (1992) Cytokines and lipopolysaccharide induce nitric oxide synthase in cultured rat pulmonary artery smooth muscle.

American Journal of Respiratory Cell and Molecular Biology, **7**, 471–6.

122. Griffiths, M.J.D., Liu, S.F., Curzen, N.P. *et al.* (1995) *In vivo* treatment with endotoxin induces nitric oxide synthase in rat main pulmonary artery. *American Journal of Physiology*, **268**, L509–18.

123. Boughton-Smith, N.K., Evans, S.M., Laszlo, F. *et al.* (1993) The induction of nitric oxide synthase and intestinal vascular permeability by endotoxin in the rat. *British Journal of Pharmacology*, **110**, 1189–95.

124. Beckman, J.S., Beckman, T.W., Chen, J. *et al.* (1990) Apparent hydroxyl radical production by peroxynitrite: implications for endothelial injury from nitric oxide and superoxide. *Proceedings of the National Academy of Sciences of the USA*, **87**, 1620–4.

125. Nguyen, T., Brunson, D., Crespi, C.L. *et al.* (1992) DNA damage and mutation in human cells exposed to nitric oxide *in vitro*. *Proceedings of the National Academy of Sciences of the USA*, **89**, 3030–4.

126. Stadler, J., Billiar, T.R., Curran, R.D. *et al.* (1991) Effect of exogenous and endogenous nitric oxide on mitochondrial respiration of rat hepatocytes. *American Journal of Physiology*, **260**, C910–6.

127. Metz, C. and Sibbald, W.J. (1991) Anti-inflammatory therapy for acute lung injury. A review of animal and clinical studies. *Chest*, **100**, 1110–9.

128. Steinberg, S.M., Rodriguez, J.L., Bitzer, L.G. *et al.* (1990) Indomethacin treatment of human adult respiratory distress syndrome. *Circulatory Shock*, **30**, 375–84.

129. Bernard, G.R., Reines, H.D., Metz, C.A. *et al.* (1988) Effects of a short course of ibuprofen in patients with severe sepsis. *American Review of Respiratory Disease*, **137**, A138 (abstract).

130. Leeman, M., Boeynaems, J.M., Degaute, J.P. *et al.* (1985) Administration of dazoxiben, a selective thromboxane synthetase inhibitor, in the adult respiratory distress syndrome. *Chest*, **87**, 726–30.

131. Maier, J.A.M., Hla, T. and Maciag, T. (1993) Cyclooxygenase is an immediate gene induced by interleukin-1 in human endothelial cells. *Proceedings of the National Academy of Sciences of the USA*, **265**, 10805–8.

132. Akarasereenont, P., Mitchell, J.A., Thiemermann, C. and Vane, J.R. (1994) Relative potency of nonsteroid anti-inflammatory

drugs as inhibitors of cyclooxygenase-1 or cyclooxygenase-2. *British Journal of Pharmacology* **112**, 183P.

133. Bone, R.C., Slotman, G., Maunder, R. *et al.* (1989) Randomized double-blind, multicenter study of prostaglandin E1 in patients with the adult respiratory distress syndrome. Prostaglandin E1 Study Group. *Chest*, **96**, 114–9.

134. Russell, J.A., Ronco, J.J. and Dodek, P.M. (1990) Physiologic effects and side effects of prostaglandin E1 in the adult respiratory distress syndrome. *Chest*, **97**, 684–92.

135. Melot, C., Lejeune, P., Leeman, M. *et al.* (1989) Prostaglandin E1 in the adult respiratory distress syndrome. Benefit for pulmonary hypertension and cost for pulmonary gas exchange. *American Review of Respiratory Disease*, **139**, 106–10.

136. Silverman, H.J., Slotman, G., Bone, R.C. *et al.* (1990) Effects of prostaglandin E1 on oxygen delivery and consumption in patients with the adult respiratory distress syndrome. Results from the prostaglandin E1 multicenter trial. The Prostaglandin E1 Study Group. *Chest*, **98**, 405–10.

137. Bihari, D., Smithies, M., Gimson, A. and Tinker, J. (1987) The effects of vasodilation with prostacyclin on oxygen delivery and uptake in critically ill patients. *New England Journal of Medicine*, **317**, 397–403.

138. Walmrath, D., Schneider, T., Pilch, J. *et al.* (1993) Aerosolised prostacyclin in adult respiratory distress syndrome. *Lancet*, **342**, 961–2.

139. Villar, J., Edelson, J.D., Post, M. *et al.* (1993) Induction of heat stress proteins is associated with decreased mortality in an animal model of acute lung injury. *American Review of Respiratory Disease*, **147**, 177–81.

140. Curzen, N.P., Griffiths, M.J.D. and Evans, T.W. (1994) The role of the endothelium in modulating the vascular response to sepsis. *Clinical Science*, **86**, 359–74.

141. Koltai, M., Hosford, D. and Braquet, P. (1993) PAF-induced amplification of mediator release in septic shock: prevention or down-regulation by PAF antagonists. *Journal of Lipid Mediators*, **6**, 183–98.

142. Levi, M., tan Cate, H., van der Poll, T. and van Deventer, S.J.H. (1993) Pathogenesis of disseminated intravascular coagulation in sepsis. *JAMA*, **270**, 975–9.

143. Branch, M., Berry, L.C., Conary, J.T. *et al.* (1993) Response of bovine pulmonary artery endothelial cells (BPAEC) to endotoxin following transfection of human manganous superoxide dismutase (MnSOD) cDNA. *American Review of Respiratory Disease*, **147**, A206 (abstract).

144. Sloane, P.J., Gee, M.H., Gottlieb, J.E. *et al.* (1992) A multicenter registry of patients with acute respiratory distress syndrome. Physiology and outcome. *American Review of Respiratory Disease*, **146**, 419–26.

INDEX

Note: page numbers in *italics* refer to tables, those in **bold** refer to figures